Praise for *Heaven's Banquet*

"Offers the kind of cooking wisdom and inspirational
recipes that even I—a reluctant cook at the best of times—
will turn to again and again."
—Jennifer Hawthorne, co-author of
Chicken Soup for the Woman's Soul

"Hospodar's heartfelt book is robust and bursting
with information and zest."
—Sue Bender, author of *Plain and Simple*
and *Everyday Sacred*

"*Heaven's Banquet* is packed with an astonishing variety
of recipes, placed in a global context of cultures,
histories, and literatures, knit together by the author's
thoughtful commitment to the Ayurvedic dietary
system. Any diet that recommends 'Eating for Bliss'
is worth exploring in some detail."
—Betty Fussell, author of *I Hear America
Cooking* and *Home Bistro*

MIRIAM KASIN HOSPODAR has worked as a chef in Ayurvedic
spas and centers in the United States, France, Switzerland,
the Philippines, Taiwan, and India. A certified teacher of the
Transcendental Meditation program, she has also served as
the director of the Maharishi Ayur-Veda Health Center in
St. Louis, Missouri, and the Health Center in Pacific Pali-
sades, California. She lives in Santa Barbara.

HEAVEN'S BANQUET

VEGETARIAN COOKING
FOR LIFELONG HEALTH
THE AYURVEDA WAY

MIRIAM KASIN HOSPODAR

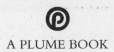
Ⓟ

A PLUME BOOK

A NOTE TO THE READER

The ideas, procedures, and suggestions contained in this book are not intended
as a substitute for medical treatment by a physician. The reader should
regularly consult a physician in matters relating to health.

PLUME
Published by the Penguin Group
Penguin Putnam Inc., 375 Hudson Street, New York, New York 10014, U.S.A.
Penguin Books Ltd, 27 Wrights Lane, London W8 5TZ, England
Penguin Books Australia Ltd, Ringwood, Victoria, Australia
Penguin Books Canada Ltd, 10 Alcorn Avenue, Toronto, Ontario, Canada M4V 3B2
Penguin Books (N.Z.) Ltd, 182–190 Wairau Road, Auckland 10, New Zealand

Penguin Books Ltd, Registered Offices: Harmondsworth, Middlesex, England

Published by Plume,
a member of Penguin Putnam Inc.
Previously published in a Dutton edition.

First Plume Printing, October 2001
10 9 8 7 6 5 4 3 2 1

Let us be together,
Let us eat together,
Let us be vital together,
Let us be radiating truth, radiating the light of life,
Never shall we denounce anyone, never entertain negativity.
—THE UPANISHADS

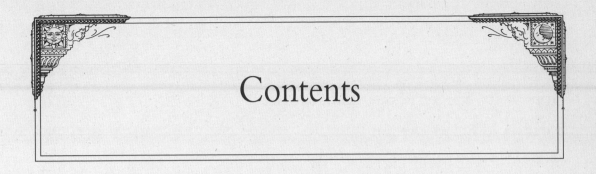

Contents

The intention of every other piece of prose may be discussed and even mistrusted; but the purpose of a cookery book is one and unmistakable. Its object can conceivably be no other than to increase the happiness of mankind.

—JOSEPH CONRAD

Acknowledgments

M any people have added their unique ingredients to *Heaven's Banquet*.
Knowing them has been deeply nourishing for me. My cup runneth over with
their generosity and also with my gratitude for it.

Infinite gratitude to Maharishi Mahesh Yogi for reviving Vedic wisdom and creating
the Maharishi Vedic Approach to Health. I hope he feels that I have represented his
knowledge well.

My dear family, including my husband, Steve, who became, among a thousand other
blessings, a beloved partner in the project: editor, proofreader, data entry person,
encourager, inspirer, and all-around angel from heaven. My beloved parents, Gerald
and Edith Kasin, who believed in and supported the project from the beginning and
have been active participants every step of the way. (My mother is the best cook anywhere, and Dad ran a close second with his Chinese feasts.) Also my incredibly wonderful brother, Peter Kasin, who can whip up a mean stir-fry.

Anand Shrivastava and Steve Barthe of Maharishi Ayur-Veda Products Interna-
tional. Mike Tompkins, whose brilliance always astounds. Robert Hensley of MAPI,
Russell Guest of MAP–Canada, and Larry Clarke of MAP–Australia. The wise vaidyas
associated with the Maharishi Vedic Approach to Health, including Dr. Balraj
Maharshi, Dr. J. R. Raju, Dr. Palakurthi Manohar, and Dr. Rama Kant Mishra. Dr.
Michael Jensen, Robert Roth, and Ken Caldwell each contributed their unique insights.

My magnificent agent, Patti Breitman—an inspiration, the best of the best. It is my
good fortune that she chose the world of publishing instead of becoming a star in
Broadway musicals. Carole DeSanti, editor extraordinaire at Dutton, who saw into the
heart of the project and nurtured its healthy growth. Many thanks to Carole's hard-
working assistant, Alexandra Babanskyj, for copious amounts of assistance, both seen

ix

and unseen. Infinite gratitude to brilliant editor Amy Mintzer and her daughter, Rosie, who added joy to the process. Sorry there's no ketchup recipe in here, Amy. Thanks to copy editor Ginny Croft, book designer Leonard Telesca for a compact yet elegant design, and Mary Ellen O'Boyle for a scrumptious cover design.

Susan Shatkin meticulously edited the material on Maharishi Ayur-Veda. Meredith Jacobsen cracked the secret code of my handwriting and translated the first drafts into coherent, neatly typed pages. Martin Zucker gave great ideas about quotations. Mona Mark, a terrific person, created terrific illustrations. Richard Barnes of the Thousand-Headed Purusha Program drew the delightful Ayurvedic symbols and decorative Vedic pillars. Gratitude to Lyn Durham and Denise Denniston Gerace. The folks at Spectrum Naturals provided detailed information about oils. Laurence Hauben gave insight into the European usage of metric measurements in cookbooks. Kudos to the ever-helpful staff of the Santa Barbara Public Library, particularly the reference department.

Thanks to the many angels of support who listened, empathized, and cheered during the book's long years of gestation, especially my dear mother-in-law, Mary Hospodar, and sister-in-law, Louise Maschek, and Judith LaMar, Anne Wright, Janice Hamilton, Jenny D'Angelo, Dana Gilbert, and the favorite auntie of the book, Sue Bender.

To all of these precious souls, and through them to the whole world, I offer the following Vedic blessing:

> *May the good belong to all the people in the world.*
> *May the rulers go by the path of justice.*
> *May the best of men and their source always prove to be a blessing.*
> *May all the world rejoice in happiness.*
> *May rain come in time and plentifulness be on earth.*
> *May this world be free from suffering and the noble ones be free from fears.*

The Banquet Is Served

*I am obsessed with the relationship between cooking and health.
When one goes to the opera, one does not expect to return having
gone deaf; one does not expect to go blind as a result of going to
the theatre. Why then, must one do oneself a damage by going
out to eat? For people who think this way there is, on one hand,
the* cuisine *for pleasure—but full of menace—and on the other,
the* diet*—for the redemption of the body. This separation is
odious, and we must find the means of reconciling pleasure and
health. I dream of a cuisine that no longer does anyone harm.*
—ALAIN SENDERENS, one of only two *chef patrons*
who have received both three Michelin stars
and four Gault-Millau toques

Cooking is a marvelous, enjoyable, and above all, necessary creative act. We could define cooking literally as an act of creation. A cook has a few basic utensils, ingredients, and cooking techniques. By combining them in different ways, he or she can create entirely new dishes or repeat old favorites. A cook is therefore a creator, a magician, the master of a territory of influence. And no matter how humble it may appear, that territory is quite a large one. Though a cook's creation doesn't end up hanging on a wall or resting in a safe-deposit box, it becomes part of something infinitely precious, another living human being. Whenever we cook we are influencing the quality of life of the people we cook for—not to mention of ourselves. Cooking is therefore a precious opportunity to enhance that quality of life.

I have always cherished a deep desire to cook and eat very good food and also to cook and eat very healthy food. These two passions have not always been compatible. Having tested the waters of vegetarianism starting at age seventeen and having worked as a professional chef, I tried, studied, and eventually discarded practically every system of diet and nutrition that I ever came into contact with. I also found myself consistently frustrated and dissatisfied with cookbooks and books on nutrition that address food as an entity in itself: its nutritional value and its sensory impact on the eater—any eater—and how a cook can exploit these features. I was far more curious about the deeper implications of that gloriously soothing and evocative word, nourishment. I was starved for wonderful cooking that would feed the mind, body, and spirit.

In the 1970s I became aware of the first expressions of an art and science of nourishment that was brought to light more fully a decade later: Maharishi Ayur-Veda. Of all the systems of health and nutrition that I have investigated over the years, Maharishi Ayur-Veda is the only one I have found to be holistic, complete, and effective. At last I had found the knowledge I had been looking for all my life—a program of health and healing from a timeless, time-tested source that included, among other things, a simple, joyous, delicious, fulfilling way of cooking and eating. I had the great good fortune to cook in professional kitchens where Ayurvedic dietary principles were practiced under the supervision of experienced Ayurvedic physicians, and to study Ayurvedic diet and nutrition with the great teachers of Maharishi Ayur-Veda in Europe, India, and the United States.

Next to eating good dinners, a healthy man with a benevolent turn of mind must like, I think, to read about them. —WILLIAM MAKEPEACE THACKERAY

In 1975 I began to write the book that I wanted to have on my own kitchen shelf, one that would explain Maharishi Ayur-Veda and offer recipes constructed according to its principles. *Heaven's Banquet* was written on three continents over a twenty-three-year period. The recipes were tested in everything from a five-star Swiss hotel kitchen to a charcoal-filled pit in the Philippines. They were sampled by many hundreds of people from around the world who passed through my various and varied kitchens and who kindly—and sometimes not so kindly but always honestly—offered their opinions and suggestions.

In these times, often anything "new" is automatically perceived as an improvement over what has come before. Many people most respect and believe the "amazing new breakthroughs" that "experts"—frequently self-proclaimed as such—have concocted themselves or have synthesized from a dozen different sources. However, there is another, more traditional method of gaining knowledge that has been practiced over the millennia by thousands of generations of seekers: that of taking guidance from ancient, time-tested sources and from wise people who are living embodiments of the knowledge they teach. As the *Rik Veda* states so simply and elegantly, "He who knows the country tells the direction to him who asks the way."

Everything I have learned about Maharishi Ayur-Veda comes from the contemporary reviver and supreme teacher of Ayurveda, Maharishi Mahesh Yogi, and from the ancient authority of traditional Ayurvedic texts. I have attempted to repeat this knowledge as precisely as I can, without coloring it with my own personal opinions.

However, the principal Ayurvedic texts do not contain much in the way of recipes or instructions for cooking, particularly for a modern kitchen. The recipes, cooking techniques, and opinions about them in *Heaven's Banquet* are my own; I have taken ancient

Ayurvedic principles and applied them to the equipment, ingredients, and techniques used in contemporary kitchens.

Therefore you must be discriminating when you evaluate the information in this book. It contains both eternal wisdom that I pass on to you just as it has been taught to me and a culinary application that I have developed from my own life experiences and training as a cook. My recipes and cooking techniques are not necessarily ancient, universal knowledge but an interpretation by one of the many students on the path. You might be able to do it better than I have—or at any rate, in a way that suits your personal tastes more closely. I hope so.

My cherished desire is that *Heaven's Banquet* provides you with tools and ideas to help you fulfill your own culinary aspirations. I wish that your table will ever be filled to overflowing with a heavenly banquet of health, happiness, and wholeness.

> *This night I hold an old accustom'd feast,*
> *Whereto I have invited many a guest,*
> *Such as I love; and you, among the store,*
> *One more, most welcome, makes my number more.*
> —WILLIAM SHAKESPEARE

Enjoy!

—Miriam Kasin Hospodar
Santa Barbara, California

AYURVEDIC SYMBOLS USED IN HEAVEN'S BANQUET

 The lotus is a symbol of transcendence, pure consciousness. Lotuses grow in lakes, with their roots in the mud and their flowers on the surface of the water, above and beyond the mud below.

 The *Amrit Kalash* is a Vedic symbol of immortality, representing the legendary vessel that contains the nectar of immortality. The Vedas state, "Ayurveda is for immortality."

 The depiction of wind represents Vata dosha, which has air and space as its essential elements.

 The sun represents Pitta dosha, which has fire as one of its essential elements.

 The moon represents Kapha dosha, which has water as one of its essential elements. The moon regulates the tides and thus has a relationship to water.

 The cornerpieces are the artist's interpretation of the traditional pillars in Vedic temples, decorated here with the symbols used in Heaven's Banquet to denote Vata, Pitta, and Kapha.

Nourishing the Mind and Body: Maharishi Ayur-Veda for Perfect Health

But what avail the largest gifts of Heaven,
When drooping health and spirits go amiss?
How tasteless then whatever can be given!
Health is the vital principle of bliss.

—JAMES THOMSON

The name *Ayurveda* comes from two Sanskrit words, *ayus,* or "life," and *ved,* meaning "knowledge" or "science." *Ayurveda* is translated as "the science of life" or, more precisely, "the knowledge of life span." Maharishi Ayur-Veda creates health by enlivening the body's own inner intelligence. Instead of focusing primarily on disease, Maharishi Ayur-Veda puts the emphasis on health. It can even be said that the programs of Maharishi Ayur-Veda do not treat disease; rather, they promote health from within. This is an extremely important distinction: Maharishi Ayur-Veda states that perfect health is a natural, normal state of life, and anything less than perfect health is abnormal.

HEALING FROM WITHIN: ENLIVENING THE BODY'S INNER INTELLIGENCE

From the perspective of Vedic science, the source of life is a unified field of infinite, pure intelligence. It is the home of all the laws of nature, the underlying, all-pervading principle that governs the entire universe in perfect harmony and without a problem. It keeps the cycle of the seasons flowing in their natural rhythm and sequence, and the planets remaining in their orbits instead of randomly flying through space and colliding with each other. Nature's intelligence creates orderly growth and change, ensuring that kittens always grow up into cats, not elephants, and that when you plant an acorn it will always blossom into an oak tree, not emerge as a cornstalk.

The pure creative intelligence that governs all of creation is found within every human being, permeating every cell of the body. It guides the orderly functioning of all

1

bodily processes perfectly and automatically, without any problems whatsoever. By enlivening the body's inner intelligence—the same intelligence that governs the entire universe—the physiology is revitalized and renewed, and healing naturally occurs from within. When we enter a dark room and flick on the light switch, darkness automatically disappears. It is the same fundamental principle at work with healing: establish health, and dis-ease and dis-order automatically disappear.

A Picture of Health: From the Individual to the Cosmos

Revere the healing power of nature.   —HIPPOCRATES

What is perfect health? A modern medical definition might be a body free of disease. A holistic health practitioner might call it a balanced body-mind system. Maharishi Ayur-Veda takes the expanded view that health not only encompasses the mind, body, emotions, and spirit of the individual but extends to the health of the entire environment. Since the intelligence within everyone is the same intelligence that governs the entire universe, each individual is not an isolated organism but is intimately connected to all of life, from the most infinitesimal subatomic particle to the entire cosmos. We are all threads in the exquisite and intricately woven fabric of creation. Another analogy would be that of a vast, lush forest: for the forest to be green and healthy, the individual trees that comprise it must be green and healthy.

The programs of Maharishi Ayur-Veda form a bridge between mind and body, consciousness and physiology, and between the individual, the environment, and the universe. They serve to help individuals live a long life in the natural state of health and harmony that is their birthright, and promote a healthy, harmonious world that is the collective birthright of all humankind.

A TIMELY REVIVAL OF ANCIENT VEDIC WISDOM

In ancient times Ayurvedic doctors, or *vaidyas*, were highly trained and greatly respected. But over centuries of foreign rule in India, Ayurvedic institutions were not supported and Ayurvedic medicine was suppressed, so that much of the ancient knowledge was lost or became distorted. Today *Ayurveda* can mean anything from a vaidya trained at an Ayurvedic medical college, to a corner pharmacy in India where a shopkeeper recommends and dispenses generalized formulations, to a Western health-care practitioner who has read a few books on the subject and purports to practice "Ayurvedic medicine."

All too often, practitioners combine Ayurveda with other systems of health care and self-development, resulting in a mishmash of Ayurvedic information that has been combined and diluted with other more recent and frequently unproven systems. Some pharmaceutical companies are capitalizing on people's regard for Ayurveda by producing products with isolated "Ayurvedic" herbs that have little to do with traditional Ayurvedic formulas.

Maharishi Mahesh Yogi, founder of the transcendental meditation program and Maharishi's Vedic science, concerned with the widespread disease in the world, recognized the inability of allopathic approaches to health care to stem the tide of illness. He knew that there was an effective, natural, cost-effective approach to health care, Ayurveda, described in the Vedic literature. In the early 1980s he began working with leading Ayurvedic scholars and vaidyas, in conjunction with medical doctors, to bring to light the complete knowledge of Ayurveda, offer it in practical programs, and to make such programs widely available. It was a heroic effort, involving identification of which among the many Ayurvedic texts represented the original, authentic authority, making accurate interpretations of those texts, and correcting the misunderstandings and misinformation that had resulted from the centuries-old suppression of indigenous health care. Vaidyas from the few remaining unbroken traditions of Ayurvedic practice lent their support and their participation to fulfill Maharishi's goal of bringing authentic knowledge of Ayurveda to humankind.

Maharishi also felt that Ayurvedic knowledge could and should be verified by modern medical science. Physicians and researchers from around the world began conducting research studies at universities and research institutions to test the effectiveness of Ayurvedic formulas and treatments. A large body of scientific research documenting the effectiveness of Ayurvedic treatments has already been published, and research is ongoing at major institutions around the world.

Last, Maharishi felt that the knowledge should be verifiable by people's experiences—in other words, people should feel better from Ayurvedic treatments, not just believe in them because they are told to by an "expert."

The names Maharishi Ayur-Veda and Maharishi Vedic Approach to Health were given to the very specific authentic system of theory and practice of Ayurveda brought to light by Maharishi and the council of vaidyas and physicians working with him.

The Mistake of the Intellect: Source of Imbalance

Maharishi Ayur-Veda describes the lack of connection with the body's inner intelligence as the primary source of human suffering. In the ancient Ayurvedic texts this condition is referred to as "the mistake of the intellect," or *pragyaparadh*. Pragyaparadh is the mistaken perception that the ever-changing display we experience through our senses is all that there is; we do not perceive the underlying wholeness of life, the home of all the laws of nature. It is as if we sailed out into the sea, looked out over the waves on the surface, and concluded that they comprised the total reality of the ocean—without perceiving that there are unfathomably vast, silent depths beneath from which those waves spring.

Wholeness is a state of perfect balance, invulnerable to disease. When we aren't living with the awareness of this reality of life, the door is opened wide for myriad imbalances at any level of the mind and body. We lack the most basic form of immunity to disease: an anchor to the stable, silent home of all the laws of nature, the source of the body's inner intelligence. We are not established in the state of perfect balance into which no imbalances can enter, the state of perfect orderliness into which no dis-orders can take root.

The Doctor Is In—Within

A unique feature of Maharishi Ayur-Veda is its nonjudgmental and nondictatorial approach. The bottom line is your own experience. The body's inner intelligence is the ultimate authority, the perfect physician. If you go to a doctor and say, "I don't feel well, I have a pain," and the doctor tells you, "There's nothing wrong with you—it's all in your head"—well, you still don't feel well! A health care practitioner trained in Maharishi Ayur-Veda recognizes that if you are experiencing discomfort, then something *must* be wrong. He or she does not view a patient in terms of a single symptom, organ, or body part that may be causing a problem, but looks at the whole person: your constitutional makeup, attitudes, lifestyle, behavior, and environment.

AYURVEDIC DIET AND NUTRITION

Let food be your medicine and medicine be your food.   —HIPPOCRATES

Most people would agree that a blissful, healthy mind and body require nutritious foods. Ayurvedic texts emphasize wholesome diet as vital for promoting health and happiness. What comprises a "wholesome diet"? There is no single formula that applies to all individuals, though there are some universal and unchanging principles that do.

Modern Nutritional Science: What's Wrong with This Picture?

From the point of view of Ayurveda, contemporary nutritional science often misses the point by searching for universal prescriptions. Nutritionists tend to identify certain foods as "bad" and others as healthy and beneficial for everyone, yet these foods fall in and out of favor, depending on the latest research "discovery." The first wave of research is widely acclaimed, sets off a fad, and then is negated by the next wave.

"Everyone should drink at least one quart of milk per day." "Everyone should reduce milk intake." "Eat margarine instead of butter for a healthy heart." "Well, maybe margarine isn't as great as we first thought." Sometimes we eat a food promoted as having wonderful health-giving properties and feel terrible afterward. Yogurt, for instance, is promoted as being a universally healthy food. However, for each person who feels nourished by it, there is one who gets an acid stomach and another who gets a stuffy nose. The modern approach to nutrition consistently produces partial answers and partial truths. Fragmented observation—seeing only one part of the picture—all too often leads to mistaken conclusions.

Each human physiology is a marvel of exquisitely individual components, relationships, and transformations that are constantly changing yet are based on eternal and unchanging laws of nature. Maharishi Ayur-Veda explains how even subtle differences in individual constitution can make what is good for one individual not necessarily good for another—and recommends how to nourish both.

How Do I Determine the Most Nourishing Foods for Me?

Ayurvedic texts identify eight overall considerations, each one a world of knowledge in itself, that determine how nourishing any particular food or meal will be for an individual. All are addressed in the following pages:

1. *Nature of the food.* This refers to a food's natural qualities, such as lightness or heaviness, whether it is heating or cooling, etc.
2. *Method of preparation.* Whether or not the food is cooked, what type of vessel it is cooked in, how it is flavored, how clean it is, etc.
3. *Combination.* How different ingredients and dishes are combined.
4. *Quantity.* The amount of food needed to thrive on. A highly individual consideration that changes with one's amount of activity, age, environment, etc.
5. *Place or habitat.* The influence of the type of environment one lives in or is eating in.
6. *Time.* Considerations such as the age of the person eating, the season, and whether it is daytime or evening.
7. *Guidelines* for the best way to partake of food.
8. *The eater.* A vital and often overlooked influence. Whether or not a food is nourishing is ultimately dependent upon the person who eats it. One's unique physiology, one's state of consciousness, and general state of health influence any food's effect.

"This sounds overwhelming! How can I figure out all that when I have 30 minutes to get a meal on the table for five hungry people?" You can't intellectually decipher all the different factors that make a particular food healthy for any individual at any given point of time. There is a saying, "Nature knows best how to organize." Only the infinite organizing power of all the laws of nature can possibly figure out all the thousands of factors that go into making a perfect decision when it comes to choosing foods to eat. When one is living in accord with the laws of nature, one's decisions are spontaneously life-supporting. All the information given here is to help us increasingly enliven our bodies' inner intelligence and from there to do the best we can to create healthy meals, without strain, and with tidings of comfort and joy.

Digestion: Key to Good Health

> *Heaven is largely a matter of digestion, and digestion is mostly a matter of mind.*   —ELBERT HUBBARD, *A Thousand and One Epigrams*

Maharishi Ayur-Veda emphasizes the vital importance of good digestion for ideal health. Food is the substance through which we bring Nature's energy and intelligence into our bodies. When we are in balance, food is fully digested; its nutrients are absorbed by the body and what is not needed is eliminated. In fact, we could say the same thing about all our experiences. When we are able to fully process, or "digest," our experiences, we absorb that which nourishes our mind, body, emotions, and spirit and let go of those experiences that do not.

Digestive Fire, or Agni

> *The Agni which digests food is regarded as the master of all agnis because increase and decrease of other agnis depend on the digestive fire. Hence one should maintain it carefully by taking properly the wholesome food and drinks, because on its maintenance depends the maintenance of life-span and strength.*
> —*CHARAKA SAMHITA*

The physiological processes used to digest food are defined by Ayurveda as *Agni*, or digestive fire. There are various Agnis with specific metabolic functions. According to Ayurveda, the digestive process starts from the moment food enters our mouth and we taste it. Digestion is similar to fueling a fire. The food is "cooked" by Agni—converted into the forms in which nutrients can be utilized by the body. When the Agnis are strong, digestion is strong. When the Agnis are weak, digestion is sluggish or incomplete. One must then "kindle" them with heating foods and spices, such as ginger and black pepper, so that they will function more efficiently.

Nourishing the Seven Vital Tissues, or Dhatus

Ayurveda defines seven basic tissues that support the body, called the *dhatus*:

Blood plasma, lymph: *rasa*
Red blood (hemoglobin): *rakta*
Muscle: *mamsa*
Fat: *medha*
Bone: *ashti*
Central nervous system and bone marrow: *majja*
Sperm and ova: *shukra*

Each vital tissue has its own metabolism that extracts and utilizes the nourishment it needs from the food we eat. When food is thoroughly digested, it nourishes, in order, the seven vital tissues, each drawing nourishment from the one before. When digestion is complete and the vital tissues are in balance, each area is completely nourished and formed, and the next in line responds accordingly and is completely nourished and formed.

The Biochemical Component of Bliss, or Ojas

> *Increase of ojas makes for contentment, nourishment of the body and increase of strength.* —ASHTANGA HRIDAYA

When all seven vital tissues are completely nourished and working in balance, a biochemical substance called *ojas* is produced from the finest essence of the food. This is a subtle substance that permeates the entire body and mind. A person with a good supply of ojas is often described as having a glow about them or as looking radiant. Indeed, ojas literally brings a glow to the skin. According to Ayurveda, ojas is responsible for nourishing the most subtle aspects of mind and body. It keeps the balance of all bodily systems and therefore creates bliss. The ultimate physiological goal of cooking, eating, and digestion is to produce ojas.

Microcirculatory Channels, or the Shrotas

Ayurvedic physiology defines the body as being filled with intricate networks of channels through which its intelligence moves through and between cells, nerves, and all the bodily systems. These microcirculatory channels are collectively known as the *shrotas*. They are the transporting passages for all tissues, the channels through which nourishment enters and wastes are removed. The shrotas take different forms in different tissues, just as cells do. There are thirteen basic types of channels, some specific to the vital tissues and others dealing with the transport of major forms of nourishment and waste matter. According to the *Charaka Samhita*, one of the principal Ayurvedic texts, as long as the circulatory channels are fully functioning, a person will not have diseases. When the body is in balance, ojas flows unobstructed through the shrotas, bringing refined nourishment to all aspects of the physiology and personality. However, when there is imbalance or the presence of impurities, the body's microcirculatory systems can become blocked, impeding the flow of intelligence and causing myriad problems.

Undigested Food, or Ama

> *Clogged with yesterday's excess, the body drags the mind down with it, and fastens to the ground this fragment of divine spirit.* —HORACE

What happens when we eat indigestible foods or food combinations or too much food? What happens if digestion is weak and the vital tissues are out of balance, so that we cannot fully process the foods we eat? Improperly digested food remains in the body and forms *ama*, a sticky substance that creates havoc wherever it goes. Ama is the functional opposite of ojas. It causes blockages, and the body's communication systems cease functioning well. When Ama disturbs the digestive process, it causes incomplete formation of the vital tissues. Ama tends to settle in areas of the body that are already weak and out of balance, bringing on disease. It can take on many forms of unwanted deposits, such as calcium deposits in the joints, plaque in the arteries, and growths such as cysts and tumors.

The same is true about all our experiences in life. When we experience something that is "indigestible"—overwhelming or traumatic—or something that overloads our senses and we cannot fully process, we can be left with emotional ama, a "clogging" of our emotions that adversely affects our emotional health and well-being.

How can you tell if you have ama? A coated tongue, particularly foul-smelling breath, dullness of the senses, loss of appetite, depression, or unclear thinking can indicate the presence of ama. An assessment by a doctor trained in Maharishi Ayur-Veda can best determine if and where there is ama present. There are numerous ways to help remove it, including dietary changes, herbal formulations, and treatments.

How can you prevent ama? Ayurveda describes the most digestible foods, food combinations, and methods of preparation to ensure that nourishment is fully accepted and utilized by the mind-body system. It also suggests methods of strengthening digestion, so that the body better utilizes the foods it is given.

Guidelines for Optimum Digestion

> *The fate of a nation has often depended upon the good or bad digestion of a prime minister.*   —VOLTAIRE

Here are some simple, enjoyable things you can do to ensure optimum digestion and assimilation. If you follow these recommendations at least some of the time, you should experience a variety of health benefits. Many people report that their weight normalizes, they have more energy, their digestion improves, and they sleep better. These are all the natural results of restoring balance.

❖ Eat in a settled atmosphere.

> *Unquiet meals make ill digestion.*   —WILLIAM SHAKESPEARE

❖ Avoid eating when you are upset.

> *Joy, temperance and repose,*
> *Slam the door on the doctor's nose.*   —HENRY WADSWORTH LONGFELLOW

❖ Sit down when you eat.

> *It isn't so much what's on the table that matters, as what's on the chairs.*
>   —W. S. GILBERT

❖ Eat only when you are hungry.

> *A good meal ought to begin with hunger.*   —FRENCH PROVERB

❖ Don't talk when chewing.   —YOUR MOTHER

❖ Eat at a moderate pace, neither too fast nor too slow.

> *Food eaten neither too slowly nor too hurriedly is uniformly digested.*
> —SUSHRUTA SAMHITA

❖ Wait until one meal is digested before eating the next (that is, an interval of two to four hours after a light meal, four to six hours after a full one).

> *Now good digestion wait on appetite, and health on both!*
> —WILLIAM SHAKESPEARE

❖ Sip warm water with your meal.
❖ Eat food that pleases all your senses.
❖ Eat to only two-thirds to three-quarters of your capacity. (Leaving one-third to one-quarter of your stomach empty aids digestion.)
❖ Don't rush through a meal. There should be no feeling of hurry, of having to wolf down the food and jump up from the table.

> *He sows hurry and reaps indigestion.*   —ROBERT LOUIS STEVENSON

❖ Eat in the most harmonious, most pleasant atmosphere possible. Options may be limited, but there are always *some* choices (like pulling over to the side of the road to eat instead of whipping out a sandwich while waiting at a red light—my old trick while in college).
❖ Eat at regular times as much as possible. Our bodies, including our digestive systems, thrive on routine. You will be surprised how good you feel by simply adopting this practice.

> *Irregularity of diet brings about ill health.*   —SUSHRUTA SAMHITA

❖ Be grateful for the food you receive. It is a gift of Nature's abundance and a human being's efforts. Taking in food is a precious link between you and everyone and everything that provided it. Gratitude is an acknowledgement of that link and sets up a positive attitude for digesting your food.
❖ Praise the cook. Yes! This is an Ayurvedic prescription for good health. It gives a positive, uplifting tone to the whole relationship that brought you the food.
❖ Sit quietly for a few minutes after your meals.

> *To eat is human, to digest divine.*   —CHARLES T. COPELAND

Don't feel guilty if you are not practicing all these points all of the time! They are general guidelines, not rigid prescriptions to dogmatically force on yourself and those you dine with. Assimilate them gradually and comfortably. As always with Ayurvedic suggestions, *see how you feel.*

MIND-BODY TYPES: THE THREE DOSHAS

❖ You are tall and willowy. Your body always seems to be in motion, mouth included. Your mind moves quickly, picking up new bits of information—and often just as quickly forgetting them. You eat erratically and it's hard to pin you down to a specific mealtime. However, you can consume mountains of the rich food you crave and never gain an ounce.

❖ Your brother is of average height and weight. His hair is graying and thinning, although he is only thirty-three. Highly intelligent and dynamic, he speaks articulately and passionately about the things he believes in and, truth be told, tends to be a bit fanatical about his causes. He loves milk shakes, chilled salads, anything cold—and has to have his meals on time, or else he gets cranky and you have to run for cover.

❖ Your sister has thick, wavy hair and a warm, friendly face with big, beautiful eyes. She hates rushing and tends to be slow walking and slow talking. She is also initially a bit slow on the uptake, but once someone has repeated his phone number to her a couple of dozen times, she'll remember it long after he's moved. She is on the *zaftig* side and feels like she only has to look at food to gain weight. However, unlike your brother, she can easily skip meals.

According to Maharishi Ayur-Veda, each of these family members contains combinations of physiological and psychological traits that can be categorized into specific groups called *mind-body types*. Each mind-body type responds differently to the same foods and to many other things, including environmental factors such as the weather. Eating the foods most suited to his or her mind-body type will help each person maintain balance and good health. Everyone has a distinct mind-body type, which is determined by the combination of three basic components, called *doshas*.

What Is a Dosha?

The three doshas are basic governing agents, or controllers, of every aspect of the universe. The Sanskrit word *dosha* literally means "impurity." Why impure? Because they no longer represent the undifferentiated wholeness of the home of all the laws of nature—they are separate entities and, as such, have potential for imbalance. The home of all the laws of nature, of creative intelligence, is without any qualities whatsoever—it is one unified, undifferentiated whole, beyond the experience of the five senses. Just as the vast, silent ocean manifests as active, moving waves on its surface, so everything in creation is unbounded wholeness at its basis, though it takes on different, active forms on the surface.

The Five Senses and Five Elements: Basis of the Three Doshas

Vedic science identifies five basic building blocks of creation through which creative intelligence expresses itself. Each has a nonmaterial aspect and a material one:

- ❖ The nonmaterial, or subtle, aspect consists of the five senses: hearing, touch, sight, taste, and smell.
- ❖ The material aspect consists of the five elements: space, or *akasha*, air, fire, water, and earth.

The three doshas, **Vata**, **Pitta**, and **Kapha**, are structured from the five senses and the five elements. They therefore each have specific qualities colored by the particular set of senses and elements of which they are comprised. It is important to understand this to make sense of the specific qualities each of the doshas possesses.

Vata is a combination of space, the essence of hearing; and air, the essence of touch.
Pitta is a combination of fire, the essence of sight; and water, the essence of taste.
Kapha is a combination of water, the essence of taste; and earth, the essence of smell.

In human beings, the three doshas regulate the thousands of different functions in the mind-body system through their basic governing activities:

Vata *governs bodily functions concerned with movement.*
Pitta *governs bodily functions concerned with heat, metabolism, and energy production.*
Kapha *governs bodily functions concerned with physical structure and fluid balance.*

Their areas of influence are generated by the elements they are made of. Space and air are related to movement; fire and water to heat and metabolism; and water and earth to structure and fluid balance.

Qualities of the Doshas

Besides controlling the basic functions in all organs and systems of the body, the doshas have specific tendencies, or qualities. These qualities can also be identified in the environment, foods, and all other material substances and conditions. The qualities are, again, based on the elements that make up each dosha.

Vata *is moving, quick, light, cold, rough, dry, and leads the other doshas.* Anything with these qualities indicates the presence of Vata—a cold, dry wind; a rough, dry, light food such as popcorn; a fast-moving, anxiety-provoking action movie.

Pitta *is hot, sharp, light, acidic, slightly oily.* Hot salsa, noontime sun in summer, a piercing trumpet note, all indicate the presence of Pitta.

Kapha *is heavy, oily, slow, cold, steady, solid, dull.* Ice cream, the gait of an elephant, the grogginess one feels following an afternoon nap, all have qualities of Kapha.

The Ten Mind-Body Types

The three doshas exhibit their qualities in specific, identifiable physical and mental traits within each individual. Every aspect of the mind and body is influenced by the combination and proportions of doshas present. Knowing which doshas are dominant in an individual gives us a psycho-physiological blueprint of his or her personality and physiology: height and weight patterns, behavior patterns, physical characteristics, likes and dislikes, sleep patterns, which diseases one is prone to develop, even such subtle traits as what one dreams about. In most people one or a combination of two doshas predominates. A small number of people have all three doshas in more or less equal amounts. The various combinations and properties give rise to ten general mind-body types. They are:

Mono-doshic:	Vata
	Pitta
	Kapha
Bi-doshic:	Vata-Pitta
	Pitta-Vata
	Pitta-Kapha
	Kapha-Pitta
	Vata-Kapha
	Kapha-Vata
Tri-doshic:	Vata-Pitta-Kapha

Characteristics of the Ayurvedic Mind-Body Types

Pure mono-doshic types show some specific characteristics reflecting the qualities of that dosha. Bi- and tri-doshic types combine some of the traits exhibited by each dosha. The people described a few pages ago are classic mono-doshic types—Vata, Pitta, and Kapha. Bi- and tri-doshic types have a combination of some of the traits of each dosha. In bi-doshic types one dosha usually dominates. A Vata-Pitta type has a higher proportion of Vata than Pitta. A Pitta-Vata type has more Pitta than Vata. These are generalities—each individual is different. Usually a person has a majority, but not all, of the characteristics of his or her mind-body type.

Characteristics of a Vata Type

Lighter, thinner build
Performs activity quickly
Tendency toward dry skin

Aversion to cold weather
Irregular hunger and digestion
Quick to grasp new information; also quick to forget
Tendency toward worry
Tendency toward constipation
Tendency toward light, interrupted sleep
Speaks quickly, with irregular speech patterns

Characteristics of a Pitta Type

Moderate build
Performs activity with medium speed
Aversion to hot weather
Prefers cold food and drinks
Sharp hunger and digestion
Can't skip meals
Medium time to grasp new information
Medium memory
Moles or freckles
Good public speaker
Tendency toward irritability and anger
Enterprising and sharp in character

Characteristics of a Kapha Type

Solid, heavier build
Great strength and endurance
Slow, methodical in activity
Oily, smooth skin
Slow digestion, mild hunger
Tranquil, steady personality
Slow to grasp new information; also slow to forget
Slow to become excited or irritated
Sleep is heavy and long
Hair is plentiful, thick, and wavy

Do Our Doshas Always Remain the Same?

Just as we are born with a specific set of genes and DNA, each individual has a unique combination of the three doshas. The proportions of the doshas we are born with is called our *prakriti*, or "nature." Our nature constitutes the ideal proportion and balance of the doshas for our particular mind-body system, and never changes throughout our life. However, our doshas tend to deviate from their original pattern of balance and become imbalanced. The impermanent, changeable pattern of imbalanced doshas is known as an individual's *vikriti*.

BALANCE OF THE THREE DOSHAS FOR PERFECT HEALTH

He whose doshas are in balance, whose appetite is good, whose tissues are functioning normally, whose elimination is in balance, whose body, mind and senses remain full of bliss, is called a healthy person.   —SUSHRUTA SAMHITA

The high ideal of health described in the *Sushruta Samhita*, one of the main classical texts of Ayurveda, is the result of maintaining our perfect balance of the three doshas. Achieving perfect balance does not mean that all three must be present in equal amounts. Rather, it means that the doshas are present in the ideal proportion for each person's individual mind-body system and that they are working in a balanced state of harmony with each other. All aspects of Maharishi Ayur-Veda are designed to bring the doshas into the correct proportion that constitutes perfect balance for that particular individual. Some indications of balanced doshas are:

Balanced Vata

Mental alertness
Proper formation of body tissues
Normal elimination
Sound sleep
Strong immunity
Sense of exhilaration

Balanced Pitta

Normal heat and thirst mechanisms
Strong digestion
Lustrous complexion
Sharp intellect
Contentment

Balanced Kapha

Muscular strength
Vitality and stamina
Strong immunity
Affection, generosity, courage, dignity
Stability of mind
Healthy, normal joints

Imbalance and Mind-Body Type

*Similarity of substances is always the cause of increase and dissimilarity is the
cause of decrease.*   —CHARAKA SAMHITA

When the doshas significantly increase or decrease in the physiology, they tip the scales
and go out of balance. The doshas increase and decrease on the principle of "like
attracts like." If you have a predominance of Vata dosha, you will have the tendency to
accumulate more Vata. A variety of physical, behavioral, and environmental factors can
cause a dosha to increase or decrease to the point of creating an imbalance. The even-
tual result of imbalanced doshas is disease. The types of symptoms or diseases that
manifest when a particular dosha goes out of balance are based on the qualities of that
dosha: light, heavy, oily, cold, etc. Some of the more common symptoms of imbalance
in the doshas are:

Imbalanced Vata

Dry or rough skin
Insomnia
Constipation
Common fatigue (nonspecific causes)
Tension headaches
Intolerance of cold
Degenerative arthritis
Underweight
Anxiety, worry

Imbalanced Pitta

Rashes, inflammatory skin conditions
Peptic ulcer, heartburn
Visual problems
Excessive body heat
Premature graying or baldness
Hostility, irritability

Imbalanced Kapha

Oily skin
Slow digestion
Sinus congestion
Nasal allergies
Asthma
Cysts and other growths
Obesity

How Do I Determine My Mind–Body Type?

1. **Appendix A contains a questionnaire to help you determine your mind-body type.** It is intended to help clarify some universal characteristics of each dosha.

2. **There is a wealth of books, pamphlets, and audio- and videotapes** describing each dosha and the characteristics of the ten mind-body types in detail. These will give you a deeper understanding of the three doshas and all their characteristics to help you better understand your own traits and tendencies. Many can be sent to you at home. Some centers offer invaluable courses in pulse diagnosis so that you can evaluate your own doshas on a daily basis. See Appendix B for addresses and telephone numbers.

3. **Have a consultation with a health-care practitioner trained in Maharishi Ayur-Veda.** He or she will use a variety of diagnostic techniques to determine your individual mind-body type. The first technique is to feel the pulse in your wrist. Pulse diagnosis is a highly accurate and sophisticated Ayurvedic science for determining your overall state of health. The proportions of Vata, Pitta, and Kapha indicating mind-body type can be identified, and imbalances and the presence of ama can be located through pulse diagnosis. The second technique is to observe your physical characteristics and ask questions about your physical and emotional makeup. The health-care practitioner can then design a personal program of diet, exercise, herbal formulas, behavioral recommendations, and any other recommendations that will help restore you to balance, keep you there, and prevent future imbalances from arising before they can give rise to disease.

   If you are already under the care of a physician, your personal Ayurvedic program will be designed to work in harmony with your present doctor's recommendations—there is no conflict between Maharishi Ayur-Veda and modern Western medicine. See Appendix B to locate a Maharishi Ayur-Veda Health Center or a health-care practitioner trained in Maharishi Ayur-Veda.

DIET AND PERFECT HEALTH:
FOODS THAT NOURISH EACH MIND-BODY TYPE

Regimen is better than physic. Everyone ought to be his own physician. We ought to assist, and not force nature. Eat with moderation what agrees with your constitution. Nothing is good for the body but what we can digest.

—VOLTAIRE

Maharishi Ayur-Veda explains that the old proverb "One man's meat is another man's poison" is literally true when it comes to diet. Foods cause specific doshas either to increase or decrease. Since we are more likely to create an imbalance by *increasing* the predominant doshas of our mind-body type, we say that foods that calm down the influence of a dosha *pacify* that dosha, and foods that increase it *aggravate* it.

THE VATA-PACIFYING DIET

	Favor	Reduce or Avoid
QUALITIES	Heavy, warm, unctuous*	Light, cold, dry
TASTES	Sweet, sour, salt	Pungent, bitter, astringent
QUANTITIES	Larger portions, but not to the point of indigestion	
DAIRY	*All dairy products*	
SWEETENERS	*All in moderation*	
OILS	*All oils*	
GRAINS	*Rice, wheat, cooked oats*	*Barley, buckwheat, corn, millet, rye, uncooked oats*
FRUITS	*Sweet, sour, heavy fruits, such as: avocados, bananas, berries, cherries, grapes, mangoes, melons, oranges, peaches, plums, pineapples*	*Light, dry fruits, such as: apples, cranberries, dried fruits, pears, pomegranates*
VEGETABLES	*Asparagus, beets, carrots, cucumbers, green beans, okra, radishes, sweet potatoes, turnips* Almost all other vegetables can be eaten in moderation, if well cooked in oil with the addition of Vata-pacifying spices	*Cabbage, raw vegetables, sprouts*
SPICES	*Almost all spices* can be used in moderation, with an emphasis on sweet, heating spices	Large quantities of pungent, bitter, and astringent spices, such as: *chilies, coriander, fenugreek, parsley, saffron, turmeric*
NUTS AND SEEDS	*All nuts and seeds*	
BEANS	*Garbanzos, red lentils (masoor dal), mung (moong dal), tofu in small quantities*	*All—except those listed*
NON-VEGETARIAN	*Chicken, turkey, seafood*	*All red meats*

*This word can have a positive connotation in Ayurveda.

THE PITTA-PACIFYING DIET

	Favor	Reduce or Avoid
QUALITIES	Cool or warm, liquid, moderately heavy	Hot
TASTE	Sweet, bitter, astringent	Salt, sour, pungent
QUANTITIES	Moderate portions	
DAIRY	*Butter, ghee, sweet lassi, milk*	*Cheese; cultured dairy products, such as buttermilk, sour cream, and yogurt except in sweet lassi*
SWEETENERS	*All—except those listed*	*Honey, molasses*
OILS	*Coconut, olive, soy, sunflower*	*Almond, corn, safflower, sesame*
GRAINS	*Barley, oats, wheat, white rice*	*Corn, millet, brown rice, rye*
FRUITS	Sweet, ripe fruits only, such as: *apples, avocados, cherries, figs, mangoes, melons, pears, pomegranates, prunes, raisins* Only if sweet and completely ripe: *green grapes, oranges, pineapples, plums*	Sour, unripe fruits, such as: *apricots, bananas, berries, cranberries, grapefruits, olives, papayas, peaches, persimmons*
VEGETABLES	*Asparagus, bell peppers, broccoli, Brussels sprouts, cabbage, cauliflower, celery, cucumbers, green beans, leafy greens—all types except spinach, okra, peas, potatoes, sweet potatoes, sprouts, summer squash, winter squash*	*Beets, carrots, chilies, eggplant, garlic, onions, radishes, spinach, tomatoes*
SPICES	Sweet, bitter, astringent, such as: *cardamom, cilantro, cinnamon, coriander, small amounts of cumin and black pepper, dill, fennel, mint, saffron*	*All pungent, heating spices; chilies should be avoided*
NUTS AND SEEDS	*Coconuts, pumpkin seeds, sunflower seeds*	*All—except those listed*
BEANS	*Garbanzos, mung (moong dal), soybeans and tofu*	*All—except those listed*

	Favor	Reduce or Avoid
NON-VEGETARIAN	Chicken, egg whites, pheasant, shrimp, turkey	Egg yolks, red meats—especially beef; seafood—except shrimp

THE KAPHA-PACIFYING DIET

	Favor	Reduce or Avoid
QUALITIES	Light, dry, warm	Heavy, unctuous, cold
TASTES	Pungent, bitter, astringent	Sweet, sour, salt
QUANTITIES	Be careful not to overeat	
DAIRY	Warm low-fat or nonfat milk, small quantities of warm whole milk with 1–2 pinches of turmeric or ginger added before boiling	All—except those listed
SWEETENERS	Honey	All—except honey
OILS	Small amounts of: almond, corn, ghee, safflower, sunflower	All—except small amounts of those listed
GRAINS	Barley, buckwheat, corn, millet, rye, all other grains—except those listed	Oats, rice, wheat
FRUITS	Light, dry fruits, such as: apples, apricots, cranberries, dried fruits, pears, pomegranates	Heavy, juicy, sweet, sour, such as: avocados, bananas, coconuts, dates, fresh figs, grapefruits, grapes, mangoes, melons, oranges, papayas, peaches, pineapples, plums
VEGETABLES	All—except those listed	Sweet, juicy vegetables, such as: cucumbers, sweet potatoes, summer squash, tomatoes
SPICES	All—except for salt	Salt
NUTS AND SEEDS	Pumpkin seeds, sunflower seeds	All—except those listed
BEANS	All—except tofu	Tofu

THE KAPHA-PACIFYING DIET *(cont.)*

	Favor	Reduce or Avoid
NON-VEGETARIAN	*Small amounts of chicken—white meat only; eggs—not fried in oil or butter; seafood*	*All red meats*

My life partner is a Kapha-Pitta, my daughter is a Vata, my son is a Pitta-Vata, and I am a Kapha. Does this mean we all have to eat different meals? We can reasonably assume that there will be a variety of mind-body types within any given group. The above charts are offered as information to help you make informed choices—it would be a misuse of them to attempt to match up every food item in every meal with each person's mind-body type. Mind-body type is only one factor out of many involved in planning healthy meals, as evidenced by the eight criteria for judging the wholesomeness of foods listed on page 5. The doshas governing each season and the time of day play a role. The way foods are cooked can alter their effects on a person's doshas, such as the fact that vegetables that are not necessarily Vata-balancing are fine for Vata types when cooked with oil. How strictly you adhere to serving only foods that specifically pacify each dosha is up to you and your own comfort. Some of the recipes in *Heaven's Banquet* are specific to one or two doshas, and many aren't. Keep some dosha-specific condiments on hand, such as Maharishi Ayur-Veda churnas, and some chutneys and sauces that balance different doshas.

Eating for Bliss: Foods to Reduce or Avoid

> *Only the use of wholesome food promotes the growth of a person, and that of unwholesome food is the cause of disorders.*   —CHARAKA SAMHITA

As long as you can fully digest a food, it is fine for you to eat it. We can safely conclude that all foods have at least some good effect on some of the people some of the time. We could also say that most foods have some untoward effects for some people some of the time. However, there are some foods whose qualities tend to bring dullness and heaviness to the mind and body and to create ama in most people most of the time. They are not included in *Heaven's Banquet*. Many are commonly eaten today, and it may seem a bit arbitrary and puzzling at first that Ayurveda identifies them as having less than life-supporting effects. Others have some good effects but are not supportive of subtler processes of consciousness. There are always trade-offs. Whether you choose to eat them or not depends on the type of functioning you wish to uphold most in your life. Keep in mind that these foods were not always held in high regard. Throughout history we see activities and practices that were prevalent at one time and later abandoned after lessons were collectively learned about them in the school of hard knocks.

❖ *Leftovers* are heavy and create ama. If you adopt no other dietary change, try this one: eat freshly cooked meals.

A warmed-up dinner was never worth much. —Nicolas Boileau-Despréaux

Many of us were brought up to feel that certain dishes "taste best the next day." However, they won't have the same good effects on your mind and body. Once you get used to the bright, lively flavors of freshly cooked foods, you won't want to eat old, stale foods again (which is exactly how leftovers will probably begin to taste to you). In the long run it costs more to restore health that has been compromised by consistently eating leftovers than it does to eat only freshly cooked foods.

The art of using up leftovers is not to be considered as the summit of culinary achievement.   —Larousse Gastronomique

❖ **Preserved, fermented, canned, and frozen foods** tend to create ama. The exceptions are dried, uncooked vegetables and fruits, and fruits cooked with sugar, such as jams. Sun-ripened fruits are considered to be "precooked" by nature, and drying them or preserving them does not injure their life-supporting qualities.

❖ **Meat, fish, and eggs:** Ancient Ayurvedic texts describe physiological effects of eating different meats—not all of them undesirable. However, the long-standing tradition and overall feeling among vaidyas is that eating animal flesh is not supportive to enlivening the mind-body system's inner intelligence—not to mention the inner intelligence of the hapless animal. Eggs can have a subtle effect of causing the mind to wander—not always overtly noticeable but perhaps not the best thing to eat before performing brain surgery or balancing your checkbook.

❖ **Onions and garlic:** In some cases these foods have a healthy effect on the body; garlic is included in some Maharishi Ayur-Veda dietary recommendations for addressing specific, temporary imbalances. However, onions and garlic are generally not recommended for universal daily use, as they have a dulling effect on refined mental activity. This may come as a surprise, as the use of garlic practically constitutes a food fad in some quarters and is touted in many herbal medical guides. However, there is plenty of historical precedent, and current practice as well, among people concerned with clear, refined mental processes. Besides being well known by traditional Vedic scholars in India, garlic was considered by the ancient Egyptian priests to be impure and unfit for eating. It might have been all right for the conscripts building the pyramids, but garlic eaters were barred from worshipping at the temple of Cybele, the earth goddess. Garlic was also a controversial food among philosophers and physicians in ancient Greece. Onions and garlic are refrained from to this day by many Chinese Buddhists. According to the Muslim tradition, when Satan stepped out of the Garden of Eden after the fall of Adam and Eve, onions sprouted in the footprints of his right foot, and garlic in the footprints of his left.

Try cooking without these ingredients for a while. You will become sensitive to the flavors of foods that are ordinarily drowned out by these strident flavors. Onions and garlic have certainly been overworked as flavoring agents. I have a particular, pardon the expression, beef about their ubiquitous presence in vegetarian recipes. Open almost any vegetarian cookbook and you will find that, with the exception of the desserts, almost every recipe calls for onions and/or garlic. The rest of the world does not cook this way! On the other hand, the role onions and garlic do play in the cuisines of the world can scarcely be denied. I suggest using the spice *hing* (asafoetida) to replace the taste they provide. Hing has an added benefit of promoting good digestion.

❖ **Mushrooms:** Mushrooms are not technically vegetables but fungi, which Ayurveda identifies as being less than nourishing and creating some negative effects.

> The cook's personal cleanliness contributes greatly to the life-supporting value of the food. Obviously it is a good idea to cook with clean hands and to tie your hair back. A common practice in the West that is unthinkable in more traditional Eastern cultures is that of tasting from the pot with the stirring spoon. Keep a separate spoon in a cup near the stove. Pour food into it from the stirring spoon so that the tasting spoon never touches the food in the pot. Traditional Ayurvedic cooks do not taste the food at all until it is served, gauging the flavor by other cues, such as smell and appearance.

❖ **Genetically engineered foods:** Potatoes with genetic material from scorpions, tomatoes with genetic material from fish—what foods these morsels be? Foods that have been "improved" by the introduction of genetic material from other species are rapidly entering our food supply. Often the alterations are intended to give them a very long shelf life. While the FDA states that they are safe, an increasing number of scientists disagree, citing that there has been woefully insufficient research on the effects of genetically engineered foods. They feel that there is no definitive proof that they really are safe to eat. Vaidyas, Western physicians, and scientists who have embraced Maharishi Ayur-Veda heartily agree. Genetically engineered foods are often difficult to identify. Organically grown foods that are grown from nongenetically engineered seeds are safe.

> A group of students of Ayurveda in ancient India were assigned to find a plant for which there was no use in Ayurvedic healing. After a long search, each came back bearing a specimen to show their teacher—except for one. When asked by his sniggering cohorts why he had returned empty-handed, he replied, "I was unable to find a plant for which there is no use." The teacher exclaimed, "You are right. There is no plant that does not have some use in Ayurveda."

Are All Foods in Heaven's Banquet *Ayurvedic?*

There are a few foods included in *Heaven's Banquet* that are considered by some to be less than ideal. Some vaidyas recommend avoiding them entirely, while others feel they can be healthfully consumed if measures are taken to neutralize their less desirable effects. In any case, many people who incorporate Ayurvedic principles into their lives eat them, while others don't. I have chosen to include these foods, accompanied by instructions for ways to help balance their less desirable qualities. Alternate ingredients are listed wherever possible.

❖ Hard cheeses that have been aged are particularly avoided by many because they can block the shrotas (microcirculatory channels).

❖ Some vaidyas do not recommend potatoes because they are digested very, very slowly. Other vaidyas feel that tomatoes do not have good effects—indeed, they aggravate all three doshas—yet some vaidyas prescribe them for other, good qualities they possess.

❖ Leavening in general and yeast in particular can create ama.

❖ Some people don't use commercial liquid seasonings, such as Dr. Bragg's Aminos or Dr. Bronner's Mineral Bouillon, because although not fermented, they aren't fresh either and are not a traditional Ayurvedic food.

❖ Chilies are sometimes found in the suggested variations for recipes. They can be eaten in small amounts by people with a high proportion of Kapha and actually aid their digestion, but generally chilies are highly incendiary and disturbing to the digestive process.

So How Strict Should I Be?

What some call health, if purchased by perpetual anxiety about diet, isn't much better than tedious disease. —GEORGE DENNISON

There are no shoulds. Do whatever brings you the most happiness, is most comfortable for your life, and speaks most meaningfully to you. Happiness, after all, is most important. People who take Maharishi Ayur-Veda to heart do so with many different levels of desire, comfort, and commitment. There is no one right way to do it.

Foods Suitable to the Individual

What is patriotism but the love of food one ate as a child? —LIN YUTANG

A "beloved" contemporary master of Maharishi Ayur-Veda was asked by his students, "What is the best food to eat?" His reply: "The food your mother makes you." The students were stunned, as visions of the now-dubious contents of their school lunch boxes danced through their heads. It is the nurturing, nourishing qualities of the love a mother might imbue in the food she serves her children that is probably the basic import of that statement. However, this statement brings to light another important Ayurvedic principle described by the Sanskrit phrase *oka satmya*. Says the *Charaka Samhita,* a principal Ayurvedic text, "Whatever is suitable to the person because of regular use is known as oka satmya." There is a strong cultural influence on what is nourishing to one person and not another; our minds and bodies are adapted to the foods we grew up eating. Entire cultures eat foods and food combinations that are inherently healthy but would be indigestible to those who grew up in another culture. Germans thrive on dairy products that would sink a Chinese; Italian wheat pasta might send a cornmeal-eating Guatemalan to the pharmacy for antacids. Furthermore, when we eat foods often and as part of our family and culture, we can become habituated to—and even thrive on—those that are described in Ayurveda as being less than ideal for health.

Another very powerful consideration is the emotional value, the deep comfort we feel when eating the foods we grew up on. How many of us who have spent time in a foreign country have felt intense relief when we encountered a dish of our native land—perhaps even one we might not enjoy so much at home? After spending a year in Taiwan, a pizza I somewhat desperately obtained from a fast food joint felt like manna from heaven.

Does this mean that we cannot change our diets if we feel they are less than ideal? Of course not. Do we accept less-than-ideal attitudes and activities we grew up with once we become aware of a better way? However, it is important to keep our culinary history in mind as we make changes in our diet and our life. We must be very gentle with ourselves, very respectful of what has come before—of the very powerful pull it has on us and of the nourishing value it has had. *Charaka Samhita* recommends making changes of habits and diet very, very gradually: "A wise person should alleviate himself from habitual malpractices gradually. Adoption of good practices should also be in a similar way. . . . Demerits given up gradually and merits adopted in the same way become ever-prevented and unshakable."

THE DOSHAS AND THE SEASONS

> *Live in each season as it passes; breathe the air, drink the drink, taste the fruit,*
> *and resign yourself to the influence of each.*   —HENRY DAVID THOREAU

The change of seasons is a major cycle that has a profound influence on health. Each season is governed by a different dosha. The weather and environmental conditions of each season express the qualities of its corresponding dosha. Each dosha has a tendency to *increase* within our bodies during its particular season. For instance, Pitta has the quality of heat. The hot summer sun of Pitta season may cause heat to increase in the body of a Pitta type person to the point of imbalance. A heat rash, digestive problems, or other Pitta-related disorders may appear as a result. On the other hand, a Vata type will feel soothed by that same hot sun, which pacifies the cold quality of Vata dosha in that individual.

The doshas correspond to three major seasonal periods. They are different from the four calendar seasons we are familiar with. Here are the approximate dates for the Northern Hemisphere; they are opposite in the Southern Hemisphere:

Vata Season is mid-October to mid-March (*when it is likely to be dry, cold, and windy*).

Pitta Season is mid-June to mid-October (*when it is likely to be hot*).

Kapha Season is mid-March to mid-June (*when it is likely to be rainy and cold*).

The principle holds even in the "seasonless" climates of places like Florida and southern California. Though the weather changes may be far less dramatic, they still affect our doshas. Also, a day in *any* season that is windy and cold will be Vata-aggravating. Cold, rainy, or damp weather will aggravate Kapha, and hot weather anytime will usually increase Pitta.

You can help counteract the seasonal effects of the doshas by eating foods that pacify the particular dosha increasing in that season. To a certain extent, we do this already. Eating hot soup on a cold winter day or a dish of ice cream during a summer heat wave are obvious choices. Ayurveda simply takes this common sense principle one step further. There are specific seasonal dietary recommendations for the different mind-body types. Following these recommendations not only affects overall well-being in the long run, but people often find great relief from the seasonal blues. Imagine escaping the flu season unscathed, feeling less irritable and tired in the summer, avoiding the depression and aching joints that come when it rains. By eating in harmony with the seasons, we can avoid symptoms of imbalance.

The following are the diets recommended for each mind-body type during the different Ayurvedic seasons.

SEASONAL DIETS FOR THE TEN MIND-BODY TYPES

	KAPHA SEASON March–June	PITTA SEASON July–October	VATA SEASON November–February
❶ VATA	► VATA DIET	VATA DIET	VATA DIET
❷ PITTA	► PITTA DIET	PITTA DIET	PITTA DIET
❸ KAPHA	► KAPHA DIET	KAPHA DIET	VATA/KAPHA (1)
❹ VATA-PITTA	► VATA/KAPHA (1)	PITTA DIET	VATA DIET
❺ PITTA-VATA	► VATA/KAPHA (1)	PITTA DIET	VATA DIET
❻ VATA-KAPHA	► KAPHA DIET	PITTA/VATA (2)	VATA DIET

(1) Balance of Vata and Kapha diets: Select equal proportions of food from the "favor" section of each diet. The "reduce or avoid" section can be ignored at this time. (2) Balance of Pitta and Vata diets: Select equal proportions of food from the "favor" section of each diet. (The "reduce or avoid" section can be ignored at this time.)

SEASONAL DIETS FOR THE TEN MIND-BODY TYPES *(cont.)*

	KAPHA SEASON	PITTA SEASON	VATA SEASON
	March–June	July–October	November–February
❼ KAPHA-VATA	▶ KAPHA DIET	VATA DIET	VATA DIET
❽ PITTA-KAPHA	▶ KAPHA DIET	PITTA DIET	PITTA/VATA (2)
❾ KAPHA-PITTA	▶ KAPHA DIET	PITTA DIET	VATA/KAPHA (1)
❿ VATA-PITTA-KAPHA	▶ KAPHA DIET	PITTA DIET	VATA DIET

If you have a bi-doshic mind-body type: Favor the routine suited to each of your doshas during its season. If you are a Pitta-Kapha type, favor the Pitta-pacifying diet during Pitta season, and the Kapha-pacifying diet during Kapha season. When Vata season comes, combine a Vata-pacifying diet, for the season, with a Pitta-pacifying diet (for your dominant dosha). Don't worry about being overly specific; these are general guidelines.

If you have a tri-doshic mind-body type: Easy! Just follow the diet to pacify each dosha during its season.

TIME CYCLES AND THE DOSHAS

 In addition to the seasons, the doshas influence other important time cycles, such as the times of day.

The hours 2:00–6:00 A.M. and P.M. are governed by Vata.
The hours 6:00–10:00 A.M. and P.M. are governed by Kapha.
The hours 10:00–2:00 A.M. and P.M. are governed by Pitta.

Your activities will be more harmonious and successful if you perform them during the time that they will be supported by each dosha. For instance, exercise pacifies Kapha and will be most effective during the Kapha hours. However, sleeping during the Kapha times will increase Kapha and make you more sluggish. The Vata times of day are best for quiet activities and rest, as quietness pacifies Vata. Digestion is most efficient during the Pitta times. Noon, when the sun is at its zenith, is the time of greatest Pitta influence and ideal for taking your main meal.

Although all three doshas are present at all times in everyone in different amounts, a general influence from one dosha is more enlivened at different times during a person's life:

Childhood is governed by Kapha.
Adulthood is governed by Pitta.
Elderhood is governed by Vata.

Some indications of the influences are that Kapha governs structure, and childhood is the time when the body's structure is growing and forming. Pitta supports the time of life where activity in society is usually the greatest. Old age is when one is more prone to Vata imbalances, such as anxiety, insomnia, and arthritis.

THE PSYCHO-PHYSIOLOGY OF TASTE

Good living is an act of our judgment by which we grant a preference to those things which are agreeable to the taste above those that have not that quality.
—JEAN-ANTHELME BRILLAT-SAVARIN

"Eat it anyway—it's good for you!" These are words you will never hear from the lips of a mother attuned to Ayurveda. Ayurveda explains that the reaction our body has to the taste on the tongue is actually the first step in the digestive process. Whether a food's flavor "makes our mouth water" or "makes our stomach churn" has a large bearing on how our body metabolizes it. For this reason it is important to prepare food that is tasty and delicious—eating foods that are to one's liking is Ayurvedic. However, a caution is in order: we can't always go by taste alone, as our tastes can be affected by imbalances in the doshas and the presence of ama. When we are out of balance, we can actually crave the foods that increase our imbalances even more.

The Six Tastes

Ayurveda describes six major tastes by which all foods can be categorized. Each taste has the effect of increasing some doshas and decreasing others. Many foods contain more than one taste. It is easy to tell which tastes some foods contain. Others are less obvious, and one has to go by the traditional designations in the Ayurvedic texts.
  The six tastes are:

Sweet: Sugar, honey, rice, milk, butter, and pasta are examples of sweet foods. *Sweet increases Kapha and decreases Vata and Pitta.*
Sour: Lemons, cheese, yogurt, tomatoes, and sour fruits are examples of sour foods. *Sour increases Pitta and Kapha and decreases Vata.*
Salt: Salt. *Salt increases Pitta and Kapha and deceases Vata.*

Bitter: Leafy greens, fenugreek, and turmeric are examples of bitter foods. *Bitter increases Vata and decreases Pitta and Kapha.*

Pungent or spicy: Cayenne and other chilies, ginger, and radishes are examples of pungent foods. *Pungent increases Vata and Pitta and decreases Kapha.*

Astringent: Beans, lentils, apples, pears, and potatoes are examples of astringent foods. *Astringent increases Vata and decreases Pitta and Kapha.*

Using the Six Tastes to Balance the Doshas

Who satisfieth thy mouth with good things; so that thy youth is renewed like eagles.
—PSALMS 103.5

To maintain perfect balance and be completely nourished, we should ideally have all six tastes at every meal. If you pay attention, you will notice after eating a meal with only one or two of the tastes, such as cottage cheese with a piece of toast, that you won't feel completely satisfied. That's because you haven't been completely nourished. Eating all six tastes strengthens your immune system, and consistently not having all six tastes can weaken your immunity to disease. In addition to including all six tastes in a meal, you can keep yourself in balance by emphasizing the tastes that pacify your doshas. These are:

Vata: *sweet, sour, and salt*

Pitta: *sweet, bitter, and astringent*

Kapha: *pungent, bitter, and astringent*

Cravings: What to Do When the Body Says Stop! and the Mind Says Go!

When we follow our natural desires, all goes well. A balanced mind and body work together. Our body lets us know when it needs food, how much it needs, and what types of foods will be most nourishing. Simple enough. However, when imbalances are present, these signals can go awry. Eating can become dissociated from our body's needs, and when toxic impurities, or ama, is present, we can develop cravings for foods that aren't good for us. That's when we start reaching for the salsa even when our irritated stomach is begging us not to. Or we find ourselves habitually taking second helpings whether we're hungry or not. Or we wind up with an eating disorder.

The usual method of dealing with these cravings is to attempt to renounce them. We make New Year's resolutions, vows to our Maker, our partner, our mirror—and end up miserable because we're continually fighting the craving. Worse, when we inevitably succumb to it, we feel both miserable *and* guilty. Too often, cravings are treated as a sign of moral weakness and attributed to lack of willpower and self-discipline. The whole thing becomes a vicious circle. What to do?

According to Ayurveda, a craving is a distress signal sent up by a mind-body system that is desperately seeking balance and misguidedly attempting to rectify its lack of balance. The approach Maharishi Ayur-Veda takes is to follow the path of comfort, of happiness, of fulfilling one's desires. Ayurveda seeks to restore balance, so that our mind is once again in tune with the true needs of our body. Here are a few techniques for dealing with cravings:

❖ **Do not force yourself to give up undesirable foods or deprive yourself by forced "dieting."** Forcing will create an even bigger conflict—and imbalance—than the craving has already.

❖ **Take the measures recommended by Maharishi Ayur-Veda to restore balance to your mind-body system.** Pay special attention to including all six tastes in each meal and to removing toxic impurities, or ama. As balance returns, negative habits will lessen of their own accord. Your desires will spontaneously begin to change in favor of the foods that support health and happiness. If your eating habits are consistently and uncontrollably off the mark, it is a very good idea to consult a health care practitioner trained in Maharishi Ayur-Veda.

❖ **Pay attention to what you are eating.** Take time to really enjoy your food. As Thoreau said, "He who pays attention to the savor of his food can never be a glutton; he who does not cannot be otherwise."

❖ **Pay attention to how you feel.** Remember that your body has within it all the intelligence it needs to maintain balance. Be receptive to what it is telling you. The voice of our deepest feelings and desires often speaks in a whisper. When we quietly listen in a receptive and nonjudgmental manner, we will hear it loud and clear.

The pleasure of eating is not in the costly flavor but in yourself. —HORACE

How Do I Get Started?

❖ **Study the information in this book and adopt it as you feel comfortable with it.** For most people the learning process continues over time. I find that you have to integrate this type of knowledge into your life and experience the results before it makes complete sense. It has taken me years to absorb and integrate the knowledge of this system, and I am still learning. Just be easy about the whole thing and enjoy it!

❖ **The suggestions should be taken as *recommendations*, not as rigid prescriptions.** If you try to follow each recommendation to the letter, you will drive yourself crazy and miss the point. It is not intellectually possible to determine exactly how a particular dish is going to affect each individual. *Sushruta Samhita* simply states, "Food which is congenial to one's temperament begets no discomfort after eating." The bottom line in Maharishi Ayur-Veda is always your own experience, how you feel. Consciousness is the greatest vaidya, the ultimate source of the perfect dietary prescriptions for any individual at any moment.

A person desirous of long life . . . should place utmost faith in the teachings of Ayurveda. —ASHTANGA HRIDAYA

Creation 101:
Let There Be Dinner

It is a fortunate thing that an obedience to the laws of nature is quite often an inherent thing in a good cook. —M. F. K. Fisher

How to Cook Wonderful Ayurvedic Food on a Terrible Schedule

Everything should be made as simple as possible, but not one bit simpler.
                                                    —Albert Einstein

Many of us have demands on our time that don't allow many hours (or minutes) for meal preparation. In fact, it is the time factor that stops many people cold when considering a switch to Ayurvedic cooking. I have rarely cooked under ideal conditions. Professional stints have been for large groups with small kitchen staffs, and cooking at home has usually been juggled with a full-time job. Here are some techniques I've developed over years of producing fresh meals in short order:

❖ Buy dry goods such as dal, beans, grains, and pasta in bulk. Your weekly shopping list will be shorter.

❖ A Crock-Pot (slow cooker) is a great time-saving tool, as it can cook foods overnight and while you are at work. Even when you are at home, you don't have to constantly keep an eye on the food—it won't boil over or burn. Crock-Pots are especially useful for cooking dal and other beans, Khichari, soups, stews, and ghee. You can use the type of timer that automatically turns lights on and off to turn on your Crock-Pot while you are out.

❖ Prepare one-pot meals in a Crock-Pot. This works particularly well for the evening meal, in keeping with the Ayurvedic recommendation for lighter dinners.

30

❖ Try Khichari, Dal Soup with Barley, Minestrone (with pasta added before serving), or any type of stew or soup containing dal, grains, and vegetables.

Alternatively, cook dal or vegetable soup in your Crock-Pot and cook a grain on the stove just before serving. Basmati rice, bulgar, quinoa, and buckwheat cook in 20 minutes, and couscous in its ubiquitous instant form cooks in no time flat.

Changing the order, cook a bean dish or a bean-and-rice dish in a Crock-Pot and make a steamed or sautéed vegetable on the stove just before serving. Chopped spinach takes 3 to 5 minutes to cook, as do corn, asparagus, summer squashes cut into small pieces, and a number of other vegetables. In any case, simple vegetable dishes generally do not take long to prepare.

❖ Pasta mixed with sautéed vegetables can be prepared quickly. Capellini, vermicelli, and extra-thin spaghetti cook in 4 to 6 minutes. A sprinkling of olive oil and fresh herbs are all that is needed to create a lovely main dish or one-dish meal. Add tofu, Panir, or nuts for a more substantial dish.

❖ Cookies, biscuits, and scones all bake quickly. You can prepare the dough in a food processor in a few seconds. For bar cookies, such as shortbread, you don't even have to take the time to form individual cookies.

❖ All the above having been said, it also helps to make a psychological shift regarding the use of time to enhance your quality of life. As Einstein proved so eloquently, time is a relative phenomenon. I feel that it is worth the time it takes to nourish your body well. Whatever time we "lose" by preparing fresh foods we may gain by adding more years to our life and more vitality and happiness to those years.

OPERATING INSTRUCTIONS FOR NOVICE COOKS

Cooking demands attention, patience, and, above all, a respect for the gifts of the earth. It is a form of worship, a way of giving thanks. —JUDITH B. JONES

Welcome to the fun! Make yourself at home. Here is a tour of the house to help you feel more confident and comfortable.

❖ Read all of "Creation 101: Let There Be Dinner." It was written for you.
❖ Before trying a recipe:

1. Read the beginning of the recipe section; for example, before preparing Herb Biscuits, read the paragraphs concerning biscuits in general—they contain information that applies to the preparation of all biscuits.
2. Read the recipe through once. Check to see if there are any ingredients that need advance preparation, such as beans that must be soaked overnight. Also make sure that the time involved in the preparation is compatible with your schedule and that you have all the ingredients on hand.

❖ Follow recipes exactly until you develop a feel for cooking. When you have gained confidence and cooking procedures become more automatic, you can begin to improvise and experiment with a better chance of success. Most recipe sections include lists of suggested variations and alternate ingredients to aid in successful improvisation. Where the heading "Variations" appears at the bottom of a recipe, specific ingredients and alternate cooking methods that work well are listed. These are only suggestions—there are many other possibilities that would prove successful and interesting.

❖ Finally, when a recipe advises the addition of an ingredient "to taste," or no specific measurement is listed, proceed cautiously. It's easy to add more and impossible to subtract—the tragedy of kitchen arithmetic.

FOR EXPERIENCED COOKS

A complete lack of caution is perhaps one of the signals of a real gourmet: he has no need for it, being filled as he is with a God-given and intelligently cultivated sense of gastronomical freedom.   —M. F. K. FISHER

❖ All the recipes have been designed to embody Ayurvedic principles. They may therefore have a different construction than you are used to. There is a value to working from the recipes, even though you may feel you could make a standard-sounding dish with your eyes closed. If you have been cooking and baking with eggs all your life, the section "Baking Without Eggs" in the "Basic Ingredients for a Heavenly Banquet" chapter may be news. In fact, an experienced cook is at a slight disadvantage here because some cooking procedures must be unlearned.

❖ Those of you who know how to get around in a kitchen probably rarely follow recipes verbatim but use them as springboards for your own creativity. The joy of cooking is when you have mastered enough skills in the kitchen to create dishes according to your desires. However, there are days when even the most fertile culinary imagination seems to poop out and whimpers for a jump start. For those times I think you'll enjoy the suggested "Variations" that follow many recipes—some of the best ideas can be found in them. There are also lists of "Additions and Variations" for major recipe groupings, such as "Muffins" and "Salad Dressings."

WORDS OF ENCOURAGEMENT FOR NEW VEGETARIANS

And God said, Behold, I have given you every herb bearing seed, which is upon the face of all the earth, and every tree, in which is the fruit of a tree yielding seed; to you it shall be for meat. —GENESIS

Although some people are vegetarian from birth, most of us have not been raised that way; we make a decision at some point to stop eating meat. It is a way of eating, cooking, and thinking about eating and cooking that has to be learned—which also means that many culinary habits also have to be unlearned.

I "became a vegetarian" several times before it stuck. My desire was great and my preference strong, but I had no idea how to prepare satisfying meals. Although the vegetarian diet offers rich advantages, people commonly have the following experiences when they are making the transition from a meat-based regime:

❖ Unless you grossly overeat you will not have the heavy, "full" feeling that comes after eating a meat meal.

❖ Many vegetarian foods don't have the dense, chewy texture of meat. You may miss that.

❖ A vegetarian meal is not constructed in the same manner as a traditional Western meat meal. There isn't necessarily one main protein-rich dish surrounded by some second-fiddle vegetables. You may feel confused about how to plan a meal.

Planning an Ayurvedic vegetarian meal is a matter not of replacing the meat in a traditional meal format but of composing a different type of meal altogether. Read the section on "Menu Planning and Menus" to get a feel for the construction of vegetarian meals. Here are some tips to help you make a smooth, happy transition to a vegetarian diet.

❖ Observe your physical sensations after a meal—you do not have to experience a heavy stomach in order to feel satisfied. You may begin to enjoy the lightness you feel after a vegetarian meal.

❖ Some vegetarian foods are dense and heavy. None of them imitate meat; however, they will help you feel more comfortable if you eat them often at first. Ayurveda recommends you eat such heavier foods at your lunchtime meal, especially "curds" such as tofu and cheese.

The "Tofu, Panir, and Seitan" chapter treats three ingredients that can all be prepared to be heavy, dense, and chewy.

Dishes made with ground nuts, such as Nut Loaf and Nut Pâté en Croûte are heavy and filling.

Thick slices or chunks of sautéed eggplant have a succulent, dense texture.

❖ Prepare dishes that are already familiar to you. *Heaven's Banquet* contains recipes for many meatless dishes commonly eaten by nonvegetarians.

❖ Above all, Ayurveda recommends changing your diet very gradually. Be comfortable and don't strain to avoid eating meat. Straining does not serve the cause of good health. Neither does guilt.

RESTRICTED DIETS

For those with food sensitivities, following an Ayurvedic program may help you become more tolerant of foods to which you are allergic. Some food sensitivities can be the result of toxic impurities, or ama, and imbalance. Others are aggravated by the way a specific food is prepared and combined with other foods, rather than by the food item itself. Most of the recipes in *Heaven's Banquet* can be successfully adapted to suit your special needs.

Low Salt and Salt-Free Diets: The Quest for F-L-A-V-O-R

Salt is good: but if the salt have lost its saltiness, where with will you season it?
Have salt in yourselves, and have peace, one with another.   —MARK 9.50

❖ Use the highest-quality ingredients. Very fresh organically grown produce, herbs, spices, etc., contain the most flavor, color, and texture.

❖ Lemon juice is your greatest Ayurvedic friend for adding flavor. You can sprinkle it over prepared dishes or add it during preparation.

❖ Become acquainted with a wide variety of herbs and spices. Fresh herbs have more flavor than dried ones. To bring out the flavor of dried herbs, sauté them in oil or lightly toast them in a dry pan before using. Indian spiced dishes are very flavorful. See "Indian-Style Spiced Vegetables and Curries" in the "Vegetables" chapter.

❖ Fresh ginger adds a wonderful kick to foods when raw and mellow flavor when cooked. Hing (asafoetida) sautéed in a little oil adds flavor to savory dishes.

❖ Use ghee and high-quality, expeller-pressed oils. Extra virgin olive oil, toasted sesame oil, walnut oil, and hazelnut oil are especially tasty.

❖ Waterless methods for cooking vegetables, such as baking, sautéing, stir-frying, or deep-frying in oil or ghee, bring out their flavors. If your use of oil is also restricted, try baking, or steaming in a steaming basket.

❖ Do not overcook foods.

❖ In addition to flavor, textural, and color contrasts add to the overall effect of an interesting meal.

Dairy-Free Cooking

Though Ayurveda recommends the consumption of dairy, almost every recipe in *Heaven's Banquet* can be prepared without the use of dairy products. The symbol ✪ in the recipes indicates a dairy-free variation.

Wheat-Free Cooking

❖ See the section on "Flours" in the "Basic Ingredients for a Heavenly Banquet" chapter to acquaint yourself with the wide variety of nonwheat flours. Many of these can be substituted for wheat flour in dishes that contain small amounts.

❖ Read the section on "Thickeners" in the "Basic Ingredients for a Heavenly Banquet" chapter. You can prepare flour-free cream sauces, cream soups, and other dishes usually thickened with a roux by using arrowroot or cornstarch. You can also experiment with rice flour, which the French consider a superior thickening agent because of its delicate flavor.

❖ Thick-textured soups and sauces can also be achieved by reducing the amount of liquid in a recipe and replacing it with puréed vegetables or grains. Dry, dense vegetables such as potatoes, winter squash, and cauliflower work well for this purpose. In earlier days finely powdered almonds and chestnuts were preferred thickening agents. Chestnut flour can sometimes be found in gourmet foods stores.

❖ Dosas (pp. 202–205), pancakes made from dal and rice, are adaptable to a wide variety of dishes. You can use them as crusts for individual pizzas, top with sandwich fillings, eat them like pancakes with jam or syrup, wrap them around fillings like crêpes, and apply dozens of other creative ideas.

❖ In recipes calling for breading, cornmeal or teff can substitute for bread crumbs.

❖ Steamed cabbage leaves and other large green leaves such as chard can be wrapped around the fillings in Crêpes (pp. 375–77), Wontons (p. 290), Pierogen (p. 268), etc. You can also use rice-flour spring roll wrappers and bean-curd skins (*yuba*), both found in Asian markets.

❖ Tortillas made from *masa harina*, a fine grind of hominy, can be used for chips, crackers, and flat breads. They can be deep-fried, toasted, or baked for a variety of textures.

Oil-Free Cooking

Ayurvedic cooking is usually done with at least a little oil. Totally oil-free cooking is recommended only during temporary, specially prescribed purification diets or when a specific medical need is established by a health-care practitioner.

❖ You can find nonstick woks, baking pans, muffin pans, and other cookware, in addition to the more common nonstick frying pans, in specialty kitchen stores. You can also line conventional baking pans with baker's parchment to render them stickless.

❖ Dishes that are usually fried or deep-fried, such as burgers, falafels, and samosas, can be baked instead. As a rule of thumb, bake them in a 350°F (180°C) oven for about 30 minutes, although times will vary a bit from recipe to recipe.

❖ Many recipes call for sautéing dried herbs or spices in oil to bring out their flavors. You can achieve a similar effect by lightly toasting them in a dry pan over low heat for a minute until they are fragrant.

❖ Prepare yeasted breads without oil by increasing the amount of water slightly. They will be a little drier and more crumbly.

❖ Read the section on "Thickeners" in the "Basic Ingredients for a Heavenly Banquet" chapter. Dishes that are usually thickened with a roux can instead be made with arrowroot or cornstarch.

THE AYURVEDIC KITCHEN: STAGE FOR THE DRAMA OF CREATION

My kitchen is a mystical place, a kind of temple for me. It is a place where the surfaces seem to have significance, where the sounds and odors carry meaning that transfers from the past and bridges to the future. —PEARL BAILEY

Organizing the kitchen means setting the stage and arranging the props for the miraculous drama of creation. How you create the stage set and the care you give to maintaining it—whether it's the most primitive campfire arrangement or a sophisticated, professionally equipped kitchen—can greatly affect the quality of your performance.

A branch of Vedic science revived as Maharishi Sthapatya Veda encompasses the field of Vedic architecture: how to construct buildings that promote the health and well-being of the people who live in them. It is a fascinating body of knowledge of building in harmony with the laws of nature, covering everything from optimum building materials to the ideal placement of each room to enhance its particular function. Sthapatya Veda prescribes the best location for the kitchen—and even of the stove within the kitchen—for healthy and harmonious cooking. If you are building or remodeling a home, you might wish to consult with an architect trained in Maharishi Sthapatya Veda to design an ideal, life-supporting environment.

❖ In the spirit of Ayurveda, it is good to help keep your extended body—the earth—healthy by recycling as much as possible, and by being alert that the materials you use in your kitchen do no harm. Commercial environmentally friendly products are available in natural foods stores. It is also remarkably simple and inexpensive to make cleaning supplies at home. An excellent source of information is *Nontoxic and Natural* by Debra Lynn Dadd (Jeremy Tarcher, 1984). An ancient technique of keeping the environment and atmosphere fresh is to periodically wash surfaces with a solution of strained lemon juice and salt diluted in plenty of water.

❖ It is important to consider what materials your tools, storage containers, and cookware are made of. All surfaces that touch your food should be either nonreactive, not cause any chemical reactions in the food, or reactive in a way that exerts a positive influence. Nonreactive materials include stainless steel and glass. Good reactive materials include unglazed clay, the most ancient and natural substance used for cooking, and cast iron.

The two most undesirable reactive surfaces are aluminum, which adds unhealthy aluminum salts to the food, and plastic, which adds various substances, including estrogens, to the food. Plastic containers and utensils can melt and can also absorb oils, which can become rancid and impart their flavor to foods. Cellophane or cellulose bags, processed from wood fibers, are a better choice than plastic bags and wrap.

❖ The most nontoxic sponges are natural sea sponges. There are also sponges made of cellulose, from wood fiber. Another option for cleaning up spills is to keep a large pile of inexpensive cotton dish towels. Reserve paper towels only for jobs that require a disposable absorber, such as draining deep-fried foods—the trees will thank you.

❖ Ayurveda does not recommend microwave ovens for the simple reason that they do not cook food by the traditional means of application of heat. It is the use of heat that transforms raw ingredients into nourishing food. All sorts of subtle transformations take place during this process that a microwave cannot begin to duplicate. The effects of microwaves on health have not been fully documented. However, it is wise to stay within the most basic laws of nature governing cooking.

All civilized nations cook their food, to improve its taste and digestibility. The degree of civilization is often measured by the cuisine.   —MARY LINCOLN

Ayurvedic Cookware

Different materials from which cookware is made have different properties; no one material seems to cover all bases. Some conduct heat well; others preserve the nutritional value of the food; and others clean easily. Some pots and pans combine several materials, utilizing the best features of each. There are many variations to choose from, even among top-of-the-line products. The following discussion of the basic components of good (and bad) cookware can help you make choices.

❖ *Stainless-steel* is nonreactive, easy to clean, and lightweight. However, it does not conduct heat particularly well. Cookware made of stainless steel combined with other metals, such as copper lined with stainless steel and stainless steel with an aluminum core, make use of the benign properties of stainless steel and the ability of the other metals to conduct heat well.

❖ *Copper* is an effective heat conductor. Most copper pots are lined with tin, but some can be found with stainless-steel linings; copper itself adversely affects acid ingredients. The lining should be checked once a year for damage or wear, and any broken or worn spots should be repaired to prevent the copper from touching the food.

❖ *Cast-iron* is heavy, slow heating, and introduces iron into the food. However, acid foods become discolored when cooked in cast iron.

❖ *Nonstick cookware:* A nonstick skillet pan is a real boon to Ayurvedic cooking, as you can sauté foods in a smaller amount of oil than in a conventional skillet. It is especially useful for foods that tend to stick to the pan, such as potatoes and tofu. A soapstone griddle, an almost extinct species, is the original nonstick cookware.

❖ *Enamel cookware* of high quality is fine. The inexpensive types tend to chip easily, exposing what is usually a less desirable material underneath.

❖ Nonmetallic cookware materials such as *treated glass* and unglazed or lead-free glazed *ceramic* are wonderful for Ayurvedic cooking; their only potential downside is their fragility relative to metal ware. Unglazed clay is great for baking bread, and it's a very Ayurvedic, close-to-nature material. Unglazed ceramic bakeware such as casserole dishes and pizza stones should heat with the oven rather than go in after it is preheated. Keep unglazed clay clean by scrubbing off baked-on food with a stiff brush when the tiles are cool. Do not use soap—it is absorbed by the clay and the flavor is released into your next dish.

❖ Wooden bowls are aesthetically beautiful for mixing and serving. However, wood absorbs oil, and the cold-pressed oils used in Ayurvedic cooking become rancid after a while and detract from the healthfulness and flavors of the foods housed in the bowl forever more.

Some Useful Tools for the Contemporary Ayurvedic Kitchen

Tools are made, but born are hands.   —WILLIAM BLAKE

Hands: Your hands are undoubtedly your best Ayurvedic tools. As long as they are clean, don't be afraid to use them for mixing, stirring, forming, and so forth. A meal is an expression of the inner qualities of the cook, and a cook's loving touch can only enhance it. Also, your hands are far more sensitive than any other instrument for detecting lumps and other textural qualities.

Blender: If you have a good food processor, you will need your blender mostly for liquids. Blenders produce smoother purées than food processors, but you must add more liquid to the mixture for the blender to handle it. Look for a blender that is powerful enough to crush ice—this indicates that it will be able to purée fruits, vegetables, and beans, make nut butters, and do dozens of other things. Whether it has three speeds or twenty is unimportant. The blender container should be glass, not plastic.

Food mill: A wonderful old-fashioned tool for puréeing soft foods such as cooked apples and root vegetables, the food mill leaves peels and other less-than-soft materials behind rather than blending them in, as food processors and blenders do.

Food processors: With a food processor, you can create an exciting variety of textures that are not easily accomplished by hand, such as purées and pâtés. You can use the processor for instant chopping, grating, and slicing, of course, but you can also prepare cake and cookie batters and pie and bread dough in it with minimal time and effort. The preparation technique that many chefs prefer to do by hand is slicing. You can be much more accurate with a knife than a slicing disc for producing uniform pieces in the shapes that you desire.

Grinders: Electric and hand grinders are available for grinding nuts, seeds, spices, and grains.

❖ A small electric coffee grinder works well for grinding spices, but a mortar and pestle brings out their flavors more. Look for a heavy, deep mortar with a slightly roughened surface for grinding spices, nuts, and seeds. Slightly roughened porcelain and stone work well—but nothing too rough, like volcanic stone. Smooth wooden, porcelain, and marble mortars are more decorative than practical.
❖ Keep a pepper grinder with your cooking spices for the freshly ground black pepper that is preferable for Ayurvedic cooking.

Knives: A good, sharp knife is the single most important kitchen utensil. Some professional chefs keep their own personal knives and carry them in a special case to wherever they are donning their toques. Forged blades are better than stamped blades. Carbon-steel blades are some of the finest. However, they must be washed and dried immediately after use.

Wok and karai: Woks, used extensively for Chinese and Japanese cooking for stir-frying, can also be used for sautéing, steaming, preparing soups and stews, and deep-frying. Buy a wok with a lid. Heavy rolled-steel woks are best for deep-frying and stir-frying. An Indian pot called a *karai* has the same basic shape as a wok but has steeper sides. Available in cast iron and stainless steel, karais can be purchased in Indian markets. They generally don't come with lids, but it's helpful to find a lid that fits.

> *Economy is a distributive virtue, and consists not in saving but in selection.*
> —EDMUND BURKE

COOKING: THE PROCESS OF TRANSFORMATION

If you aren't up to a little magic occasionally, you shouldn't waste your time trying to cook.
—COLETTE

Ayurveda recommends eating mostly cooked foods. Cooking transforms raw ingredients into better-tasting, more easily digested foods. Some nutrients are lost during any cooking process. However, in the final analysis the foods are rendered more digestible by cooking, and therefore the body is able to absorb *more* nutrients from them. I think of cooking as a process mirroring that of creation itself: all the variety in the universe comes out of different combinations of the five elements. In cooking, we select from a handful of ingredients, and by combining them in different ways and applying different cooking methods to our mixtures, we are able to conjure up an infinite variety of dishes. For instance, zucchini and flour—with a little help from a few accompanying ingredients—can be fried into zucchini pancakes, deep-fried into zucchini tempura, baked into zucchini bread, or boiled into cream of zucchini soup.

MENU PLANNING AND MENUS: CREATING AYURVEDIC MEALS FOR HEALTH, HARMONY, AND HAPPINESS

In a menu you have to succeed at harmony, and then your stomach is proud of you. It says, "You're intelligent. What you've done is right."
—JEAN BAPTISTE TROISGROS

When we prepare a meal, we become responsible for contributing to the health and well-being of those who eat it. It is a privilege, a blessing really, to be allowed to care for others—and for oneself—in such a manner, and it can be done with great dignity, creativity, and fun. The flow of an Ayurvedic meal from start to finish is designed to promote optimum digestion and maximum pleasure. Naturally, one is hungriest and the digestive powers are poised to pounce at the commencement of a meal. Therefore an ideal Ayurvedic meal begins with the heaviest foods first, then progresses to increasingly light dishes, ending with the lightest to digest, such as lassi or fruit. As always, these are guidelines to be aware of—not rigid decrees.

❖ For optimum digestion, it is best to eat your main meal at lunch and lighter fare for dinner. Until the Industrial Revolution this was the way of the world. When people began working at jobs away from home, families began to eat their main meal at dinnertime, when everyone was more likely to be together. This is a purely *sociological* phenomenon. The *physiological* reasons for eating the main meal at lunch remain unchanged: one has more hours of activity to digest the meal, and the metabolism works most efficiently during the day. It may be a major change of habit to make lunch your larger meal, but you will ultimately feel much healthier for it. Soups, breads, pasta, and milky grains such as Rice Pudding are all good evening fare.

❖ Try to include all six tastes in each meal.

❖ In general, cooked foods are more easily digested and metabolized than raw ones, and warm or room-temperature foods easier to digest than ice-cold ones. Mind-body types and the season play a role here (e.g., Pitta types and people during

Pitta season appreciate cooler foods, such as salads), but all types generally do better with a majority of warm, cooked foods.

❖ Sweet and unctuous foods are usually the heaviest dishes in a meal. Translation: Eat heavy desserts first! It is said that when the first bite you take has a sweet taste, the sweetness literally nourishes your feelings and inspires a sense of fulfillment that permeates the entire meal. When you think about it, it makes no sense whatsoever to eat something heavy and difficult to digest as a finale. However, if the dessert you are taking is light, such as a piece of fruit, it is more appropriate at the conclusion of a repast.

❖ Serve curds at the noontime meal rather than in the evening. Curds include cheeses, yogurt, buttermilk, and tofu. These foods are harder to digest and are more fully metabolized during the day, when we are more active. At night, when we are sleeping and the system is operating at a lower metabolic rate, they may not be fully digested. This creates toxic impurities, or ama. Furthermore, these foods increase Pitta and may keep you awake at night.

❖ Combinations of complementary yet contrasting elements create graceful, harmonious meals. Balance a heavy, filling dish with a light one, a complex dish with a simple one, a spicy food with a bland or cooling food, a crisp texture with a soft texture, a light color with a bright color.

❖ If you are serving a new and unusual dish to your family for the first time, perhaps the rest of the meal could be composed of old favorites.

❖ Plan a meal that can be prepared in the time available. If preparation of one dish takes most of your available time, the other dishes should be ones that can be assembled quickly.

❖ Plan dishes that will not need the same equipment at the same time; for example, bake the apples at 350°F (175°C) earlier in the day so that the pizza can go in later at 500°F (260°C).

One Week of Main Meals

Not on emerald but on cookery let us build our empire.
—CARMICHAEL, 18TH-CENTURY DIPLOMAT

Black Bean Cakes with Avocado-Pecan Salsa
New World Chopped Salad
Cilantro-Pumpkin Seed Corn Muffins with Herb-Flavored Ghee
Coffee-Almond Cheesecake

Asian-Cajun Eggplant Gumbo
Basmati Rice
Fennel Cole Slaw with Pecan Dressing
Louisiana Pralines

Dal I
Mixed Vegetable Curry (Sabji Tarkari)
Sudarshan Rice
Cilantro Chutney (Haridhania Chatni)
Cucumber Raita (Khira Raita)
Farina Halva (Sooji Halva)

Vegetable Soup with Lemon Pistou
Saffron Potato Cakes with Hazelnut Crust
Summer Squash with Fennel and Dill in Sour Cream
Blueberry Tea Cake

Spring Pasta for Pitta sprinkled with toasted almonds
The Vaidya's Salad
'Swonderful Shortbread

Mixed Vegetables Simmered in Coconut Milk (Sayur Manis)
Eggplant Salad with Crispy Tofu (Yum Mekeyau)
Golden Rice Simmered in Coconut Milk (Nasi Kuning)
Prasad Fruit Salad

Creamy Zucchini-Cashew Soup
Squash Stuffed with Wild Rice Succotash
Applesauce Gingerbread with Applesauce

He that will enter into Paradise must have a good key.　　—George Herbert

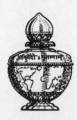

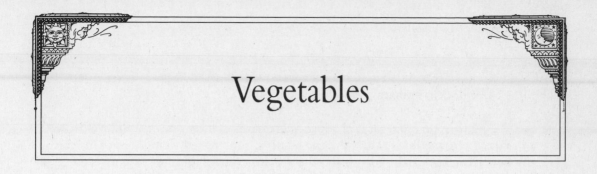

Vegetables

The essence of all beings is earth.
The essence of earth is water.
The essence of water is plants.
The essence of plants is human beings.

—*CHANDOGYA UPANISHAD*

Beautifully prepared, flavorful vegetable dishes are one of the glorious highlights of an Ayurvedic meal. Most vegetables are balancing for Kapha, many for Pitta, and a handful for Vata. However, vegetables cooked in ghee or oil with Vata-pacifying spices, when eaten in moderation, are balancing for Vata as well. The addition of herbs and spices and ingredients such as nuts and beans also affects a dish's overall effect on the doshas.

FIVE EASY PIECES OF ADVICE FOR AYURVEDIC VEGETABLE COOKERY

❖ It is good to add salt while the vegetables are cooking rather than shaking it on at the table, so that it can dissolve and become absorbed into the vegetables. This makes salt more easily absorbed by the body, lessening the chances of any problems caused by salt intake.
❖ Slower cooking methods and a lower heat are recommended for Ayurvedic vegetable cooking, as generally it is beneficial to heat foods slowly as an assist to the numerous nutritional transformations that take place during the cooking process.
❖ In Ayurvedic cuisine, vegetables are more thoroughly cooked than is presently in fashion. Not overcooked, but not crunchy, warmed-up raw. Generally, vegetables that are well cooked with a little oil or ghee are the most digestible and nutritious.
❖ Harder-to-digest vegetables, including potatoes, broccoli, cauliflower, Brussels sprouts, and cabbage, are recommended for daytime repasts rather than evening.

SELECTION

Vegetables have been improved until they're downright poisonous.

—JOSEPH MITCHELL

For those who have concluded that a good vegetable is hard to find—you are right! You have to be careful, discriminating, and knowledgeable.

❖ According to Ayurveda, ideal produce is grown *in season*, *locally,* and by *organic*, *soil-sustaining* methods. These are the ancient, time-tested techniques of nurturing the best from the earth. Obviously, the way to control all these factors is to grow your own. But for those who don't have a garden plot or the time or desire for one, here are some guidelines for selection.

In Season

How many things by season seasoned are. —WILLIAM SHAKESPEARE

FWhen you support Natural Law, Natural Law supports you. The laws of Nature that create the seasons dictate which plants are fruitful during each one. It is all part of a larger ecological plan of life, and eating foods when they are in season helps keep the individual in harmony with Nature's Big Picture. This is simply and amply evidenced by the fact that no matter how hard we try to circumvent those laws, fruits and vegetables always *taste* best when they are grown in their natural season.

Locally Grown

Our bodies are intimately connected with our entire environment. The air we breathe, the water we drink, the climactic conditions we encounter, all literally become part of us. For this reason we are better nourished by produce grown in the same geological and climactic conditions that we are exposed to. In order to transport produce over long distances, a lot of artificial procedures must be applied to circumvent nature, such as harvesting unripe produce, applying coatings to it, and later "ripening" it with gasses.

Does this mean we should never eat a mango if we live in Toronto, or subsist solely on potatoes and beets in a Nebraska winter of our discontent? Not quite. It means that when there is a choice between purchasing a Toronto-grown green bean and one that has just gotten off the plane from Tierra del Fuego, we know which one is the wiser Ayurvedic choice. It is not always possible to obtain produce from exclusively local sources, but do it when you can. Farmers' markets and produce stores that buy directly from nearby farmers are good bets.

Organically Grown by Soil-Sustaining Methods

*O pure Earth, may that we utilize your soil well without causing you injury or harm and disturbing any vital element in you. —*ATHARVA VEDA, PRITHIVI SUKTA

By "organically grown," I mean undyed, unsprayed, untreated vegetables grown from ungenetically engineered seeds with natural fertilizers. Organically grown produce may be more expensive and difficult to obtain for a number of complex political and societal reasons, none of which are worth compromising your health and world ecology for. The precious soil that our Mother Earth wears and shares with us so generously has sustained countless generations of living beings. It is the responsibility of each generation to care for the land properly during its short time of stewardship so that it remains unpolluted and fertile for the next generation. As consumers, we can support wise and enlightened farmers who practice soil-sustaining agriculture.

COOKING WITH WATER: BOILED AND STEAMED VEGETABLES

Ayurveda recommends preparing foods with a little oil of some type, except when following temporary prescribed purification diets or while ill. However, many people are joined at the hip to their vegetable steamers and get, uh, steamed at the thought of using any other method. No problem. Think about perhaps adding a dab of ghee or oil to the vegetables as they steam or dressing them lightly with an unctuous sauce before serving.

* ❖ A steaming basket is the best tool. Cooking vegetables directly in water leaches away nutrients and flavor.
* ❖ All vegetables can be steamed. Long-cooking root vegetables such as potatoes, beets, and turnips can be cut into small pieces so that they finish cooking in your lifetime.
* ❖ Add salt to vegetables while they are steaming to help keep them firm and to allow the salt to dissolve and become absorbed.
* ❖ Most vegetables fare better with steaming than with boiling. However, long-cooking vegetables that keep their jackets on during cooking, such as potatoes, yams, artichokes, turnips, and beets, can be boiled without loss of flavor and nutrients.

THE WAY OF SAUTÉING

Slow sautéing is an excellent method that is frequently employed in Ayurvedic vegetable preparation. Sautéing greatly enhances the flavor of most vegetables. It also enables you to add health- and flavor-enhancing herbs and spices to the vegetables as they cook.

* ❖ A technique I use that cooks vegetables more quickly and thoroughly than conventional sautéing is to keep the heat fairly low and cover the skillet, lifting the lid to stir occasionally.
* ❖ For best results, sauté vegetables in ghee or oil. Butter is fine for shorter-cooking

vegetables but may burn during a long haul. I usually sauté vegetables in a non-stick pan, which allows the use of less oil and prevents them from sticking and burning.

❖ For long-cooking vegetables such as winter squash, potatoes, beets, and turnips, boil whole until partially cooked, then drain, peel, and slice into small pieces for sautéing. Alternatively, cut into tiny pieces and sauté very slowly for a long time.

❖ Use flavored ghee and oils for subtle enhancement. Dried herbs can be added at the beginning of cooking. With the exception of rosemary and sage, fresh green herbs lose their flavors with long cooking and are best chopped and tossed in just before serving.

❖ Drizzle in a small amount of tahini or Taratoor Sauce (pp. 512–13) just before serving, or stir one or two spoonfuls of nut butter into sautéed vegetables and thin with stock or water to a sauce consistency.

❖ To heft up sautéed vegetables, add any of the following at the end of cooking, just before removing from the stove. Add a grain and a salsa or chutney, and you have a lovely meal.

Sautéed pieces of firm tofu, seitan, or panir (p. 209)
Toasted nuts, or toasted sesame, sunflower, or pumpkin seeds (pp. 545–46)
Plain Pakoras (pp. 291–92)
Plain Vadas (pp. 295–96)
Wheat Balls for Spaghetti (p. 256)

ROASTING VEGETABLES TO INTENSIFY FLAVOR

Roasting magnifies vegetables' natural flavors. They cook slowly, with little or no water added to remove their natural juices, and the sugars in long-cooking vegetables such as beets and carrots caramelize and intensify their flavors. Although most vegetables, with the exception of leafy greens, can be roasted, root vegetables and squash respond especially well. Add dried green herbs, citrus juice, liquid seasoning, or salt and pepper while roasting for increased flavor.

❖ Most vegetables can be baked whole. Halve or quarter them to reduce cooking time, which may be desirable in the case of rutabagas, turnips, and winter squash.

Method:
1. Coat a baking pan and the prepared vegetables generously with oil or melted ghee. If you wish to avoid oil, place prepared vegetables in a baking dish with a little water to prevent scorching.
2. Cover and bake in a 400°F (200°C) oven until very tender, 30 to 40 minutes for most.

*There are many ways to love a vegetable. The most sensible way is to love it
well treated. Then you can eat it with the comfortable knowledge that you will
be a better man for it, in your spirit and in your body too.* —M. F. K. FISHER

DEEP-FRIED VEGETABLES

People love the appearance of deep-fried vegetables with their crisp brown edges, and
cooking in oil always enhances flavor better than water cooking. However, the trade-off
is that they are more difficult to digest than vegetables cooked by any other method and
are recommended by Ayurveda only for occasional occasions.

 ## TEMPURA

JAPAN   *4 servings*

Tempura was invented in sixteenth-century Japan to please Portuguese traders, who rel-
ished batter-dipped, deep-fried foods. However, Japanese artistry created something
light, delicate, and vegetarian from a concept that usually produced greasy, heavy fare.
The Catholic Portuguese named the dish from their word for the vegetarian "ember
days" of Lent. The secret to crisp, nongreasy tempura is to have the oil very hot and the
batter chilled.

*¾ cup (110 g) unbleached white or
  whole wheat flour
¾ cup (90 g) soy or besan (chickpea)
  flour
1 teaspoon salt*

*1 cup plus 2 tablespoons (270 ml)
  water
Oil for deep-frying
4 to 5 cups (1 to 1.2 l) sliced vegetables*

1. Combine the flours, salt, and water in a blender or beat until smooth. Chill. Add
   more water if necessary.
2. Heat the oil for deep-frying. Have a platter covered with paper towels nearby.
3. Pat the vegetables dry with a towel. Dip each piece into the batter to coat thoroughly.
4. One at a time, gently drop the pieces into the hot oil. Deep-fry until golden and
   crisp, turning once or twice as necessary. Drain and serve immediately.

VARIATIONS

Urad and other dal flours can substitute for the soy or chickpea flour.

Fruit Fritters: Prepare tempura with firm, fairly dry fruits such as apple and
pineapple rings, banana chunks, and apricot halves. (Juicy, squishy types dilute the

batter and fall apart during cooking.) After draining on paper towels, dust with confectioner's sugar.

Tempura Kebabs: For a dramatic presentation, prepare tempura from skewered foods.

1. Thread foods prepared for tempura on small wooden skewers. (You can find them in most supermarkets.) Leave plenty of room at each end of the skewer for holding.
2. Heat oil for deep-frying in a wide pot or 10-inch (26 cm) skillet with high sides. Have a platter covered with paper towels nearby.
3. Pour the tempura batter into a wide, shallow receptacle, such as a cake pan. Dip the entire skewer into the batter and coat all the food thoroughly.
4. Deep-fry the kebabs. Turn gently once or twice during the frying as necessary. Drain and serve immediately.

STIR-FRIED VEGETABLES

By Ayurvedic standards, vegetables stir-fried for the classical 2 minutes emerge undercooked and difficult to digest. I suggest cooking vegetables in a wok on a medium rather than high flame for a few minutes more than the traditional stir-fry. Or use the *kinpura* method described below. Vegetables should emerge crisp-tender rather than hard and crunchy—a degree or two past warmed-up raw. This pleasant compromise provides the flavors and most of the textures of traditional stir-fried vegetables but is kinder and gentler to the stomach.

❖ Most vegetables can be stir-fried or kinpura-fried, though the techniques work best for those that cook quickly. Longer-cooking vegetables should be cut into tiny pieces, and root vegetables can be grated.

Kinpura-Fried Vegetables

The kinpura technique was developed in Japan to combine steaming and stir-frying. It cooks all vegetables more thoroughly and is especially useful for longer-cooking varieties.

Method:
1. Begin to stir-fry.
2. After about 10 seconds, sprinkle a little water over the vegetables and cover immediately. The water creates steam, which will further cook them. Avoid adding so much water that it collects in the bottom of the wok.
3. After the water has evaporated, sprinkle on a little more water. Continue sprinkling and stir-frying until the vegetables are sufficiently cooked.

It is dangerous to heat, cool, or make a commotion all of a sudden in the body . . . because everything that is excessive is an enemy to nature.   —HIPPOCRATES

STIR-FRIED VEGETABLES WITH ALMONDS (CHAO SUCAI XINGREN)

CHINA *4 servings*

Here is a basic stir-fry, which is delicious as is or can be used as the starting point for many variations.

STEP ONE

2 tablespoons mild-flavored oil
Pinch of hing (optional)

1 to 2 tablespoons minced fresh ginger

STEP TWO

6 cups (1.4 l) thinly sliced mixed
vegetables (8 cups/2 l if large
amounts of greens are included)
Liquid seasoning

⅓ cup (45 g) blanched almonds, toasted
Toasted sesame oil
White pepper
Chopped fresh cilantro

1. Heat the oil in a wok. Add the hing and ginger and sauté for 30 seconds over medium heat.
2. Add the vegetables, sprinkle on a little liquid seasoning, and stir-fry over medium heat until crisp-tender. Add the almonds. Garnish with a few drops of toasted sesame oil and white pepper and cilantro to taste.

VARIATION
   Stir-Fried Vegetables with Tofu (Chao Sucai Doufu): Replace the almonds with 1 cup (220 g) sautéed cubed tofu. You can also use both almonds and tofu together.

THROW A ZUCCHINI ON THE BARBIE: GRILLED VEGETABLES

Columbus reported that the West Indies natives cooked foods on a grate made of green sticks set over a fire. The name of such fare? *Barbacoa.* This may be the origin of the name for a certain backyard activity. Grilling imparts its unique, irresistible smoky flavor and, like roasting, intensifies vegetables' natural flavors.

❖ Consider the grill. Vegetables are smaller than the foods that grills are customarily designed to accommodate. You might want to obtain one of the screenlike affairs used to grill delicate fish.
❖ Before grilling, coat vegetables with oil to keep them from drying out and shriveling. Try olive oil and flavored oils to go the extra mile on flavor. You can also use Citrus Vinaigrette (p. 318).
❖ Preheat the grill and brush the grate with oil to prevent sticking. Grill vegetables

on one side until halfway cooked, then turn them over and leave them alone until done. The less you move them around, the better the sear marks will look.

❖ Serve grilled vegetables at room temperature as part of a salad or an antipasto platter. They are also a delicious addition to sandwiches. The mock mayonnaises go well with grilled vegetables, as do spoonfuls of pesto, Guacamole (pp. 279–80), and Sambal (pp. 515–16). Or keep it simple with just a spritz of citrus juice.

❖ Chop or purée grilled vegetables into soups, stews, and sauces. There is a substantial difference in flavor when you prepare a cream soup with a base of grilled—rather than sautéed—vegetables. Adding some chopped grilled peppers to a simple vegetable medley dresses it up considerably.

Vegetables to Grill

❖ *Asparagus:* Yes! It works! Just be careful to not let the spears fall through a widely spaced grate.

❖ *Artichokes:* Steam or boil artichokes until just barely done. Drain, but leave a little water on to further steam them on the grill. Halve lengthwise and cut out the chokes. Place on the grill cut side down until they are seated by the grate.

❖ *Root vegetables such as celeriac, beets, carrots, parsnips, potatoes, and yams:* Steam or boil root vegetables until just barely tender, then slice and finish them on the grill. Be careful with potatoes and yams; they should be underdone and cut into large, thick slices. Handle gingerly. Carrots and parsnips can be grilled whole.

❖ *Corn:* Peel back the husk but do not remove it. Pull out the cornsilk as best you can, then smooth the husk back over the corn. Thoroughly immerse the ears in cold water. (The water helps steam the corn while it grills.) Gently shake off the excess water. Grill, husk and all, for about 25 minutes, turning the corn several times. Be careful when removing the husks—they're hot.

❖ *Eggplant:* A real winner. Cut into slices ¼-inch (5 mm) thick. Lightly prick or score with a fork and brush particularly well with oil. The skin will become charred, so remove it before serving.

❖ *Fennel:* Slice lengthwise so that the stalks remain attached to the bulb. Steam until halfway cooked, then finish on the grill, cut side down.

❖ *Bell peppers:* A natural for grilling. Remove the seeds and cut into halves or quarters. Flatten as much as possible.

❖ *Tomatoes:* Grilled tomatoes don't hold their shape well; however, their smoky flavor adds an unusual touch to sauces and soups. Grill firm tomatoes, such as Romas, whole, then chop or purée.

❖ *Zucchini and other summer squash:* Halve small squash lengthwise. Slice large squash lengthwise into three or four pieces or into long diagonals.

Kebabs

Also called *shish kebabs* and *shashlik,* kebabs provide an attractive, if theatrical, presentation. Pile up kebabs on a serving platter or bring them to the table on individual plates atop beds of grain. Bulgar Pilaf and couscous are traditional. I have also presented kebabs atop Curried Pasta with Apricots and Pine Nuts.

❖ Aim for a contrast of colors, flavors, and textures. Generally, two pieces each of four or five different foods are sufficient for each kebab. Cut into chunks large enough to be skewered. Either brush with oil or marinate in Citrus Vinaigrette (p. 318) for an hour.

❖ Carefully thread on skewers. You can use metal skewers or the little wooden skewers available in supermarkets. For a rustic, aromatic presentation, thread foods on fresh rosemary branches. Leave room at each end of the skewer for picking it up. Alternatively, broil by placing the skewers over a roasting pan to catch the dripping marinade. Lower the broiler rack and turn the kebabs every few minutes until done.

Vegetable Purées

Besides the familiar potatoes and squash, most vegetables can be transformed into delightful purées. Try puréed peas, carrots, cauliflower, Jerusalem artichokes, broccoli, or beets—it can be like discovering entirely new vegetables. Vegetable purées can be used to replace part of the water in soups and stews for thickness and flavor and can also be thinned to create sauces.

Method: Cook about twice the amount of vegetables as the amount of purée you desire (for example, 6 cups/780 g of raw peas will produce approximately 3 cups/720 ml of purée). Vegetables can be puréed in a food mill, food processor, blender, or for a lumpier rendition, with a potato masher. Food mills separate the pulp from the skin and any tough bits. Food processors and blenders mix everything together, so you must peel vegetables and remove all their tough parts before puréeing. *Never, never* purée potatoes in a food processor unless you are partial to glue.

Once you have processed, blended, mashed, or otherwise beaten your vegetables to a pulp, you can enhance the purée with citrus juice, ghee, crème frâiche, a little mint in pea purée, dill or grated orange zest in carrot purée, cinnamon in rutabaga or parsnip purée, and so forth.

Vegetables au Gratin

Gratin means "crust" in French, and refers to a dish topped with a sprinkling of bread crumbs and baked until the crumbs are browned. French gratins are light and delicate, with just a smattering of sumptuous, golden crust. They do not necessarily include the heavy cheese sauce featured in made-in-the-U.S.A. versions. A *gratin dish* is an unlidded shallow casserole that is designed for both baking and serving.

❖ *Vegetables á la Polonaise:* A more rapidly prepared alternative to a gratin is to serve a dish in the Polonaise, or Polish, style. Top cooked vegetables with bread crumbs that have been sautéed in a little ghee or oil for a few minutes until toasty brown. The treatment works wonderfully well with crucifers such as cauliflower, broccoli, and Brussels sprouts.

 # PISTACHIO GRATIN OF ASPARAGUS

6 servings

A light gratin that you can apply to all the vegetables of the rainbow. For a more standard coating, replace the ground nuts with more bread crumbs and omit the ginger and lemon zest.

	STEP TWO
1½ *pounds (750 g) asparagus*	*Salt*
Ghee or oil	*Black pepper*
Lemon juice	

	STEP THREE
3 *tablespoons fine*	1 *teaspoon finely grated lemon zest*
dry bread crumbs	1 *tablespoon melted ghee or oil*
3 *tablespoons ground pistachios*	*Salt*
½ *teaspoon ground ginger*	

1. Butter a gratin dish or an oven-to-table baking dish.
2. Trim the tough ends off the asparagus. Steam until just barely tender and no more. Place in the gratin dish and toss with a little ghee and lemon juice and a sprinkling of salt and pepper. Arrange evenly.
3. Toss the bread crumbs with the pistachios, ginger, lemon zest, ghee or oil, and a sprinkling of salt. Sprinkle evenly over the asparagus.
4. Place in the broiler for a minute or two, until the topping is lightly browned. Be very alert not to burn the crumbs.

VARIATION
Add ½ cup (120 ml) crème frâiche or thick coconut milk to the asparagus before adding the crumbs.

INDIAN-STYLE SPICED VEGETABLES AND CURRIES

The spices and seasonings associated with Indian cooking are essential elements of Ayurvedic cooking. Your entire mind-body system sings a joyful song when it is offered vegetables sumptuously flavored with aromatic spices. Spices help ensure that the six tastes are present and accounted for, and individual spices offer many different health-enhancing effects. Furthermore, the techniques by which Indian vegetable dishes are prepared tend to follow sound Ayurvedic principles: they are well cooked and contain a little oil.

> All the dishes lumped under the title of "curry" in the West are not considered as such in India, where *karhi* or *kadi* is a thin, yogurt-based sauce. In India spiced vegetables are usually categorized as either "wet" or "dry." Wet dishes contain a liquid sauce in which the vegetables are usually braised, and dry dishes are vegetables sautéed with spices. Within these loosely descriptive categories is a wide range of regional variations.

Preparing Indian–Style Vegetables

The following describes a general *style* of preparing vegetables. You can use spices quite subtly if you wish, and the dish will certainly not be hot unless you deliberately add chilies or large amounts of warming spices such as pepper and mustard seeds.

Method:
1. Heat a little ghee or mild-flavored oil in a lidded skillet, wok, or heavy pot. Add spices that require sautéing and cook for about 1 minute over low heat.
2. Stir in the vegetables, salt, and remaining spices, turmeric last.
3. *For a dry dish:* Cover and sauté until the vegetables are tender, stirring occasionally. *For a wet dish:* Pour in just enough water to steam the vegetables: ½ to ¾ cup (120 to 180 ml) for 4 cups vegetables. Cover and simmer until the vegetables are tender.

Ingredients:
- ❖ *Oils:* Ghee and mild-flavored oils, such as sunflower and sesame, are most appropriate.
- ❖ *Spices* are the most distinctive feature of this style of cooking. To get acquainted with their flavors, try adding one or two spices while sautéing vegetables or preparing a stew. Add a little fresh ginger when sautéing spinach, some mustard seeds sautéed in oil to a stew, a little cumin and turmeric to sautéing vegetables. Conservative bravery brings success. Here is a list of spices to choose from. Do not attempt to use all of them in one dish!

To sauté in oil in Step 1 before adding the vegetables:
Hing
Whole cumin seeds

Whole brown mustard seeds
Peeled and minced fresh ginger
Whole or ground fenugreek
Whole fennel seeds

To add in Step 2 with the vegetables:
Ground coriander
Whole or ground cloves
Ground cinnamon
Crushed cardamom seeds
Ground black pepper
Ground turmeric (always add last—it is somewhat heat sensitive)

To add in Step 3, just before serving:
Chopped fresh cilantro
Garam masala

Flavorings:
❖ Grated coconut is used in south Indian and Gujarati dishes. Sauté in Step 1 with the other spices.
❖ Split, hulled urad dal is employed as a seasoning in south Indian cooking. Sauté a tiny amount in Step 1 along with the other spices until it is a light reddish brown. Add it to the oil first so that it cooks the longest.
❖ Sprinkle on a little lemon or lime juice just before serving.
❖ A small amount of chopped tomato, about one medium tomato per dish, is added as a flavoring in north India and Pakistan. Sauté in Step 1 for a few minutes after adding the spices and before adding the vegetables.

Sauces: The "wet" vegetable dishes of India tend to have more sauce than Western dishes; they often resemble soup. Sauces are cooked in the pot with the vegetables rather than served as a separate entity.

❖ Stir in yogurt or buttermilk at the end of cooking, and heat just to serving temperature. One to 2 cups (240 to 480 ml) sauce is enough for vegetables to serve 4 to 6 people. You can also use a mixture of chopped tomatoes, added first, as described above, and buttermilk or yogurt added at the end of cooking. Use approximately 1 cup (240 ml) of each.
❖ Stir a small amount of crème fraîche or sour cream into a finished dish. In earlier times the cream that rose to the top of yogurt made from unhomogenized milk was employed.
❖ Add tamarind water and a little sugar for a sweet-and-sour dish.

You can create a more substantial main course dish by adding any of the following, alone or in combination:

Vadas (add just before serving to a "wet" vegetable dish)
Pakoras (add just before serving to a "wet" vegetable dish)
Cubes of pan-browned Panir (add during the last minute of cooking)
Toasted cashews or almonds

❖ *The Ultimate Addition:* For festivals, weddings, and other celebratory occasions, Indians serve dishes topped with edible pure silver foil. Just before serving, place 2 to 3 leaves of silver on top of the food. Don't worry about proper arrangement or about breaking the leaves—it doesn't matter. Silver foil is available in gourmet kitchen supply stores and Indian markets.

 # MIXED VEGETABLE CURRY I

INDIA   *4 servings*

A somewhat moist curry. You can omit the tomatoes and water for a drier dish.

STEP ONE

2 tablespoons ghee or mild-flavored
  oil
Pinch of hing (optional)
1 to 2 tablespoons minced fresh
  ginger

1 teaspoon cumin seeds
3/4 teaspoon brown mustard seeds
2 medium tomatoes, chopped

STEP TWO

1 cup (100 g) finely cut cauliflower
2/3 cup (25 g) peeled and finely cubed
  eggplant
2/3 cup (40 g) finely cut green beans
2/3 cup (90 g) peas
1 medium zucchini, quartered
  lengthwise and sliced

1 medium potato, peeled and diced,
  or 1 cup (110 g) peeled and diced
  winter squash
1 teaspoon turmeric
Salt
1 teaspoon sugar
1/2 cup (120 ml) water
Chopped fresh cilantro

1. Heat the ghee or oil in a pot. Add the hing, ginger, cumin, and mustard seeds, and sauté over low heat until the mustard seeds "dance," about 1 minute. Add the tomatoes and cook for 2 to 3 minutes, stirring frequently.
2. Add the vegetables, turmeric, a sprinkling of salt, the sugar, and water. Bring to a boil. Cover, reduce the heat, and simmer until the vegetables are tender, 20 to 30 minutes. Stir in the cilantro and adjust the salt.

❀ MIXED VEGETABLE CURRY II

INDIA   *4 servings*

The legacy of an Indian monk visiting America, this rich curry in a buttermilk sauce is served over rice or with Indian flat breads. It is especially sumptuous topped with Vadas or Pakoras.

STEP ONE

⅓ cup (75 g) ghee
½ teaspoon salt
1 teaspoon cumin seeds
½ teaspoon ground fenugreek
½ teaspoon ground cinnamon

¼ teaspoon ground cardamom
1 to 3 whole cloves
½ teaspoon turmeric
2 medium tomatoes, chopped

STEP TWO

2 tablespoons besan (chickpea flour)   *2 cups (480 ml) buttermilk*

STEP THREE

*¾ cup each: peas (110 g),
finely cut cauliflower
(75 g), zucchini, quartered
lengthwise and sliced (75 g),
thinly sliced carrots (90 g),
and finely cut green beans (85 g)*

Chopped fresh cilantro

1. Heat the ghee in a pot over low heat. Add the salt. Add the spices in order at 30-second intervals. When all the spices have been added, add the tomatoes and cook for 2 to 3 minutes. Mash with a fork while cooking.
2. Stir in the besan. Cook for 1 minute, stirring constantly. Slowly add the buttermilk, stirring constantly.
3. Add the vegetables. Cover and simmer until the vegetables are tender, about 20 minutes. Stir in the cilantro and adjust the salt.

VARIATION

❂ Replace the buttermilk with coconut milk for a more cooling influence for Pitta.

VEGETABLE STEWS

A well-prepared stew fulfills all the recommendations of Ayurvedic vegetable preparation: it is warm, well cooked, and moist. Stews can be prepared from almost any vegetable and make excellent use of small amounts of beans and grains that may be languishing in the cupboard. You can prepare hearty winter stews with root vegetables, which benefit from the long cooking this method provides.

- ❖ Heavy lidded soup pots and casseroles are ideal. You can also perform the initial cooking steps on the stove, then transfer the stew to a Crock-Pot to simmer.
- ❖ Braising is the most common method of preparing stews; the preliminary sautéing helps bring out the flavors of herbs and vegetables before liquid is added to "stew" the mixture.
- ❖ Beans and grains add thickening. You can also use less water to cook the stew and add Béchamel Sauce, vegetable purées, or Nut or Pan Gravy toward the end of cooking.
- ❖ Employ everything and anything from your repertoire to flavor your stew. Vegetables cooked in liquid tend to taste a tad washed out. Miriam's Sofrito, liquid seasoning, and vegetable broth granules can be useful. The suggestions at the beginning of the "Soups" chapter are helpful, since a stew is essentially a very thick soup.

 # VEGETABLE GOULASH

HUNGARY   *4 to 6 servings*

One man may yearn for fame, another for wealth, but everyone yearns for paprika goulash.   —HUNGARIAN PROVERB

Goulash has been prepared in eastern Europe since the ninth century, originally seasoned with caraway and saffron. Paprika, the spice usually associated with the dish, was developed in Hungary from New World capsicums in the sixteenth century. If you like heat, use hot rather than sweet paprika and add to taste—1 tablespoon of hot paprika might induce global warming. Serve over wide, flat pasta.

STEP ONE

¼ cup (55 g) ghee or butter
Pinch of hing (optional)
1 bell pepper, cut into chunks
2 medium potatoes, peeled and cubed

1 stalk fennel or celery, thinly sliced
2 cups (210 g) shredded cabbage
1 carrot, thinly sliced
1 teaspoon dried marjoram or oregano

STEP TWO

¾ cup (180 ml) water
3 cups (700 g) chopped tomatoes

1 teaspoon finely grated lemon zest

STEP THREE

1 teaspoon caraway seeds
1 tablespoon sweet paprika

Liquid seasoning or salt
¼ to ½ teaspoon black pepper

STEP FOUR

2 tablespoons ghee or butter

2 tablespoons flour

1. Heat the ghee or butter in a heavy lidded pot or casserole. Add the hing, vegetables, and marjoram or oregano. Sauté for 5 minutes over low heat, stirring frequently.
2. Stir in the water, tomatoes, and lemon zest. Cover and simmer until all the vegetables are tender, 20 to 30 minutes.
3. Add the caraway seeds, paprika, salt, and plenty of black pepper to taste.
4. Melt the ghee or butter in a small skillet over low heat. Add the flour and cook for 1 minute, stirring rapidly with a whisk to remove lumps.
5. Beat into the goulash and simmer until thickened, 2 to 3 minutes.

 # TAGINE OF FAVA BEANS, ARTICHOKE HEARTS, AND EGGPLANT WITH APRICOT COUSCOUS

MOROCCO   *4 servings*

A springtime dish. A tagine is a stew prepared in a *couscousière*, an ingenious double-boiler-type arrangement in which the tagine cooks in the lower vessel and the couscous sits over it in a steamer-like chamber, cooking in the fragrant steam from the tagine. You can use lima or other fresh beans instead of favas—you don't need to blanch and peel other beans. The carrots and couscous add more balance to the vegetables for Vata and Pitta. See page 65 for how to prepare fresh artichoke hearts.

STEP ONE

3 tablespoons olive oil
Pinch of hing (optional)
2 tablespoons minced fresh
   ginger
1½ teaspoons cumin seeds

⅔ cup (80 g) chopped fennel or
   celery
1 medium red bell pepper, coarsely
   chopped

STEP TWO

3 cups (210 g) peeled and cubed
   eggplant
6 artichoke hearts
2 carrots, quartered lengthwise
   and cut into 2-inch (5 cm) pieces

1 tomato, chopped (optional)

STEP THREE

2 cups (300 g) shucked,
   blanched, and peeled fava beans
1 cup (240 ml) stock or water
¼ teaspoon saffron threads
½ teaspoon turmeric

½ teaspoon paprika
¼ teaspoon ground cinnamon
1 teaspoon sugar
Salt

STEP FOUR

1 tablespoon lemon juice

⅔ cup (160 ml) chopped fresh cilantro

1. Heat the oil in a large pot. Add the hing, ginger, and cumin seeds and sauté over low heat until fragrant, about 1 minute. Add the fennel or celery and the bell pepper and sauté, stirring frequently, for 5 minutes.
2. Add the eggplant, artichoke hearts, carrots, and tomato. Continue to sauté, stirring frequently, until the eggplant begins to become tender.
3. Stir in the fava beans, stock or water, spices, and sugar. Sprinkle with salt. Cover and simmer until the beans and vegetables are tender.
4. Stir in the lemon juice and cilantro. Adjust the salt. Serve with couscous.

 # APRICOT COUSCOUS

4 to 6 servings

Substitute quinoa for couscous and dried cranberries for apricots to provide more balance for Kapha.

STEP ONE

3 tablespoons ghee or olive oil
Pinch of hing (optional)

¾ cup (90 g) chopped fennel or
celery

STEP TWO

1 cup (185 g) couscous
2 cups (480 ml) stock or water
½ teaspoon salt
½ cup (60 g) thinly sliced dried
apricots

½ teaspoon ground cinnamon
½ teaspoon crushed cardamom seeds

STEP THREE

⅓ cup (45 g) blanched almonds, toasted

1. Heat the ghee or oil in a saucepan. Add the hing and sauté until fragrant, about 30 seconds. Add the fennel or celery and sauté over low heat for 5 minutes.
2. Add the couscous. Sauté, stirring, for 2 minutes. Add the stock or water, salt, dried apricots, cinnamon, and cardamom. Bring to a boil, cover, reduce the heat, and simmer until all the water is absorbed and the couscous is tender.
3. Stir in the almonds and fluff up the couscous with a fork.

MIDDAY AT THE OASIS

Tagine of Fava Beans, Artichoke Hearts, and Eggplant
Apricot Couscous
Cucumbers with Yogurt, Dill, and Mint (p. 305)
Lemon–Mint Sorbet (p. 481)

VEGETABLES STROGANOFF

RUSSIA   *4 to 6 servings*

This version, with a tomatoey vegetable sauce, must have come from some Italian branch of the Stroganoff family. Actually, its creator is American; Penelope Winslow described her invention to me while strolling through the Swiss Alps. She cooks it for 8 hours, something I've never managed to do. Serve over wide flat pasta.

STEP ONE

2 tablespoons olive oil
Pinch of hing (optional)
1 cup (240 ml) minced fresh
  parsley
1 teaspoon dried basil leaves

½ teaspoon dried thyme
¼ teaspoon rosemary
½ bell pepper, finely chopped
1 carrot, grated
1 medium zucchini, grated

STEP TWO

3 cups (700 g) chopped ripe
  tomatoes
½ cup (120 ml) vegetable stock or
  water

1 bay leaf

STEP THREE

⅔ cup each: sliced carrots (80 g),
  zucchini (60 g), and
  cauliflower (70 g)

½ cup (65 g) peas

STEP FOUR

½ to ¾ cup (60 to 120 ml)
  sour cream

Liquid seasoning or salt
Black pepper

1. Heat the olive oil in a heavy lidded pot. Add the hing and herbs and sauté over low heat for about 30 seconds. Add the bell pepper, grated carrot, and zucchini and sauté for 5 minutes more.
2. Add the tomatoes, stock or water, and bay leaf. Cover and simmer over very low heat, stirring occasionally, until the sauce is very thick, 1½ to 2 hours.
3. Steam the carrots, zucchini, cauliflower, and peas until tender. Drain thoroughly and add to the sauce.
4. Add the sour cream. Season to taste with liquid seasoning or salt and pepper.

VARIATIONS
   Stir in cubes of sautéed tofu, seitan, or Panir at the end of cooking.
   ✿ Replace the sour cream with Tofu Mayonnaise (p. 503).

VEGETABLE PIES

"Vegetable pie" is a somewhat loose term that covers a broad range of possibilities, particularly when it comes to the crust. Besides encasing vegetables in pastry, you can sandwich them between layers of grains, bread crumbs, cheeses, and even wide, thin slices of other vegetables to serve as bottom and top crusts. Consult the index under "Pies" for a complete listing of recipes for vegetable pies.

 ## VEGETABLE PIE WITH A DOUBLE CRUST

One 9-inch (23 cm) pie

STEP ONE

Pastry Crust (pp. 406–407)

STEP TWO

3 tablespoons ghee or oil	*½ teaspoon dried oregano*
1 tablespoon minced fresh	*½ teaspoon dried thyme*
ginger	*1 potato, peeled and finely diced*
Pinch of hing (optional)	*½ bell pepper, chopped*
½ teaspoon dried basil	*1 carrot, thinly sliced*

STEP THREE

4 cups (940 ml) finely cut mixed	*¼ cup (20 g) slivered dried tomatoes*
vegetables	*(optional)*

STEP FOUR

¾ cup (165 g) ricotta	*Black pepper*
cheese or crumbled panir	
Liquid seasoning or	
seasoned salt	

1. Line a 9-inch (23 cm) buttered pie pan with half the dough. Preheat the oven to 350° F (180°C).
2. Heat the ghee or oil in a large lidded skillet. Add the ginger, hing, herbs, potato, bell pepper, and carrot and sauté for 7 minutes over low heat, stirring frequently.
3. Add the mixed vegetables and dried tomatoes. Cover and cook over low heat, stirring occasionally, until the vegetables are tender.
4. Stir in the ricotta or panir. Season to taste with liquid seasoning or seasoned salt and pepper.
5. Spoon the vegetable mixture into the crust. Spread evenly. Put on the top crust, seal, and prick in a few places with a fork.
6. Bake until the crust is golden brown, about 1 hour.

VARIATION

❂ Replace the ricotta cheese with sautéed crumbled tofu or chopped seitan.

SHEPHERD'S PIE WITH VEGETABLES
ENGLAND   *6 servings*

Add sautéed crumbled tofu or panir or chopped seitan to the filling to make it heartier.

STEP ONE

2 tablespoons ghee or oil	*½ teaspoon dried thyme*
Pinch of hing (optional)	*1 large tomato, chopped (optional)*
½ teaspoon dried basil	

STEP TWO

6 cups (1.4 liters) finely cut mixed vegetables	*Liquid seasoning or salt*
	Black pepper
¾ cup (180 ml) vegetable stock or water	

STEP THREE

Mashed Potatoes (pp. 123–24)

STEP FOUR

Paprika	*Minced fresh parsley*

1. Preheat the oven to 350°F (180°C). Heat the ghee or oil in a heavy lidded soup pot or casserole. Add the hing and herbs and sauté for 1 minute over low heat, stirring frequently. Add the tomato and cook for 2 minutes, stirring frequently.
2. Add the vegetables and the stock or water. Bring to a boil. Cover, reduce the heat, and simmer until the vegetables are tender. Season to taste with liquid seasoning or salt and pepper.
3. Place the vegetables in a buttered baking dish. Spread evenly. Completely cover the vegetables with an even layer of the mashed potatoes.
4. Bake for 30 minutes. Garnish with sprinklings of paprika and minced parsley.

 ## CORNISH PASTIES
ENGLAND   *10 to 11 pasties*

An adaptation of the classic English savory pastry. I've filled the pasties with vegetables and ricotta; you can also use other cheeses or tofu or seitan.

STEP ONE

1 tablespoon ghee or oil	*2½ cups (600 ml) finely cut mixed vegetables*
Pinch of hing (optional)	
½ teaspoon rosemary	

STEP TWO

½ cup (120 g) ricotta cheese   **Black pepper**
Liquid seasoning or salt

STEP THREE

Pastry Crust (pp. 406–407)

1. Heat the ghee or oil in a large skillet. Add the hing, rosemary, and vegetables and sauté over low heat until tender, about 10 minutes.
2. Mix in the ricotta and season to taste with liquid seasoning or salt and pepper.
3. Preheat the oven to 375°F (190°C). Roll out the dough ⅛-inch (3 mm) thick on a floured board. Cut out 5-inch (15 cm) rounds.
4. Place a large spoonful of filling on half of each circle. Fold the dough over to make a half moon and seal the edges thoroughly. Press the tines of a fork along each edge and prick the crust once.
5. Place the pasties on a buttered baking sheet. Bake until golden, about 25 minutes.

VARIATIONS
Add chopped toasted nuts to the filling.
Add sesame seeds to the crust.

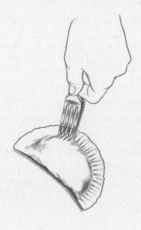

ARTICHOKES

Eating an artichoke is like getting to know someone really well.
—WILLI HASTINGS

Legend has artichokes originating in Zinari, an Aegean island where a jealous goddess turned a gorgeous maiden into the thistly plant. To this day, artichokes remain a lesser-known vegetable outside Europe and coastal California—French and Italians consume two hundred times the amount of artichokes as Americans.

❖ If the leaves are tightly closed, the artichoke is likely to be young and fresh. If the leaves spread like an opening flower, it is an older model.

❖ An artichoke's delicate flavor is best appreciated with a simple sauce for dipping. When serving it hot, accompany with melted ghee or Ghee and Lemon Sauce, a mock mayonnaise, Cream Cheese Hollandaise, or Citrus Vinaigrette.

Steamed or Boiled Artichokes

Slice or snip off the thorny tops of the leaves. Break off the tiny leaves close to the stem and cut off the browned stem end. Steam for 30 to 50 minutes or boil in water to cover (although the artichokes will float on top) for 20 to 40 minutes. Pull off an inner leaf. If it comes off easily, the artichoke is done. To add extra flavor, add a little olive oil, lemon juice, and green herbs to the cooking water.

 # ARTICHOKES À LA GRECQUE

GREECE   *4 servings*

Serve with rice to soak up the fennel- and dill-laced sauce.

STEP ONE

4 artichokes

STEP THREE

*1 cup (100 g) quartered lengthwise   1 cup (110 g) thinly sliced fennel or
and thinly sliced carrots*   *celery*

STEP FOUR

¼ cup (60 ml) olive oil   *Pinch of hing* (optional)
¼ cup (60 ml) melted ghee or   *½ teaspoon salt*
*   butter*   *Black pepper*
¼ cup (60 ml) lemon juice
1 teaspoon fennel seeds
*2 tablespoons or more chopped
   fresh dill or 1 teaspoon dried
   dill*

1. Trim the tips of the leaves and cut off the stems so that the artichokes can sit upright. Place in a large pot, add water to cover, and bring to a boil. Cover, reduce the heat, and simmer until just barely tender, about 15 minutes. Drain.
2. Preheat the oven to 350°F (180°C).
3. Mix the carrots and fennel or celery. Spread evenly in a lidded baking dish. Place the artichokes upright on top of the vegetables.

4. Mix the oil, ghee or butter, lemon juice, fennel seeds, dill, hing, salt, and a sprinkling of pepper. Pour over the vegetables.
5. Cover and bake until all the vegetables are tender, about 45 minutes.

Artichoke hearts, the fully edible part of the vegetable, can be put to all sorts of uses. Marinate them for salads; slice and use for tempura; tuck into crêpes; add to pasta, pizza, grain dishes, and vegetable medleys. Freshly prepared artichoke hearts have not only more life-supporting effects but also superior flavor and texture compared to their unfortunate relatives, which, through no visible fault of their own, have been ruthlessly bottled or frozen.

If you have access to tiny young artichokes, you only need to cook them briefly until tender, remove their tough outer leaves, and trim off the top portion of the inner leaves if they are tough. Cook mature types just until tender. Drain well and allow to cool until you can handle them. Remove the leaves gently, taking care not to pull away too much of the heart. Carefully trim off the chokes. Peel the stems and trim off the tough ends.

 # ARTICHOKE FILO PIE

10 to 12 servings

It is a funny thing about life; if you refuse to accept anything but the best you very often get it.
                                                        —SOMERSET MAUGHAM

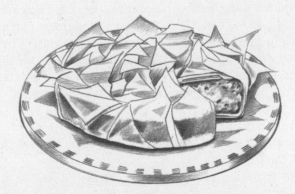

Serve this when you really want to bowl 'em over. If you don't have a springform pan, you can arrange the pie in a rectangular baking dish. The addition of the small amount of chopped broccoli strengthens the flavor of the artichokes. Note that the artichoke hearts must be cooked in advance.

STEP ONE

2 tablespoons olive oil
Pinch of *hing* (optional)
2 cups (200 g) *thinly sliced fennel
or celery*

1 cup (90 g) *finely chopped
broccoli florets*
½ cup (120 ml) *minced fresh parsley*
Liquid seasoning or salt

STEP TWO

2 pounds (1 kg) *ricotta cheese*
2 cups (200 g) *grated Gruyère
or Swiss cheese*
½ cup (50 g) *grated Parmesan
cheese*
2 tablespoons *arrowroot or
cornstarch*

2½ cups (415 g) *sliced cooked
artichoke hearts*
Salt
Black pepper

STEP FOUR

½ cup (110 g) *ghee
or butter*

½ cup (120 ml) *olive oil*

STEP FIVE

1 pound (320 g) *filo pastry*

To prepare the filling:

1. Heat the olive oil in a skillet. Add the hing, fennel or celery, broccoli, and parsley. Sprinkle with liquid seasoning or salt, cover, and sauté over low heat until tender, stirring occasionally.
2. Mix together the ricotta, grated cheeses, and arrowroot or cornstarch. Mix in the sautéed vegetables and the artichoke hearts. Add salt and pepper to taste. Set aside.

To assemble the pie:

3. Preheat the oven to 300°F (150°C).
4. Melt the ghee or butter with the olive oil over low heat. Using a pastry brush, coat the bottom and sides of a 10-inch or 12-inch (28 cm) springform pan with the oil mixture.
5. Lay a sheet of filo in the pan, draping the edges of the pastry over the sides. Brush with a few gentle swipes of the oil. Lay another sheet of filo in the pan with the long edges draped in another direction. Continue to fill the pan with filo, brushing each sheet with the oil, until half the pastry has been used up.
6. Spoon in the filling and spread evenly.
7. Lay the remaining sheets of filo on top, brushing each sheet with the oil. Turn up all the edges over the pie. It should look rough and rustic. If there is any remaining oil, pour a little over the top.
8. Bake until the filo is golden brown, 1 to 1¼ hours. Allow to stand at room temperature for about 15 minutes. Remove to a plate, using 2 spatulas. To serve, cut into wedges with a serrated knife.

VARIATION

The hard cheeses can be replaced with an additional cup of ricotta or crumbled Panir and 1 cup (230 g) of cream cheese. The filling will not be as firm as with the hard cheeses.

THE IN-LAWS ARE COMING! THE IN-LAWS ARE COMING!

Artichoke-Filo Pie
Mediterranean Spinach (pp. 125–26)
Pistachio, Fig, and Anise Bread with Mango-Flavored Butter (p. 328)
Raspberry Sorbet (p. 481)

ASPARAGUS

I stick to asparagus which still seems to inspire gentle thought. —CHARLES LAMB

Succulent asparagus is happily a tri-doshic vegetable—good for all and at all times of day. In addition to the usual green variety, there is white asparagus, a delicacy in Europe, grown beneath mulch to prevent chlorophyll from developing.

- ❖ Steaming is the usual method for cooking this delicate vegetable. Asparagus can also be sautéed, stir-fried, or grilled. Serve either hot or at room temperature. Asparagus is so delicious in its own right that it deserves undivided attention. If you do combine it with other vegetables, try to make it the star attraction.
- ❖ Serve hot in Chinese-style dishes or with a sprinkling of ghee and lemon juice and a grating of pepper. Creamy sauces such as Crème Fraîche and Cream Cheese Hollandaise also enhance asparagus. For room-temperature renditions as an antipasto or salad, serve tossed with Citrus Vinaigrette or topped with a mock mayonnaise. Remember that asparagus loses its color when marinated.

Steamed Asparagus

The steaming of asparagus has been a subject of discussion for centuries—the challenge is to cook the tougher stalks until tender without overcooking the delicate tips. Other than using a steaming basket, here are two methods that work well.

Method I: Snap off the white part of the stalks and lightly peel the lower inch of the remaining stalks. Lay flat in ½ inch (1.3 cm) of boiling water in a wide skillet. Cover, reduce the heat, and simmer until bright green and crisp-tender, about 5 minutes. Young, thin asparagus may take less time.

Method II: Snap off the white part of the stalks and lightly peel the lower inch of the remaining stalks. Tie into a bundle. Stand upright in a deep pot filled with 1 inch (2.5 cm) of boiling water. Invert another pot over the top to serve as a lid. Reduce the heat and simmer until bright green and crisp-tender, about 5 minutes. The water cooks the stalks while the steam cooks the tips.

ASPARAGUS TORTE

6 servings

Epicure: One who gets nothing better than the cream of everything but cheerfully makes the best of it.   —OLIVER HEREFORD

Torta di sparagi, the original dish described in an Italian cookbook from 1622, was flavored with cinnamon and rose water.

STEP ONE

1 pound (230 g) asparagus

STEP TWO

½ cup (120 ml) sour cream
⅛ teaspoon ground nutmeg
¾ teaspoon salt
¼ cup (32 g) arrowroot or
*   cornstarch*

3 tablespoons unbleached white
*   flour*

STEP THREE

1 cup (235 g) ricotta cheese
1 cup (100 g) grated mild cheese,
*   such as Gruyère or Monterey*
*   Jack*

Partially Baked Crust (p. 409)

1. Preheat the oven to 350°F (180°C). Peel the asparagus stems. Steam the asparagus until just barely tender, about 3 minutes. Drain. Slice off the tips and set aside.
2. Place the stems in a food processor or blender with the sour cream, nutmeg, salt, arrowroot or cornstarch, and flour. Purée thoroughly.
3. Beat in the ricotta and grated cheese. Gently stir in the asparagus tips. Pour the mixture into the pie shell and spread evenly.
4. Bake until the crust is lightly browned and the top of the filling has browned in a few spots, about 30 minutes.

BEETS

Beets are Vata-balancing and therefore a boon during the winter Vata season for both lunch and dinner. Some people can't quite get past beets' intense color to their culinary charms. Ancient varieties were yellow-orange, like today's *mangel-wurzel* type, available in farmers' markets. In my experience they can be less flavorful than the standard red varieties. There are also white and pink beets. Look for small, fresh, brightly colored young beets; large, brownish ones can be old, bitter, and hard.

❖ Baking is a superior way to cook beets. It gives them a meltingly soft texture, and their sugars caramelize and add intensity and complexity to the flavor. Beets can also be boiled or sliced and steamed, but they lose some flavor to the cooking water. Beets tend to share their color with their neighbors, so it is best to cook them separately and combine with other vegetables before serving.

❖ Beets can be used in virtually any recipe calling for carrots, though they take longer to cook. Slice them to bring them closer to the cooking time for whole carrots. Cube and cool cooked beets and add to salads. Marinate in Citrus Vinaigrette for antipasti and composed salads.

Baked Beets

Scrub beets with a vegetable brush. Bake whole for best flavor and to prevent the color from bleeding. Rub with ghee or oil or place in a baking dish with a little water. Sprinkle with salt. Cover and bake in a 350°F (180°C) oven until tender, 1 hour or longer. Trim the root and stem ends, peel, and slice.

Boiled Beets

To prevent beets from spreading their red color around during cooking, leave all the usual preparation procedures, such as cutting off the stem and root ends, peeling, and slicing, until *after* they have been fully cooked. Scrub with a vegetable brush. Cook whole in water to cover until quite tender, for 30 to 40 minutes or longer. You can quarter or slice them to shorten the cooking time, but they will bleed their color.

 # BEETS WITH ORANGE, GINGER, AND MINT

4 to 6 servings

Beets' flavor is complemented by sweet-and-sour treatments, which also enhance their Vata-balancing quality. Orange is a particularly wonder flavor for beets. Add orange juice and zest to other beet-adorning sauces such as Sweet-and-Sour Sauce and sour cream.

STEP ONE

6 small beets

STEP TWO

1 tablespoon ghee or butter *1 tablespoon minced fresh ginger*
Pinch of hing (optional)

STEP THREE

2 teaspoons sugar *2 tablespoons minced fresh mint*
2 teaspoons arrowroot or *or 2 teaspoons crumbled dried*
   cornstarch   *mint*
1 cup (240 ml) orange juice

1. Trim and quarter the beets. Bake or steam until tender. Peel.
2. Melt the ghee or butter in a saucepan. Add the hing and ginger and sauté over low heat, stirring frequently, for about 1 minute.
3. Stir the sugar and arrowroot or cornstarch into the orange juice until dissolved. Stir into the saucepan and cook until thickened, stirring constantly. Toss the beets and mint with the sauce.

BROCCOLI

Broccoli is a Pitta- and Kapha-balancing member of the cabbage family that is best eaten at the noontime meal. Eaten daily in ancient Rome, broccoli remained unknown outside Italy until introduced into France by Catherine de' Medici's chefs. Today broccoli is common not only throughout much of the Western world but also in Southeast and East Asia. It is an extremely versatile vegetable, taking on different characteristics depending on how it is sliced and which parts are used. It can be left whole, cut into spears or small florets, chopped, or puréed.

❖ The main consideration with broccoli is not to overcook it. There is a point at which it is tender yet still retains its brilliant green color. Before that point it is too crunchy, while after it, it is too limp and gray. To achieve perfect doneness, take into account that the flowery tops are delicate and the stalks are hard and require longer cooking. I deal with this by either peeling the stalk or not using it at all and saving it for purées and chopped broccoli dishes.

❖ Since overcooking increases broccoli's sulphurous flavor, long-cooking soups and stews don't do it much justice. Use in more quickly cooked dishes. It is delicious gratinéed and makes a lovely purée mixed with ghee, lemon, and cream cheese or crème fraîche. It is at home at room temperature in antipasti and composed salads. Toss with a dressing just before serving—its brilliant green color goes the way of all good things when you marinate it.

 ## BROCCOLI WITH PEPPERS AND CASHEWS

4 servings

You can substitute pecans, pine nuts, and other nuts, but I think that toasted cashews are particularly tasty. Save the stems for Creamy Broccoli Soup.

STEP ONE

2 tablespoons ghee or olive oil
Pinch of hing (optional)
½ teaspoon rosemary

1 tablespoon fresh or
½ teaspoon dried thyme
2 tablespoons minced fresh or
1 teaspoon dried basil

STEP TWO

1 red bell pepper, cut into strips
5 cups (450 g) small broccoli florets

1 cup (240 ml) chopped fresh parsley
Liquid seasoning or salt

STEP THREE

¼ cup (40 g) toasted cashew
   pieces

1 teaspoon lemon juice
Black pepper

1. Heat the ghee or oil in a 10-inch (26 cm) lidded skillet. Add the hing, rosemary, and if using dried herbs, the thyme and basil, and sauté over low heat for 30 seconds, stirring constantly.
2. Add the bell pepper strips, broccoli, and parsley and sprinkle lightly with liquid seasoning or salt. Stir, cover, and sauté, stirring occasionally, until the vegetables are tender.
3. Stir in the cashews, and if using fresh herbs, the thyme and basil. Add the lemon juice, adjust the salt, and add pepper to taste.

BROCCOLI BURRITOS WITH GOLDEN RICE AND WARM CORN SALSA

MEXICAN AMERICAN   *4 burritos*

Burritos, "little burros," are found more in the United States than in Mexico. There is a lightness to this version, yet it contains all the elements of a full lunchtime meal. I like to use black-eyed peas because they don't have to be soaked. However, you can substitute tri-doshic aduki or the more usual beans for Mexican dishes, such as black, pinto, and kidney. Chutneys make a luscious accompaniment instead of salsa and give you options for adding more balance for different doshas.

STEP ONE

½ cup (80 g) dried black-eyed peas

STEP TWO

1 tablespoon ghee or oil
Pinch of hing (optional)
1 carrot, grated
½ cup (100 g) basmati rice
1⅛ cups (270 ml) water

1 tablespoon chopped dried tomatoes
   (optional)
½ teaspoon salt
¼ teaspoon paprika
¼ teaspoon turmeric

STEP THREE

2 tablespoons ghee or oil
Pinch of hing (optional)

3 cups (300 g) chopped broccoli
Liquid seasoning or salt

1 teaspoon cumin seeds
1 tablespoon minced fresh ginger
½ cup (70 g) coarsely chopped
   bell peppers

Black pepper

STEP FOUR

1 cup or more panir (220 g),
   ricotta cheese (220 g), or
   shredded Monterey Jack cheese
   (100 g)

Chopped fresh cilantro
4 large flour tortillas (the kind
   specified for burritos, about 10 inches/
   26 cm in diameter)

1. Clean the beans and place in a pot with 6 cups (1.4 l) of water. Bring to a boil, reduce the heat, and simmer until tender, 1½ to 2 hours. Drain.
2. Meanwhile, heat the ghee or oil in a saucepan. Add the hing and sauté for 30 seconds, until fragrant. Add the carrot and sauté for a minute or two. Add the rice and sauté for a minute, stirring constantly. Stir in the water, dried tomatoes, salt, paprika, and turmeric. Bring to a boil. Cover, reduce the heat, and simmer until all the water is absorbed and the rice is tender, about 20 minutes. Keep covered until ready to use.

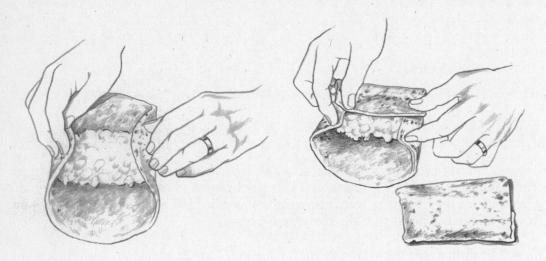

3. Heat the ghee or oil in a skillet. Add the hing, cumin seeds, and ginger and sauté over low heat for 1 minute, until fragrant. Add the bell peppers and broccoli. Sprinkle with liquid seasoning or salt and some pepper. Cover and cook, stirring occasionally, until the broccoli is tender. Stir in the beans. Adjust the seasonings.
4. *To assemble:* Lay each tortilla flat on a plate. Divide the rice evenly among them, spreading in a rectangle in the middle of each tortilla and leaving the sides uncovered for folding. Cover the rice with the broccoli-bean mixture. Sprinkle the cheese on top and sprinkle cilantro over the cheese. Bring up 2 sides so that they partially cover the filling. Roll up from a third side to form a thick package. Serve with salsa.

Warm Corn Salsa

About 2 cups (480 ml)

To add a little balance for Vata, toss in ½ avocado, cubed.

STEP ONE

2 tablespoons mild-flavored oil
Pinch of hing
1 teaspoon cumin seeds

½ cup (70 g) chopped green bell
   peppers
1½ cups (225 g) fresh corn kernels

STEP TWO

1 tablespoon minced fresh ginger
1 small tomato, chopped
2 tablespoons lime juice

Chopped fresh cilantro
Salt
Black pepper

1. Heat the oil in a skillet over low heat. Add the hing and cumin seeds and sauté until fragrant, about 1 minute. Add the bell peppers and cook for 1 minute. Add the corn kernels, cover, and cook until crisp-tender, 3 to 5 minutes.
2. Remove from the heat. Stir in the ginger, tomato, lime juice, and chopped cilantro. Season to taste with salt and pepper.

VARIATIONS

Grill the corn and peppers over coals and briefly sauté the spices in oil.
Add finely chopped green chilies.

Brussels Sprouts

Brussels sprouts are a somewhat recent addition to the planet's repertoire of lunchtime Pitta- and Kapha-balancing vegetables. They are believed to have been developed in the thirteenth century, but they were first written about in 1587 and nobody who's talking is sure whether or not they really come from Brussels.

❖ The dislike that many people harbor toward Brussels sprouts is usually due to a strong sulphurous flavor caused by overcooking, using old Brussels sprouts, or— for a double whammy—both at once. Lightly cooked, young, fresh sprouts tossed with a delicious sauce are a different story entirely. For best results, steam, kin-pura-fry, or sauté whole Brussels sprouts. You can also sauté or stir-fry halved or shredded sprouts. Since overcooking brings out their sulphurous flavor, soups, stews, and other long-cooking preparations are not suitable to Brussels sprouts.

SHREDDED BRUSSELS SPROUTS WITH CREAM

4 to 6 servings

Here is a method of preparing Brussels sprouts that usually pleases even those who profess not to like them. It is a great side dish for a Thanksgiving or other holiday dinner.

STEP ONE
1½ pounds (685 g) Brussels sprouts

STEP TWO
2 tablespoons ghee or butter   *Pinch of hing* (optional)

STEP THREE
1 cup (240 ml) thick coconut   *Salt*
  milk or crème fraîche   *Black pepper*

1. Trim the stem ends from the Brussels sprouts. Shred by slicing crosswise across the leaves. Remove any thick parts of the stem.
2. Melt the ghee or butter in a large skillet or wok. Add the hing and the shredded sprouts and sauté over medium heat, stirring constantly, until just barely tender.
3. Add the coconut milk or crème fraîche. Cook over high heat for 1 to 2 minutes, stirring constantly, until the cream is distributed and slightly reduced. Season to taste with salt and plenty of pepper.

VARIATIONS
  Add cooked peeled chestnuts or toasted cashews to the finished dish.
  Add a little rosemary to the ghee or butter in Step 2.
  Replace the Brussels sprouts with shredded cabbage.

CABBAGE

In the night the cabbages catch at the moon, the leaves drip silver, the rows of cabbages are series of little silver waterfalls in the moon.   —CARL SANDBURG

Green cabbage, the scion of the mustard family, is a lunchtime vegetable that balances Pitta and Kapha. The Romans considered it an antidote for melancholia. Indeed, depression is often caused by a Kapha imbalance. Cabbage is happily always in season, versatile, and inexpensive. Unfortunately, its accessibility has given it the air of something that is a little too ordinary. However, there are many uncommon dishes that you can create with cabbage. It responds beautifully to spices and sauces, and besides the Germanic and Russian treatments we associate it with, cabbage appears in Indian, Chinese, and African dishes.

In addition to tightly packed white-green and purple heads, cabbage comes in loose-leafed varieties such as Savoy, Napa, and a variety of Asian species. Loose-leafed cabbages are especially handy for steaming lightly and using to prepare stuffed cabbage rolls and cabbage-wrapped dolmathes. They can also be steamed and wrapped around the fillings for Spring Rolls (pp. 284–86).

❖ Cabbage can be steamed, sautéed, stir-fried, or kinpura-fried. It combines well with most other vegetables in soups, stews, East Asian–style dishes, Indian-style spiced vegetables, and casseroles. The only thing to watch for is overcooking, which brings out the sulphurous qualities of cabbage, especially when it is cooked in liquids. Try not to cook longer than 30 minutes in soups and stews.

 # CABBAGE-TOMATO CURRY (BANDHGOBHI TAMATAR SABJI)

INDIA   *3 to 4 servings*

This is a popular vegetable dish in south India. A visiting Indian couple requested it every day of their ten-day stay with us! Their version contained much more oil and both of the suggested variations.

STEP ONE

2 tablespoons mild-flavored oil	*1 teaspoon cumin seeds*
Pinch of hing (optional)	*½ teaspoon brown mustard seeds*

STEP TWO

1½ cups (350 g) chopped ripe tomatoes

STEP THREE

¾ cup (180 ml) water	*1 teaspoon turmeric*
Pinch of ground cloves	*Salt*
4 cups (420 g) shredded green cabbage	*Chopped fresh cilantro*

1. Heat the oil in a pot. Add the hing, cumin seeds, and mustard seeds and sauté over low heat until the mustard seeds "dance."
2. Add the tomatoes and cook for a few minutes, stirring frequently, until they begin to become mushy.
3. Add the water, cloves, cabbage, turmeric, and a sprinkling of salt. Bring to a boil. Cover, reduce the heat, and simmer until the cabbage is very tender, 20 to 30 min-

utes. Uncover toward the end of cooking to let a little of the water boil off. Adjust the salt. Sprinkle with cilantro before serving.

VARIATIONS

For heat, add 1 teaspoon or more black pepper in Step 4, or add crumbled red chilies to the oil in Step 1.

Add a sprinkling of urad dal to the oil in Step 1 before adding the spices. Sauté the spices until light brown before adding the tomatoes.

 # SPICY RED CABBAGE WITH APPLES (ROTKOHL MIT ÄPFELN)

GERMANY   *4 to 5 servings*

A wonderful lunchtime dish for balancing Kapha.

STEP ONE

5 cups (525 g) shredded red cabbage	*¾ cup (180 ml) apple juice or water*
1 red-skinned apple, chopped	*¼ cup (60 ml) lemon juice*
	2 teaspoons sugar

STEP TWO

1 tablespoon mild-flavored oil	*1½ teaspoons cumin seeds*
Pinch of hing (optional)	*½ teaspoon yellow mustard seeds*

STEP THREE

½ teaspoon ground cinnamon	*⅛ teaspoon ground cloves*
	Salt

1. Place the cabbage, apple, apple juice or water, lemon juice, and sugar in a pot and bring to a boil. Cover and reduce the heat to a simmer.
2. Meanwhile, heat the oil in a small skillet. Add the hing, cumin seeds, and mustard seeds and sauté over low heat until the mustard seeds "dance."
3. Add the sautéed spices to the cabbage. Add the cinnamon, cloves, and a sprinkling of salt. Cover and simmer until the cabbage is tender.
4. Adjust the seasoning. If using water instead of apple juice, you may need to add another teaspoon of sugar.

VARIATIONS

Add ⅓ cup (45 g) raisins in Step 1.

After cooking, drain and stir in a little sour cream, crème fraîche, or yogurt.

GOLUBSTI (STUFFED CABBAGE ROLLS) WITH MULTIPLE-CHOICE FILLINGS AND SAUCES

RUSSIA   *8 rolls—4 servings*

The Eastern Orthodox church proscribes eating meat on holy days—of which there are upward of two hundred per year—making dishes such as this vegetarian golubsti quite welcome. Here is a version filled with tiny orzo pasta, your choice of tofu, seitan, or panir, and three different sauces with which to anoint the rolls. Loose-leafed cabbages such as Napa or Savoy are the easiest to work with—you'll need two or three cabbages from which to pluck only the largest outer leaves. Step 7, which involves dredging the rolls in flour and browning them, is traditional and makes the rolls especially tasty, but it can be skipped by those avoiding extra oil or extra work.

STEP ONE

12 whole green cabbage leaves

STEP TWO

2 tablespoons ghee or oil   *Liquid seasoning or salt*
Pinch of hing (optional)
1½ cups finely chopped seitan
   (200 g), firm tofu (330 g),
   or panir (300 g)

STEP THREE

1 tablespoon minced fresh ginger   *½ cup (60 g) chopped fennel or celery*
½ cup (65 g) chopped bell pepper   *1 grated carrot*

STEP FOUR

½ cup (100 g) orzo

STEP FIVE

¼ cup (70 g) roasted cashew butter   *2 tablespoons finely chopped*
1 teaspoon sweet paprika   *fresh dill*
¼ cup (120 ml) finely   *Black pepper*
   chopped flat-leaf parsley

STEP SIX

Flour   *Ghee or mild-flavored oil*

STEP SEVEN

2 to 3 cups (500 to 700 ml)
   Carrot-Pepper Sauce (p. 255),
   tomato sauce, or Sour Cream
   Dill Sauce (page 78)

1. Blanch the cabbage leaves, 2 or 3 at a time, just until tender. Drain gently, taking care not to break them. Set aside.
2. Heat the ghee or oil in a skillet. Add the hing and the seitan, tofu, or panir, sprinkle with liquid seasoning or salt, and sauté over medium-high heat, stirring frequently, until browned.
3. Add the ginger, bell pepper, fennel or celery, and grated carrot. Reduce the heat, cover, and sauté, stirring frequently, until the vegetables are tender.
4. While the vegetables are cooking, cook the orzo until al dente. Drain.
5. Mix the cashew butter, paprika, parsley, and dill into the vegetables. When well mixed, gently stir in the orzo. Sprinkle with pepper and adjust the salt.
6. Preheat the oven to 350°F (180°C). Place the cabbage leaves, curling upward, on a work surface. Spoon some of the filling onto each leaf. Roll up the leaf, tucking the edges in, to make a package enclosing the filling.
7. Place the flour in a shallow bowl. Dredge each cabbage roll in it. Sauté in a generous amount of ghee or oil on each side until lightly browned.
8. Place the cabbage rolls in a buttered baking pan, seam side down. Pour one of the sauces over them. Bake for 30 minutes.

 ## SOUR CREAM DILL SAUCE

2 cups (480 ml)

This also makes a lovely dip, salad dressing, or topping for baked potatoes.

2 cups (480 ml) sour cream   *¼ cup (60 ml) minced flat-leaf parsley*
*¼ cup (60 ml) finely chopped fresh
   dill*

Beat the ingredients together until the sour cream has the texture of a thick liquid.

CARROTS

Balancing for Vata, carrots can always be eaten at lunchtime and occasionally for dinner. The way carrots are sliced provides a variety of different effects. Sautéed shredded carrots provide a very different experience from sautéed sliced carrots.

❖ Whenever possible, buy baby carrots (a.k.a. Belgian or French carrots)—they are the sweetest and most tender. Large, impressive-looking carrots usually have an unimpressively hard texture. Little wonder—they have been bred deliberately to be sturdy for withstanding long-distance travel. Don't store carrots next to apples—there is literally a case of bad chemistry between them that mars their flavors.

❖ The universality of carrots extends to cooking them. Almost any cooking method can be applied, but baking especially brings out their sweet flavor. Carrots can be added to just about any type of ethnic vegetable combination.

 ## SESAME-GINGER CARROTS

4 servings

STEP ONE

3 tablespoons ghee or oil
Pinch of hing (optional)
2 tablespoons minced fresh ginger or
  ¼ teaspoon ground ginger

3 cups (360 g) *thinly sliced carrots (slice
  on the diagonal)*

STEP TWO

¼ cup (35 g) sesame seeds   *Salt*

STEP THREE

2 tablespoons raw or brown sugar

1. Melt the ghee or oil in a wok or large skillet. Add the hing and sauté over low heat for 30 seconds, until fragrant. Add the ginger and carrots and sauté over low heat, stirring frequently, until the carrots start to become tender.
2. Add the sesame seeds and a sprinkling of salt and continue sautéing, stirring constantly, until the carrots are tender.
3. Sprinkle with the sugar, adjust the salt, and stir just until the sugar dissolves but not long enough to caramelize it.

VARIATION
Replace the carrots with green beans or snap peas. Omit the sugar.

 ## CARROT CRUMBLE

4 to 6 servings

A light main dish. You can make a squash or a yam crumble by substituting 3½ cups (800 g) puréed cooked winter squash or yams for the carrots.

STEP ONE

7 (840 g) *cups sliced carrots*

STEP TWO

3 to 4 tablespoons ghee or butter
½ teaspoon ground cardamom
½ teaspoon ground ginger

1½ tablespoons raw or dark brown
    sugar
Salt

STEP THREE

¼ cup (30 g) wheat germ
¼ cup (35 g) sunflower seeds
¼ cup (30 g) rolled oats
½ cup (75 g) whole wheat flour

¼ teaspoon salt
3 tablespoons ghee or melted butter
1 tablespoon water

1. Preheat the oven to 350°F (180°C). Steam the carrots until very tender. Drain well.
2. Purée the carrots in a food processor or food mill with the ghee or butter, spices, and sugar. Add salt to taste.
3. Place the wheat germ, sunflower seeds, and oats in a blender or food processor and blend to a powder. Mix with the flour and salt. Add the ghee or butter and the water and mix to a crumbly texture.
4. Spread the carrot mixture in a buttered baking dish. Sprinkle the crumbly topping evenly over it. Bake until the topping is browned, 40 to 45 minutes.

 # CARROTS VICHY (CAROTTES À LA VICHY)

FRANCE   4 servings

STEP ONE

1 pound (230 g) baby carrots or halved mature carrots

STEP TWO

2 tablespoons ghee or butter
4 teaspoons sugar

¼ teaspoon salt

1. Trim the ends and lightly scrape the carrots.
2. Place ½ inch (1.3 cm) of water in a saucepan. Add the ghee or butter, sugar, salt, and carrots. Bring to a boil. Cover and reduce the heat to medium-high.
3. Cook until the carrots are tender and all the water has evaporated. Watch very closely during the last few minutes of cooking to make certain that the liquid doesn't scorch. A light syrup will remain in the bottom of the pan. Roll the carrots in it to coat.

CAULIFLOWER

Cauliflower is nothing but cabbage with a college education. —MARK TWAIN

My college roommate, Annie Joachim, made a weekly purchase of a cauliflower. Each time, without fail, she would solemnly intone over her prize, "Cauliflower is an elegant vegetable." It's not easy being white: Pitta- and Kapha-balancing cauliflower does not come by its color without a little help from its friends. When small, broccoli-like flowers form, farmers gather up the leaves around them to prevent chlorophyll from developing. The flowers then grow into milk-white "curds."

❖ Cauliflower can be steamed either whole or in pieces or cut into florets and sautéed. Cook cauliflower just until tender; overcooking ruins its delicate flavor and accentuates its sulphurous quality. It doesn't generally work well in long-cooking soups and stews.

❖ Cauliflower has a particular affinity for toasted accompaniments, such as nuts and bread crumbs. Toss with Sauce Noisette or Salsa di Noci or sprinkle with toasted almonds, cashews, hazelnuts, or walnuts or serve gratinéed.

Sesame-Pistachio Cauliflower Quesadillas

4 large quesadillas

Oscar Wilde declared, "Consistency is the last refuge of the unimaginative." Here is an Indian variation on a Mexican theme, with a choice of adding dried tomatoes and mozzarella for a somewhat Italian influence.

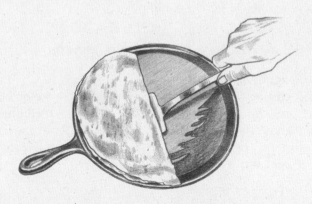

STEP ONE

2 tablespoons ghee or oil	1 tablespoon minced fresh ginger
2 tablespoons sesame seeds	1 teaspoon brown mustard seeds
Pinch of hing (optional)	2 teaspoons cumin seeds

STEP TWO

4 cups (420 g) finely chopped
cauliflower
1 cup (140 g) slivered red bell
peppers
Liquid seasoning or salt

¼ cup (20 g) slivered dried tomatoes
(optional)
¼ cup (30 g) pistachio halves
Black pepper

STEP THREE

4 large flour tortillas (the kind
specified for burritos, about
10 inches (26 cm) in diameter

1 cup (200 g) or more crumbled panir
or chopped fresh mozzarella cheese
Chopped fresh cilantro

1. Heat the ghee or oil in a large skillet. Add the sesame seeds, and sauté over medium-low heat until lightly browned. Stir in the hing, ginger, mustard seeds, and cumin seeds and sauté for 30 seconds.
2. Stir in the cauliflower and bell peppers. Sprinkle with liquid seasoning or salt, cover, and sauté until tender. Stir in the dried tomatoes and pistachio halves, sprinkle with black pepper, and adjust the salt.
3. Place a tortilla flat on a plate. Spoon one-fourth of the cauliflower mixture onto half of it, leaving the edges uncovered. Sprinkle the cauliflower with one-fourth of the cheese, then with cilantro. Fold in half. Repeat with the remaining tortillas.
4. Coat a large griddle or skillet with a generous amount of ghee. Cook each quesadilla until golden brown. Carefully turn and cook the other side. You may need to use 2 spatulas to grip each side of the quesadilla and flip it over. Serve with salsa.

VARIATIONS

✪ Omit the cheese.
Substitute broccoli or cabbage for the cauliflower.

Of all flowers, I like the cauliflower best. —SAMUEL JOHNSON

CAULIFLOWER AND COCONUT (PHULGOBHI NARIYAL SABJI)

INDIA   4 to 6 servings

STEP ONE

½ cup (110 g) ghee or butter
Pinch of hing (optional)

1 tablespoon minced fresh ginger
½ teaspoon brown mustard seeds

STEP TWO

½ cup (40 g) grated unsweetened coconut, fresh or dried

STEP THREE

1 cauliflower, cut into very small
  pieces

¾ teaspoon turmeric
Salt

1. Heat the ghee or butter in a large skillet. Add the hing, ginger, and mustard seeds and sauté over a low heat until the mustard seeds "dance."
2. Add the coconut and sauté, stirring constantly, until golden, about 1 minute.
3. Add the cauliflower, turmeric, a sprinkling of salt, and just enough water to steam the cauliflower. Stir, cover, and cook over low heat until the water has evaporated and the cauliflower is tender. Adjust the salt.

VARIATIONS

Add a handful of chopped fresh cilantro just before serving.
For heat, add 1 teaspoon or more black pepper in Step 3 or add chilies in Step 1.

 # TENDER LOVING CAULIFLOWER

RUSSIA *4 servings*

I have no idea what they call this dish in Russia. It consists of meltingly soft pieces of cauliflower in a whisper-light, crusty coating. You can prepare Brussels sprouts and broccoli in the same manner.

STEP ONE

1 large head cauliflower

STEP TWO

½ cup (70 g) flour
½ teaspoon salt

Pinch of hing (optional)

STEP THREE

3 tablespoons ghee or butter

1. Cut the cauliflower into small florets. Steam until almost tender. Drain well.
2. Mix the flour, salt, and hing together in a large bowl. Add the cauliflower and toss until thoroughly coated with the flour mixture.
3. Melt the ghee or butter in a large skillet over medium heat. Add the cauliflower and immediately stir to coat with the oil. Sauté, stirring frequently, until the cauliflower is tender and has a nicely browned crust.

VARIATIONS

Add dried green herbs such as basil, thyme, and sage to the flour in Step 2.
Add toasted cashews or almonds to the finished dish.

Cauliflower and Peas with Tomato (Phulgobhi Matar Tamatar Sabji)

INDIA   *4 to 6 servings*

A feast for the eyes—red tomatoes and green peas on a field of turmeric-golden cauliflower, with accents of black mustard seeds.

STEP ONE

⅓ cup (80 ml) ghee or oil
Pinch of hing (optional)
1 tablespoon minced fresh ginger

¾ teaspoon brown mustard seeds
1 teaspoon cumin seeds

STEP TWO

2 tomatoes, chopped

STEP THREE

1 large head cauliflower, cut into small pieces
¼ teaspoon ground fenugreek

1 teaspoon turmeric
½ cup (120 ml) water
Salt

STEP FOUR

¾ cup (100 g) peas

Chopped fresh cilantro (optional)

1. Heat the ghee or oil in a pot. Add the hing, ginger, mustard seeds, and cumin seeds and sauté over low heat until the mustard seeds "dance."
2. Add the tomatoes and cook for 2 minutes, stirring frequently.
3. Add the cauliflower, fenugreek, and turmeric. Stir in the water. Sprinkle lightly with salt, cover, and simmer for 10 minutes.
4. Add the peas and more water if necessary. Cover and continue to simmer until the vegetables are tender, 5 to 10 minutes more. Adjust the salt. Sprinkle with chopped cilantro before serving.

VARIATION

For heat, add 1 teaspoon or more black pepper in Step 3 or add minced chilies in Step 1.

Celeriac, Celery Root, or Celeri-Rave

> *Looks can be deceiving—it's eating that's believing.*   —James Thurber

Celeriac, a large, knobby, root vegetable developed during the Renaissance, has been used in fine French cooking for centuries. In the raw it looks like a creature from outer space. However, its rough outer appearance belies its subtle, exquisite flavor.

❖ Celeriac must be peeled, a project that can fast become a major wrestling match. It is easier to peel after it has been sliced and easier yet after it has been cooked.

❖ Celeriac can be steamed or baked. It also can be grated, blanched, and marinated for antipasti and composed salads.

❖ Steam slices of celeriac until tender, 20 minutes or longer.

Baked Celeriac

Slice celeriac into ½-inch pieces. Peel the slices before or after cooking. Brush both sides with melted ghee or oil and sprinkle with salt. Place on a baking sheet. Bake in a 350°F (180°C) oven until tender, 30 to 40 minutes. Turn over once or twice during the baking.

 # CELERIAC PANCAKES

About 14 small pancakes

Somewhat resembling latkes, but with the special subtle flavor of celeriac. You can also substitute grated parsnips to create a medieval European favorite: parsnip fritters. Serve with one of the mock mayonnaises or with a chutney or salsa.

STEP ONE

4 cups (350 g) grated celeriac
½ cup (120 ml) finely chopped
  flat-leaf parsley
1 cup (65 g) fresh bread
  crumbs
1 tablespoon arrowroot or
  cornstarch

3 tablespoons unbleached white flour
1 teaspoon salt
½ teaspoon turmeric
2 tablespoons lemon juice
¼ cup (60 ml) water

STEP TWO

Ghee or oil

1. Toss the celeriac and parsley together. Add the bread crumbs, arrowroot or cornstarch, flour, salt, and turmeric and toss until blended. Stir in the lemon juice and water.

2. Heat a skillet and add a generous amount of ghee for pan-browning. Take a small handful of the celeriac mixture and squeeze it into a ball, then flatten it to form a pancake. Place in the pan and flatten as much as possible with the back of a spatula. Cook on both sides until browned and slightly crispy. Repeat until all the pancakes are cooked. Serve immediately.

CHAYOTE, CHRISTOPHINE, OR MIRLITON

Chayote is actually a fruit, sometimes called a *vegetable pear* or *mango squash* in a slightly schizophrenic acknowledgment of the fact. Chayotes can be peeled and cooked in the manner of summer squash. In the Caribbean they are grated and served au gratin with cheese. Their one large seed can either be eaten or discarded.

 ## GINGER-COCONUT CHAYOTES

4 to 6 servings

You can prepare summer squash or kohlrabi in this manner, but it is a really good way to cook chayotes. The coconut milk enhances their sweetness and gives a nod to chayote-appreciating Caribbean shores.

STEP ONE

2 tablespoons ghee or oil
Pinch of hing (optional)
2 tablespoons minced fresh ginger
½ cup (70 g) chopped red bell peppers

4 cups (580 g) peeled and diced chayotes
½ teaspoon turmeric

STEP TWO

1 cup (240 ml) coconut milk
Salt or liquid seasoning

½ cup (120 ml) chopped cilantro

1. Heat the ghee or oil in a large skillet. Add the hing and ginger and sauté over low heat for 1 minute. Add the bell peppers, chayotes, and turmeric. Stir, cover, and sauté until the chayotes are almost tender, stirring occasionally.
2. Stir in the coconut milk. Cover and simmer until the chayotes are tender and the coconut milk is slightly thickened. Season to taste with liquid seasoning or salt. Stir in the cilantro just before serving.

VARIATION

For a main dish, sauté 1½ cups (330 g) cubed firm tofu in ghee or oil until browned and stir into the mixture in Step 2 along with the coconut milk.

CORN

*I believe in the forest, and in the meadow, and in the night in which the corn
grows.*   —HENRY DAVID THOREAU, "Walking"

Since ancient times Kapha-balancing corn has been a staple of the Americas. To the
natives it was an emblem of life. The one becoming the many was symbolized by the
many kernels coming out of a single ear of corn and also by the many colors and varieties existing within one species.

- ❖ Eat corn that is fresh, *Fresh*, FRESH. There are hybrids that maintain their sugars
  for a few days, but generally sugars in corn convert to starch soon after picking.
  Look for fresh green husks and golden cornsilk—no brown at the ends. The kernels should be juicy when pierced with a fingernail.
- ❖ Corn is usually steamed or boiled but can also be grilled. It is so wonderful on its
  own that often it is best to leave well enough alone. Steamed corn on the cob with
  plenty of melted ghee or butter, a sprinkling of salt, and a grinding of pepper
  occupies its own little corner of gastronomical heaven. Salvadorans add a sprinkling of lime juice.
- ❖ You can, however, also remove the kernels and serve them creamed and add them
  to all manner of Western-style vegetable medleys. Corn is also grown in north
  India, and the kernels can be added to Indian-style spiced vegetables and curries.

Steamed Corn

Remove the husks and cornsilk. Break off the stem. Break in half, if necessary, to fit in
your steamer, or steam in a small amount of water in a covered large skillet for 3 to 5
minutes. (The Shakers timed a minute by one recitation of the Lord's prayer.) For corn
off the cob, scrape off the kernels and steam for no more than a couple of minutes.

BOCOLES (FRESH CORN PANCAKES)

MEXICO   *4 to 5 servings*

Aztec farmers were required by law to plant corn by the roadside to provide sustenance
for hungry travelers. Here is an adaptation of an Aztec dish. Serve with Salsa Cruda.

STEP ONE

*3 cups (450 g) yellow corn
 kernels*
½ cup (65 g) yellow cornmeal
*2 tablespoons toasted besan
 (chickpea flour)*

½ teaspoon salt
*2 tablespoons melted ghee or
 mild-flavored oil*
Water to blend

STEP TWO

Ghee or oil

1. Process all the ingredients in a food processor or blender, adding just enough water to make a very thick batter.
2. Melt ghee or oil in a skillet over medium heat. Spoon in the batter to make 2-inch (5 cm) pancakes, and cook on both sides until they are a crusty, deep golden brown. Do not flip the bocoles until they are completely done on one side, or they will fall apart in midair.

 # CORN FRITTERS

UNITED STATES   *18 to 20 fritters*

I've added herbs to make a savory dish. You can also omit the herbs and serve the fritters southern style with sorghum syrup.

STEP ONE

1 cup (140 g) flour	*⅛ teaspoon crumbled dried sage (optional)*
1 teaspoon salt	
2 teaspoons baking powder	*3 tablespoons melted ghee or mild-flavored oil*
¼ teaspoon baking soda	
2 tablespoons arrowroot or cornstarch	*¾ cup (180 ml) water*
	¾ cup (180 ml) yogurt
½ teaspoon dried thyme (optional)	

STEP TWO

2 cups (300 g) corn kernels

STEP THREE

Mild-flavored oil, such as sesame or corn

1. Mix the dry ingredients together. Add the ghee or oil, water, and yogurt. Mix well. (Use a blender or food processor for best results.) Chill for 1 hour.
2. Mix the corn kernels into the batter.
3. Heat oil ¼ inch (5 mm) deep in a heavy skillet over medium heat. Have a platter covered with paper towels nearby. Spoon in the batter to make 2-inch (5 cm) pancakes. Cook on each side until golden and crisp. Drain.

VARIATION

Add a little chopped bell pepper to the batter.

THAI CORN FRITTERS (TOD MAN KHAO POHD)

THAILAND   *12 medium or 18 small fritters*

Traditionally, these crisp fritters are small puffs, perfect for appetizers or a side dish. You can also make them a bit larger in the manner of Western corn fritters to serve as a main dish. Accompany with Sweet-and-Sour Sauce (p. 514).

STEP ONE

½ cup (70 g) rice flour
½ cup (70 g) unbleached white
 flour
1½ teaspoons sugar

¾ teaspoon salt
¾ teaspoon baking powder
½ teaspoon black pepper
Pinch of hing (optional)

STEP TWO

¾ cup (180 ml) water
¼ cup (60 ml) minced fresh cilantro

1 cup (150 g) fresh corn kernels

STEP THREE

Mild-flavored oil, such as sesame or corn

1. Mix all the dry ingredients together.
2. Stir in the water to make a thick batter. Stir in the cilantro and corn.
3. Heat oil ½ inch (1.3 cm) deep in a large skillet over medium heat. Have a platter covered with paper towels nearby. Drop either large or small spoonfuls carefully into the oil. Fry on each side until lightly browned. Drain.

ATOL DE ELOTE: A SONG, A DANCE, AND A CORN PUDDING

EL SALVADOR   *5 cups (1.2 liters)*

Estamos muy contentos y alegres
moviendo el rico atol de elote.
Solamente son tres pasos y los
vamos a enseñar:
Uno, todo mundo agachadito,
dos, agarrando la paleta, y
tres, moviendo el atol de elote
todo el día y toda la noche.
    Jája!

We are happy and content
stirring the rich corn pudding.
There are only three steps
we are going to teach you:
One, everybody ready,
two, holding the stirring stick, and
three, stirring the corn pudding
all day and all night.
    Aha!

Every day throughout El Salvador, elderly women and young girls alike sway their hips and sing this song as they stir a pot of smooth, sweet, soup-pudding. Atol de elote is traditionally served as a main course. You can also feature it as a gentle dessert or serve it for breakfast. The charming Ana Cecilia Rosales taught me the song, the dance—and the corn pudding to go with them.

STEP ONE

6 cups (900 g) fresh corn kernels   3½ cups (840 ml) nondairy milk
(about 8 ears)

STEP THREE

⅓ cup (70 g) sugar

1. Purée the corn kernels and milk together in a blender or food processor.
2. Line a sieve with a piece of clean muslin or cheesecloth and place over a soup pot. Pour the corn mixture in several batches into the cloth. Bring up the edges of the cloth and carefully squeeze and wring out all the liquid. Discard the corn solids.
3. Add the sugar. Set the pot over low heat. Stir constantly with a whisk until the mixture thickens and is just barely simmering, about 10 minutes. Serve hot.

VATA-BALANCING VEGETABLES YOU MIGHT NOT HAVE THOUGHT TO COOK BUT MIGHT CHANGE YOUR MIND ABOUT

Cucumbers are one of the handful of vegetables that are intrinsically balancing to Vata; they are most balancing when served cooked and warm. Some Europeans have an appreciation for steamed or sautéed cucumbers dressed in the manner of summer squash, whereas many Americans would rather suffer a tax audit than touch a cooked cucumber. If you are willing to give cooked cukes a chance, add them to sautéed vegetable medleys, Indian-style vegetables, and stews.

Radishes cooked with ghee or oil are balancing to Vata. Their sharpness mellows quite a bit when cooked, and a tiny amount of grated radish adds surprisingly good flavor when cooked for a long time in soups and vegetable mixtures. Daikon and icicle radishes can be sautéed with Indian spices.

EGGPLANT OR AUBERGINE

Eggplant's dense texture makes it a satisfying and versatile palette for a variety of flavors and treatments. Persian cooking boasts a thousand eggplant recipes. Eggplant in itself is light and dry, making it balancing to Kapha. However, it has a seemingly insatiable lust for oil, which adds heaviness to prepared eggplant dishes. Its ability to absorb oil can be checked to a degree by cooking it slowly in a nonstick pan and giving it a planned feeding of a set amount of oil and no more.

❖ Ayurveda recommends young eggplants with undeveloped seeds. This ideal is best fulfilled by long, thin Asian varieties. There are also white-skinned varieties and small, round, green-skinned types to be had at farmers' markets.

❖ Eggplant peel is difficult to digest, and though many people eat it happily, Ayurvedic cooks generally remove it from all except very young Asian eggplants.

❖ Eggplant does not cozy up to water cooking. Bake or sauté in Western, Indian, and Middle Eastern dishes and add to Chinese and Southeast Asian–style stir-fries. It is also an ideal vegetable for grilling and for preparing Pakoras and Tempura. It responds beautifully to a wide variety of herbs and spices. While eggplant purée is not gorgeous on its own—its grayish color can be off-putting—it provides a tasty basis for dips and spreads; can be adorned with olive oil, lemon juice, and green herbs for antipasti; or mixed with yogurt and spices for Meze.

❖ Eggplants can occasionally be bitter. When you seem to have latched onto a bitter crop, soak the slices in cold water for 15 minutes and then gently squeeze out the moisture, or sprinkle with a generous dose of salt and press with a weight for 30 minutes.

Broiled or Grilled Whole Eggplant

Eggplant loses much of its moisture—and therefore its bulk—in this treatment, so double the number you think you'll need. When broiling, place the whole eggplant in a baking pan to catch moisture. Grill or broil on one side for about 10 minutes. Turn over and continue to cook until tender, about 5 minutes. The skin will blacken during the process, but this adds wonderful smoky flavor. Peel. The finished result will be a soft pulp especially good for purées.

EGGPLANT SLICES

Slices of cooked eggplant present many enticing possibilities. They can be served solo with a sauce, but the doors of creativity really fly open when they are treated as a receptacle for toppings in the manner of pizza, pie crust, or crêpes. Eggplant slices can be fried or baked, plain or breaded.

 ## BAKED EGGPLANT SLICES

Eggplant slices baked without a coating shrink when cooked; therefore, slice them thicker than your intended final size. Also, make sure they are thoroughly coated with oil, or they will shrivel unattractively. Allow 2 slices per person.

1. Preheat the oven to 350°F (180°C). Peel the eggplant and cut crosswise into ¾-inch (2 cm) rounds.
2. Place on a well-oiled baking sheet (nonstick sheets allow you to use less oil). Brush the top of each piece with oil. Sprinkle with salt and pepper.
3. Bake until tender, 30 to 40 minutes. Turn each piece over after 15 minutes.

 ## BREADED EGGPLANT SLICES

The ability to choose what food you must eat, and knowingly, will make you able to choose other less transitory things with courage and finesse.
—M. F. K. FISHER

Buttermilk and yogurt are ideal mediums for affixing breading. There are, however, other ways and means: use nondairy milk if you want a very light coating of crumbs; for a heavier crust, use Tempura batter (p. 48) instead of a dairy coating. Allow 2 slices per person.

1. Peel the eggplant and cut into ½-inch (1.3 cm) slices.
2. Place buttermilk or yogurt in a bowl. If using thick yogurt, whisk it with a little water to the consistency of thick cream. Place bread crumbs or other breadings, such as cornmeal or semolina, in another shallow bowl. If you like, you can season the breading with salt, hing, and spices or dried green herbs.
3. Dip *one slice at a time* in the buttermilk or yogurt mixture to coat thoroughly. Next, dredge in the breading until coated on all sides. Rinse your fingers when they become gummy, or they will pull the breading off the slices.
   To bake: Preheat the oven to 350°F (180°C). Liberally oil a baking pan. You must have a good deal of oil in the pan to thoroughly coat the crumbs. Place the eggplant slices in the pan, then turn them over. The breading should be lightly coated with oil. Bake until the eggplant is tender and the coating is nicely browned, 30 to 40 minutes.
   To pan-brown: Heat oil ½-inch (1.3 cm) deep in a large skillet over medium heat. Have a tray covered with paper towels nearby. Gently place several slices in the oil, allowing room to maneuver a spatula. Cook until the coating is golden brown, then carefully turn over and repeat on the other side, checking to make sure the eggplant is tender before removing. Drain. Repeat until all the eggplant is fried, replenishing the oil as necessary.

❖ *Classic Eggplant Parmesan:* Here, there, and everywhere, this is the mainstay company dish that nonvegetarians serve when entertaining vegetarians and vice versa. A real crossover hit. Layer slices of pan-fried breaded eggplant with tomato sauce and grated mozzarella. You can alternatively use Carrot-Pepper Sauce (p. 255) and spoonfuls of ricotta or panir. Bake in a 350°F (180°C) oven for 30 minutes.

❖ *Eggplant Florentine:* Top baked, breaded, or grilled eggplant slices with mounds of creamed spinach.

❖ *Eggplant Pizza:* Top baked, breaded, or grilled eggplant slices with anything you would use on a pizza. Place under the broiler for a minute or two to finish.

❖ *Eggplant Cannelloni:* Peel 2 eggplants and slice lengthwise into 10 pieces. Bread and pan-brown as described above. Roll the slices around the following filling. Place in a baking pan, top with tomato sauce or Carrot-Pepper Sauce (p. 255), and bake in a 350°F (180°C) oven for 30 minutes. For the filling, beat together:

1½ cups (355 g) ricotta cheese	*1 tablespoon arrowroot or*
½ cup (60 g) fine dry bread crumbs	*cornstarch*
1 cup (100 g) shredded	*Salt*
mozzarella cheese	*Black pepper*

NEW ORLEANS ROUX

Cajun joke: Q: How do you make gumbo?
  A: First you make a roux . . .
Not roaring with laughter? Then you probably didn't know that the roux in question is prepared by mixing equal parts of oil and flour in a cast-iron skillet and baking it for eight hours. You must stir the mixture every hour and spend the time in between fervently praying that it doesn't burn! Vegetarian Louisiana chef Bucky Black suggests the following streamlined procedure:

Toast unbleached white flour in a dry skillet over medium heat. Stir frequently until it is caramel brown for Creole dishes and chestnut brown for Cajun dishes.

To season gumbo, mix together 1 tablespoon toasted flour with 1 tablespoon ghee or oil for each cup of liquid. Beat into simmering gumbo.

ASIAN-CAJUN EGGPLANT GUMBO

UNITED STATES   *6 servings*

Great is the meal which brings together people who are distant to each other.
                                                    —THE TALMUD

Yet another ethnic influence thrown into the big, black Cajun gumbo kettle? The flavors and spirit of the dish are genuine bayou, with ginger and tofu or seitan replacing foods less appealing to Ayurvedic vegetarians. Exported Cajun fare is inevitably highly spiced with cayenne and hot sauce, but true, homemade Cajun food may or may not be hot, according to the family's taste.

STEP ONE

1 tablespoon ghee or oil	Liquid seasoning or salt
Pinch of hing (optional)	
4 cups firm tofu (880 g) or seitan (520 g), cut into 1-inch (2.5 cm) chunks	

STEP TWO

¼ cup (60 ml) ghee or mild-flavored oil	1 teaspoon dried oregano
Pinch of hing (optional)	1 cup (110 g) finely chopped fennel or celery
2 tablespoons minced fresh ginger	1 cup (140 g) finely chopped bell peppers
1½ teaspoons dried thyme	

STEP THREE

½ cup (120 ml) minced fresh parsley	1 large eggplant, peeled and cut into 1-inch (2.5 cm) chunks

STEP FOUR

3 tablespoons toasted flour (see sidebar, p. 93)	1 teaspoon black pepper
2½ cups (600 ml) vegetable stock	Salt
2 bay leaves	Cooked rice
1 teaspoon sugar	Filé powder or crumbled fresh sassafras leaves (optional)

1. Heat the ghee or oil and the hing in a nonstick skillet. Pat the tofu or seitan dry with paper towels and add. Sprinkle with liquid seasoning or salt. Sauté over medium-high heat, stirring frequently, until nicely browned. Set aside.
2. Heat the second amount of ghee or oil in a large, heavy-bottomed pot. Add the hing and sauté until fragrant, about 30 seconds. Add the ginger, thyme, oregano, fennel or celery, and bell peppers. Cover and sauté over low heat, stirring occasionally, for 5 minutes.

3. Stir in the parsley and eggplant. Cover and continue sautéing, stirring occasionally, until the eggplant is almost tender, 7 to 10 minutes.
4. Sprinkle the roux flour over the vegetables and stir in well. Stir in the stock, bay leaves, sugar, and pepper. Bring to a simmer, stirring frequently. Add the tofu or seitan, cover, and simmer until the vegetables are tender, 15 to 20 minutes. Add salt to taste. To serve, place a mound of rice in the center of an individual bowl for each diner and pour the gumbo over it. Pass filé at the table to sprinkle onto the gumbo

VARIATION
Add Tabasco sauce or cayenne to taste.

 # EGGPLANT-POTATO CURRY (BAIGAN ALU SABJI)

INDIA   *4 servings*

STEP ONE
2 tablespoons mild-flavored oil
Pinch of hing (optional)
1 tablespoon minced fresh ginger

1½ teaspoons cumin seeds
¾ teaspoon brown mustard seeds

STEP TWO
1 medium eggplant,
   peeled and cut into tiny cubes

2 medium potatoes, peeled and cut
   into tiny cubes

STEP THREE
Salt
1 teaspoon turmeric

Chopped fresh cilantro

1. Heat the oil in a large skillet. Add the hing, ginger, cumin seeds, and mustard seeds and sauté over low heat until the mustard seeds "dance."
2. Add the eggplant and potatoes. Sauté for 5 minutes, stirring constantly.
3. Add a sprinkling of salt and the turmeric. Cover and sauté until the vegetables are tender, 20 to 30 minutes. Stir occasionally. Adjust the salt. Sprinkle with chopped cilantro before serving.

VARIATIONS
For heat, add 1 teaspoon or more black pepper in Step 4 or add cayenne or crumbled red chilies to the oil in Step 2.

Add 2 chopped tomatoes to the oil after sautéing the spices in Step 2. Cook for 2 minutes, stirring frequently, before adding the vegetables.

For a more substantial lunchtime main dish, add cooked garbanzos (chickpeas) or sautéed panir cubes to the finished dish.

MOUSSAKA

MIDDLE EAST   *4 servings*

Moussaka was originally a dish of central Asia. This version, one of the most popular recipes in the book, is Turkish style, as opposed to the Greek nonvegetarian version. It can also be cooked like a stew rather than baked. Serve with couscous, bulgar, or rice. Note that the garbanzos must be prepared in advance.

STEP TWO

¼ cup (60 ml) olive oil
Pinch of hing (optional)
1 tablespoon minced fresh ginger

1½ teaspoons cumin seeds
1 large eggplant, peeled, quartered, and sliced

STEP THREE

2 cups (460 g) chopped ripe tomatoes
Liquid seasoning or salt
1 teaspoon ground cinnamon

½ teaspoon sugar
1 cup (160 g) cooked garbanzos (chickpeas)
Black pepper

1. Preheat the oven to 350°F (180°C). Oil a covered casserole.
2. Heat the oil in a skillet. Add the hing, ginger, and cumin seeds and sauté over low heat for 30 seconds. Add the eggplant and sauté for 5 minutes, stirring frequently.
3. Add the tomatoes, sprinkle with liquid seasoning or salt, and continue cooking for 3 to 4 more minutes. Stir in the cinnamon, sugar, and garbanzos. Adjust the liquid seasoning or salt and add black pepper to taste.
4. Place in the casserole, cover, and bake for 1 hour.

May this Earth, whose surface . . . sustains an abundant variety of herbs and plants of different potencies and qualities, support all human beings, in all their diversity of endowment, in mutually supportive harmony and prosperity.
                                        —PRITHIVI SUKTA, ATHARVA VEDA

EGGPLANT PÂTÉ

2 cups (480 ml)

Eggplants are usually cooked in oil, but here the use of ghee adds to the suave, luxurious flavor and texture of this unusual pâté. There's a whole lot of toasting going on (nuts, bread crumbs, crostini), which you might wish to do before assembling all the ingredients. If you are planning to serve the pâté in the evening, replace the cream cheese with mashed avocado. Serve with crostini or other crackers.

STEP ONE

3 tablespoons ghee
Pinch of hing (optional)
1 tablespoon minced fresh ginger
1 stalk celery

4 cups (280 g) peeled and coarsely
*   chopped eggplant*
Liquid seasoning or salt

STEP TWO

½ cup (60 g) dry bread crumbs

STEP THREE

½ cup (70 g) blanched almonds,
*   toasted*
½ cup (65 g) hazelnuts, toasted
¼ cup (60 g) cream cheese or
*   creamy chèvre*

1 tablespoon lemon juice
Black pepper

1. Heat the ghee in a large skillet. Add the hing and ginger and sauté over low heat for 1 minute. Add the celery and eggplant and sprinkle with liquid seasoning or salt. Cover and cook until tender, stirring occasionally. Allow to cool to room temperature.
2. Toast the bread crumbs in a dry pan or toaster oven until lightly browned.
3. Place the eggplant in a food processor with the toasted bread crumbs, toasted nuts, cream cheese or chèvre, and lemon juice. Process for several minutes, until completely smooth. Add black pepper to taste and adjust the liquid seasoning or salt.

ENDIVE, BELGIAN

Belgian endives were developed in the 1800s by botanists experimenting with ways to grow vegetables during cold northern winters. You can break off the leaves to add to salads or use them as scoops for dips. Steam them or, for a more interesting treatment, braise them with the following recipe. Look for small, young endives. Older ones can be unpleasantly bitter.

BRAISED BELGIAN ENDIVE, CELERY, OR FENNEL

6 servings

STEP ONE

¼ cup (55 g) ghee or butter
12 small Belgian endives or celery
   stalks, trimmed at both ends, or
   pieces of fennel, quartered
   lengthwise

STEP TWO

1 cup (240 ml) salted vegetable stock   2 teaspoons sugar
1 tablespoon lemon juice   Black pepper

1. Heat the ghee or butter in a wide, lidded skillet. Add the vegetables and turn to coat on all sides.
2. Add the stock, lemon juice, and sugar. Sprinkle with pepper. Bring to a boil, cover, reduce the heat, and simmer until the vegetables are tender, about 10 minutes.
3. Transfer the vegetables with a slotted spoon to a warm serving platter. Turn the heat to high and boil the sauce, stirring frequently, until cooked down to about ¼ cup (60 ml). Pour over the vegetables.

FENNEL OR FINOCCHIO

The fennel is beyond any vegetable delicious. It greatly resembles . . . celery,
perfectly white, and there is no other vegetable equals it in flavor.
   —THOMAS APPLETON TO THOMAS JEFFERSON, 1824

It is a shame that fennel is so underutilized. Besides offering a unique licorice-like flavor coupled with a celery-like texture, it is balancing for all doshas. It can be eaten morning, noon, or night. Technically a fruit, fennel was known in ancient China, India, and Egypt. Called *marathon*, it was a symbol of success in ancient Greece.

❖ Look for fresh green tops on firm, tightly packed bulbs. The tops can be used as an herb. Sautéed fennel is an excellent textural substitute for cooked onions and can be added to dishes in the same manner as celery. Marinate cooked fennel for antipasti and composed salads. You can also bake or grill partially cooked halves.

Fennel Baked with Fennel

6 servings

STEP ONE

3 large fennel bulbs

STEP TWO

⅓ cup (80 ml) olive oil   *Salt*
1 tablespoon lemon juice   *Pepper*
1 teaspoon fennel seeds
2 tablespoons chopped fennel
  tops

1. Preheat the oven to 425°F (220 °C). Coat a 9 × 13-inch (23 × 33 cm) baking dish with olive oil. Trim the stalks off the fennel bulbs, reserving the tops. Quarter the bulbs lengthwise. Place in the baking pan, cut side up.
2. Drizzle with the olive oil and lemon juice. Sprinkle with the fennel seeds, fennel tops, salt, and pepper. Bake until tender, about 30 minutes.

 # Fennel Stuffed with Ricotta

6 servings

STEP ONE

6 large fennel bulbs

STEP TWO

2 tablespoons olive oil   *1 tablespoon lemon juice*
1 teaspoon fennel seeds   *2 teaspoons sugar*
1 cup vegetable stock

STEP FOUR

1½ cups (355 g) ricotta   *Salt*
  cheese   *Black pepper*
¼ cup (60 g) cream cheese
2 tablespoons chopped fennel
  tops

STEP FIVE

3 tablespoons ground walnuts   *1 tablespoon olive oil*
¼ cup (30 g) fine dry bread   *Salt*
  crumbs

1. Preheat the oven to 350°F (180°C). Coat a 9×13-inch (23 × 33 cm) baking dish with olive oil. Trim the stalks off the fennel bulbs. Cut in half lengthwise along the broader side of the bulb, so that you have 2 wide fennel halves. Reserve the tops for the filling.
2. Heat the olive oil in a wide, lidded skillet. Add the fennel seeds and sauté over low heat for a minute. Add the vegetable stock, lemon juice, and sugar. Bring to a boil. Add the fennel bulbs, cut side down, cover, reduce the heat, and simmer until the bulbs are tender, about 10 minutes. Transfer the fennel to the baking dish, cut side up.
3. Bring the cooking liquid to a boil and cook down until ⅓ cup (80 ml) remains.
4. While the liquid is boiling, mix the ricotta, cream cheese, and fennel tops together. Season to taste with salt and pepper. Spread evenly on the fennel bulbs, making sure a little gets between the stalks.
5. Toss the ground walnuts, bread crumbs, olive oil, and a sprinkling of salt together. Sprinkle over the ricotta mixture on each bulb. Bake until the crumbs are lightly browned, about 20 minutes.

GREEN BEANS OR SNAP BEANS AND OTHER EDIBLE-POD BEANS

Standard green beans—The Vegetable Formerly Known as String Beans—are balancing for Pitta and Kapha, while French beans, a.k.a. *haricots verts*, are happily tri-doshic. Edible-pod beans grow both on meandering vines and on short bushes. The Omaha tribe distinguished them as "walking beans" and "beans not walking."

❖ Fresh pod beans can be green, yellow, or purple, and short or long. Chinese long beans are actually a relative of black-eyed peas rather than green beans. However, they can be prepared in the manner of their nonrelative.

Steaming and sautéing are generally the best methods of cooking edible-pod beans. Slicing edible-pod beans in different ways gives them a variety of roles to play: leave them whole, serve them julienned, cut into large or small pieces, or chop or purée them for entirely different effects. Cut into tiny pieces and replace summer-only peas in recipes during autumn, winter, and spring.

GREEN BEANS AND COCONUT (BARBATTI NARIYAL SABJI)

INDIA   *4 servings*

STEP ONE

2 tablespoons ghee or oil
Pinch of hing (optional)

1 tablespoon minced fresh ginger
½ teaspoon brown mustard seeds

STEP TWO

¼ cup (20 g) grated coconut, fresh or dried

STEP THREE

3 cups (300 g) green beans,
   trimmed and snapped in half

½ cup (120 ml) water
Salt

1. Heat the ghee or oil in a pot. Add the hing, ginger, and mustard seeds and sauté over low heat until the mustard seeds "dance."
2. Add the coconut. Sauté, stirring constantly, until lightly browned, about 1 minute.
3. Add the green beans, water, and a sprinkling of salt. Bring to a boil, cover, and reduce the heat. Cook over medium-high heat until the water is gone and the green beans are tender. Adjust the salt.

VARIATION

For heat add 1 teaspoon or more black pepper in Step 3, or add minced chilies in Step 1.

 # GREEK-STYLE GREEN BEANS

4 to 6 servings

STEP ONE

3 tablespoons olive oil
Pinch of hing (optional)

1 cup (110 g) chopped fennel or
   celery

STEP TWO

4 cups (400 g) green beans, cut into
   2-inch (5 cm) lengths
Liquid seasoning or salt
2 tablespoons lemon juice

1½ tablespoons chopped fresh dill
   or fennel tops
Black pepper

1. Heat the oil in a large skillet. Add the hing and sauté over low heat for 30 seconds, until fragrant. Add the fennel or celery, cover, and sauté until it is limp, about 5 minutes.

2. Add the green beans. Sprinkle with liquid seasoning or salt, cover, and cook until the beans are tender, stirring occasionally. Stir in the lemon juice, dill or fennel tops, and a sprinkling of liquid seasoning, and adjust the salt.

 # GREEN BEAN CURRY (BARBATTI TARKARI)

INDIA   *4 servings*

Lemon Rice and Pakoras are colorful accompaniments.

STEP ONE

1 tablespoon ghee or oil	*1 tablespoon minced fresh ginger*
Pinch of hing (optional)	*2 tomatoes, chopped*
¾ teaspoon brown mustard seeds	

STEP TWO

1 teaspoon turmeric	*Salt*
3 cups (350 g) green beans,	*½ cup (120 ml) water*
cut into ½-inch (1.3 cm)	*Chopped fresh cilantro* (optional)
pieces	

1. Heat the ghee or oil in a pot. Add the hing, mustard seeds, and ginger and sauté over low heat until the mustard seeds "dance." Add the tomatoes and sauté for a few minutes, stirring frequently, until they become mushy.
2. Stir in the turmeric, green beans, a sprinkling of salt, and the water. Cover and simmer until the beans are tender, 12 to 15 minutes. Adjust the salt. Sprinkle with chopped cilantro before serving.

VARIATION

For heat, add 1 teaspoon or more black pepper in Step 3 or add cayenne or crumbled red chilies to the ghee or oil in Step 1.

BITTER GREENS

Bitter to the mouth, sweet to the heart.   —GERMAN PROVERB

The old saying is quite literally true, for many bitter greens balance Pitta dosha and thus are good for the heart. A number of greens balance Kapha and are fine for both the noon and evening meals. Many cultures have a tradition of "spring tonic": eating the first tender leaves of wild spring greens and drinking their cooking water to clean and purify the body after a long winter spent without fresh vegetables. Luckily, in less snow-bound areas greens thrive in the winter, providing the tonic of their wonderful flavors and nutritious attributes throughout many months of the year.

From a culinary standpoint, there are essentially two types of greens: tender, milder-flavored greens such as spinach and chard, which cook exceptionally quickly, and hardy, strong-flavored greens such as collard and kale, which require a leisurely cooking time to be rendered tender and mild flavored. Hardy bitter greens can be boiled—don't be afraid to do it! The first time I encountered turnip greens, I steamed them for a few minutes and served them forth to forty hungry people. Shouts of distress echoed through the dining room as the victims encountered their sinus-clearing bitterness.

❖ Look for bright, crisp leaves without yellow or brown spots. If very young, tender greens are available, go for them.

Individual Bitter Greens

It would be impossible to list all the greens that our dear Mother Earth provides. Those who enjoy foraging for wild foods could probably find hundreds of varieties in any area that supports verdant growth—I've even encountered greens gatherers along the urban hillsides of Los Angeles. Here is a handful of common bitter greens available for the plucking in farmers' markets, produce stores, and occasionally in supermarkets.

Arugula, aka rucola, rocket, or roquette, is balancing for Kapha. Once called "white pepper" in England, arugula's smoky-bitter leaves, now associated with Italian cooking, are tender and commonly added to salads. When cooked, arugula's flavor softens a bit. Chop and add small amounts to soups or sauté for pasta dishes just until barely wilted. Arugula cooks almost instantaneously, like spinach.

Beet greens, balancing for Pitta and Kapha, are quite flavorful and can be used in recipes calling for cooked spinach. Some people like them uncooked in salads, but I find them too tough to eat raw.

Broccoli rabe, or broccoli di rapa, is a bitter flavored relative of broccoli that forms mostly into leaves and stems and sports a few flowers rather than full-blown florets. Eaten mostly in Italy, it can be steamed or sautéed and is good tossed with pasta.

Chard, a Pitta and Kapha-balancing type of beet, sprouts leaves rather than a large root. There are two common varieties: *Swiss chard*, with brilliant green leaves and thick white stems, and *red chard*, with thinner red stems. Chard can be prepared in the same manner as spinach, although its cooking time should be slightly increased to deal with the stem. Go easy on the salt—chard has plenty of sodium on its own. Chard leaves can replace cabbage leaves in Golubsti (Stuffed Cabbage Rolls) and grape leaves in Dolmáthes.

Collard greens are widely eaten in Ethiopia, Kenya, and neighboring parts of Africa. They came to the United States from Africa and are now associated with the southern states. Young collards do not need to be boiled within an inch of their life but can be sautéed over low heat for about 10 minutes or steamed until tender. However, their elders do get tough and bitter, and cooking for 20 to 30 minutes is in order. Collards are often served with a sour flavor such as lemon juice and can also be creamed.

Cresses: While a wide variety of cresses grow wild or can be cultivated in a home garden, *watercress* is usually the only type commercially available. It makes delicious cream soup and is often served creamed. Cresses add flavor to soups and stews, and can be added to dishes in the manner of parsley. You can also replace basil or spinach with cress in pesto.

Dandelion greens harvested in early spring are tender and can be used raw in salads or lightly sautéed. Later in the season they become tough and bitter. Commercially grown dandelion leaves are available over a longer period but can also be quite bitter.

Kale is balancing for Pitta and Kapha. In the British Isles it was said that faeries plucked kale leaves to fly on at night, so if a farmer found his kale patch disturbed in the morning, it was a good omen. Kale is quite hardy and requires long sautéing or stewing to become tender.

Mustard greens are a hardy green eaten throughout much of the world. Their flavor can be quite sharp and stinging and less balancing for Pitta.

Nettles: The tops and young, tender shoots of wild nettles are cooked like spinach in the British Isles. Only touch the leaves with the hairs facing downward to avoid their sting. When cooked, their prickly nature is tamed.

Pea vine leaves, used in Chinese cooking, are wonderfully sweet and are best sautéed or stir-fried and dressed very simply.

Radicchio, a type of chicory, begins its life with full intentions of becoming as green as the next bitter green. However, when the plants are half grown, farmers shield them from sunlight to prevent photosynthesis, causing them to retain a rich red and white coloration. *Radicchio di Verona* and *radicchio di Castelfranco* form rounded heads like cabbage, while *radicchio di Treviso,* considered the best by connoisseurs, has elongated leaves. Radicchio is usually added to green salads for color contrast. While it loses some of its color when cooked, it is delicious added to dishes in the manner of cabbage or braised like Belgian endive. According to Marcella Hazan, slicing the leaves on the diagonal brings out their sweetness.

Sorrel, from the French *surele,* "sour," is a relative of rhubarb and buckwheat. Gaius Laelias pronounced it as having "philosophic superiority." Its very sour flavor is popular in soup and as a purée. For best flavor, stack the leaves and slice across them. Sorrel leaves melt into a purée after about 15 minutes of cooking. You may want to tone down its assertive sourness by combining it with milder greens.

Turnip greens are balancing for Kapha and are treated in the same manner as collard greens. When old and tough, turnip leaves must be boiled. Young turnip greens can be steamed or sautéed.

ASIAN GREENS

 The subject of Asian greens is virtually endless, as my father discovered when he made inquiries on my behalf in Chinese markets and restaurants in the United States and Taiwan. Not only are there gazillions of varieties, but their names change within the same language so that even neighboring villages can have their own names for a particular green. Asian greens are usually stir-fried or sautéed, or sliced and added to soups. Although described here as Chinese, most are common to countries throughout Southeast and East Asia. Here are some of the most common greens with their most widely accepted Mandarin monikers, courtesy of the efforts of Jerry Kasin.

Bok-choy is first mentioned in fifth-century literature and is used extensively in Chinese cooking. With luck you can find *qing gang cai* or *qing jiang cai*, "baby bok-choy," the young green stems packed tightly like a bulb and topped with tender green leaves, and *cai xin*, "baby bok choy hearts." *Shanghai bai cai* closely resembles baby bok choy. All can be cooked whole.

Da bai cai or shandong bai cai, "Napa cabbage," can be shredded raw into salads as well as cooked.

Jie lan, "Chinese broccoli," resembles broccoli rabe, with a profusion of green leaves and a few flowers and buds. The stalks look tough but cook very quickly.

Tianjin bai cai, "celery cabbage" or "Chinese cabbage," has pale, elongated, tender leaves assembled in a tightly packed head.

Xue cai, "Chinese mustard greens," are quite pungent and require longer cooking.

⚜ SAG (SPICED GREENS)

INDIA   *4 servings*

Sag is traditionally served with cornmeal chapatis (see Tortillas) in north India and Kashmir and prepared with whatever greens are handy.

2 tablespoons ghee or mild-flavored
  oil
Pinch of hing (optional)
1 tablespoon minced fresh ginger
½ teaspoon whole fenugreek seeds
4 cups (360 g) turnip, collard, or
  other greens, chopped

2 pounds (1 kg) spinach, chopped
1 teaspoon lemon juice
Salt
Black pepper

Heat the ghee or oil in a large pot or wok. Add the hing, ginger, and fenugreek seeds, and sauté over low heat until fragrant, about 1 minute. Add the greens and spinach, cover, and cook, stirring frequently, until tender, about 10 minutes. Season with the lemon juice, salt, and pepper.

VARIATION

For heat, increase black pepper to 1 teaspoon or more or add crumbled red chilies to the oil.

 # GUMBO Z'HERBES

UNITED STATES   8 to 10 servings

A Cajun contraction of *gumbo aux herbes*, this dish is meatless for Lent and traditionally eaten on Maundy Thursday. It is supposed to contain seven green vegetables to bring seven new people to you who will bring you luck. However, it is a project to find seven greens at the market, so feel free to substitute other greens or to shorten the list. Lengthy cooking time is a feature of Cajun cookery; I have more than halved the time this gumbo spends on the stove in a Cajun household. Hopefully, it still brings luck.

STEP ONE

6 cups (570 g) coarsely chopped
  spinach
6 cups (570 g) coarsely chopped
  collard greens
4 cups (380 g) coarsely chopped
  turnip or beet greens
4 cups (420 g) coarsely chopped
  green cabbage

2 cups (190 g) coarsely chopped
  watercress
2 cups (190 g) coarsely chopped
  dandelion greens or chicory
1 cup (240 ml) coarsely
  chopped flat-leaf parsley
8 cups (1.9 l) vegetable
  stock

STEP TWO

1/4 cup (55 g) ghee or butter
2 healthy pinches of hing
 (optional)
2 tablespoons minced fresh
 ginger
2 cups (220 g) finely chopped
 celery or fennel

1 cup (140 g) finely chopped
 green bell peppers
2 teaspoons dried thyme
2 to 3 bay leaves

STEP FIVE

1/4 teaspoon ground cloves
1/2 teaspoon ground allspice
1 teaspoon black pepper

Salt
Cooked rice

1. Place all the chopped leafy vegetables and the vegetable stock in a large soup pot. Bring to a boil. Partially cover, reduce the heat, and simmer very slowly for 30 minutes.
2. Meanwhile, melt the ghee or butter in a large skillet over low heat. Add the hing, ginger, celery or fennel, bell peppers, thyme, and bay leaves. Cover and cook, stirring occasionally, until the vegetables are tender. Set aside.
3. Drain the green vegetables in a large sieve held over a bowl to catch the pot liquor (stock). Press out all the liquid with the back of a spoon. Coarsely grind—but do not purée—the vegetables in a food processor.
4. Add the greens to the skillet containing the celery and bell peppers. Cover and cook over low heat, stirring occasionally, for 10 minutes.
5. Meanwhile, measure 6 cups (1.4 liters) of the pot liquor back into the soup pot. Add the greens, cloves, allspice, and pepper. Bring the mixture to a boil. Partially cover, reduce the heat, and simmer for 45 minutes to 1 hour. Add salt to taste. To serve, place a mound of rice in the center of an individual bowl for each diner and pour the gumbo over it.

JERUSALEM ARTICHOKES, OR SUNCHOKES

In salad, they have the taste of artichoke hearts, a little less firm, however; fried in fritter-dough, they evoke salsify; boiled whole they resemble, but from afar, potatoes. —NICHOLAS DE BONNEFONS, GENTLEMAN-IN-WAITING TO LOUIS XIV

First spotted in Canada by Samuel de Champlain in 1603, samples of this New World tuber were later shipped to Paris from Brazil, and Parisians surmised that Canada and Brazil occupied the same region. Italians inadvertently added to the general European confusion by giving the vegetable their word for sunflower, *girasole*, which was garbled into "Jerusalem artichoke." Today American marketers are attempting to popularize the vegetable by giving it a snappier handle, "sunchoke."

❖ The slices tend to discolor quickly, so sprinkle with lemon juice if they must stand more than a few minutes when raw. Stir-fry, sauté, or steam until crisp-tender, or steam or boil like potatoes until soft. It is not 100 percent necessary to peel them, but most people prefer to do so. Use slices for tempura, serve au gratin, or purée. Jerusalem artichokes have a delicate flavor. I wouldn't suggest much beyond a little ghee or butter and lemon juice.

Steamed Jerusalem Artichokes

Scrub with a vegetable brush. Peel if desired. Steam whole until tender but still a little crisp, 15 to 20 minutes, or steam a little longer until soft, then mash.

CLOSE ENCOUNTERS WITH ALIEN VEGETABLES

Kohlrabi is a member of the cabbage family, making it balancing for Pitta and Kapha and best eaten at lunchtime. It looks like a creature from a Dr. Seuss book. Both the leaves and stem are edible, and kohlrabi can be cooked in the same manner as turnips. Like turnips, older kohlrabis can be fibrous. *Steamed kohlrabi:* Trim the ends and peel. Steam kohlrabis whole until tender, about 45 minutes. Sliced, they take about 25 to 30 minutes.

> *Having the pungency of a high-born radish bred to a low-brow cucumber.*
> —ALICE B. TOKLAS, ON KOHLRABI

Lotus root, used in Chinese cooking, is an especially beautiful vegetable, revealing delicate, lacy patterns when sliced crosswise. Stir-fry in Chinese-style vegetable combinations, add to Chinese-style soups, or slice thin, blanch, and dress with oil and lemon juice as a salad. The raw slices discolor easily, so sprinkle them with lemon juice if they must stand more than 10 minutes.

Marrows: Well known in England and other parts of Europe but not found much elsewhere, marrows can be treated in the manner of a winter squash or a long-cooking zucchini. Peel and remove the seeds before cooking.

Sea vegetables: Agar agar is used in Ayurvedic cooking as a gel-like thickener. Otherwise, there is some question surrounding the nourishing value of sea vegetables, especially since many, such as *arame*, *hijiki*, and some forms of kelp, are precooked. Even the staunchest supporters agree that the present polluted condition of the oceans makes use of wild sea vegetables somewhat dicey. There are some that have been farmed in controlled water sources. Go by your own feelings about eating them.

Plantains: Though related to bananas, they are not sweet and are treated as vegetables. Plantains can be boiled until tender and peeled and mashed, or boiled until almost tender and pan-browned in the manner of home fries. Deep-fried plantain chips are made virtually everywhere plantains grow. Called *tostones* and *banana pesé* in the Caribbean, the chips are sprinkled with salt like potato chips. Among the Ethiopian Falasha Jews, they are cut into 1-inch (2.5 cm) chunks, deep-fried, and sprinkled with salt, pepper, and ground ginger.

Salsify, or oyster plant, can be prepared in the same manner as parsnips. Look for the type that has a blackish skin and peel before cooking. Salsify is hard to digest, so it is advisable to eat it in small amounts.

OKRA

Tri-doshic okra is definitely a popularity-challenged vegetable. As all challengers know, it develops a slimy texture when it touches water, a feature diplomatically referred to as "roping" by agriculturalists. Sliminess is a nutritive quality mentioned in Ayurvedic texts, but there are many whose doshas go out of balance just thinking about eating slimy okra. There are ways and means of taming roping: wipe okra dry before slicing, use a dry cutting board, a dry knife, and handle with dry hands. Lightly cooked dishes that do not contain water or juicy vegetables will not be slimy. Some people eliminate roping by carefully trimming most of the stems off but leaving the pods whole so that the inner juices are not exposed to water. If you use okra in a soup or stew, sauté and add to the dish just before serving.

 ## OKRA AND CORNMEAL

UNITED STATES *4 to 6 servings*

A classic southern dish you can prepare two ways. Stop at the end of Step 1 and you'll have tender pieces of okra with a crispy coating. Add the tomatoes and herbs, and the cornmeal softens and the dish takes on a different character.

STEP ONE

⅓ cup (80 ml) ghee or mild-flavored
  oil
Pinch of hing (optional)
3 cups (400 g) okra, cut into ½-inch
  (1.3 cm) slices

½ cup (65 g) yellow cornmeal
Salt

STEP TWO

1 cup (230 g) chopped tomatoes
  (optional)

⅓ cup (80 ml) minced fresh herbs,
  such as parsley or basil (optional)

1. Heat the ghee or oil in a large skillet. Add the hing and sauté until fragrant, about 30 seconds. Add the okra and cornmeal. Sprinkle lightly with salt and sauté over medium heat, stirring frequently, until the cornmeal is lightly browned and the okra is tender, about 5 minutes.
2. If desired, stir in the tomatoes and herbs. Cook until the tomatoes are warmed through and have lost their crispness, 1 to 2 minutes.

 # OKRA CURRY (BHENDI SABJI)

INDIA   *4 servings*

STEP ONE

2 tablespoons ghee or oil
Pinch of hing (optional)
1 tablespoon minced fresh ginger

1½ teaspoons cumin seeds
½ teaspoon black mustard seeds

STEP TWO

6 cups (800 g) okra,
  halved lengthwise and cut into
  1-inch (2.5 cm) pieces

1 teaspoon turmeric
Salt

STEP THREE

⅓ cup (25 g) grated coconut,
  fresh or dried

Chopped fresh cilantro (optional)

1. Heat the ghee or oil in a pot. Add the hing, ginger, cumin seeds, and mustard seeds and sauté over low heat until the mustard seeds "dance."
2. Add the okra, turmeric, and a sprinkling of salt and sauté over low heat, stirring frequently, until the okra is tender.
3. Add the coconut and sauté, stirring constantly, for a minute until lightly browned. Adjust the salt. Sprinkle with chopped cilantro before serving.

VARIATIONS

For heat, add 1 teaspoon or more black pepper in Step 2 or add crumbled red chilies to the oil in Step 1.

Omit the coconut for a more Kapha-balancing dish.

 ## OKRA GUMBO

UNITED STATES   *6 servings*

Jardin loin, gumbo gâté.
When the garden is far, the gumbo is spoiled.   —CREOLE SAYING

Gumbo comes from the West African words for okra, *ngombo* or *kingombo*. This version gives you the option to prevent the okra from getting viscous, a boon to those not to the gumbo born.

STEP ONE

2 tablespoons ghee
Pinch of hing (optional)
1½ cups (175 g) finely chopped celery
1 cup (140 g) finely chopped green bell peppers

½ cup (120 ml) minced fresh parsley
1½ teaspoons dried thyme
1 teaspoon dried oregano

STEP TWO

1½ cups (350 g) chopped tomatoes
2½ cups (600 ml) vegetable stock

2 bay leaves
1 to 2 teaspoons black pepper
2 teaspoons sugar

STEP THREE

1 tablespoon ghee
Pinch of hing (optional)
2 cups diced seitan (260 g) or tofu (440 g)

Salt

STEP FOUR

1 tablespoon ghee
Pinch of hing (optional)
3 cups (400 g) okra, cut into ½-inch (1.3 cm) pieces

Salt

STEP FIVE

Cooked rice

1. Melt the ghee in a soup pot. Add the hing and sauté over low heat until fragrant, about 30 seconds. Add the celery, bell peppers, parsley, thyme, and oregano. Cover and cook until very tender, stirring occasionally, about 20 minutes.
2. Process the tomatoes and stock in a blender until smooth. Add to the cooking vegetables. Stir in the bay leaves, pepper, and sugar. Bring to a boil. Cover, reduce the heat, and simmer for 20 to 30 minutes.
3. While the broth is simmering, heat the second amount of ghee in a nonstick skillet over medium-high heat. Add the hing and the seitan or tofu. Sprinkle with salt and sauté, stirring frequently, until nicely browned. Set aside.
4. Heat the third amount of ghee in the skillet over medium heat. Add the hing and sauté until fragrant, about 30 seconds. Add the okra, sprinkle with salt, and sauté, stirring frequently, until tender.
5. Stir the okra into the broth. At this point, if you are To the Gumbo Born, you will want to cover and simmer the mixture for up to an hour. If you are anyone else, which means you don't enjoy slimy okra, stir in the seitan or tofu, and adjust the salt and pepper. To serve, place a mound of rice in the center of an individual bowl for each diner and spoon the gumbo over it.

VARIATION
Add Tabasco sauce or cayenne to taste.

PARSNIPS

Fine words butter no parsnips.   —SIR WALTER SCOTT

Parsnips enjoyed immense popularity in old Europe, especially appreciated during vegetarian Lenten days. The rise of the potato signaled the fall of the parsnip's fortunes. Pity. They are delicious and, Ayurvedically speaking, more balancing than potatoes.

❖ Parsnips shine with water-free slow cooking, in which their sugars caramelize and they brown a little around the edges. Baking particularly enhances their sweetness. Their delicate flavor does well with simple flavorings: ghee, lemon juice, and some minced fresh herbs or sweet spices are usually enough.
❖ Anything you can do to a carrot, except eat it raw, you can perpetrate on a parsnip.
❖ For an approximation of parsnip fritters, a medieval delight, prepare Latkes (pp. 121–22) or Celeriac Pancakes (p. 85) using parsnips.

Glazed Parsnips or Carrots

6 servings

STEP ONE

12 parsnips or carrots

STEP THREE

⅓ cup (70 g) raw or packed brown sugar
3 tablespoons (45 ml) melted ghee or butter

½ teaspoon ground cinnamon
1 tablespoon orange or apple juice

1. Preheat the oven to 400°F (200°C). Trim the ends and peel the parsnips or lightly scrape the carrots.
2. Steam until almost tender. Drain. Place in a buttered baking pan.
3. Mix the sugar, ghee or butter, cinnamon, and juice. Pour over the carrots or parsnips and roll them in the mixture to coat.
4. Bake for 20 minutes.

VARIATION

Add a little ground ginger and finely grated orange zest in Step 3.

Peas

Every good cook, from Fannie Farmer to Escoffier, agrees on three things about these delicate messengers to our palates from the kind earth-mother: they must be very green, they must be freshly gathered, and they must be shelled at the very last second of the very last minute.
—M. F. K. Fisher

A Pitta- and Kapha-balancing vegetable, peas have been cultivated in Asia for millennia. The name is from the Sanskrit *pis*, also origin of "piece."

❖ Among the many varieties of peas are those that must be separated from their pods, including standard garden peas, and *mange tout*, "eat all" or edible-pod peas, including *snap peas* and *snow peas*.

❖ For those that must be podded, 2 pounds of pea pods yield about 2 cups of peas. For best results, lightly steam shucked peas or cook them slowly in a large quantity of ghee or butter. Podded peas make a particularly delicious purée. Edible-pod peas can be steamed, sautéed, or stir-fried.

❖ Peas create a sweet, flavorful broth from their cooking water, making them a desirable addition to soups, stews, and other vegetable mélanges. Don't be afraid to slice edible-pod peas—it makes them more versatile, and at times eating sliced pieces can be more enjoyable than attempting to maneuver the entire pod.

❖ The season for podded peas is regrettably short. Try substituting green beans cut into pea-sized pieces during the rest of the year.

PEAS AND LETTUCE (PETIT POIS AUX LAITUES)

FRANCE   *4 servings*

The original recipe, hundreds of years old, calls for ½ pound (230 g) of butter plus a drenching of heavy cream. This treatment, which is a little more circumspect with the fats, brings out all the special flavor and sweetness of peas.

STEP ONE

3 tablespoons ghee or butter
Pinch of hing (optional)
1 stalk celery with leaves,
*   thinly sliced*

¼ cup (60 ml) minced fresh
*   parsley*
2 cups (180 g) shredded
*   lettuce*

STEP TWO

½ cup (120 ml) water
1 teaspoon sugar
2 cups (260 g) peas

1 tablespoon minced fresh mint
*   (optional)*
Liquid seasoning or salt

1. Melt the ghee or butter in a saucepan. Add the hing and celery and sauté over low heat until the celery begins to become tender. Add the parsley and lettuce and sauté for 5 more minutes.
2. Add the water, sugar, peas, mint, and a sprinkling of liquid seasoning or salt. Cover and simmer until the peas are tender. Drain. Add more ghee or butter if desired. Adjust the salt.

PEAS AND PANIR (MATAR PANIR)

INDIA   *4 servings*

STEP ONE

Firm panir prepared from
½ gallon (1.9 l) milk

Ghee or oil

STEP TWO

2 tablespoons ghee or oil
Pinch of hing (optional)
1 tablespoon minced fresh ginger

2 cups (460 g) chopped tomatoes

STEP THREE

1 teaspoon turmeric
2 cups (260 g) peas
¼ cup (60 ml) water

Salt
Large pinch sugar

STEP FOUR

¼ teaspoon garam masala

Chopped fresh cilantro (optional)

1. Slice the panir into 1-inch (2.5 cm) pieces. Coat a skillet with a generous amount of ghee or oil. Sauté the panir cubes on both sides until lightly browned. Set aside.
2. Heat the ghee or oil in a saucepan. Add the hing and ginger and sauté for 1 minute over low heat, stirring frequently. Add the tomatoes and cook, stirring frequently, until slightly mushy, 2 to 3 minutes.
3. Add the turmeric, peas, water, a sprinkling of salt, and the sugar. Cover and simmer until the peas and tomatoes are completely tender, about 15 minutes.
4. Stir in the garam masala and the panir. Adjust the salt. Cook 1 more minute for the flavors to blend. Sprinkle with chopped cilantro before serving. Serve over rice or with Indian flat breads.

VARIATION

For heat, add 1 teaspoon or more black pepper in Step 4 or add chopped green or red chilies to the ghee or oil in Step 1.

 # PEAS AND POTATO CURRY (MATAR ALU SABJI)

INDIA   *4 servings*

This curry is also used in the preparation of Biryani. Serve over rice or with Indian flat breads.

STEP ONE

¼ cup (60 ml) ghee or
   mild-flavored oil
Pinch of hing (optional)
1 tablespoon minced fresh ginger

1½ teaspoons cumin seeds
5 cups (700 g) potatoes,
   peeled and cut into small cubes

STEP TWO

1 cup (240 ml) water	1 cup (130 g) peas
1 teaspoon turmeric	Salt
¼ teaspoon ground fenugreek	Chopped fresh cilantro (optional)

1. Heat the ghee or oil in a pot. Add the hing, ginger, and cumin seeds and sauté for 1 minute over low heat, stirring frequently. Add the potatoes and sauté for 5 minutes, stirring constantly.
2. Add the water, turmeric, fenugreek, peas, and a sprinkling of salt. Cover and simmer until the vegetables are tender, 15 to 20 minutes. Adjust the salt. Sprinkle with chopped cilantro before serving.

VARIATION

For heat, add 1 teaspoon or more black pepper in Step 4 or add chopped green or red chilies to the oil in Step 1.

> *How luscious lies the pea within the pod.*   —EMILY DICKINSON

PEPPERS

To the end of his days, Columbus believed that he had sailed to Asia and brought back pepper. Asia it was not; pepper it was not. Within a couple of decades, the genus he did find, *capsicum* or chilies, had been introduced 'round the world in a world that, until then, few Europeans had even suspected was round. Some chilies are mild enough to be used as a vegetable with a slight kick, notably *New Mexican* chilies such as *Anaheim* and *pasilla (poblano)*. Others were bred into milder forms, now known collectively as *sweet peppers: bell peppers, sweet yellow Hungarian wax peppers* (not to be confused with the hot variety), *pimientos*, and *Italian frying peppers*. Bell peppers are the most common and come in glorious colors.

❖ Peppers are more digestible when peeled. Remove the seeded portion and stem. Peel with a sharp vegetable peeler or use the method described in the recipe in Method I for Roasted Peppers, below. Peppers are a natural for grilling.

Roasted Peppers

A deceptively simple recipe for the wonderful flavor, texture, and appearance that peppers acquire through this treatment. Mix different colored bell peppers and serve in antipasti and composed salads.

Bell peppers, cut into quarters or eights
Olive oil
Salt

Method I:

1. Peel the peppers with a vegetable peeler before slicing. Drizzle on a little olive oil, sprinkle with salt and a little hing, and toss until they are lightly coated with the oil.
2. Place the peppers on a baking sheet. Bake in a 350°F (180°C) oven for 30 minutes, turning them over once or twice to roast evenly. Serve at room temperature, sprinkled with lemon juice.

Method II: The classic technique. It takes a little time, but has some entertainment value—it's fun to purposely burn something in order to get it right! You can grill the peppers instead of broiling them.

1. Place the peppers in a single layer in an oiled baking pan, skin side up. Place in the broiler about 2 inches (5 cm) from the heat source. Broil until the skins are puffy and blackened. If necessary, turn the peppers to thoroughly blacken the skins.
2. Remove the peppers, place in a heavy brown paper bag, and close tightly. Allow them to sit for a few minutes to "sweat." This helps loosen their skins.
3. Quickly peel and rub off the skins. They should come right off. If the peppers are allowed to cool, you will find it difficult—if not impossible—to remove the skins.
4. Drizzle with olive oil and lemon juice. Serve at room temperature.

PEPPERS STUFFED WITH SICILIAN EGGPLANT

4 servings—2 peppers each

The bread crumb–laced eggplant filling, with the complex sweet-savory flavors favored in Sicily, can also be used to stuff cabbage rolls, and when the eggplant is chopped fine, even ravioli. Alternate green, yellow, and red bell peppers for color contrast.

STEP ONE

8 large, firm, unbruised bell peppers

STEP TWO

1 tablespoon olive oil   *1 cup (70 g) fine dry bread crumbs*

STEP THREE

2 tablespoons olive oil   *4 cups (280 g) peeled and cubed*
Pinch of hing   *eggplant*
1 tablespoon minced fresh   *Liquid seasoning or salt*
ginger
½ cup (65 g) coarsely chopped
fennel or celery

2 teaspoons finely grated
 lemon zest
1 teaspoon sugar
¼ cup (30 g) raisins

STEP FOUR

⅓ cup (45 g) pine nuts
½ cup (20 g) finely chopped
 flat-leaf parsley
Black pepper

STEP FIVE

3 cups (700 ml) Carrot-
 Pepper Sauce (p. 255) or
 Tomato Sauce (pp. 505–506)

1. Preheat the oven to 350°F (180°C). Slice off the stem ends of the peppers and remove the seedy portions. Steam for a few minutes until *almost* tender. Drain well. Set aside.
2. Heat the olive oil in a skillet. Add the bread crumbs and sauté over medium-low heat, stirring constantly, for a few minutes, until the crumbs are toasted. Set aside.
3. Heat the second amount of oil in the skillet. Add the hing and ginger and sauté over low heat for a minute. Add the fennel and the eggplant, sprinkle with liquid seasoning or salt, cover, and sauté until the eggplant is tender, stirring frequently.
4. Stir in the lemon zest, sugar, raisins, pine nuts, parsley, and toasted bread crumbs. Sprinkle with black pepper and adjust the seasoning.
5. Gently fill the pepper cases with the stuffing. Pour a little of the sauce into a baking pan and place the peppers upright in the pan. Pour the remaining sauce over them.
6. Bake until the sauce and peppers are thoroughly heated through, 20 to 30 minutes.

POTATOES

Pray for peace and grace and spiritual food,
For wisdom and guidance, for all these are good,
But don't forget the potatoes. —J. T. PETTEE, "Prayer and Potatoes"

Potatoes have been surrounded by one controversy or another throughout much of their history, including in Ayurveda. Some vaidyas feel that they are the least valuable vegetable because they digest slowly. They encourage people to avoid them. Other vaidyas do not feel strongly against them if you procure as fresh a product as possible, cook them with digestive spices such as hing, cumin, ginger, and black pepper, and cook or dress them with unctuous ingredients such as ghee and sour cream to counteract their dryness. Potatoes are most balancing to Kapha; however, the addition of butter, ghee, sour cream, etc. will add a note of balance for Vata. Because they are so heavy, it is kinder to the tummy to eat them at the noon meal rather than in the evening.

❖ There are many varieties of potatoes. The main division is between thin-skinned, "waxy" types and thick-skinned, dry, "mealy" ones. Waxy types are good for boiling. The small ones are often called *new potatoes* and are prized for their delicate flavor and texture. *Yukon gold* and *yellow Finn* varieties have yellow flesh and are particularly creamy textured. Thick-skinned *russet potatoes*, also called *Idaho* and *baking potatoes*, are drier, often more mature, and are preferable for baking and making French fries.

❖ Thick-skinned potatoes store much longer than the thin-skinned varieties, for which reason I usually use thin-skinned ones. Nonorganically grown potatoes are often genetically engineered, sprayed with sprout inhibitors, and kept in storage before they see the light of day in a grocery store. Farmers' markets are good places to seek out fresh, unsprayed potatoes.

❖ Look for firm potatoes without sprouts or green spots. Once sprouted, they contain small amounts of toxic alkaloids. Peel very deeply or, better yet, toss 'em. Store potatoes in a cool, dark, ventilated area in paper or cloth bags that allow them to breathe.

STAND-INS FOR POTATOES

Here are a few vegetables that are waiting in the wings to stand in for potatoes. None completely mimic potatoes' uniquely soothing texture—let's face it, potatoes they're not. However, they do have the advantages of possessing more nourishing Ayurvedic effects. They also don't require as heavy an application of butter or ghee, nor do they turn to glue in a food processor the way potatoes do.

Sweet potatoes and yams are the obvious choices. Anything you can do to a potato you perpetrate on a sweet potato or yam, and their sweetness can be de-emphasized by using savory seasonings.

Chestnuts are used interchangeably with potatoes in Europe. It is necessary to cook and peel chestnuts, making dishes containing large amounts a labor of love.

Parsnips cook quite quickly, make fabulous latkes and hash browns, and produce a flavorful purée.

Rutabagas make a golden purée to dress like mashed potatoes, and they can also be used to make French fries.

Taro root can be cooked like home fries and French fries—and who can resist a mottled-purple French fry?

Cauliflower: Puréed cauliflower has an appearance and texture that heads in the general direction of mashed potatoes.

Plantains can be prepared like mashed potatoes and home fries.

Jerusalem artichokes can be prepared like mashed potatoes.

HAZELNUT-CRUSTED SAFFRON POTATO CAKES

SWEDEN   *8 to 10 cakes*

Serve these delicately flavored lunchtime cakes with a creamy sauce such as crème fraîche, sour cream, or tofu mayonnaise. Yellow Finn or Yukon gold potatoes enhance the golden saffron color. You can replace the hazelnuts with blanched almonds, cashews, or for glorious color, pistachios.

STEP ONE

3 medium potatoes   *Salt*
¼ teaspoon saffron soaked
  in 2 tablespoons hot water

STEP TWO

⅔ cup (110 g) coarsely ground   *Pinch of hing* (optional)
  hazelnuts   *1½ teaspoons cumin seeds*
½ cup (60 g) fine dry bread   *½ teaspoon salt*
  crumbs

STEP THREE

Ghee or oil

1. Boil the potatoes in water to cover until very tender. Drain very well. As soon as they are cool enough to handle, peel and mash thoroughly with the saffron water. Add salt to taste. Allow to cool.
2. Toss the ground nuts with the bread crumbs, hing, cumin seeds, and salt. Place in a shallow bowl.
3. Scoop up a handful of potato mixture and form into a sphere the size of a tennis ball. Press into the hazelnut mixture to coat on both sides, flattening into a thin patty. Repeat with all the remaining mixture. Coat a skillet generously with ghee or oil. Pan-brown the cakes on both sides over medium-low heat until browned and crusty.

PAN-BROWNED OR
OVEN-ROASTED POTATOES

4 to 6 servings

There are many ways to prepare these brown, crusty potatoes with tender, buttery centers. My favorite is to use yellow Finn potatoes and to add sliced red bell peppers and rosemary after they have browned halfway. Dollops of sour cream and Salsa Cruda add unctuousness and digestive spices.

STEP ONE

6 medium potatoes

STEP TWO

¼ cup (60 ml) ghee or oil   *Salt*
Pinch of hing (optional)   *Black pepper*

1. Boil the potatoes in water to cover until halfway done, about 10 minutes. Drain. Peel when cool enough to handle.
2. *To pan-brown:* Cut the potatoes into ½-inch (1.3 cm) chunks. Heat the ghee or oil in a large skillet. Using a nonstick skillet helps keep the crust on the potatoes instead of sticking to the pan. Add the hing and potatoes and sprinkle with salt and plenty of black pepper. Cook over medium-high heat, stirring only occasionally so that a crust can form. The potatoes should be nicely browned and crusty on the outside and tender inside.
3. *To oven-roast:* Preheat the oven to 425°F (220°C). Leave the potatoes whole or cut them lengthwise into quarters or eighths. Place in a baking pan and toss the potatoes with enough ghee or oil to coat them thoroughly. It is important that they be generously coated or they won't brown properly. Sprinkle with salt and pepper. Bake until nicely browned on the outside and tender on the inside. Wedges take about 30 minutes, and whole potatoes can take up to 1 hour. Turn once or twice during the baking so they brown on all sides.

VARIATIONS

Use unpeeled new potatoes, 2 to 4 per person, depending on their size.

Before serving, toss with finely chopped fresh herbs: parsley, chervil, basil, cilantro, and tarragon are all nice.

About halfway through cooking, sprinkle with dried green herbs or fresh rosemary. Stir the potatoes so the herbs also become coated with oil.

To give oven-roasted potatoes a wonderful crispy coating, after thoroughly coating the potatoes with ghee or oil, roll in fine dry bread crumbs and bake in a well-buttered pan.

 LATKES (POTATO PANCAKES)

JEWISH   *4 servings*

What is not well known about these Jewish delicacies, traditionally served on Hanukkah, is that they are also a traditional Swedish dish. A nonstick pan is an asset for preparing the pancakes. Serve with sour cream and/or applesauce.

STEP ONE

4 cups (550 g) peeled, grated   *⅓ cup (45 g) unbleached white flour*
  potatoes   *½ teaspoon baking powder*
1 teaspoon salt

STEP TWO

Ghee or oil

1. Drain the potatoes well. Place in a bowl and mix with the salt, flour, and baking powder.
2. Melt 1 tablespoon ghee or oil in a nonstick skillet over medium heat. Working in batches, plop the potato mixture into the pan in small handfuls. Press and spread out with the back of a spatula to form thin pancakes.
3. Cook on both sides until golden brown. If not using nonstick cookware, the first batch may stick to the pan, but the following batches won't stick as much. Add more ghee or oil as needed.

VARIATIONS

For a savory version, add a pinch of hing and minced fresh herbs, or hing, minced fresh ginger, and curry spices to the batter in Step 1.

Add corn kernels and/or sautéed sliced fennel or celery to the batter in Step 1.

 # RÖSTI

SWITZERLAND   *4 to 6 servings*

One could call rösti a Swiss national dish—a crusty, buttery potato cake.

STEP ONE

6 medium potatoes

STEP THREE
Salt

¼ cup (60 ml) ghee

STEP FOUR

2 tablespoons water

1. Boil the potatoes in water to cover until half cooked, 10 to 15 minutes.
2. Drain and peel. Slice into ¼ inch (5 mm) thick rounds, then cut the rounds into ½ inch (1.3 cm) wide strips.

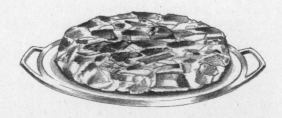

3. Melt the ghee in a small nonstick skillet over medium heat. Add the potatoes, sprinkle with a little salt, and cook, stirring, for a minute or two.
4. Press the potatoes into the pan. Sprinkle with the water, cover, and cook over medium heat for about 15 minutes, shaking the pan occasionally to keep the potatoes from sticking.
5. Check the sides to see if the potatoes are browned. When they are, uncover the skillet and invert an ovenproof plate over it. Turn the skillet and plate over so that the potatoes come out in a cake on the plate. If they have not browned, place them in a 400°F (200°C) oven until they are golden brown. Cut into wedges.

MASHED POTATOES, A WARM BLANKET, AND WINNIE THE POOH

4 to 6 servings

What I say is that, if a fellow really likes potatoes, he must be a pretty decent sort of fellow.
　　　　　　　　　　　　　　　—A. A. MILNE, *Winnie the Pooh*

Ah, the ultimate comfort food—warm, creamy, mild. A potato masher does a good job, but the ultimate lump buster is a food mill. Under no conditions ever use a food processor on lump-impaired potatoes. After beating the potatoes to a pulp, apply an electric mixer or beat rapidly with a wooden spoon and a strong arm to fluff them up. There are also those who are most comforted by the slightly lumpy, dense, fork-mashed variety.

STEP ONE
6 medium thin-skinned potatoes or *10 to 12 new potatoes*

STEP TWO
2 to 6 tablespoons (30 to 90 ml) ghee, butter, or olive oil　　　*¼ cup (60 ml) nondairy milk, buttermilk, or crème fraîche*

STEP THREE
Salt　　　　　　　　　　　*Black pepper*

1. Boil the potatoes in their jackets in water to cover. Cook until very tender so that there are no hard, intractable pieces that will resist mashing. Drain. Peel when just cool enough to handle.
2. Melt the ghee, butter, or oil in a small saucepan. Mix with the nondairy milk, buttermilk, or crème fraîche.
3. Mash the potatoes thoroughly with the liquid mixture. Season to taste with salt and pepper. Beat until fluffy.

DRESSING UP MASHED POTATOES

❖ Combine potatoes with equal amounts of puréed rutabaga, carrot, or
  cauliflower.
❖ Replace the milk with Dip with Three Fennels and Three Peppers, Tar-
  ragon–Pistachio Dressing, Herbed Chèvre Sauce, a pesto, or Creamy
  Horseradish Sauce. You may need to beat in a few tablespoons of liquid
  for a fluffy texture.
❖ Beat into the potatoes before serving:
  Caraway seeds
  Finely grated orange or lemon zest
  A few drops of toasted sesame oil
  Sautéed finely chopped vegetables, such as Miriam's Sofrito (page 000),
     cabbage, bitter greens, steamed peas or corn kernels
  A minute amount of finely grated horseradish
  Cream cheese or chèvre

SPINACH, INCLUDING AMARANTH AND LAMB'S QUARTERS

"Eat your spinach!" It's difficult to imagine the bad rap this marvelous, Kapha-balancing vegetable once had among children—but then again, it's hard to imagine the
travesty that came out of a can during a brief period of infamy. Catherine de' Medici
popularized the vegetable in France; any dish labeled "Florentine" is so named after her
home turf and contains spinach.

❖ American spinach is grown from an ancient variety with spiny seeds while European spinach comes from a tastier strain developed in the 1700s. Fellow members
  of the goosefoot family include multicolored *amaranth*, of which hundreds of
  varieties exist in the Himalayas and the Andes, and *lamb's quarters*, which grows
  wild and prolifically throughout the United States. Both can be substituted for
  spinach in any recipe.
❖ *New Zealand spinach* is botanically unrelated to spinach but often sold beside it
  in supermarkets. It is slightly coarser than spinach but, like chard, can be substituted in any spinach recipe with a minute or two extra cooking time.
❖ Spinach cooks in almost no time. It can be *lightly* steamed, sautéed, or stir-fried.
  When cooking spinach by any method, there are a few features to be alert to:

1. Sand gets trapped in the leaves, making spinach unpleasantly gritty if it is not
   fanatically rinsed before cooking. The only effective method I have ever found is
   to place it in a clean sink filled with water—lukewarm is kindest to your hands—

and swish it around for a minute to loosen the dirt. Leave alone for 5 minutes for the grit and dirt to settle to the bottom of the sink. Skim the spinach off the top without stirring up the water too much. Repeat if the spinach is especially dirty.

2. Dry rinsed spinach leaves as much as possible, or you will end up with Lake Baikal in the bottom of your cooking vessel. Small amounts can be dried in a salad spinner. For larger amounts, don't be afraid to squeeze them between towels—they almost need to be wrung out. After cooking, you may need to drain the spinach yet again.

3. What appears to be a humongous amount of uncooked spinach reduces down to a subatomic amount. To this day I am still fooled by an enormous mound of leaves piled up on my cutting board. Use a large pot and cook 2 to 3 pounds (1 to 1.5 kg) of spinach for 4 to 6 people. Employ a stupefyingly large amount of raw spinach for puréeing, a method that spinach has an affinity for.

❖ The French use the term *cire vierge*, "virgin beeswax," to describe spinach's bland flavor, meaning it takes on any impression. It is strange, then, that nutmeg is the only Western spice commonly used with it, and chervil about the only green herb. Spinach certainly works well with curry spices.

❖ Spinach goes well with creamy sauces, such as Cream Cheese Hollandaise, crème fraîche, and the mock mayonnaises. You can also simmer spinach Thai style in coconut milk.

Steamed Spinach

Wash spinach thoroughly and remove the hard stems. Usually the water clinging to the leaves after washing is sufficient moisture for steaming—don't add more than 1 to 2 tablespoons extra. Steam until tender, 2 to 4 minutes. Drain very well.

 # MEDITERRANEAN SPINACH

4 servings

The spices are intended to be quite subtle, offering an almost indefinable nuance of flavor.

STEP ONE

¼ cup (60 ml) olive oil   *¼ cup (35 g) pine nuts*
Pinch of hing (optional)

STEP TWO

2 pounds (1 kg) spinach, chopped   *Salt*

STEP THREE

¼ cup (30g) zante currants
1 tablespoon lemon juice
½ teaspoon sugar

⅛ teaspoon ground nutmeg
⅛ teaspoon ground cinnamon

1. Heat the olive oil in a large pot. Add the hing and pine nuts and sauté over low heat, stirring constantly, until the pine nuts are lightly browned. Be alert—pine nuts burn easily.
2. Add the spinach. Sprinkle with a little salt, stir, cover, and cook just until the spinach is wilted, 2 to 3 minutes. If necessary, drain the spinach in a colander, pressing out excess moisture with the back of a spoon. Return to the pot.
3. Stir in the currants, lemon juice, sugar, nutmeg, and cinnamon. Adjust the salt.

VARIATIONS

Replace the spinach with 8 cups (700 g) chopped chard and sauté until tender.
Add cubes of pan-browned panir to the finished dish.

 # SPINACH AND PANIR (PALAK PANIR)

INDIA   *4 servings*

I first witnessed the preparation of spinach and panir in India, where a lovely young woman squatted on the floor and unhurriedly ground the cooked spinach a little bit at a time with a coarse stone pestle in a large, shallow stone mortar. A nonstick pan works best for sautéing the panir cubes for this very popular dish. Drain and dry the spinach extremely well before cooking, or the spices will be lost when you drain off excess liquid later.

STEP ONE

1 cup (200 g) firm panir

1 tablespoon ghee or oil

STEP TWO

3 tablespoons ghee or mild-
  flavored oil
Pinch of hing (optional)

1½ teaspoons cumin seeds
2 tablespoons minced fresh ginger
½ teaspoon fenugreek seeds

STEP THREE

2 pounds (1 kg) spinach, coarsely
  chopped
Salt

Pinch of sugar
Crème fraîche (optional)

1. Slice the panir into cubes. Sauté in the ghee or oil over medium heat, stirring frequently, until lightly browned. Set aside.

2. Heat the ghee or oil in a large wok or pot. Add the hing, cumin seeds, ginger, and fenugreek seeds and sauté for 1 minute over low heat, stirring constantly.
3. Add the spinach and sprinkle lightly with salt. Sauté until tender. Drain off any excess water and finely chop. Some people purée the spinach. Return the spinach to the pot. Adjust the salt, add the sugar, and gently stir in the panir pieces. Serve with a decorative drizzle of crème fraîche if desired.

VARIATION

For heat, add 1 teaspoon or more black pepper in Step 3 or add cayenne or red chilies to the ghee or oil in Step 2.

 # SPINACH-CHEESE TART

One 9-inch (23 cm) pie—6 servings

Serve hot or at room temperature. It is lovely accompanied by an antipasto for a summer lunch.

STEP ONE

2 pounds (1 kg) spinach

STEP TWO

*2 tablespoons arrowroot or
   cornstarch*
1 tablespoon flour
*¼ cup (60 ml) sour cream or
   crème fraîche*
½ cup (120 g) ricotta cheese

¼ teaspoon freshly grated nutmeg
½ teaspoon salt
*1½ cups (150 g) grated mild cheese,
   such as Monterey Jack or
   mozzarella*
Partially Baked Crust (p. 409)

1. Preheat the oven to 350°F (180°C). Wash the spinach and remove the stems. Steam very lightly, just until the leaves are wilted. Drain thoroughly and chop while draining.
2. Mix the arrowroot or cornstarch and flour thoroughly into the sour cream or crème fraîche. Mix with the spinach, ricotta, nutmeg, and salt. Beat in the grated cheese. Spread evenly in the pie shell.
3. Bake until the crust and topping are lightly browned, about 30 minutes.

VARIATION

For individual tarts, line buttered muffin tins with pastry crust. Do not partially bake. Fill and bake as above.

SPANAKÓPITA (SPINACH-FILO PIE)

GREECE   *8 to 10 servings*

The Greek version of spinach pie, using filo pastry.

STEP ONE

½ cup (110 g) ghee or butter
Pinch of hing (optional)

½ cup (120 ml) olive oil

STEP TWO

Pinch of hing (optional)
1 cup (110 g) finely chopped
  fennel or celery (fennel
  is preferable)

1 cup (140 g) finely chopped green
  bell peppers
1 tablespoon minced fresh ginger
Liquid seasoning or salt

STEP THREE

3 pounds (1.5 kg) spinach, coarsely chopped

STEP FOUR

1 pound (500 g) filo pastry (24 sheets)

STEP FIVE

1 pound (500 g) feta cheese or panir

1. Melt the ghee or butter in a small saucepan. Add the hing and sauté over low heat until fragrant, about 30 seconds. Mix in the olive oil. Pour ¼ cup (60 ml) into a large wok or soup pot and set the rest aside.
2. Add the hing to the pot and sauté over low heat for 30 seconds, until fragrant. Add the fennel or celery, bell pepper, and ginger. Sprinkle with liquid seasoning or salt, cover, and cook slowly until very soft.
3. Add the spinach and sauté just until the leaves are wilted. Adjust the seasoning, remembering that the feta you may be adding later is quite salty. Drain again if necessary.
4. Brush a 10 × 14-inch (26 × 36 cm) pan with the reserved butter-oil. Lay down a sheet of filo pastry. Brush with butter-oil. Add another sheet and brush again with butter-oil. Repeat until 12 sheets are used.
5. Spread the spinach evenly over the filo. Crumble the cheese over the spinach.
6. Preheat the oven to 300°F (150°C). Lay down 12 more sheets of filo, brushing each with butter-oil. Pour any remaining butter-oil over the top. Score the top few sheets of filo with a sharp knife to make squares approximately 2½ inches (6.5 cm) wide. Sprinkle the top lightly with water.
7. Bake until the filo is *lightly* browned, just turning golden, 1 to 1¼ hours.

VARIATION

✿ Omit the feta and substitute 1 more pound (230 g) of spinach, or replace the feta with crumbled firm tofu.

Summer Squash, Including Zucchini

All summer squash, including *zucchini*, *golden zucchini*, *crookneck*, *Italian*, and *pattypan*, though varying in shape and size, are particularly balancing for Pitta and can be eaten at both lunch and dinner.

❖ Summer squashes can all be prepared in basically the same manner. They contain a great deal of moisture, and when they are cooked in water, their flavor leaches out and their texture dissolves. If steam you must, steam whole and slice *after* cooking to preserve their flavor. Waterless cooking methods such as baking, sautéing, and grilling best enhance summer squashes' flavor and texture.

❖ Summer squashes' mild flavor is particularly receptive to a wide variety of sauces, spices, and seasonings. Indian and Mexican spices, fresh green herbs, and Chinese and Southeast Asian flavorings all enhance summer squashes. They marinate beautifully for antipasti and composed salads.

Squash blossoms can be stuffed and baked. Seasoned and buttered bread crumbs are the usual stuffing, being fine enough to fill the delicate blossoms without breaking them. Use male blossoms (the ones not attached to the squash). They also can be dipped in tempura batter and deep-fried: cut open and gently press to flatten, then dip in batter and deep-fry.

Baked Summer Squash

A highly recommended technique. Baked summer squash has a wonderful, meltingly soft texture. Though it hardly needs more than a sprinkling of salt and possibly a dash of lemon juice, you can also anoint with finely chopped fresh green herbs, such as basil, dill, and parsley, before serving.

1. Slice summer squash in half lengthwise. Rub with ghee or oil and place on an oiled baking sheet. Sprinkle with salt.
2. Bake in a 325°F (160°C) oven until tender, 40 to 60 minutes. Be careful not to burn the underside.

The near end of the street was rather dark and had mostly vegetable shops. Abundance of vegetables—piles of white and green fennel, like celery, and sheaves of young, purplish, sea-dust-coloured artichokes, nodding their buds, piles of great radishes, scarlet and bluey purple, carrots, long strips of dried figs, mountains of big oranges, scarlet large peppers, a large slice of pumpkin, a great mass of colours and vegetable freshnesses. . . . How the dark, greasy, night-stricken street seems to beam with these vegetables, all this fresh, delicate flesh of luminous vegetables piled there in the air. . . . —D. H. Lawrence, *Sea and Sardinia*

GRATED SUMMER SQUASH

4 servings

Grated summer squash is almost like a new vegetable. Serve on toast or over rice or as a side dish. The delicate flavor is very nice on its own, but you could also add curry spices and minced fresh ginger while sautéing or stir in minced fresh green herbs before serving.

STEP ONE

6 cups (630 g) grated summer squash

STEP TWO

2 tablespoons ghee or butter   *Salt*
Pinch of hing (optional)   *Black pepper*

1. Sprinkle the grated squash with salt and toss. Allow to stand for 10 minutes, then drain very well, squeezing out excess moisture.
2. Melt the ghee or butter in a wok or large skillet. Add the hing and sauté over low heat until fragrant, about 30 seconds. Add the squash and sauté until tender, about 5 minutes. If there is more than a tablespoon of water left in the pan, drain it off. Season to taste with salt and pepper.

 # SUMMER SQUASH BOATS

4 servings

Given the market fare and your maritime persuasions, you can make elongated canoes or pirogues with zucchini, or round inner tubes or lifeboats with pattypan squash.

STEP ONE

6 large summer squash

STEP TWO

3 cups (700 ml) Carrot-Pepper Sauce (p. 255) or Tomato Sauce (pp. 505–506)

STEP THREE

¼ cup (60 ml) olive oil   *1 stalk celery or fennel, thinly*
Pinch of hing (optional)   *   sliced*
1½ teaspoons dried basil   *1 cup (120 g) fine dry bread crumbs*
¼ teaspoon dried rosemary   *½ cup (50 g) finely chopped walnuts*
2 tablespoons minced fresh   *Salt*
*   parsley*   *Black pepper*
1 carrot, grated

STEP FOUR
1 cup (200 g) chopped fresh mozzarella or crumbled feta (optional)

1. Preheat the oven to 350°F (180°C). Oil a baking pan. Halve the squash lengthwise and hollow out by carefully removing the seedy portion. (If you wish, you can finely chop the seedy portion and add to the sauce.)
2. Place the squash boats side by side in the baking pan and bake for 15 minutes. Remove but do not turn off the oven. Bring the sauce to a simmer.
3. Heat the olive oil in a skillet. Add the hing, basil, rosemary, and parsley, then the carrot and celery or fennel. Sauté over low heat, stirring frequently, until tender. Add the bread crumbs and walnuts. Season to taste with salt and pepper.
4. Fill the hollows in the squash with the bread crumb mixture. Pour the sauce over the boats. Sprinkle the cheese on top if desired. Bake until the squash are tender, about 20 minutes.

 # SUMMER SQUASH IN SOUR CREAM WITH DILL AND FENNEL

4 to 6 servings

This exquisite dish created by Tom Torpy works well as either a luncheon main dish or rich side dish. It also makes a delicious pasta sauce. Fennel is a wonderful tri-doshic spice badly in need of a publicist.

STEP ONE

2 tablespoons olive oil
Pinch of hing (optional)

3 medium tomatoes, cut into
*   thin wedges*

STEP TWO

6 cups (720 g) summer squash,
*   cut into ½-inch (1.3 cm)*
*   pieces*
1 teaspoon dried dill

1 teaspoon fennel seeds
Salt
Black pepper
½ teaspoon sugar

STEP THREE

½ cup (120 ml) sour cream
¾ cup (125 g) or more grated
*   Parmesan cheese* (optional)

1. Heat the olive oil in a large skillet. Add the hing and sauté over medium heat until fragrant, about 30 seconds. Add the tomatoes. Sauté until softened, 4 to 5 minutes.
2. Add the squash, dill, and fennel seed. Stir to blend. Sprinkle lightly with salt, pepper, and the sugar. Cover and simmer until the squash are just tender. Stir occasionally.
3. Stir in the sour cream and Parmesan. Heat to serving temperature—do not boil.

VARIATIONS

Replace the squash with green beans cut into ½-inch (1.3 cm) pieces.

Replace the Parmesan with crumbled feta cheese or panir.

✪ Omit the sour cream and cheese entirely, or replace the sour cream with Tofu or Cashew Mayonnaise (pp. 503–504).

Winter Squash

Winter squash are available year-round, with the exception of pumpkins, which are autumnal. Avoid pumpkins grown for jack-o'-lanterns; the smaller, *sugar pumpkin* variety is excellent. Although squashes have different flavors and amounts of moisture, with the exception of spaghetti squash, they can be used fairly interchangeably in cooking. Winter squash can also be used in recipes calling for yams and sweet potatoes. Boil or bake whole or in slices, slice and steam, or cut into tiny pieces and slowly sauté. Roundish-shaped squashes, such as pumpkin, kabocha, and acorn, are good containers for stuffings.

❖ Winter squash is very sensitive to salt—add judiciously. Butter and raw or brown sugar are standard Western accompaniments. Cinnamon, nutmeg, allspice, and ginger—"pumpkin pie" spices—all suit winter squashes. I like to use chopped crystallized ginger for a change of pace. Indian spices are quite effective for non-sweet squash dishes.

❖ *Spaghetti squash* is in a class by itself. When you run a fork through the flesh of the cooked vegetable, it separates into spaghetti-like strands. Boil whole in water to cover until tender on the inside when pierced with a knife, 40 to 60 minutes. Cut in half lengthwise and scrape a fork lengthwise along the squash to make the "spaghetti" strands. You can serve it like spaghetti with any sauce for pasta.

Baked Winter Squash

1. Bake squash whole, halved, quartered, or sliced. If quartered or sliced, remove the stringy portion and seeds and brush exposed surfaces with oil or melted ghee. Always bake spaghetti squash whole.
2. Bake in a 350°F (180°C) oven until completely tender. Sliced squash takes 30 to 45 minutes; whole squash takes 1 to 1½ hours.

Stuffed Winter Squash

Halve round-shaped squashes, seed, and bake *before* stuffing. Grain mixtures go particularly nicely.

SQUASH-PECAN CASSEROLE WITH DRIED CRANBERRIES

4 to 6 servings

A good Thanksgiving dish that I serve in hollowed-out squash shells. Squashes with drier, denser flesh, such as kabocha, lend the best texture to this dish. You can also substitute "yam"-type sweet potatoes. For a more pumpkin pie–like flavor, substitute cinnamon for the allspice.

4 cups (840 g) puréed cooked
    winter squash
¼ cup (60 ml) melted ghee or
    butter
½ cup (100 g) raw or packed
    brown sugar

STEP TWO

1 teaspoon allspice
1 tablespoon lemon juice
⅓ cup (55 g) finely chopped crystallized
    ginger
½ cup (50 g) dried cranberries
Salt

STEP THREE

½ cup (50 g) pecan halves

1. Preheat the oven to 350°F (180°C). Butter a baking dish or place hollowed-out squash shells on an oiled baking sheet.
2. Purée the squash, ghee or butter, sugar, allspice, and lemon juice together in a food processor. Stir in the crystallized ginger and dried cranberries. If you feel it's warranted, cautiously add salt to taste.
3. Spoon into the baking dish or squash shells and spread evenly. Decorate the top with the pecan halves. Bake for 30 minutes.

 # PUMPKIN OR SQUASH CURRY (KADDU SABJI)

INDIA   *4 to 6 servings*

¼ cup (60 ml) ghee or oil
Pinch of hing (optional)

STEP ONE

2 teaspoons cumin seeds
2 tablespoons minced fresh ginger

STEP TWO

¼ cup (60 ml) water
8 cups (880 g) peeled, cubed
    pumpkin or other squash

¼ teaspoon ground nutmeg
Salt
1 tablespoon sugar

1. Melt the ghee or oil in a pot. Add the hing, cumin seeds, and ginger and sauté over low heat for 1 minute, until fragrant.
2. Add the water, pumpkin, nutmeg, a sprinkling of salt, and the sugar. Cover and simmer until the pumpkin is tender. Adjust the salt and sugar.

VARIATIONS

For heat, add 1 teaspoon or more black pepper in Step 2 or add cayenne or red chilies to the ghee or butter in Step 1.

Sprinkle on a little garam masala (pp. 565–66) after cooking.

SQUASH STUFFED WITH WILD RICE SUCCOTASH

UNITED STATES   *4 servings*

Native North Americans understood squash to be the third corner of their sacred triangular nutritional foundation of beans, corn, and squash. They were grown together, with cornstalks serving as bean poles, and squash vines meandering between the stalks. The Iroquois described the beans-corn-squash trinity as three lovely celestial damsels who wandered the fields at night. Here, the trinity is combined with wild rice. You can substitute zanté currants or dried cranberries for the blueberries. Note that the beans must be soaked in advance.

STEP ONE

½ cup (95 g) dried kidney or Anasazi beans

STEP TWO

1 medium sugar pumpkin or 2 acorn squashes

STEP THREE

3 cups (720 ml) water   *½ teaspoon salt*
¾ cup (135 g) wild rice

STEP FOUR

3 tablespoons ghee or oil   *½ cup (65 g) coarsely chopped fennel*
Pinch of hing (optional)   *or celery*
1 tablespoon minced fresh ginger   *Kernels from 1 ear of corn*
⅓ cup (45 g) coarsely chopped
  red bell peppers

STEP FIVE

⅓ cup (50 g) dried blueberries   *Black pepper*
Liquid seasoning or salt

1. Rinse the beans and soak in at least 2 cups (500 ml) of water for 4 to 6 hours or overnight. Drain and simmer in 4 cups (1 l) water until tender, about 1½ hours. Drain and set aside.
2. Preheat the oven to 350°F (180°C). While the beans are cooking, cut the top off the pumpkin or halve the acorn squash and remove the seeds. Place in a baking pan, brush the cut surfaces with oil, and bake until tender.
3. While the squash is baking, bring the water to a boil. Add the wild rice and salt, cover, and cook until all the water is absorbed and the wild rice is tender, about 45 minutes.
4. Heat the ghee or oil in a skillet. Add the hing and ginger and sauté over low heat for a minute. Add the bell peppers and fennel and sauté for a few minutes, stirring frequently. Add the corn, cover, and cook for another 2 to 3 minutes or until tender.
5. Mix the corn mixture with the wild rice and the beans. Add the dried blueberries and season to taste with liquid seasoning or salt and pepper. Sprinkle the inside of the squash lightly with salt. Spoon in the stuffing. Return to the oven for 10 to 15 minutes so that everything is heated through. To serve, scoop out the flesh of the squash along with the stuffing.

SWEET POTATOES AND YAMS

Let the sky rain [sweet] potatoes.
—WILLIAM SHAKESPEARE, *The Merry Wives of Windsor*

The saga of Vata-balancing yams and sweet potatoes is an international historical-botanical tangle on which the final curtain has not yet fallen. Yams are a staple food in West Africa, so much so that their name means "food." A variety of true yams with white flesh and brown, barklike skin is also found in the Caribbean and is sometimes available in Hispanic markets. The New World tuber Columbus encountered was *batatas*, "sweet potatoes." However sweet potatoes came to be known as yams, a moist, orange-colored variety of sweet potato is commonly called a "yam," and the drier, starchier, golden-fleshed type is known as a "sweet potato." Papua New Guineans perhaps have the jump on all besieged tuber botanists: if a man plants it, it's a yam. If a woman plants it, sweet potato it is.

❖ Yams and sweet potatoes can be boiled or baked whole, or sliced and steamed. Add slices to soups, stews, Japanese-style and Indian-style vegetables, and other vegetable combinations.
❖ Yams and sweet potatoes can be used in most recipes calling for winter squash and for carrots in Carrot Crumble. The purée is also a delicious thickener for soups.

Boiled Sweet Potatoes or Yams

Boil in water to cover until very tender when pierced with a knife, about 40 minutes.

Baked Sweet Potatoes or Yams

Prick the skins and bake in a 450°F (230°C) oven until completely tender, 50 to 60 minutes. To hasten the process, embed the tongs of a fork deeply into each sweet potato to send heat into the center while baking.

 # CANDIED SWEET POTATOES

4 to 6 servings

STEP ONE

4 to 5 sweet potatoes, the "yam" type

STEP FOUR

3 tablespoons ghee or butter
1 cup (210 g) raw or packed dark
  brown sugar

1 tablespoon lemon juice
1 tablespoon orange juice or water

1. Boil the sweet potatoes until almost tender. Drain well.
2. Preheat the oven to 375°F (190°C). Butter a baking pan.
3. When the sweet potatoes are cool enough to handle, peel and quarter lengthwise. Place in the baking pan.
4. Melt the ghee or butter in a saucepan. Add the sugar, lemon juice, and orange juice or water. Bring to a boil. Pour over the sweet potatoes.
5. Bake for 20 to 25 minutes, basting and turning the sweet potatoes over once.

VARIATIONS

Sprinkle with ½ cup (50 g) chopped pecans or walnuts before baking.

Add a sprinkling of chopped crystallized ginger and/or crushed pineapple and/or grated coconut before baking.

TOMATOES

Tomatoes, unfortunately, aggravate all the doshas. Some vaidyas recommend avoiding them entirely, while others feel they have nutritional value when balanced with other ingredients.

❖ Part of the dosha-aggravating quality of tomatoes is their acidity. *Yellow tomatoes* are less acidic than red ones. *Dried tomatoes* are much less acidic than fresh ones and can be used all year.

❖ Supermarket offerings are generally picked when green, given a chlorine bath and a rinse, blow-dried, and oil-coated. They are then chilled to halt any—God forbid—ripening, and treated with gases that redden them without ripening. What you get is a bright red, unripe, and understandably tasteless Thing. Just Say No! Tomatoes should be fragrant and, optimally, just turning from green to red. Beefsteak and similar varieties should be somewhat soft to the touch but not squishy. Roma tomatoes should be firm. Ripen at room temperature but not in the sun. Store tomatoes above 55°F (13°C) for best flavor.

❖ For optimum kindness to the tummy and for aesthetics as well, when you have the time, remove the skins before cooking. Make small scrapes on the tops of your tomatoes with the tines of a fork to cut the skin, then drop them into boiling water for 30 seconds. Drain and peel.

 # PROVENÇAL STUFFED TOMATOES (TOMATES FARCIES À LA PROVENÇALE)

FRANCE   *6 servings*

These elegant tomatoes that my mother makes shine as a first course or side dish and can be served either hot or at room temperature.

STEP ONE

6 large, firm tomatoes

STEP TWO

1 cup (120 g) fine dry bread crumbs
½ cup (120 ml) olive oil
¼ cup (60 ml) minced fresh parsley
¼ cup (60 ml) minced fresh basil

¼ teaspoon fresh or dried thyme leaves
Pinch of hing (optional)
¼ teaspoon salt

STEP THREE

Salt

Black pepper

1. Preheat the oven to 350°F (180°C). Oil a baking sheet with olive oil. Slice the tops off the tomatoes. Carefully scoop out the insides, leaving a firm case. Turn the tomatoes upside down to drain the cases while preparing the filling.
2. Toss the bread crumbs, olive oil, herbs, and seasonings together.
3. Sprinkle the tomato cases with salt and pepper, then carefully fill with the mixture. Place the tomatoes on the baking sheet and bake until they are tender but still hold their shape and the filling is lightly browned, 10 to 20 minutes.

TOMATOES STUFFED WITH VEGETABLE HASH

6 servings

The name "hash" comes from the French *hache*, "to chop." Topped with dollops of sour cream and guacamole, these tomatoes are worthy of a brunch for company.

STEP ONE

6 *medium, firm tomatoes*

STEP TWO

3 *potatoes*

STEP THREE

2 *tablespoons ghee or oil*	2 *cups (180 g) chopped broccoli*
Pinch of *hing* (optional)	*florets*
1 *teaspoon rosemary*	½ *bell pepper, finely chopped*
1 *carrot, quartered lengthwise*	1 *stalk celery or fennel, thinly sliced*
and cut into ½-inch	*Liquid seasoning or salt*
(1.3 ml) pieces	*Black pepper*

STEP FIVE

1 *medium avocado*	*Black pepper*
2 *tablespoons lemon juice*	*Sour cream*
Liquid seasoning or salt	*Minced parsley or fresh cilantro*

1. Halve the tomatoes crosswise. Carefully scoop out the insides and turn the tomatoes upside down to drain. Set aside.
2. Boil the potatoes until half cooked, about 15 minutes. Drain, peel, and cut into ½-inch (1.3 cm) cubes.
3. Melt the ghee or butter in a skillet. Add the hing, rosemary, potatoes, and remaining vegetables. Sprinkle with liquid seasoning or salt, cover, and cook over low heat, stirring frequently, until the vegetables are tender. Sprinkle with black pepper and adjust the seasoning.
4. Preheat the oven to 350°F (180°C). Sprinkle the tomato cases with salt and pepper.

Fill with the vegetable mixture. Place in a baking pan with a little water to keep the tomatoes from scorching. Bake until the tomatoes are tender, 10 to 20 minutes.

5. While the tomatoes are baking, prepare guacamole by mashing the avocado with the lemon juice and adding liquid seasoning or salt and pepper to taste. Top each tomato with a spoonful each of sour cream and guacamole. Sprinkle with minced parsley or cilantro.

TURNIPS

> *I give you these roots, friends of winter and of rime;*
> *Romulus ate of them at the Table of the Gods.* —MARTIAL

Although they look hardy, turnips last for only about a week in the refrigerator. Turnips can be baked, boiled, or sliced and steamed. They can also be sliced and deep-fried. They are used often in French dishes, particularly in soups and stews. In China turnips are dried in strips and used as a meat substitute in Buddhist vegetarian cuisine.

Baked Turnips

Trim the ends and bake whole or sliced in an oiled, covered baking dish at 400° F (200° C) for about 40 minutes for sliced turnips to 1 to 1½ hours for whole ones.

 # DIM SUM TURNIP FRITTERS (LUOBO GAO)

CHINA   *12 fritters*

In the Chinese Buddhist tradition of mimicking nonvegetarian dishes, these fritters are somewhat like fish cakes. Serve as part of a Chinese-style meal, or—why not?—on a sandwich with eggless mayo.

STEP ONE

3 cups (270 g) finely grated turnips
1 carrot, finely grated
¾ cup (110 g) unbleached white
  flour

1 teaspoon baking powder
1 teaspoon salt

STEP FIVE

Oil for deep-frying

1. Mix all the ingredients for Step 1 together well. Spread evenly in an oiled 9-inch (23 cm) square pan.

2. If you have a Chinese bamboo steamer, set it up for steaming. If not, place a rack or an inverted bowl in a large wok or pot, and fill the wok with water to ½-inch (1.3 cm) below the rack. Bring the water to a boil.
3. Place the pan with the turnip mixture on the rack and cover the pot. Steam over medium heat for 20 minutes.
4. Remove the pan and let the turnip mixture cool completely. Carefully cut the mixture into 12 rectangular pieces.
5. Heat the oil. Have a tray covered with paper towels nearby. Deep-fry the cakes on both sides until golden. Drain.

MIXED VEGETABLES

MIXED VEGETABLES SIMMERED IN COCONUT MILK (SAYUR MANIS)

INDONESIA   *4 to 6 servings*

Lemon grass and kaffir lime leaves can be found in Thai markets. Serve over rice.

STEP ONE

1 stalk fresh lemon grass (optional)　　*2 tablespoons minced fresh ginger*
4 kaffir lime leaves, minced
  (optional)

STEP TWO

3 tablespoons mild-flavored oil　　*Pinch of hing* (optional)

STEP THREE

1 carrot, thinly sliced　　　　　　*1 cup (115 g) sliced green beans*
½ bell pepper, coarsely chopped　　*2 cups (210 g) coarsely chopped*
1 cup (100 g) small cauliflower florets　　*cabbage*

STEP FOUR

1½ cups (360 ml) Coconut　　　*Liquid seasoning*
　Milk (p. 494)　　　　　　　*½ to 1 teaspoon black pepper*
¼ teaspoon sugar

STEP FIVE

*⅔ cup (160 ml) coarsely chopped fresh basil (**Thai basil if available**)*

1. Crush the lower third of the lemon grass stalk, the lime leaves, and ginger together with a mortar and pestle. The lemon grass will remain whole, but not to worry—that's as it should be.

2. Heat the oil in a large lidded skillet or wok. Add the hing and the pounded mixture and sauté over low heat until the ginger begins to darken.
3. Add the vegetables and stir to coat with the oil and spices.
4. Add the coconut milk, sugar, a sprinkling of liquid seasoning, and the pepper. Bring to a boil. Cover, reduce the heat, and simmer until the vegetables are tender.
5. Remove the lemon grass stalk. Adjust the seasoning and stir in the basil.

VARIATION

Replace the pepper with minced fresh chilies, added in Step 1.

 # KOFTA (VEGETABLE BALLS IN SPICED TOMATO SAUCE)

I N D I A   *4 to 6 servings*

Different varieties of kofta, also called *kefta* and *kibbe*, are served from Armenia to India. Here is one of the many Indian versions, a unique and striking dish to serve over rice.

STEP ONE

½ head cauliflower, cut into pieces
2 medium potatoes, peeled and cubed

1 cup (130 g) peas

STEP TWO

2 tablespoons ghee or mild-flavored oil
Pinch of hing (optional)
1 teaspoon cumin seeds
1 tablespoon minced fresh ginger
½ cup (120 ml) water
3½ cups (820 g) chopped ripe tomatoes

½ teaspoon ground cinnamon
⅛ teaspoon ground cloves
1 teaspoon turmeric
1 teaspoon sugar
Salt

STEP THREE

1 teaspoon salt
1 teaspoon turmeric
⅓ cup (40 g) besan (chickpea flour)
⅓ cup (60 g) farina (Cream of Wheat)

1 tablespoon melted ghee or mild-flavored oil
Salt

STEP FOUR

Oil for deep-frying

1. Steam the cauliflower and potatoes for 15 minutes. Add the peas and steam until the vegetables are tender. Drain very well.
2. *To prepare the sauce:* While the vegetables are steaming, heat the ghee or oil in a pot. Add the hing, cumin seeds, and ginger, and sauté for 1 minute. Add the water, tomatoes, remaining spices, and sugar. Simmer, covered, stirring occasionally, for 30 minutes. Add salt to taste. Set aside.
3. *To prepare the kofta balls:* While the sauce is simmering, mash the vegetables with the remaining ingredients. Do not use a food processor, which will reduce the potatoes to glue. Add salt to taste. Roll into 1-inch (2.5 cm) balls.
4. Heat the oil for deep-frying. Have a platter covered with paper towels nearby. Deep-fry the kofta balls until well browned, turning once or twice. Drain.
5. Place in a serving bowl. Pour on the sauce and allow to stand for 1 minute before serving.

VARIATIONS

Malai Kofta (Kofta with Cream): Stir a few spoonfuls of crème fraîche or sour cream into the sauce just before serving.

For heat, add 1 teaspoon or more black pepper or add dried crumbled chilies to the sauce in Step 2.

 # VEGETABLE KUGEL

JEWISH   *6 servings*

A *kugel* is a baked pudding. Here is a purée of vegetables baked until the inside is tender and the outside is brown and crusty. For best results, use a glass baking dish so that the kugel can brown all over. Matzoh meal is available in the kosher or ethnic section of most supermarkets.

STEP ONE

6 medium potatoes

STEP TWO

¼ cup (55 g) ghee or butter	*4 carrots*
Pinch of hing (optional)	*1½ cups (200 g) peas*
2 stalks fennel or celery, thinly sliced	*2 cups (230 g) sliced green beans*

STEP THREE

⅓ cup matzoh meal (30 g) or whole wheat flour (40 g)	*Liquid seasoning or seasoned salt*
3 tablespoons arrowroot or cornstarch	*Black pepper*

1. Boil the potatoes in water to cover until tender. Drain well. Peel when cool enough to handle.
2. While the potatoes are boiling, melt the ghee or butter in a small skillet. Add the hing and sauté over low heat for 30 seconds, until fragrant. Add the fennel or celery, carrots, peas, and green beans, cover, and cook until very tender, stirring occasionally.
3. Preheat the oven to 400°F (200°C). Using a potato masher, mash the vegetables to a rough paste. Beat in the matzoh meal or flour and the arrowroot or cornstarch. Season to taste with liquid seasoning or salt and pepper.
4. Spoon the mixture into a well-buttered casserole dish and spread evenly. Bake until the top is well browned, 1 to 1½ hours.

The plants, falling from heaven, said, "The man, whom living we pervade, will not perish."   —RIK VEDA X.8.7, "Hymn to the Medicinal Plants and Herbs"

Grains and Cereals

All flesh is grass.   —ISAIAH 40.6

Grains are a staple Ayurvedic food, often eaten in much the same way today as throughout history. When you sit down to your bowl of oatmeal or rice, your ancient ancestors could join you in your repast with familiarity and fraternity.

Grains and grain products have increasingly been eaten only in their most highly refined forms. In reaction, health food advocates have promoted only unrefined and whole grains as worth eating. According to Ayurveda, whole grains, processed grains, and refined grains all have a place in our diet. The important things to look for are, first, as always, that the grains are organically farmed and, second, how and why they have been processed.

Some grains are refined to make them more digestible, making their nutrients more accessible. Grains with a heavy husk, such as barley and rice, are hard to digest, and their pearled counterparts are the better Ayurvedic choice. In other instances, the methods of refinement are simply intended to increase the shelf life of the product. The nutritious germ, for instance, is removed because it becomes rancid when exposed to steel grinders in the mill, which heat up during use.

Most grains are enveloped by an inedible *husk* or *hull*. Within the hull lies a second layer, the *bran*. The hull and bran protect the grain's *aleurone layer*, which contains oil and nutrients and its embryo, the *germ*, which germinates and sprouts. At the core is the *endosperm*, made mostly of starch that nourishes the sprouting germ.

❖ *Whole grains,* such as wheat berries, have only the hull removed by threshing. They can be broken into pieces called *groats* or *grits,* such as buckwheat groats and Scottish oatmeal. Other grains are coarsely ground, such as cornmeal and semolina. Still others are steamed and dried, such as bulgar; or steamed, dried, and flattened, such as rolled oats or wheat flakes. Many grains have the hull, bran, and germ polished off by a process known as *pearling*, leaving only the endosperm. White rice and pearl barley are treated in this manner.

❖ *Stone-ground* grains, such as stone-ground cornmeal, can contain the germ because stone grinders remain cool.

Storing Grains

Grains vary widely in shelf life, depending on the amount of processing they've undergone and their own natural longevity. However, all grains must be protected against rancidity, insects, and mold.

❖ Many grains pick up moths and other insects during storage, often appearing to make a great case for spontaneous generation. Airtight nonreactive containers such as glass jars isolate any grains that suddenly teem with entomological life. Moths move fast. After my husband and I spent a morning sorrowfully discarding sack after sack of infested grains from a storeroom alive with fluttering white wings, I have never again made the mistake of relying on paper bags or boxes.

❖ A cool, dry shelf is sufficient for short-term storage of most grains. However, the refrigerator or, better yet, the freezer provides better and longer protection against rancidity for short-lived grains and against moths for all grains.

Cooking Grains

There are absolutely no foolproof, exact measurements. Different batches of the same type of grain can contain different amounts of moisture, and you may have to add or subtract as much as ⅓ cup of water to cook 1 cup of grain.

GRAIN COOKING TIMES AND YIELDS

1 Cup Grain	Water (cups)	Salt (teaspoons)	Cooking Time (minutes)	Yield (cups)
Amaranth (165 g)	2½–3 (600–720 ml)	½	20	3 (720 ml)
Barley, hulled & hull-less (205 g)	3–3½ (600–720 ml)	½	1 hr. 20 min.	4½ (1.1 l)
Barley, pearl (205 g)	2½–3 (600–720 ml)	½	45	3½ (840 ml)
Barley grits (170 g)	4 (940 ml)	½	20	3 (720 ml)
Buckwheat (170 g)	2–2½ (480–600 ml)	½	10	2½–3 (600–720 ml)
Bulgar wheat (175 g)	2 (480 ml)	½	20	3 (720 ml)
Couscous (185 g)	2 (480 ml)	½	10–15	3 (720 ml)
Cracked wheat (175 g)	3 (720 ml)	½	55	3½ (840 ml)
Job's Tears (200 g)	3 (720 ml)	½	1 hr. 40 min.	3½ (840 ml)
Millet (195 g)	3 (720 ml)	½	30	3½ (840 ml)
Oats, whole (185 g)	4 (940 ml)	½	60	3 (720 ml)

GRAIN COOKING TIMES AND YIELDS *(cont.)*

1 CUP GRAIN	WATER (cups)	SALT (teaspoons)	COOKING TIME (minutes)	YIELD (cups)
Oats, Scottish (175 g)	4 (940 ml)	½	60	3 (720 ml)
Oats, rolled (115 g)	2¾ (660 ml)	½	10	3 (720 ml)
Quinoa (180 g)	2 (480 ml)	½	20	3 (720 ml)
Rice, white (205 g)	2 (480 ml)	½	20	3 (720 ml)
Rice, basmati (205 g)	2¼ (540 ml)	½	20	3⅔ (880 ml)
Rice, brown (200 g)	3 (720 ml)	½	45	3 (720 ml)
Rice flakes	1¼ (300 ml)	¼	5–7	2 (480 ml)
Rye, whole (200 g)	3 (720 ml)	½	60+	2½ (600 ml)
Rye, cracked (175 g)	3 (720 ml)	½	40–50	2½ (600 ml)
Rye flakes (105 g)	2 (480 ml)	½	20	2 (480 ml)
Semolina or farina (170 g)	4 (940 ml)	1	20	4 (940 ml)
Teff (165 g)	3 (720 ml)	½	20	3 (720 ml)
Triticale* (200 g)	2½ (600 ml)	½	1 hr. 45 min.	2½ (600 ml)
Triticale flakes (100 g)	2½ (600 ml)	½	20	2⅓ (560 ml)
Wheat flakes (95 g)	2 (480 ml)	½	15–20	2 (480 ml)
Wheat berries* (200 g)	2½ (600 ml)	½	2 hrs.	2⅔ (640 ml)
Wild rice (180 g)	4 (940 ml)	¾	50–60	4 (940 ml)

* Soak overnight in the amount of water given here first.

❖ Some grains taste better if they are dry-toasted or sautéed in oil before the liquid is added. Use any of the following methods:

Cook grains in a dry skillet over medium heat, stirring constantly, until they are fragrant and darken slightly. This usually takes about 5 minutes.

Scatter on a dry baking sheet and place in a 325°F (160°C) oven. Stir every 5 minutes until fragrant and slightly darkened, 10 to 15 minutes.

Pilaf or pilau-style: Sauté in 1 to 2 tablespoons ghee or oil per 1 cup (240 ml) grain over low heat, stirring constantly, for 5 minutes.

❖ Always allow grains to rest for a few minutes in the covered pot after removing from the heat. The steam will finish the cooking, making whole grains drier and more separate and porridges creamier and devoid of unappetizing little pockets of water.

❖ You can cook grains in a Crock-Pot by first boiling the water on the stove, then placing it in the Crock-Pot and stirring in the grain. Grains tend to absorb less water than with stovetop cooking, but it is not consistent enough to formulate a general rule. Drain off any excess water from finished grains.

The destiny of nations depends on what and how they eat.
—JEAN-ANTHELME BRILLAT-SAVARIN

Kapha-Balancing Grains

Kaphas need to look a little farther afield for balance in countries where wheat and rice are the most common grains to appear on the table. There is a world of interesting grains to be explored on the road less traveled.

Amaranth

The name *amaranth* comes from the Greek *amarantos*, "unfading" or "immortal." The leaves were sacred to the Greek goddess Artemis, and the grain was believed by the Aztecs to be the source of their strength. Whole grain amaranth keeps indefinitely when stored in airtight containers.

❖ Amaranth cooks up to a bland, sticky porridge, making it best suited for use as a hot cereal, in grain burgers, and for adding to baked goods. It can also be substituted in dishes based on cornmeal mush or polenta, but only if you really like amaranth—its texture is stickier.

❖ Uncooked amaranth makes a crunchy topping when sprinkled onto breads and rolls before baking and can be used as a breading for burgers.

❖ Amaranth can be popped like popcorn and is served this way in Mexico and South America. Serve for snacks or use like croutons in soups and salads.

Barley

May we escape all hunger by means of our barley.   —Rik Veda

Note: Barley is balancing for Pitta as well as Kapha.
The name *barley* is derived from the Sanskrit root *bhu*, "to be," the basis of the primitive German word *bheu*, "to grow." Hence, its very name is associated with both pure being and its manifestation. Barley was one of the primary Vedic grains. Barley plants are always fresh and green; when one stalk is gone, another shoots up to take its place. Barley therefore symbolizes abundance and renewal, living up to its name of pure being and growth.

Barley is an excellent addition to soups and stews, as it has a light thickening effect on the water. It has a slightly sticky quality, making it ideal for grain burgers and loaves and as a substitute for rice in rice puddings. Barley is available in varying stages of processing, of which the hull-less and pearled varieties are best for Ayurvedic cooking. Since the hull is indigestible, there are no advantages I can see to voluntarily putting yourself through the rigors of the lengthy soaking and boiling that unhulled barley requires.

❖ *Pearl barley* has most of the bran and part of the germ polished off. It is a good choice, as it takes less time to cook and is still quite nourishing. *Hull-less barley* is a newly developed grain that separates from its hull without polishing. *Hulled barley,* sometimes called *Scotch barley* or *pot barley*, has all the hull and part of the bran removed. It is also a good choice, although it takes a long time to cook.

Barley grits are broken-up grains that cook in about half the time as whole barley. They make a sticky porridge that is appropriate as a hot cereal and can be used to thicken soups and stews.

Buckwheat

Buckwheat is not technically a grain but the fruit of a plant related to rhubarb. Ancient Chinese records describe valleys, mountains, and lakes that were formed by the footsteps of buckwheat-eating giants.

Kasha or buckwheat? Both words are generically—and confusingly—applied to toasted and untoasted buckwheat groats, which are decidedly unidentical twins. Both are hulled and broken into pieces. However, untoasted buckwheat, sometimes called *white buckwheat*, has a mild flavor completely unlike the more assertive taste of the more commonly toasted groats. You can tell the difference by the color: toasted buckwheat is nut brown. *Whole buckwheat*, with its curious triangular shape, can be used for sprouting but not for cooking.

❖ Use buckwheat in burgers and loaves and in grain-based stuffings. Replace bulgar with buckwheat in Nut Pâté en Croûte and in Wheat Balls for Spaghetti.

> In Russia and northern Asia, until recently *kasha* meant a "banquet" or "feast." Today in the Baltic areas, kasha refers to all cereals. It connotes toasted buckwheat to the world at large, thanks to the use of the word by migrating Baltic Jews in the nineteenth century—perhaps because at the time they left, buckwheat was the only type of "kasha" ever available.

Cornmeal and Dried Corn

Corn was the staple grain of the Americas. Ancient North and Central America scriptures trace the birth of corn close to the birth of creation itself. Scientific and archaeological views of history also place corn in close relationship with humankind: corn is not found in the wild, but seems to have always been a cultivated grain.

❖ Look for organically grown, stone-ground cornmeal. It contains the whole grain and is far superior in flavor and texture to "enriched degerminated" or "bolted" cornmeal, which has everything removed but the endosperm. Store stone-ground cornmeal in the refrigerator for no more than three months and in the freezer for up to six months.

❖ Cornmeal's color—yellow, white, red, or blue—depends on the color of the corn from which it is ground. *Blue cornmeal,* or *atol de maiz azul,* is used in the cuisine of the American Southwest, where it is sacred to the Hopis. It is slightly moister than its white and yellow sisters but essentially can be substituted for them cup for cup. Add a little baking soda to keep the color from turning pinkish.

❖ Cornmeal is a versatile addition to baked goods, added either cooked or dry. Very slightly increase the liquid when pouring dry cornmeal into a batter. Use cornmeal instead of bread crumbs to coat burgers and fried foods.

❖ *Pozole, nixtamal, or hominy:* Native Americans process dried corn by soaking it with wood ash, slaked lime, or lye, which causes the hulls to expand and slough off. The Algonquin tribe called it *rockahominie*, which the Pilgrims interpreted as "hominy groats." Such processing has a sound nutritional basis; it balances corn's amino acids and renders its niacin available to the human physiology. You can substitute cooked pozole in any dish calling for corn kernels, such as Succotash and Corn Fritters. Look for stone-ground grits and store in the refrigerator for no more than a year.

Millet

> O *thou cereal deity, we worship thee. Thou hast grown very well this year, and thy flavor will be sweet. Thou art good. The goddess of fire will be glad, and we also shall rejoice greatly. O thou god, O thou divine cereal, do thou nourish the people. I now partake of thee. I worship thee and give thee thanks.*
>
> —Millet prayer of the Ainos, Japan

Millet is a whole grain with the hull removed. The Bible describes millet as "the grain of endurance." Indeed, when millet lands on arid soil, it goes into a sort of hibernation, springing back to life when touched with water. It was one of the "five sacred crops" of ancient China. There are many species of millet. *Job's tears* are mentioned in the Vedic literature. The name refers to the clusters of tear-shaped grains that form on the stalk. *Teff,* or *t'ef,* is an ancient African grain resembling millet, of which it may be a species. It is a staple crop of Ethiopia. Teff is a whole grain, for the individual grains are so tiny that nothing much can be done to them. Teff cooks into a bland, purplish brown porridge possessing the texture of amaranth. Use teff in any recipe calling for cooked cornmeal or amaranth.

Millet's lack of gustatory popularity is probably due to its flavor and texture: bland and blander. Both can be improved by toasting in a dry skillet or by sautéing in ghee or oil for a few minutes before cooking.

> *I am the one whose praise echoes on high.*
> *I adorn all the earth.*
> *I am the breeze that nurtures all things green.*
> *I encourage blossoms to flourish with ripening fruits.*
> *I am led by the spirit to feed the purest streams.*
> *I am the rain coming from the dew*
> *that causes the grasses to laugh with the joy of life.*
> *I am the yearning for good.*
>
> —Hildegard of Bingen

Quinoa

Quinoa (KEEN-wah), the sacred "mother grain" of the Incas, is classified as an herb. When Pizarro attempted to conquer Peru, one step of suppression was to forbid the cultivation of quinoa and to steer Peruvians toward a meat-based diet. The formidable Andes and hardy Incas proved too much for Pizarro, and legend has it that quinoa plants sprouted up the day Spanish boots marched away from Peru.

Quinoa is quick and easy to cook and is absolutely delicious, with a fluffy, almost weightless texture. You can substitute quinoa for white rice or bulgar. Quinoa is very perishable because of its high oil content. Store in the refrigerator for about one month or in the freezer for two months.

Rye

Rye insinuated itself into the common diet of Europe through the back door: it proliferated as a weed in wheat fields. Farmers made the best of it by harvesting and threshing the two grains together. The resultant flour, called *maslin*, was the staple flour in Europe for four centuries. Rye is hardy and generally stores well. However, being susceptible to the infamous mold ergot, rye should be purchased in small amounts and used within a month or so.

❖ *Whole rye berries* are hulled whole grains with a mild, nutty flavor. Rye berries maintain their individual shape and are best used in side dishes, stuffings, and long-cooking soups and stews. *Cracked rye* cooks faster and has a porridgey texture.

Wild Rice

Wild rice is not rice, but the seed of a grass that grows in water. The main crop comes from the middle northern United States—the domains of the Chippewa, Winnebago, and Ojibwa tribes, who called their beloved grain *manomin*, "the good berry." In earlier years the harvested grain was either sun- or smoke-dried, then thrust into pits, and young men wearing soft moccasins went "jigging"—dancing on it to loosen the hulls.

❖ Most "wild" rice today is cultivated, then harvested and processed mechanically. It is black, unbroken, and cooks in about an hour. Hand-harvested rice is lighter in color, cooks in less time, and many feel has superior flavor. Wild rice has a high moisture content, making it susceptible to mold. Purchase small quantities and store in the refrigerator or freezer.

Vata- and Pitta-Balancing Grains

Oats

> *The oat is the Horatio Alger of cereals, which progressed, if not from rags to riches at least from weed to health food.*   —Waverly Root

The origin of the name *oats* is from the Sanskrit *ad*, also the source of the word *eat*. All oats are husked, cleaned, polished, and then toasted to remove a bad-tasting enzyme. They contain a natural antioxidant, making them a long-laster on the shelf.

❖ *Scottish oats*, also called *Irish oats* and *steel-cut oats*, are oat grains cut into pieces. They take a longer time to cook, but connoisseurs consider them to make superior oatmeal. *Rolled oats* are whole grains that have first been steamed, then flattened by rollers. They are the best choice for a quicker-cooking cereal. *Quick oatmeal* is prepared like rolled oats, having first been cut into smaller pieces. *Instant oatmeal* is partially cooked, dried, then subjected to the same process as quick oatmeal. Unless you have a penchant for soggy cardboard, I don't recommend it.

Rice

> *Mother feed me, I am hungry.* —Filipino prayer, recited while planting rice

The origin of the word *rice* is *vrihih*, Sanskrit for "life-giving seed." It is mentioned innumerable times in the Vedas. The present Japanese words for rice have alternate meanings of "fulfillment" and "main food." The Chinese credit its cultivation to the celestial Emperor Shen Nung, who named it one of "the five sacred crops." Rice has consistently been used as a temple offering in the myriad religions of Asia—something of this earth worthy of returning to the gods. The Asian tradition has been adopted in the West in the practice of showering rice on a newly married couple to fructify their union.

You may have noticed the abundance of rice recipes in *Heaven's Banquet*. This is because the ancient Ayurvedic texts repeatedly refer to the nourishing value of "rice well cooked with ghee."

Selection and Storage
❖ All of the hundreds of varieties of rice come from two main strains:

Japonica, short-grained rices that become moist and mushy when cooked. Sushi rice and risotto rices are examples.

Indica rices have longer grains that retain their individual shape and are drier and fluffier when cooked. Basmati rice is an example.

White Rice or Brown—Which Is Healthier?

White rice has the hull, bran, and germ polished off, while brown rice has only the hull removed. While brown rice undeniably contains more nutrients, it is much harder to digest, making white rice, particularly basmati, the preferred grain of Ayurveda. The best white rices have been aged and can be stored on a cool, dark shelf. Brown rice contains the germ and is therefore more perishable and should be stored in the refrigerator or freezer.

❖ *Basmati rice* is the finest, most delicate, most delicious rice in the world—it spoils you for any other type. Basmati is the only type of rice in which the grains elongate when cooked. The finest basmati is grown in the Himalayas, labeled *Dehra Dun* after the Himalayan city. Unfortunately, so far nothing that is exported is organic. Less expensive hybrids of basmati and Carolina rices, called *Texmati and Calmati*, are grown respectively in Texas and California. There is also Thai basmati. However, to date absolutely nothing equals the flavor of basmati rice grown in India.

❖ *Parboiled rice* is washed, soaked, and then steamed before it is milled by an ancient process that preserves the rice's nutrition—even after the bran is polished off. Parboiled rice is slightly yellow in color and takes about 10 minutes longer to cook than long-grain white rice. It is a grain of a different stripe from "converted" rice and instant-type rices, whose delicate flavors and textures have been steamed and processed out of existence.

❖ *Short-grain white rice* is stickier than long-grain varieties. It is used for puddings and molds in the West and for congee and sweets in Asia, particularly Japan. There are several Italian short-grain rices, including *arborio*, used in the preparation of risotto.

❖ *Rice flakes* made from brown rice are sold in natural foods stores for cooking as a hot cereal. Their white rice counterpart, *phoa or poha*, can be found in Indian markets and is sautéed with nuts and spices as a breakfast dish. Phoa comes in thick and thin flakes. The thick ones must be soaked in water for a few minutes, while the thin ones are rinsed in running water to be soft and pliable enough for sautéing. Both can also be cooked as a Western-style hot cereal.

Triticale

A cross between wheat and rye, triticale (tri-ti-KAY-lee) was developed in hopes of creating a wonder grain to eradicate famine throughout the world. It has not as yet lived up to the ideal for which it was developed. It is a whole, hulled grain with both Vata- and Kapha-balancing qualities.

Wheat and Wheat Products

Harness the ploughs, fit on the yokes, now that the womb of earth is ready to sow the seed therein, and through our praise may there be abundant food; may the grain fall ripe toward the sickle. —RIK VEDA

Wheat is symbolic of abundance, of life itself. In English heraldry a wheat sheaf represents the earth's harvest. Indeed, today wheat is the most widely grown food in the world. Not surprisingly, it is most commonly consumed as white flour. Here are a few other ways to eat your wheat.

Wheat berries are hulled whole wheat kernels. They are quite chewy, and each grain maintains its shape when cooked. When cooked and then ground in a food processor, wheat berries have a chewy, meaty texture that is ideal for burgers and loaves. The ground mixture can also be added to bread dough. Because each grain holds its shape, whole cooked wheat berries are excellent for stuffings and grain salads.

Bulgar, or burghul, or ala, or bulgor, boulgar, boulghour, burghoul . . . By any name, bulgar is hulled wheat berries that have been steamed and then cracked. It was eaten in ancient China and has been found in Egyptian and Etruscan burial remains. Today bulgar is associated with Middle Eastern cuisines, the Caucasus Mountain regions, and Armenia. Because bulgar is processed, it is perishable. Store in the refrigerator or freezer for no more than several months.

❖ American-made bulgar is produced from *durum*, hard winter wheat, which is steamed, then dried in a large rotating drum (like a clothes dryer) and then pearled and cracked. Middle Eastern–made bulgar starts with soft summer wheat, which is boiled, then dried in the sun, then polished and cracked. It has a lighter, beige color and a different flavor that is prized by bulgar aficionados. It is available in Middle Eastern markets, usually in a fine grind.

Semolina and farina are essentially coarsely ground flours made from the wheat's endosperm. Farina is often marketed as *Cream of Wheat*. To-day semolina, ground from durum wheat, is widely used in Italy to make pasta, in India both as a savory grain and for making sweets, and in North Africa as the basis of couscous.

❖ Semolina has a superior texture to farina—it is the one to choose, whenever possible. You can purchase semolina most inexpensively in Indian markets, where it goes by the name of *sooji*. However, it probably won't be organic. Semolina and farina are best purchased in small amounts and stored in the refrigerator or freezer.

BRAN AND WHEAT GERM

A health promoting constituent of wheat, which nature puts in and man takes out. —WAVERLY ROOT

Look for unprocessed *wheat bran* in natural foods stores to add in small amounts to baked goods. It is dry, crisp, and tastes like cardboard. However, it is the real thing—processed bran is refined and precooked, and often contains additives to make it more palatable and therefore more marketable. Store wheat bran on a cool, dry shelf for up to a year.

Wheat germ can be served as a breakfast cereal, added to hot cereals, used in granola, and added to baked goods. It can also be used to replace bread crumbs for coating burgers and other fried or baked foods. Wheat germ is a "live" food and is therefore best when it is completely fresh. It is difficult to find fresh wheat germ—natural foods stores are the best bets. Store in the freezer. Bran's and wheat germ's flavors improve by toasting, either in a dry skillet over medium heat or in a 325°F (160°C) oven until lightly browned. Stir frequently for 5 to 10 minutes.

Couscous is not a grain in itself but a delicate pasta used extensively in Morocco. The traditional process, which involves forming the tiny pellets by hand, is an art requiring considerable skill that is practically extinct today. Because couscous is a processed food, it is perishable. Purchase in small amounts and store in the refrigerator or on a cool shelf for a month or so. Instant couscous, which is everywhere, has been cooked and then dried. Its flavor and texture are gone with the wind—and couscous cooks quickly anyway, so what's the hurry?

❖ Couscous has such a delicate flavor and texture that it is best served simply in its traditional role as a side dish and foil for flavorful stews and other dishes. You can add cooked couscous to burgers, loaves, baked goods, etc., but its unique qualities are overshadowed in such settings.

Cracked wheat is hulled wheat berries that have been broken into pieces. However, something is lost in the translation. Cracked wheat lacks the chewy texture of whole wheat berries yet retains their lengthy cooking time. It takes on a sticky texture. Most people prefer the drier, fluffier quality and short cooking time of bulgar and the convenience of other wheat porridges to give them the good things that cracked wheat delivers. However, it is a whole grain, which bulgar and many brand-name wheat cereals are not.

HOT CEREALS

Today we can enjoy a second childhood with the Ayurvedic recommendation of having "milky grain" dishes for supper. Most grains and cereals can be cooked in an increased amount of water to a soft, mushy consistency. Beyond oatmeal and the other old standbys are barley, amaranth, polenta, quinoa, and a variety of cereal flakes— something for every taste and dosha.

GRANOLA

7 cups (1.7 l)

First called "granula" in 1865, the original article was a twice-baked mixture of graham flour and water that required an overnight soaking in milk. Needless to say, it was not an overnight sensation. Health food advocate John Kellogg created his own mixture, changing the name to "granola" to circumvent the patent office. Here is a basic formula. Vary the grains, nuts, seeds, and sweetener to create different flavors. Ayurveda recommends eating cold cereals not so cold. The best policy is to serve them with warm or room-temperature milk.

STEP ONE

1½ cups (165 g) rolled oats
1½ cups (180 g) wheat germ
¼ cup (35 g) sunflower seeds
3 tablespoons sesame seeds
⅔ cup (80 g) chopped nuts

¾ cup (60 g) dried unsweetened grated coconut
½ teaspoon salt
¾ cup (150 g) raw or packed brown sugar

STEP TWO

⅓ cup (80 ml) water or fruit juice
¼ cup (60 ml) ghee, melted butter, or oil

1. Preheat the oven to 350°F (180°C). Mix the dry ingredients together.
2. Combine the water or juice with the ghee, melted butter, or oil. Mix into the dry ingredients.
3. Scatter the mixture on a baking sheet. Toast in the oven, stirring every 5 minutes, until golden brown, 20 to 30 minutes. Let cool. Store in the refrigerator in an airtight container.

VARIATION

Add raisins or other dried fruits *after* toasting. Dried berries and cherries are especially nice.

GRAIN BURGERS
10 to 12 burgers

As with all burger recipes, the ingredients and proportions are highly flexible. As long as everything holds together enough to be shaped into patties, in the all-encompassing words of the immortal Cole Porter, anything goes. Grains that mush together work best here: quinoa, millet, barley, bulgar, and couscous are all good choices.

STEP ONE

2 tablespoons ghee, butter, or oil   *1 carrot, grated*
Pinch of hing (optional)   *½ bell pepper, chopped*
1 stalk celery, thinly sliced   *¼ cup (60 ml) minced fresh parsley*

STEP TWO

3 cups (700 ml) cooked grains,   *½ cup (130 g) or more nut butter*
  thoroughly cooled   *Seasoned salt*
1 tablespoon or more flour   *Black pepper*

STEP THREE

Bread crumbs

STEP FOUR

Oil or ghee

1. Heat the ghee, butter, or oil in a skillet. Add the hing and the vegetables and sauté over low heat, stirring frequently, until the vegetables are tender.
2. Mix the sautéed vegetables into the grains. Add the flour and nut butter, adding more if necessary to make a firm, sticky mixture. Season to taste with seasoned salt and pepper.
3. Place a liberal amount of bread crumbs in a shallow bowl. One at a time, shape the burger mixture into balls, roll in the bread crumbs to thoroughly coat, and press into a burger shape. Moisten your hands with water to keep the mixture from sticking, and rinse them frequently.
4. *To bake:* Preheat the oven to 350°F (180°C). Very liberally coat a baking sheet with oil or ghee. Place each burger on the baking sheet, then immediately *turn it over*. This coats the breading with oil so that it browns nicely. Bake until golden brown, about 30 minutes.
   To pan-brown: Coat a skillet liberally with oil or ghee. Fry the burgers on both sides over medium heat until nicely browned. Add more oil or ghee as necessary.

VARIATION
   Add well-drained cooked lentils or puréed cooked beans in Step 2.

THE WELL-DRESSED BURGER

 Whether served solo or as sandwiches on burger rolls, burgers are somewhat dry and cry out to be paired with a sauce. Here are some suggestions for more exciting—and more Ayurvedic—dance partners than the ketchup-mustard-and-a-soggy-pickle routine.

Pesto (pp. 509–12)

Salsa (pp. 506–509)

Mock mayonnaise (pp. 502–504)

Cream Cheese
  Hollandaise (p. 501)

Dip with Three Fennels and
  Three Peppers (pp. 281–82)

Guacamole (pp. 279–80)

Dried Tomato Paste (p. 506)

Sweet Red Pepper Purée (p. 513)

Nut Gravy (p. 499)

Béchamel Sauce and
  Variations (pp. 498–99)

Sambal (pp. 515–16)

Salsa di Noci (p. 514)

Carrot-Pepper Sauce (p. 255)

THREE-IN-ONE GRAIN MEDLEY

4 to 6 servings

"Three-in-one" is an expression used to describe reality as one underlying holistic value uniting the means of perceiving reality: the knower, the process of knowing or perceiving, and the known, or object of perception. These grains, when cooked together, have an intriguing flavor unlike any of the individual components.

*2¼ cups (550 ml) vegetable stock
  or water*
*2 tablespoons ghee
  (optional)*
½ teaspoon salt

*⅓ cup (70 g) basmati rice,
  rinsed*
⅓ cup (60 g) quinoa
⅓ cup (55 g) bulgar wheat

Bring the stock or water, ghee, and salt to a boil. Pour in the grains. Stir, cover, and reduce the heat as low as possible. Cook until all the water is absorbed and the grains are tender. Remove from the heat and allow to stand, covered, for 5 minutes.

BARLEY WITH ROASTED WINTER VEGETABLES
6 to 8 servings

The beets lend a rosy color to the grain. You can substitute other cooked grains for barley, and substitute turnips or celeriac for one of the vegetables.

STEP ONE

2¼ cups (550 ml) vegetable stock
  or water
¾ teaspoon salt

¾ cup (150 g) pearl or hull-less
  barley

STEP TWO

2 large carrots
2 large parsnips
2 medium beets

Ghee or oil
Salt

STEP THREE

Minced fresh parsley

1. Bring the stock or water and salt to a boil. Pour in the barley, cover, reduce the heat, and simmer until the water is absorbed and the barley is tender, about 45 minutes.
2. Meanwhile, preheat the oven to 400°F (200°C). Generously coat a lidded baking dish with ghee or oil. Trim the carrots and peel and trim the parsnips. Trim the roots off the beets and cut them in half. Generously coat the vegetables with ghee or oil and place in the baking dish. Sprinkle with salt. Cover and bake for 30 to 35 minutes, until the vegetables are tender.
3. When the vegetables are cool enough to handle, slip the skins off the beets and dice them, and slice the carrots and parsnips. Toss with the barley. Add 1 to 2 more tablespoons ghee or oil and adjust the seasoning. Garnish with minced parsley.

 # BULGAR WITH VERMICELLI (ARISHDAOV TZAVARI YEGHINTZ)

ARMENIA/MIDDLE EAST   *4 to 6 servings*

An Armenian celebration dish. Vata and Pitta are both balanced by these two wheat-based ingredients. Substitute long-grain white rice for the bulgar, and you have a traditional Persian pilau.

STEP ONE

3 tablespoons ghee or butter
Pinch of hing (optional)

½ cup (40 g) vermicelli, broken into
  1-inch (2.5 cm) lengths

STEP TWO

1 cup (175 g) bulgar

STEP THREE

*2 cups (480 ml) vegetable stock or
water*

*1 teaspoon salt (if using stock containing
salt, reduce to ½ teaspoon)*

STEP FOUR

¼ cup (35 g) pine nuts, toasted (optional)

1. Melt the ghee or butter in a small saucepan. Add the hing and vermicelli. Sauté over low heat, stirring constantly, until the vermicelli is golden brown.
2. Add the bulgar and sauté for 1 minute, stirring constantly.
3. Pour in the stock or water. Add the salt. Stir to distribute the bulgar and vermicelli. Bring to a boil. Cover, reduce the heat, and simmer until the liquid is absorbed and the bulgar is tender, about 20 minutes.
4. Remove from the heat and allow to stand, covered, for 5 minutes. Fold in the toasted pine nuts if desired.

VARIATIONS

Add raisins, dried cherries, or dried cranberries.

Replace the bulgar with ⅓ cup each: long-grain white rice (70 g), quinoa (60 g), and bulgar (55 g).

 # NUT PÂTÉ EN CROÛTE

10 to 12 servings

An elegant dish featuring bulgar wheat that is perfect to serve for a holiday dinner or to impress future in-laws—the reason I invented it. You can serve it hot or at room temperature. A cheeseless version follows in the Variation.

STEP ONE

2 cups (200 g) walnut or pecan pieces

STEP TWO

*2 tablespoons ghee or mild-flavored
oil*
Pinch of hing (optional)
¼ teaspoon rosemary
1 teaspoon dried basil

1 teaspoon dried thyme
*½ cup (65 g) thinly sliced celery,
with leaves*
1 carrot, grated

STEP THREE

½ cup (85 g) bulgar

1 cup (240 ml) vegetable stock or water

STEP FOUR

¼ cup (30 g) *fine dry bread crumbs*

¼ cup (35 g) *slivered almonds*

⅓ cup (40 g) *shelled pistachios*

½ cup (4 ounces/115 g) *cream cheese*

1½ cups (150 g) *grated sharp Cheddar cheese*

Salt

Black pepper

STEP SIX

Pastry Crust (pp. 406–407)

To prepare the filling:

1. Preheat the oven to 350°F (180°C). Scatter the nuts on a baking sheet and toast, stirring every 5 minutes, until browned, 20 to 30 minutes. Grind to a powder in a blender or food processor. Set aside.
2. While the nuts are toasting, heat the oil in a small skillet. Add the hing, rosemary, basil, and thyme and sauté over low heat for 30 seconds. Add the celery and carrot and sauté for another 2 to 3 minutes, stirring frequently.
3. Add the bulgar and stock or water. Bring to a boil. Cover, reduce the heat, and simmer until the water is absorbed and the bulgar is tender, about 15 minutes. Place in a mixing bowl and allow to cool to room temperature.
4. When the bulgar mixture is cool, add the bread crumbs, almonds, pistachios, cream cheese, Cheddar, and the ground nuts and mix together thoroughly. The pâté should be thick and sticky. Season to taste with salt and pepper.
5. Take a 1-quart (1 l) casserole dish or bowl with rounded sides. Dust lightly with flour. This will serve as a mold for the pâté.

To prepare the crust:

6. Cut off ⅓ of the pie dough and set aside. Roll out the remaining dough ¼-inch (5 mm) thick, and wide enough to fill and slightly overlap the sides of the mold. Place in the mold.
7. Spoon the pâté into the crust. Press to distribute evenly and smooth the top. Bring the overlapping edges of crust over the pâté.
8. Roll out the remaining pie dough ¼-inch (5 mm) thick, and wide enough to cover the pâté and the edges of the top crust. Place over the pâté and pinch to seal thoroughly to the other crust.
9. Invert the mold onto a baking sheet and shake gently to release the pâté. The crust should thoroughly cover the filling. Gently brush off as much flour as possible.
10. Preheat the oven to 375°F (190°C). While the oven is heating, place the pâté in the freezer or, if it doesn't fit, in the refrigerator for 10 to 15 minutes to chill the crust.
11. Bake until the crust is lightly browned, about 45 minutes. There may be some excess oil on the baking sheet; don't worry about it.
12. Gently slide the pâté onto a serving plate. Allow to stand at room temperature for 20 minutes to allow the filling to set; otherwise, it will crumble when sliced. To serve, cut into wedges.

VARIATION

✿ Omit the cheeses. Add 3 tablespoons arrowroot or cornstarch and ½ cup (120 ml) Tofu Mayonnaise (p. 503) to the mixture in Step 5.

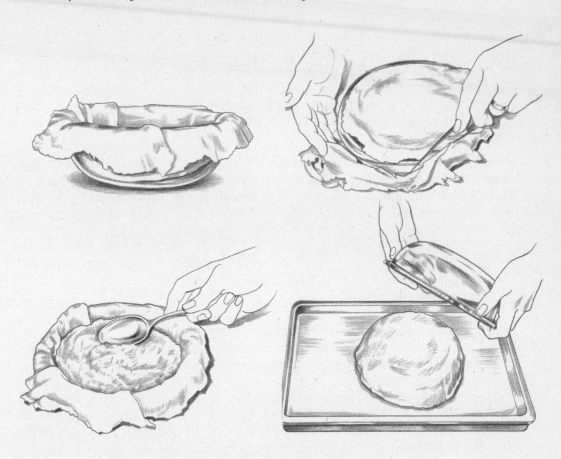

THANKSGIVING DINNER

Creamy Gingered Carrot Soup
   with Wild Rice (p. 237)
Nut Pâté en Crôute (Nut
   Pâté Baked in a Crust)
Sage Dressing (pp. 337–38)

Shredded Brussels Sprouts
   with Cream (p. 74)
Cranberry Sauce (pp. 210–11)
Pumpkin Pie and
   Apple Pie (pp. 422–23; 413)

Polenta Nera (Black Polenta)

ITALY　　4 to 6 servings

An unusual buckwheat polenta from the Valtellina region of Lombardy, Italy. The Valtellinese embellish it with their rich mountain dairy products, beating in huge amounts of butter and often grating a zesty cheese over it for good measure. Polenta Nera's color is not everyone's idea of gustatory inspiration—it resembles a tweedy taupe men's suit. It is perhaps best suited (pardon me) to being baked under a layer of vegetables and/or cheese, as in Polenta con Vegetali and Polenta Pizza, or otherwise covered with sautéed vegetables.

STEP ONE

2 cups (480 ml) stock or water

1½ teaspoons salt (less if using salted stock)

STEP TWO

1½ cups (195 g) buckwheat flour

1¾ cups (420 ml) vegetable stock or water

STEP THREE

2 tablespoons ghee or butter

1. Bring the stock or water and salt to a boil.
2. Meanwhile, whisk the buckwheat flour into the second amount of stock or water until smooth. Add the mixture in a slow, steady stream to the boiling liquid, stirring constantly with a whisk.
3. Reduce the heat, add the ghee or butter, and continue to cook, stirring constantly, for a full 20 minutes, when the polenta will begin to pull away from the sides of the pot. This takes muscle, and you will probably have to switch to a wooden spoon. You do need to keep up the stirring; Polenta Nera can lump up or burn if neglected for more than a half minute.

   For pan browning or baking with toppings: Pour into a buttered 9 × 13-inch (23 × 33 cm) baking pan and spread evenly. It will cool and harden in 45 to 60 minutes at room temperature.

VARIATIONS

Beat in up to 4 more tablespoons (55 g) ghee or butter in Step 2. (This will make the polenta soft and not suitable for cutting into squares or frying.)

Beat up to ½ cup (50 g) grated cheese—Parmesan or other melting cheeses—into the finished polenta. (This will make the polenta soft and not suitable for cutting into squares or frying.)

A CORNMEAL CORNUCOPIA: CREATING DELICIOUS DISHES WITH MUSH, POLENTA, AND GRITS

Vasudhaiv Kutumbakam—The World Is My Family.   —*MANU SMRITI* 11.12.22

Cornmeal is a food that has spread far and wide among the world family. Each culture has given it a slightly different culinary spin, and yet *plus ça change, plus c'est la même chose*—the more things change, the more they stay the same. In an international Ayurvedic kitchen, cornmeal mush, polenta, and grits can often be treated and adorned interchangeably.

❖ There is an international choice of liquids to cook the cornmeal in: Besides water or vegetable stock, try the mixture of nondairy milk and water that Italians use for polenta, the mixture of buttermilk and water employed in the Baltic, or coconut milk, a Caribbean addition. The nondairy milk and buttermilk will help the dish become more balancing to Vata, and coconut milk and other nondairy milks help balance Pitta.

Once it is cooked, there are two basic ways to serve cornmeal:

1. As a porridge, which can be either sweetened and served as a hot cereal, or treated as a savory dish in the manner of mashed potatoes: with ghee or butter and salt or with a sauce or gravy.
2. Hardened so that it can be cut into pieces. Spread the porridge in a buttered baking pan and cool. It will harden into a mass that can be baked with toppings or cut into pieces and pan-fried, grilled, or deep-fried. The pieces can be served as breakfast or light dinner fare, like pancakes, or topped with sauces, vegetables, beans, and cheeses for sumptuous savory dishes.

 ## CORNMEAL MUSH

4 to 6 servings

This rather inelegantly named porridge is enjoyed largely in the central Western Hemisphere, from the southern United States to the Caribbean to Mexico and Central America. It also constitutes African "mealies."

1 cup (130 g) cornmeal   Salt
3 cups (720 ml) water

1. Mix the cornmeal into 1 cup (240 ml) of the water until free of lumps. Bring the remaining water to a boil.
2. Whisk the cornmeal mixture into the boiling water. Add a pinch of salt. Return to a boil, then reduce the heat, stirring almost constantly until the mixture is thick. A whisk is a good stirring tool to prevent lumps.

 # GRITS

4 to 6 servings

The pride of the American South, grits are served at breakfast with syrup or as a side dish for lunch or dinner with a pat of butter or a drizzling of gravy. You can use this recipe for both plain corn and hominy grits. The true, creamy southern style is to cook grits on the lowest heat possible for 1 to 2 hours and then beat in plenty of butter to make the mixture creamy. If you wish to attempt such a treatment, a heat diffuser is handy, plus a Southerner who owes you a lot of money to stir it. Or you could use a Crock-Pot.

¾ cup (105 g) grits
3¾ cup (900 ml) water
½ teaspoon salt

3 tablespoons ghee
or butter (optional)

Bring the grits, water, and salt to a boil in a saucepan, stirring constantly. Cover, reduce the heat, and simmer until all the water is absorbed, 15 to 20 minutes. Or cover and cook on the lowest heat possible for at least 1 hour. Beat in the butter or ghee. Remove from the heat and allow to stand, covered, for 2 to 3 minutes.

 # POLENTA

ITALY   *3 cups (720 ml)*

A harvest moon in a mist.   —ALESSANDRO MANZONI, 19TH-CENTURY
NOVELIST, DESCRIBING POLENTA BEING POURED OUT

The word *polenta* comes from the Latin *pulmentum*, a staple grain dish of ancient Rome and an integral part of the rations for the Roman legions that was adapted to cornmeal after 1492 by Renaissance inheritors of the concept.

1 cup (150 g) polenta
4 cups (950 ml) water or stock

½ teaspoon salt
Black pepper

Mix all the ingredients together in a pot and bring to a boil, stirring constantly. Reduce the heat and simmer, uncovered, stirring almost constantly, until thickened, usually 15 to 20 minutes. However, coarsely ground cornmeal can take up to 1 hour and is best prepared in a double boiler.

VARIATIONS

Mamaliga: (Romania) Vigorously beat ⅓ cup (75 g) butter into cooked Polenta to make it as smooth as possible. Serve as a side dish with a flavorful stew.

Baked Mamaliga: Beat 1⅓ cups (265 g) feta cheese into Mamaliga. Spread evenly in a buttered baking pan and bake for 30 minutes at 350°F (180°C).

 ## POLENTA CON VEGETALI (POLENTA WITH VEGETABLES)

9 × 13-inch (23 × 33 cm) pan

Made with Polenta or Polenta Nera, this baked cornmeal dish festooned with stripes of colorful vegetables has an Italian accent. However, Cornmeal Mush and Grits work just as well. For a lunchtime main dish, add cheese to either the cornmeal mixture or the topping. Serve with a bowl of pesto passed at the table.

STEP ONE

Polenta (opposite),
   Polenta Nera (p. 162),
   Cornmeal Mush (pp. 163–64),
   or Grits (opposite)

STEP TWO

2 cups (70 g) very finely diced eggplant
1½ cups (200 g) very finely diced red or yellow bell peppers
1½ cups (175 g) very finely diced zucchini

Pinch of hing (optional)
Olive oil
Salt
Black pepper

1. Cook the cornmeal as thick as possible. Pour into a buttered 9 × 13-inch (23 × 33 cm) baking pan and spread evenly. Chill to harden, 45 to 60 minutes.
2. Preheat the oven to 350°F (180°C). Sauté each of the vegetables separately with a pinch of hing in a minimum amount of olive oil (about 2 tablespoons for the eggplant and 1 teaspoon each for the peppers and zucchini). Cook until just barely tender, 5 to 7 minutes. Season with a sprinkling of salt and pepper. (I sauté one vegetable while dicing the next.)
3. Sprinkle the vegetables in stripes on the cornmeal. There should be enough for three 9-inch (23 cm) stripes of each vegetable, completely covering the cornmeal.
4. Bake for 30 minutes. Cut into squares to serve.

PAN-FRIED CORNMEAL SQUARES

Up from the meadows rich with corn. Clear is the cool September Morn.
—JOHN GREENLEAF WHITTIER

Fried squares of polenta, an Italian dish, can be sauced with dollops of pesto or flavored Panir Mayonnaise. I like to beat some chopped dried tomatoes, pine nuts or pumpkin seeds, and chopped herbs into the cooked cornmeal before pouring it into the pan to set. However, fried cornmeal mush is a Yankee dish that makes a delicious breakfast or light dinner accompanied by sweet syrup or fruit sauce.

STEP ONE
Cornmeal Mush (pp. 163–64), Polenta (p. 164), or Grits (p. 164)

STEP TWO
Flour or bread crumbs (optional)   **Ghee or olive oil for frying**

1. Cook the cornmeal as thick as possible. Spread evenly in a buttered 9 × 13-inch (23 × 33 cm) baking pan. Chill to harden, 45 to 60 minutes.
2. Cut into squares. (Italians slice it with a tautly pulled string.) If desired, dredge the squares in flour or bread crumbs for more even browning. Generously coat a skillet with the ghee or olive oil and heat. Fry the squares on both sides until lightly browned and crusty.

VARIATIONS
❖ **French-Fried Cornmeal Pieces:** Cut the cooled cooked cornmeal into small rectangles, half moons, or thick strips. Don't make the pieces wider than 2 inches (5 cm) at any point or they might break. Dredge in flour for more even browning. Deep-fry until browned and crusty at the edges. Drain on paper towels. Serve like French fries with a dip or mock mayonnaise or pesto to dunk them in.
❖ **Grilled Cornmeal Pieces:** Cornmeal pieces are a bit delicate and can fall apart when you attempt to turn them over on the grill. Grill on a small grate and use a spatula to flip them. Cut the cooled cooked cornmeal into squares or rectangles no more than 3 inches (7.6 cm) wide. Brush with ghee or oil. Brush the grill grate with ghee or oil, and grill the squares on both sides until sear marks are left on the surface.
❖ **Deep-Dish Cornmeal Pizza:** Use the cooled cooked cornmeal as a "crust" to cover with your favorite toppings for pizza. Bake in a 350°F (180°C) oven until done, about 30 minutes.

RANCH HOUSE POZOLE CHILI

4 to 6 servings

This is the kind of hearty, Kapha-balancing lunch you'll want to come home to after driving a herd of buffalo down the entire Old Chisholm Trail or some similar activity. Note that the beans and pozole must be soaked overnight.

STEP ONE

½ cup (95 g) dried kidney,
   pinto, or Anasazi beans

1½ cups (160 g) pozole

STEP TWO

6 cups (1.4 l) water

1 bay leaf

STEP THREE

2 tablespoons ghee, butter, or
   oil
Pinch of hing (optional)
2 tablespoons minced fresh
   ginger
1½ teaspoons dried oregano

1 cup (110 g) finely chopped fennel
   or celery
1 cup (140 g) finely chopped bell
   peppers
2 medium tomatoes

STEP FIVE

1 tablespoon oil
Pinch of hing (optional)
2 teaspoons cumin seeds

1 cup ½-inch (1.3 cm)
   cubes of seitan (130 g) or tofu (220 g)

STEP SIX

½ teaspoon ground allspice
1 teaspoon sugar
½ teaspoon black pepper
1 teaspoon paprika
1 cup (240 ml) chopped fresh
   cilantro

Salt
Salsa Cruda (p. 507)
Sour Cream
Grated Monterey Jack cheese
   (optional)

1. Clean the beans and pozole thoroughly. Place in a bowl with at least 6 cups (1.4 liters) water and soak overnight.
2. Drain and rinse. Place in a soup pot with the water and bay leaf. Bring to a boil, then reduce the heat and simmer.
3. Meanwhile, heat the ghee, butter, or oil in a large skillet. Add the hing, ginger, and oregano and sauté over low heat until fragrant, about 30 seconds. Add the fennel or celery and bell peppers and sauté until almost tender, stirring occasionally. Add the tomatoes and cook for another minute.
4. Add the vegetable mixture to the simmering beans and pozole. Continue to simmer until the beans and pozole are tender and the water is mostly evaporated, leaving a rich gravy remaining, 2½ to 3 hours.

5. Meanwhile, heat the oil in the skillet. Add the hing and cumin seeds and sauté until fragrant, about 30 seconds. Add the seitan or tofu and sauté over medium heat until browned, stirring frequently.
6. Add the sautéed seitan or tofu, allspice, sugar, pepper, paprika, and cilantro to the finished beans and pozole. Add salt to taste. Serve topped with Salsa Cruda, sour cream, and cheese.

VARIATIONS

If you like your chili hot, add ¼ to ½ teaspoon more black pepper in Step 6 or replace the black pepper with chilies in Step 5.

If you can't stand the heat, before you get out of the kitchen, reduce the pepper in Step 6.

 # Persian-Style Millet with Dried Cherries

4 to 6 servings

A dish that makes millet taste good! This interpretation of an old Persian treatment for rice works astoundingly well with millet, which responds to sweet flavors. It is also, of course, delicious with Persian rice (Chelo, see opposite) and would be equally intriguing with steamed couscous.

STEP ONE

¼ cup (55 g) ghee
Pinch of hing (optional)

⅓ cup (40 g) chopped celery or
fennel

STEP TWO

¾ cup (150 g) millet
2½ cups (600 ml) water

¾ teaspoon salt
⅛ teaspoon saffron

STEP THREE

⅓ cup (45 g) dried cherries
¼ cup (60 ml) water
1 teaspoon sugar

½ teaspoon ground cinnamon
¼ cup (30 g) pistachio halves

1. Heat the ghee in a saucepan. Add the hing and sauté over low heat for 30 seconds until fragrant. Add the celery or fennel and cook for a minute or two until it begins to soften.
2. Add the millet and sauté, stirring constantly, for about 5 minutes, until the millet darkens slightly. Add the water, salt, and saffron. Bring to a boil, cover, reduce the heat, and simmer until the millet is tender and the water is absorbed. Stir a few times and be careful that it doesn't stick to the bottom or burn. Remove from the heat and allow to stand, covered, for 5 minutes.
3. While the millet is cooking, combine the cherries, water, sugar, and cinnamon in a small saucepan. Bring to a boil, cover, reduce the heat, and simmer for about 5 minutes, until most of the water is absorbed and the cherries are tender. Fold the cherry mixture and the pistachios into the millet.

BAKED RICE

4 to 6 servings

Some recipes are all in their ingredients, while others are a triumph of technique. Although these ingredients may not look particularly interesting on first glance, baked rice has a uniquely wonderful flavor and texture.

STEP TWO

¼ *cup (55 g) ghee*
1 *cup (205 g) long-grain white rice, preferably basmati*

STEP THREE

2 *cups (480 ml) water* or   ½ *teaspoon salt*
  2¼ *cups (540 ml) for basmati*

1. Preheat the oven to 375°F (190°C). Butter a covered 1-quart (1l) baking dish.
2. Melt the ghee or butter in a saucepan. Add the rice and sauté over low heat for 1 to 2 minutes, stirring constantly.
3. Add the water and salt. Bring to a boil. Pour mixture into the baking dish.
4. Cover and bake until the liquid is absorbed, 20 to 30 minutes.

VARIATION
Stir in sautéed vegetables or chopped fresh herbs before baking.

 # CHELO (PERSIAN RICE)

I R A N   *6 servings*

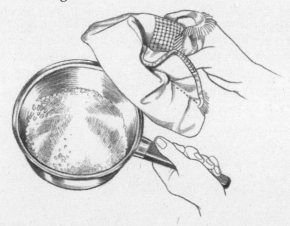

People who have visited Iran universally wax poetic about the perfect rice they were served there—the separate, fluffy grains fragrant with butter and the irresistible golden crust that forms in the bottom of the often waist-high cooking cauldrons. Here is a home-sized version. Plain rice doesn't get any better than this. Note the soaking time in Step 1.

STEP ONE

1¼ cups (255 g) long-grain white rice,   3 cups (700 ml) water
    preferably basmati   1 tablespoon salt

STEP TWO

4 cups (950 ml) water   1 tablespoon salt

STEP THREE

¼ cup (55 g) ghee or unsalted butter

1. Wash the rice very thoroughly. Place in a bowl with the water and salt, stir to distribute, and if time permits, allow to soak at least 3 hours—overnight for best results. Soaking is not absolutely necessary but makes the fluffiest rice. Drain and rinse.
2. Bring the 4 cups water and the salt to a rolling boil. Add the drained rice. As soon as the water begins to move as it returns to a boil, time the boiling at 4 minutes. Drain the rice in a sieve and rinse with cold water to stop the cooking.
3. Melt 2 tablespoons of the ghee or butter in a medium saucepan. Swirl the pan to distribute evenly. Mound up the rice in a cone shape to completely cover the bottom. Sprinkle 2 tablespoons water over the rice. Distribute the remaining 2 tablespoons ghee or butter evenly over the top. Drizzle the ghee if semiliquid, or cut the butter into small pieces.
4. Wrap the lid with a dish towel to absorb the steam. Fit as tightly as possible over the pot. Place over medium heat for 5 minutes. Reduce the heat to low and cook for 25 minutes. Remove from the heat and allow to stand, covered, for 5 minutes.

VARIATION

Ta-Dig (Rice Crust): Add ¼ cup (50 g) more rice in Step 1. Cook over medium heat for 10 minutes in Step 4, then reduce the heat to very low and cook for 40 minutes. Spoon out the rice without disturbing the crust. Loosen the crust with a spatula and serve separately. If the crust is stubborn, partially immerse the pot in a bowl of cold water for a minute, then try again. Ta-Dig is the true test of a Persian cook's skill, so don't be discouraged if it takes a few tries to master it.

RICE WITH DILL AND LIMA BEANS (BAGALI SHEVID POLOW)

IRAN   *4 to 6 servings*

You can prepare this sumptuous pilau using other fresh beans, such as blanched and peeled fava beans. Add ½ cup (75 g) more beans and you have a main dish. This dish works only with *fresh* dill, and upon occasion I've substituted fennel tops from our bounteous backyard supply of the ubiquitous southern California weed.

STEP ONE

1 cup (205 g) long-grain white rice,
preferably basmati

3 cups (700 ml) water
1 tablespoon salt

STEP TWO

4 cups (940 ml) water
1 tablespoon salt

1 cup (150 g) fresh lima beans

STEP THREE

1 large baking potato

2 tablespoons ghee or butter

STEP FOUR

1 cup (240 ml) chopped fresh dill
2 tablespoons ghee or butter

2 tablespoons water

STEP FIVE

Salt

Black pepper

1. Rinse the rice well. Combine the rice, water, and salt in a bowl. Soak for at least 2 hours or at most overnight.
2. Drain the rice. Bring the second amount of water and salt to a boil in a medium saucepan. When boiling merrily, stir in the rice and lima beans. Return to a boil and, as soon as the water starts to bubble, boil for exactly 4 minutes. Drain and rinse immediately.
3. Peel the potato and cut into ¼-inch (5 mm) rounds. Clean any stray rice kernels out of the saucepan, and melt the ghee or butter in it. Remove from the heat and line with the potato rounds. Do not overlap.
4. Toss the dill with the rice. Mound up the rice mixture over the potatoes in the shape of a mountain (something symmetrical, like Mount Fuji, though Mount Ararat is more geographically correct). Drizzle the ghee, if semiliquid, or cut the butter over the rice and sprinkle with the water.
5. Wrap the saucepan lid with a dish towel to absorb the steam. Cover and cook over medium heat for 8 minutes. Reduce the heat and cook on low for 35 minutes. Remove from the heat and allow to stand, covered, for 5 minutes. Season to taste with salt and pepper. Serve the rice garnished with the potato slices, which should be beautifully browned.

VARIATION

Persians would use much more butter. If desired, top the rice with up to 4 tablespoons more ghee or butter in Step 4.

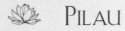 ## PILAU

INDIA   *4 to 6 servings*

Pilaus have been prepared in India since ancient times. Some are sweet, some savory, some spicy. Here is a simple, Vata-balancing offering. You could substitute pistachios for cashews to make the dish balancing for Pitta, and quinoa for rice to give more balance to Kapha.

STEP ONE

1 cup (205 g) long-grain white rice,   *2 to 4 tablespoons ghee*
   preferably basmati

STEP TWO

2 cups (480 ml) water or   *¼ cup (35 g) blanched almonds,*
   2¼ cups (540 ml) for basmati   *toasted*
½ teaspoon salt   *¼ cup (30 g) raisins*
⅛ teaspoon saffron threads
¼ cup (40 g) cashew halves,
   toasted

1. Melt the ghee in a small saucepan. Add the rice and sauté over low heat for 2 to 3 minutes, stirring constantly.
2. Add the remaining ingredients, water first. Bring to a boil. Cover, reduce the heat, and simmer until the water is absorbed and the rice is tender. Remove from the heat and allow to stand, covered, for 5 minutes.

 ## SUDARSHAN RICE

4 to 6 servings

An Indian cook visiting the Maharishi Ayur-Veda Health Center in Los Angeles prepared this pilau utilizing Western ingredients. The crunchy fried walnuts and the contrast of the green broccoli to the yellow rice add greatly to the dish. If you wish to avoid the oil, you can sauté or steam the vegetables and dry-toast the nuts, but a little something will be lost in the translation.

STEP ONE

2 tablespoons ghee	*1 cup (205 g) long-grain*
Pinch of hing (optional)	*white rice, preferably basmati*

STEP TWO

2 cups water (480 ml) or	*½ teaspoon turmeric*
2¼ cups (540 ml) for basmati	*1 teaspoon salt*

STEP THREE

Oil for frying	*1 cup (90 g) julienned carrots*
1 cup (90 g) small broccoli florets	*1 cup (110 g) julienned zucchini*

STEP FOUR

¼ cup (25 g) walnut pieces	*¼ cup (40 g) cashew pieces*

STEP FIVE

½ cup (120 ml) chopped fresh cilantro   *1 medium tomato, coarsely chopped*

1. Heat the ghee in a medium saucepan. Add the hing and sauté over low heat until fragrant, about 30 seconds. Add the rice and sauté, stirring constantly, for 1 to 2 minutes.
2. Add the water, turmeric, and salt. Bring to a boil. Cover, reduce the heat, and simmer until the water is absorbed and the rice is tender. Remove from the heat and allow to stand, covered, for 5 minutes.
3. While the rice is cooking, heat oil 1 inch (2.5 cm) deep in a skillet. Have a platter covered with paper towels nearby. Add the broccoli, carrots, and zucchini and fry, stirring occasionally, until the vegetables are tender and their edges are browned. Remove with a slotted spoon and drain on the paper towels.
4. Fry the walnuts and cashews in the heated oil until lightly browned. Remove with a slotted spoon and drain on the paper towels.
5. Gently toss the fried vegetables and nuts with the cilantro and tomato. Add the mixture to the cooked rice and gently toss. Cover and allow to stand for 2 to 3 minutes before serving.

 # FRIED RICE (CHAO FAN)

CHINA   *4 to 6 servings*

In ancient Chinese worship, three grains of rice signified the upsurge, awakening, and increase of the life force. Basmati rice does not hold up well to the long sautéing and stirring required for this dish; it is better to substitute a sturdier type of white rice.

STEP ONE

Liquid seasoning	*1 cup (205 g) long-grain white rice*
2 cups (480 ml) unsalted stock	
or water	

STEP TWO

3 tablespoons sesame or other
  mild-flavored oil
Pinch of hing (optional)
1 tablespoon minced fresh ginger

¼ green bell pepper, cut into
  matchstick slivers
¾ cup (90 g) thinly sliced celery
¾ cup (55 g) mung sprouts

1. Add enough liquid seasoning to the water to give it a brownish color and the flavor of a soup stock. Bring to a boil. Add the rice, cover, reduce the heat, and simmer until the liquid is absorbed and the rice is tender.
2. Heat the oil in a wok or skillet. Sauté the hing, ginger, bell pepper, and celery over low heat for 5 minutes, stirring constantly. Add the sprouts and sauté just until they are wilted.
3. Add the cooked rice. Sauté for about 6 minutes, stirring constantly. Adjust the salt.

VARIATIONS

Stir in a drizzle of toasted sesame oil after cooking.
Stir in a handful of chopped fresh cilantro.
Add cubes of stir-fried tofu after cooking.

 # LEMON RICE (NIMBU BHAT)

INDIA   4 to 6 servings

A tart, flavorful dish from south India. For a true south Indian touch, add a tiny sprinkling of urad dal and flaked red chilies to the ghee in Step 1 and sauté until the urad dal is golden brown.

STEP ONE

2 tablespoons ghee or butter
Pinch of hing (optional)

½ teaspoon cumin seeds

STEP TWO

1 cup (205 g) long-grain white rice, preferably basmati

STEP THREE

2 cups (480 ml) water or
  2¼ cups (540 ml) for basmati
½ teaspoon turmeric
½ teaspoon salt

½ cup (80 g) cooked garbanzo
  beans (chickpeas) (optional)

STEP FOUR

¼ cup plus 2 tablespoons (90 ml) lemon juice

1. Heat the ghee or butter in a saucepan. Add the hing and cumin seeds and sauté for 1 minute over low heat.
2. Add the rice and sauté for 2 to 3 minutes, stirring constantly.
3. Pour in the water. Add the turmeric, salt, and garbanzos. Stir and bring to a boil. Cover, reduce the heat, and simmer until the water is absorbed and the rice is tender.
4. Gently fold in the lemon juice. Cover and allow to stand for 2 to 3 minutes.

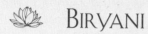 # BIRYANI

INDIA   *6 servings*

There are many types of Biryani: rice-based dishes with additions that can include fruits and vegetables, nuts, beans, and dairy.

STEP ONE

2 cups (480 ml) water or
  2¼ cups (540 ml) for basmati
1 cup (205 g) long-grain
  white rice, preferably basmati

⅛ teaspoon saffron
½ teaspoon salt

STEP FOUR

Peas and Potato Curry
  (pp. 115–16)
1¼ cups (300 ml) yogurt

⅓ cup (45 g) cashews, pistachios,
  or pine nuts
3 tablespoons raisins

1. Combine the water, rice, saffron, and salt in a small saucepan. Allow to stand for 20 to 30 minutes.
2. Bring the mixture to a boil. Cover, reduce the heat, and simmer until the water is absorbed and the rice is tender.
3. Preheat the oven to 350°F (180°C). Butter a baking dish.
4. Spread the rice evenly in the baking dish. Drain any excess liquid from the Peas and Potato Curry. Spread it evenly over the rice. Cover the curry evenly with the yogurt. Sprinkle with the nuts and raisins.
5. Bake until the yogurt has set, 30 to 40 minutes.

VARIATION
  Substitute other vegetable curries for the Peas and Potato Curry.

RICE WITH CARAMELIZED COCONUT MILK (ARROZ CON COCO)

COLOMBIA   *4 to 6 servings*

Rice cooked in fresh coconut milk is ubiquitous in Central America. The first batch of coconut milk is boiled down until only the rich oil and caramelized solids remain, which give the dish its unique flavor. Various foods can be added, such as chunks of plantain or pumpkin; this Colombian version is slightly sweetened with the addition of raisins.

STEP ONE

1 large coconut

STEP THREE

1 cup (205 g) long-grain white rice, preferably basmati

STEP FIVE

1½ teaspoons sugar   *½ teaspoon salt*
½ cup (65 g) raisins

To prepare the coconut milk:

1. Remove the coconut meat according to the directions on page 549. Set aside the liquid for some other use. Cut the coconut into pieces and place in a blender or food processor with 1 cup (240 ml) hot water. Purée as thoroughly as possible.
2. Line a strainer with a piece of clean cheesecloth or muslin that has been dampened and wrung out. Strain the coconut milk through it, then draw up the edges of the cloth to form a bag and squeeze out any remaining liquid. Add water to make 1 cup (240 ml) liquid.
3. Return the coconut to the blender or food processor. Add 2¼ cups (540 ml) hot water and purée again. Keeping the first batch of coconut milk separate, strain the second batch through the cloth, squeezing out all the liquid. Place the rice in it to soak.

To prepare the rice dish:

4. In a small saucepan, bring the first batch of coconut milk to a boil. Allow it to boil over medium-high heat until a golden oil and some solids remain. Reduce the heat and cook, stirring constantly, until they are golden brown.
5. Immediately add the second batch of coconut milk containing the rice. Add the sugar, raisins, and salt. Stir once and bring to a boil. Cover, reduce the heat, and simmer until the liquid is absorbed and the rice is tender. Remove from the heat and allow to stand, covered, for 5 minutes.

GOLDEN RICE SIMMERED
IN COCONUT MILK (NASI KUNING)

THAILAND/INDONESIA/MALAYSIA   *3 cups (720 ml)*

Turmeric-colored rice is traditionally served at Indonesian weddings. A gentle dish, it tastes most sumptuous when you use a flavorful stock. Kaffir lime leaves can be found in Thai markets but are not absolutely necessary. I've purchased lemon grass from ordinary supermarkets upon occasion, as well as in Thai groceries. An easy method of mincing the lime leaves and ginger is to combine them in a blender with the stock.

STEP ONE

1 lemon grass stalk

STEP TWO

*1 cup (205 g) long-grain white rice,
preferably basmati*
*1 cup (240 ml) vegetable stock or
water or 1¼ cups (300 ml) for
basmati*
*1½ cups (360 ml) Coconut Milk
(p. 494)*

1 tablespoon minced fresh ginger
Pinch of hing (optional)
4 kaffir lime leaves, minced (optional)
½ teaspoon turmeric
½ teaspoon salt
Finely chopped cilantro (optional)
Toasted coconut shreds (optional)

1. Crush the lemon grass stalk using a mortar and pestle.
2. Combine all the ingredients except the cilantro and coconut in a small saucepan. Allow to soak for 20 minutes.
3. Bring to a boil. Cover, reduce the heat as low as possible, and simmer until the liquid is absorbed, about 20 minutes.
4. Remove from the heat and allow to stand, covered, for 5 minutes. Remove the lemon grass stalk before serving and garnish, if desired, with the cilantro and coconut.

PAELLA

SPAIN   *4 to 6 servings*

The Moors of North Africa planted Asian rice in the Valencia region of southern Spain and prepared the saffron-scented rice dishes of their native lands using local ingredients. Paella is a Spanish pronunciation of *pilau*. Paella is traditionally served in an oval copper pan. For a beautiful presentation, serve paella on an oval platter, surrounded by whole cooked artichokes. The Spanish use saffron lavishly—up to 1 teaspoon. For best texture, choose a sturdy long-grain rice; basmati doesn't withstand the mixing process well.

STEP ONE

¼ to ½ teaspoon saffron
  soaked in ¼ cup (60 ml)
  hot water

2 cups (480 ml) water
1 teaspoon salt
1 cup (205 g) long-grain white rice

STEP TWO

⅓ cup (45 g) peas

STEP THREE

3 tablespoons olive oil
Pinch of hing (optional)

½ green bell pepper, cut into chunks
1 red bell pepper, cut into chunks

STEP FOUR

1 tomato, chopped
½ cup (85 g) sliced cooked artichoke
  hearts

½ cup (80 g) cooked garbanzo beans
  (chickpeas)
2 tablespoons lemon juice

1. Bring the saffron water, water, and salt to a boil. Add the rice. Cover, reduce the
   heat, and simmer for 10 minutes.
2. Add the peas. Cover and simmer until the water is absorbed and the rice is tender.
3. While the rice is cooking, heat the olive oil and hing in a skillet. Add the bell peppers and sauté over low heat, stirring frequently, until tender.
4. Gently toss the peppers, tomato, artichoke hearts, garbanzos, and lemon juice with
   the rice. Add more salt if necessary.

VARIATION
   Add pan-fried tofu, panir, or seitan cubes.

 RISI E BISI (RICE AND PEAS)

ITALY   4 to 6 main-dish servings

On the feast day of St. Mark, April 25, Risi e Bisi was traditionally eaten by the *doges* of
Venice. Unless there is a doge in your *palazzo*, feel free to substitute other vegetables,
such as asparagus tips or French beans. To produce the best texture, cook very slowly.

STEP ONE

5⅓ cups (1.3 l) vegetable stock
¾ teaspoon salt (less if stock is salted)

1 bay leaf

STEP TWO

3 tablespoons ghee or butter
Pinch of hing (optional)
1 cup (110 g) finely chopped celery or
  fennel

½ cup (70 g) finely chopped yellow
  bell pepper

STEP THREE

1⅓ cups (275 g) arborio rice

STEP FOUR

1 cup (130 g) peas

STEP FIVE

2 tablespoons ghee or butter   *White pepper*
½ cup (50 g) grated
  Parmesan cheese (optional)

1. Bring the stock, salt, and bay leaf to a boil. Reduce the heat so that the stock is barely simmering.
2. Meanwhile, melt the ghee or butter in a heavy-bottomed casserole or soup pot. Add the hing and sauté over low heat until fragrant, about 30 seconds. Add the celery or fennel and bell pepper and sauté, stirring frequently, until almost tender, about 5 minutes.
3. Add the rice and sauté for 1 to 2 minutes, stirring constantly. Add ½ cup (120 ml) of the heated stock. Simmer, stirring constantly, until all the liquid is absorbed. Continue to add the stock in approximately ½-cup (120 ml) increments, stirring and simmering until each addition is absorbed before adding the next. The process will take about 30 minutes.
4. Stir in the peas with the last addition of stock. Cook until the rice and peas are tender but the risotto is still somewhat soupy. Add a small amount of stock or water if necessary.
5. Remove from the heat. Add the ghee or butter and the Parmesan. Beat for 1 minute. Add pepper to taste, adjust the salt, and serve immediately.

 # RISOTTO VERDE (GREEN RISOTTO)

ITALY   *4 to 6 main-dish servings*

Risotto was the Renaissance Italian's response to the succulent rice dishes they were tasting from points both west and east: Spanish Paella and Middle Eastern pilaus, experienced through lively trade relations with Constantinople. Here is an herb- and fennel-laced risotto.

STEP ONE

1 cup (90 g) loosely packed   *½ cup (120 ml) chopped flat-leaf*
  chopped spinach   *parsley*
1 cup (240 ml) loosely packed   *5⅓ cups (1.25 l) vegetable stock*
  chopped basil leaves
½ cup (120 ml) loosely packed
  chopped fennel tops

STEP TWO

¾ teaspoon salt (less if stock is salted)

STEP THREE

2 tablespoons ghee or butter   *1 cup (110 g) finely chopped fennel*
Pinch of hing (optional)   *½ cup (70 g) finely chopped green
                                            bell peppers*

STEP FOUR

1⅓ cups (275 g) arborio rice

STEP SIX

½ cup (120 ml) crème fraîche or   *White pepper*
  sour cream
*½ cup (50 g) grated Parmesan
  cheese* (optional)

1. Purée the spinach, basil, fennel tops, and parsley with ⅔ cup (160 ml) of the vegetable stock in a blender or food processor. Set aside.
2. Bring the remaining stock and salt to a boil. Reduce the heat so that it is barely simmering.
3. Meanwhile, melt the ghee or butter in a heavy-bottomed casserole or soup pot. Add the hing and sauté over low heat until fragrant, about 30 seconds. Add the fennel and bell peppers, and sauté, stirring frequently, until almost tender, about 5 minutes.
4. Add the rice and sauté for 1 to 2 minutes, stirring constantly. Add ⅔ cup (160 ml) of the heated stock. Simmer, stirring constantly, until all the liquid is absorbed. Continue to add the stock in approximately ½-cup (120 ml) increments, stirring and simmering until each addition is absorbed before adding the next. The process will take about 25 minutes.
5. Add the herb purée, including all the liquid. Simmer and stir until the rice is tender and the liquid is absorbed.
6. Stir in the crème fraîche or sour cream and return to a simmer. Add the Parmesan and beat for 1 minute. Season to taste with pepper and adjust the salt. Serve immediately.

VARIATIONS

Replace the crème fraîche or sour cream with 2 tablespoons ghee or butter in Step 6. Replace the chopped fennel with celery and the fennel tops with fresh tarragon.

❂ Replace the ghee or butter with olive oil, and the crème fraîche or sour cream with thick coconut milk.

TRADITIONAL STEAMED COUSCOUS

MOROCCO   *3 cups (720 ml)*

Longer-cooking (is 20 minutes *long* cooking?) couscous is an endangered species; survival of the fittest seems to have fallen into the hands of insipid instant couscous. Pity. If you can find the real thing, try this traditional cooking method—it's also the real thing. In lieu of a *couscousière*, couscous can be prepared in a steamer or in a colander that fits completely within a large pot. If your steaming apparatus has large holes, line it with cheesecloth.

STEP ONE

1 cup (185 g) noninstant   *2 cups (480 ml) water*
  couscous   *½ teaspoon salt*

STEP TWO
2 to 4 tablespoons olive oil or melted ghee (optional)

1. Soak the couscous in the water and salt for 10 minutes.
2. Drain thoroughly. Toss with the oil or ghee if desired.
3. Place the couscous in the steamer or colander. Place in a pot above boiling water. Cover and cook until the couscous is tender, about 10 minutes.

 ## UPMA

INDIA   *4 servings*

In this breakfast and snack dish from south India, farina and semolina come into their own. Upma often is made with whole black peppercorns.

STEP ONE
1 cup (180 g) farina (Cream of Wheat) or coarsely ground semolina

STEP TWO
¼ cup (60 ml) ghee or mild-flavored oil   1½ teaspoons cumin seeds

STEP THREE
1 cup (130 g) peas   *1 teaspoon salt*
1 cup (110 g) green beans, cut into   *Whole black peppercorns*
  1-inch (2.5 cm) pieces   *(optional)*
2 cups (480 ml) water   *3 curry leaves* (optional)

1. Toast the farina in a dry pan over a medium-low heat until it is slightly darkened. Remove from the heat and set aside.
2. Heat the ghee or oil in a pot. Add the cumin seeds and sauté for 1 minute.
3. Add the peas, green beans, water, salt, a conservative sprinkling of whole black peppercorns, and the curry leaves. Cover and simmer until the vegetables are tender.
4. Uncover and add the farina, a little at a time, stirring constantly to avoid lumps. Cook until very thick, stirring constantly. Serve immediately.

VARIATION

Omit the vegetables or replace the green beans with bell pepper or zucchini.

Though He had commanded the clouds from above and opened
the doors of heaven,
And had rained down manna upon them to eat, and had given
them the grain of heaven.
Man did eat angel's food; He sent them food to the full.

—PSALMS 78.23–25

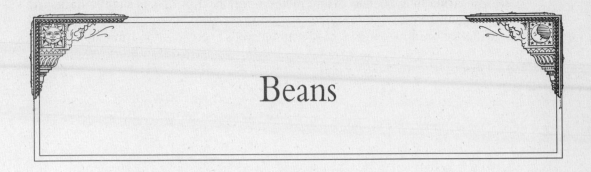

Beans

If pale beans bubble for you in a red earthenware pot, you can often decline the dinners of sumptuous hosts.

—Martial, A.D. 85

Beans, also known as *legumes*, *pulses*, and *dal*, are good, nourishing food that has helped sustain the world since time immemorial. Not only has nearly every generation of humankind benefitted, but so has the environment, for bean plants enrich and replenish the soil. Beans and grains served together provide the staple nourishment for many cultures—good, sound, Ayurvedic food combining. In Asia beans have always been served with rice. Throughout the Americas bean plants were grown next to corn, the cornstalks serving as living bean poles. As they were sown, so were they reaped and eaten: beans and corn together.

People with predominantly Kapha mind-body types often feel they must count their culinary blessings where they may because so many foods are off their list. Start counting—the bean universe is your playground, where most beans are Kapha friendly. In addition, mung beans, lauded in Ayurvedic texts for their supreme digestibility and health-giving qualities, can be eaten by everyone. Garbanzos balance Vata and Pitta in addition to Kapha; lentils are also balancing for Vata; and Pitta types can eat soybeans. With the exception of mung, most beans have heavy, dry, and rough qualities that require stronger Agni to digest. It is therefore more desirable to serve them at the midday repast, when Agni is most powerful, rather than for the evening meal.

Digestion: the conversion of victuals into virtues. —Ambrose Bierce

- ❖ It is a kindness to your tummy to eat beans that are well cooked. Well cooked means *very* soft. An undercooked bean is crunchy or crumbly when you bite into it.
- ❖ Ginger, cumin, hing, black pepper, and chilies are all good friends to beans because they stimulate the digestive fire, Agni. These spices are traditionally

sautéed in ghee or oil before being added to a dish, and they should be added to beans that are already fully cooked so that their flavors don't diminish. Beans are also delicious with green herbs. Savory is called "the bean herb" and is a customary seasoning in Europe. Sauté dried herbs in a little oil before adding. Fresh herbs should be stirred in just before serving.

The Bean Universe

Ethnic markets, natural foods stores, and farmers' markets are fertile hunting grounds for stalking unusual beans. Beans of "a certain age" take a long time to cook and never get as tender as you'd like them. It's hard to tell young'uns apart from their elders, but if you see dried-up, broken, wrinkly beans, or a bin that obviously has not been touched for months, steer clear. Store beans away from extreme heat and cold, which make them tougher, and away from moisture, mold, and insects. Airtight containers, such as glass jars, are ideal.

The Common Bean

Most beans belong to one botanical family, *Phaseolus vulgaris,* known as *common beans.* Literally hundreds of varieties exist. Here are some more readily available varieties:

Aduki or azuki: Tiny red tri-doshic beans used in Chinese and Japanese cuisines. Cooked with white rice, they lend the rice an attractive pink hue.

Black, or turtle, beans are found in dishes throughout the cuisines of the Western hemisphere, from black bean soup in the United States to various combinations with rice in the Caribbean and South America.

Anasazi: Archaeologists exploring the Mesa Verde cliff dwellings in Colorado, built by the Anasazis, a mysterious lost tribe, discovered a pot filled with beans. They were identified by botanists as a unique strain of the common bean, slightly sweeter than other common beans and happily containing 75 percent less oligosaccharides, the component that causes flatulence. Use like pinto and kidney beans.

Haricots are the dried seeds of mature *haricots verts*—green beans. The large haricot brood includes cannellini, great northern, navy, and other white beans. Haricots are somewhat interchangeable in cooking, although some have taken on distinct ethnic connotations. Italians, particularly from Tuscany, adopted *cannellini* as their own. The adoptees, the Tuscans, came to be known as *mangia fagioli,* "bean eaters." White beans are a signature ingredient of dishes from Brittany. Navy beans received their military calling when they were served to the navy in the nineteenth century, probably far more often than the sailors cared for.

Kidney: Kidney beans come in well-known red, lesser-known white, and little-known brown varieties. They are standard issue in foods of the American South and Central America and are also popular in India and in Europe. Fresh, very young kidney beans, known as *flageolets*, are a delicacy in Italy and France.

Lima, or butter, beans: Although the beans were named for Peru's capital, somehow the "L" got relegated to lowercase and the pronunciation altered. They are a staple in parts of Africa and are one of the few beans enjoyed in China, where they are deep-fried as a garnish for *congee*, breakfast rice porridge. Fresh limas are green, and dried limas can be green or white. There is also a smaller bean from Mexico called *sieva*, or *baby lima*.

Pinto beans are a staple throughout Central and South America and the southern United States. *Pink beans*, or *pinquitos* and *cranberry beans* are close relatives. Alas, the beautiful bright colors and markings on all these beans disappear when they are cooked.

Lentils

Transported from India along the westerly trade routes, lentils settled into the cuisines of the Middle East, Africa, and Europe.

- ❖ *Brown lentils,* the most common type, are a classic in soup. They are also excellent in burgers and loaves, to which they give the best flavor and texture of all the beans. In France brown lentils are dressed very simply with butter and salt, and in the Middle East, with olive oil.
- ❖ *Red lentils,* also called *masoor, or mansoor, or mussouri dal,* are balancing to Vata as well as Kapha. They are bright orange when uncooked but become a mellow gold when fully cooked. *Brown masoor dal* has the seed coat intact; *red masoor* has been skinned. A larger variety of red lentils used in Egyptian cooking can be employed in the same manner as brown lentils.
- ❖ *Green lentils* are smaller and firmer than their brown brothers. The French dress and serve them as a salad.

Garbanzos, Chickpeas, Ceci, or Kabli Chana

Native to South and Southeast Asia, garbanzo beans were cultivated in the Middle East and Africa as far back as 5000 B.C. Today they are prevalent in the cuisines of India, the Middle East, and the Mediterranean countries.

Fava, Broad, Windsor, or Horse Beans

Daily rations for pyramid construction crews, fava beans remain a staple in Egypt and are popular in North Africa, the Middle East, and Mediterranean countries. Favas are often served fresh. They must be podded, cooked, and their thick skins removed.

Black-eyed Peas, Pigeon Peas, Cowpeas, or Lobya

Relatives of mung beans, black-eyed peas hail from India and are world travelers that left a few family members behind to take root on whatever shores they touched. Hence, black-eyed pea dishes turn up in the most unexpected places, and you can add them to the dishes of many lands. There is even a stronghold of black-eyed pea champions in the south of France: the gastronomic order of the *Taostos Moungetos*, the "black-eyed pea tasters."

Mung beans, moong dal, yellow cram, or kalamata beans are the most nourishing and digestible legume and, along with aduki beans, the only widely available tri-doshic legume. They can be served to people when sick or otherwise in need of very light food and can be eaten by all on a daily basis. Their most desirable form for Ayurvedic cooking is split and hulled. Split, hulled mung beans can be found in Indian markets, where they are called *moong dal*. They are cooked to a soft, porridgey texture, like lentils. Whole mung beans can be found in natural foods stores.

Yellow and Green Split Peas

"Pease porridge" sustained many generations of Europeans through many a long, cold winter. Split peas completely lose their shape when cooked and are most suitable for soups and sauces.

Soybeans

A variety of descriptive names show the importance of soybeans in the East Asian diet, including "king of beans" and "meat of the soil." The only time Westerners ever attempted to eat whole soybeans regularly was during a brief health food movement in the 1960s—and even then, the legume didn't win many gustatory converts. More people enjoy products processed from soybeans, such as *tofu, soy flour,* and *dried bean curd* or *yuba*. Because soybeans take so long to cook, they have been processed into quick-cooking forms, soy grits, and soy flakes.

Dal

Dal means "beans," and there are some types used frequently in Ayurvedic cooking that are well worth becoming acquainted with. They can be found in Indian markets. *Toor* or *toovar dal* is particularly nourishing and digestible. It comes in two forms: plain and oily. Oily toor dal is coated with castor oil for protection against insects and has a very pleasant taste despite what you might think! Rinse thoroughly before cooking to remove the oil. *Urad dal* or *black gram* is a staple of south India. It is most commonly split and hulled but can also be found whole and split with its black skins intact. *Chana dal* comes in several varieties, all kissin' cousins to garbanzos. *Black chana* looks like a small brown garbanzo. *Yellow chana,* which is much smaller than garbanzos, is split and husked and has a light golden color.

THE TEN COMMANDMENTS OF BEAN COOKERY

I. *Rinse thy beans before cooking.* This helps help banish beans' main source of flatulence and indigestibility, the dread *oligosaccharides.* Soaking also reduces cooking times by approximately 30 minutes.

II. *Sort thy beans, so that thy teeth may live long.* Spread uncooked beans on a platter and carefully check for pebbles. A minute or two or sorting is a valuable exercise in preventative dentistry!

III. *Soak those beans that needeth soaking, so that they shall finish cooking in thy lifetime.* Place beans in 3 to 4 times the amount of water as beans. Most beans absorb all the water they can in about 4 hours, but it is often more convenient to soak them overnight. Fava beans and older beans can require up to 24 hours of soaking. Discard any beans that float to the top; they have an air pocket between the skin and the bean that may contain mold.

   Quick soaking method: When in a pinch for time, bring the water and beans to a boil, remove from the heat, and allow to soak for 1 hour.

IV. *Simmer beans in fresh water—never the soaking water.* I use 6 times as much water as beans because the water boils off during long cooking. Bring to a boil, partially cover, then reduce the heat and simmer until they are cooked. It is important to *simmer* the beans, not boil them. When rushed, they become tough and hard to digest. During cooking, a foamy scum made of starches, proteins, and minerals can form on the top. Not to worry—cooking beans in a partially covered pot prevents scum from forming. If it does anyway, just skim it off.

V. *Thou shalt not add cold water to simmering beans.* Cold water interrupts the cooking process, and the beans may not soften. Add boiling water if you must add more.

VI. *Thou shalt not add salt to simmering beans,* for it toughens beans' skins and prevents them from absorbing more water.

VII. *Thou shalt not add acid ingredients while thy beans are cooking,* such as large amounts of tomatoes or lemon juice, which toughen the skins and inhibit further water absorption.

VIII. *Thou shalt not add baking soda.* Although sometimes recommended to reduce flatulence, the alkalinity of baking soda weakens beans' cell structure, and both nutrients and flavor disappear into the cooking water.

IX. *Honor thy beans' different cooking times,* which vary for different types of beans. They can also vary dramatically depending on the mineral content of the cooking water and the beans' age—older ones can take literally hours longer than younger ones.

X. *Thou shalt use a Crock-Pot if thy feet wandrest from the kitchen.* A practical way to deal with long cooking times on busy schedules. Bring presoaked beans to a boil on the stove with the same amount of cooking water you would use for stovetop cooking. Place the boiling mixture in a Crock-Pot set on high. Cooking times are about the same as for stovetop simmering. I have never had much success with the low setting because the beans sometimes ferment during the extra-long time it takes to cook them.

BEAN SOAKING AND COOKING TIMES

One cup (240 ml) of dried beans cooks into approximately 2 to 2½ cups (480 to 600 ml) cooked beans.

1 CUP (240 ML) BEANS	SOAK	COOKING TIME	COMMENTS
Aduki	yes	2 hrs.	
Anasazi	yes	2 hrs.	
Black or turtle	yes	2½ hrs.	
Black-eyed peas	no	2½ hrs.	
Chana dal, split	no	2½ hrs.	
Chana dal, whole	yes	2½–3 hrs.	
Fava	24–36 hrs.	2–2½ hrs.	Peel after soaking; cook very well to avoid possible allergic reaction in people of Mediterranean heritage.
Garbanzo	yes	3+ hrs.	
Haricot	yes	2–2½ hrs.	
Kidney, cannellini, navy, and other white beans	yes	2½ hrs.	Cook very slowly.
Lentils, brown	no	1½ hrs.	Less time for firm lentils for salad.
Lentils, red	no	45–60 min.	
Lima	yes	2+ hrs.	Cook in an uncovered pot to release tiny amounts of cyanide.
Mung, whole	no	2½–3 hrs.	
Mung, split	no	1½–2 hrs.	Stir occasionally to avoid scorching.
Peas, split	no	3–4 hrs.	
Pinto	yes	2½ hrs.	

1 Cup (240 ml) Beans	Soak	Cooking Time	Comments
Soybeans	24 hrs.	5–6 hrs.	
Soy flakes	no	40 min.	
Soy grits	no	45–60 min.	
Toor or toovar dal	no	3–4 hrs.	Wash oil off "oily toor dal" thoroughly.
Urad dal	no	2–3 hrs.	Burns easily; stir occasionally.

 # KHICHARI (SAVORY DAL AND RICE)

INDIA   *4 to 6 servings*

A basic, important Ayurvedic dish. Mung bean Khichari is balanced for all doshas. Unadorned Khichari is served in cleansing diets and while undergoing *Panchakarma*, the supreme Ayurvedic rejuvenation treatment. It is also suitable when people are ill and for the delicate digestions of the very young and very old.

STEP ONE

1 cup (205 g) basmati rice   *5 cups (1.2 l) water*
⅔ cup (200 g) mung or toor dal,
  lentils, or split peas

STEP TWO

2 tablespoons   *¾ teaspoon black mustard seeds*
  ghee or oil   *¼ teaspoon ground fenugreek*
Pinch of hing (optional)   *1 teaspoon turmeric*
2 tablespoons minced fresh   *Salt or liquid seasoning*
  ginger   *Sugar* (optional)
1½ teaspoons cumin seeds   *Chopped fresh cilantro*

1. Bring the rice, beans, and water to a boil in a pot. Cover, reduce the heat, and simmer until the dal is tender, all the water is absorbed, and the mixture resembles a thick porridge, about 1½ hours. Stir occasionally and be alert toward the end of the cooking so that the mixture doesn't stick. Add more water if necessary.
2. Heat the ghee or oil in a small skillet. Add the hing, ginger, cumin seeds, mustard seeds, and fenugreek. Sauté over low heat until the mustard seeds "dance." Add to the Khichari. Stir in the turmeric. Add salt or liquid seasoning and a pinch of sugar to taste. Garnish with chopped cilantro.

VARIATIONS

Cook finely cut vegetables in the Khichari. Try green beans, carrots, peas, and zucchini.
To balance Kapha, add black pepper to taste or add chilies to taste to the ghee or oil.
Garnish with toasted unsweetened coconut shreds or chopped toasted almonds or
cashews.

Stir in a small amount of coconut milk before serving to further balance Pitta.
Replace the Basmati rice with barley to further balance Kapha. Add 1 cup water.

No illness which can be treated by diet should be treated by any other means.
—MOSES MAIMONIDES

 # PONGAL (TOASTED DAL AND RICE)

INDIA   *4 servings*

Eaten in south India as a breakfast food, Pongal is close in concept to Khichari but with
a tiny bit more texture from the dry-roasted grains. It also cooks more quickly. The
black pepper is traditional; reduce or omit if you'd like a milder flavor. Curry leaves are
small aromatic leaves used in South Indian cooking. They can be used fresh or dried,
and are sometimes available in Indian markets. Curry leaves are not eaten, but set aside
on the diner's plate.

STEP ONE

½ cup (100 g) split hulled mung dal   *1 cup (205 g) basmati rice*

STEP TWO

5 cups (1.2 l) water   *8 curry leaves* (optional)

STEP THREE

¼ cup (60 ml) melted ghee   *1 teaspoon coarsely ground black*
Pinch of hing (optional)   *pepper*
2 tablespoons minced fresh ginger   *Liquid seasoning or salt*
2 teaspoons cumin seeds   *Toasted whole cashews* (optional)
½ teaspoon turmeric   *Toasted grated coconut* (optional)

1. Separately toast the mung dal and rice in a dry skillet over medium heat, stirring constantly, for about 5 minutes each. Both will darken very slightly and look quite dry.
2. Rinse the toasted dal and rice and place in the water with the curry leaves. Bring to
   a boil, cover, reduce the heat, and simmer until the water is absorbed and the mixture has the texture of oatmeal porridge, about 40 minutes.

3. Heat the ghee in a small skillet. Add the hing, ginger, and cumin seeds, and sauté over low heat for about 1 minute, until fragrant. Stir into the Pongal. Add the turmeric and black pepper. Season to taste with liquid seasoning or salt. If desired, garnish with a sprinkling of toasted cashews and coconut.

 # BLACK BEAN CAKES WITH AVOCADO-PECAN CHUTNEY

10 burgers

Myriad varieties of bean cakes—and also bean loaves—can be created from this recipe. Use any type of common bean your heart desires: Anasazi, pinto, kidney, etc. This recipe calls for quinoa, but you can substitute other grains, such as bulgar or couscous, to make a more balanced dish for Vata or Pitta. To create a bean loaf, press the mixture into an oiled loaf pan and bake for 30 to 40 minutes in a 350°F (180°C) oven. Serve with Avocado-Pecan Chutney (recipe follows), which is friendly to Vata and Pitta. Add a dollop of sour cream or crème fraîche to make Vata's smile even wider.

STEP ONE

1 cup (185 g) *dried black beans*

STEP THREE

1 tablespoon ghee or oil   1 carrot, grated
Pinch of hing (optional)   1 stalk fennel or celery, thinly sliced
1 tablespoon minced fresh ginger   ½ bell pepper, minced
1 teaspoon cumin seeds

STEP FIVE

1 cup (185 g) cooked quinoa   ⅓ cup (40 g) dry bread crumbs
¼ cup (40 g) whole wheat   Salt
   flour   Black pepper

STEP SIX

Ghee or oil

1. Clean the beans. Place in a bowl with a least 3 cups (720 ml) of water and soak overnight.
2. Drain, rinse, and place the beans in a pot with 6 cups (1.4 l) of water. Bring to a boil, reduce the heat, and simmer until tender.
3. Meanwhile, heat the ghee or oil in a small skillet. Add the hing ginger, and cumin seeds and sauté over low heat until fragrant, about 30 seconds. Add the carrot, celery, and bell pepper and sauté until tender, stirring frequently.
4. Drain the beans. Purée in a food processor, adding just enough water to mash them thoroughly. Allow to cool to room temperature.

5. Mix together the beans, sautéed vegetables, quinoa, flour, and bread crumbs. Season to taste with salt and pepper.
6. Shape the mixture into patties. Heat a little ghee or oil in a nonstick skillet or griddle. Fry the cakes on both sides over low heat until a golden-brown crust forms.

AVOCADO-PECAN CHUTNEY

1¾ cups (500 g)

STEP ONE

2 medium avocadoes, cubed
⅓ cup (30 g) chopped pecans, toasted

¼ cup (60 ml) lemon juice
¼ cup (40 g) chopped crystallized ginger
2 teaspoons raw sugar or honey

STEP TWO

1 teaspoon oil
Pinch of hing (optional)
1 teaspoon cumin seeds
½ teaspoon brown mustard seeds

Salt
Black pepper
Chopped fresh cilantro

1. Toss the avocado cubes with the pecans, lemon juice, crystallized ginger, and sugar or honey.
2. Heat the oil in a small skillet. Add the hing, cumin seeds, and mustard seeds and sauté over low heat until the mustard seeds dance. Add to the chutney. Season to taste with salt and plenty of black pepper. Garnish with chopped cilantro.

VARIATIONS

Replace the pecans with ¼ cup (20 g) toasted unsweetened coconut shreds.
Add minced green chilies.

 ## MOORS AND CHRISTIANS (MOROS Y CRISTIANOS)

CUBA   *4 servings*

Named by some culinary humorist, the Moors and Christians of this Cuban national dish are black beans served over white rice. It is served on New Year's Day to bring good luck. Prepared with black-eyed peas the dish becomes Hoppin' John, the New Year's Day good-luck dish of the southern U.S. Note that the beans must be soaked ahead of time.

STEP ONE

1 cup (185 g) black beans

STEP TWO

6 cups (1.4 l) water   1 bay leaf

STEP THREE

3 tablespoons ghee, butter, or oil   ½ cup (70 g) finely chopped bell
Pinch of hing (optional)   peppers
1 teaspoon dried thyme   1½ cups (350 g) puréed fresh
1 cup (110 g) finely chopped celery   tomatoes

STEP FOUR

Salt   Cooked rice
Black pepper   Lemon wedges

1. Clean the beans. Place in at least 3 cups (700 ml) water and soak for 4 to 6 hours, or overnight.
2. Drain, rinse, and place the beans in a medium saucepan with the water and the bay leaf. Bring to a boil. Reduce the heat, partially cover, and simmer until tender, about 2½ hours. At this point, the water should just cover the beans.
3. Melt the ghee, butter, or oil in a large skillet. Add the hing and thyme, and sauté over low heat until fragrant, about 30 seconds. Add the celery and bell peppers and sauté for 10 minutes, stirring constantly. Add the tomato purée and cook for 2 to 3 minutes more.
4. Add the vegetable mixture to the beans. Simmer until the sauce surrounding the beans is thick and gravylike, about 45 minutes. Season to taste with salt and pepper. Serve over rice, garnished with lemon wedges to squeeze over the beans.

VARIATIONS

Add a sprinkling of liquid seasoning with the salt and pepper in Step 4.

Moros y Cristianos is often given a sour flavor with vinegar. Add more lemon juice or stir in a little tamarind paste in Step 4 if you desire such a flavor.

 # ACARAJÉ (BLACK-EYED PEA FRITTERS)

BRAZIL/AFRICA/CARIBBEAN   *About 30*

Street food that hails from Nigeria, Acarajé migrated to the Caribbean, where it is made from soybeans on some islands, and to Brazil, where it is sometimes prepared from chickpea flour. All the above are fried in *dendê*, palm oil, with its characteristic golden color.

STEP ONE

1 cup (160 g) dried black-eyed peas

STEP TWO

1 teaspoon salt   *¼ teaspoon baking powder*

STEP THREE

Besan (chickpea flour) or soy flour

STEP FOUR

Oil for deep-frying

1. Clean the beans. Place in a bowl with at least 3 cups (700 ml) of water and soak overnight.
2. Drain, rinse, and process the beans in a blender or food processor with the salt and baking powder. Add water a little at a time while processing, just until they are ground to a smooth paste.
3. If necessary, beat in besan or soy flour, a teaspoon at a time, until the batter is thick enough to be dropped in rough teaspoonfuls from a spoon.
4. Heat oil for deep-frying. Have a plate covered with paper towels nearby. Test the temperature by deep-frying a heaping teaspoonful of the mixture, turning once or twice, until golden brown. Drain on paper towels. Check to see if it is cooked through. If not, lower the temperature of the oil. If the fritter still doesn't cook, add more flour. When everything is well and wisely put, deep-fry the rest of the mixture in the same manner in several uncrowded batches. Serve immediately.

 # FALAFEL

MIDDLE EAST   *About 24*

Falafel sandwiches are popular Israeli street food, served in a halved piece of pita bread with shredded lettuce and chopped tomatoes, and drizzled with Taratoor Sauce (pp. 512–13). Across the way in Egypt the dish is called *ta' a mia*, and is prepared from fava beans, another bean option. You will need the finely milled bulgar available in Middle Eastern markets. If you only have access to the coarser American bulgar, you must cook it rather than soak it.

STEP ONE

1 cup (190 g) dried garbanzo beans (chickpeas)

STEP THREE

½ cup (85 g) bulgar

STEP FOUR

¼ *cup (60 ml) minced fresh*
  parsley
2½ *teaspoons toasted ground*
  cumin
Pinch of hing (optional)

2 *tablespoons minced fresh*
  ginger
1 *teaspoon salt*
¼ *cup (60 ml) lemon juice*

STEP FIVE

*Besan (*chickpea flour*), soy, or whole wheat flour*

STEP SIX

Sesame seeds (optional)

STEP SEVEN

Oil for deep-frying

1. Clean the garbanzos. Place in at least 3 cups (700 ml) of water and soak overnight.
2. Drain, rinse, and place the garbanzos in a pot with 6 cups (1.4 liters) of water. Bring to a boil. Reduce the heat and simmer until very tender, about 2½ hours.
3. Meanwhile, soak the bulgar in 1 cup (240 ml) water for at least 1 hour.
4. Drain the garbanzos and the bulgar. Mash the garbanzos to a paste with the parsley, cumin, hing, ginger, salt, and lemon juice. Beat in the bulgar. (You can also simply throw everything into a food processor and purée.)
5. Attempt to form a little of the mixture into a 1-inch (2.5 cm) ball. If it does not hold together completely or feels wet, beat the flour, a tablespoon at a time, into the mixture until it holds together well. If the mixture is too wet, the falafels will disintegrate when fried. However, do not attempt to make them firm and dense, like bread dough, or they will be dry and rock-hard.
6. Form 1-inch (2.5 cm) balls. If desired, roll in sesame seeds to coat. Flatten each ball slightly. For best results, allow the falafels to dry in the sun for an hour.
7. Heat oil for deep-frying. Have a tray covered with paper towels nearby. Deep-fry the falafels, turning gently once or twice, until golden brown. Drain on paper towels.

 ## THE PURITAN'S FEAST: BOSTON BAKED BEANS WITH BOSTON BROWN BREAD

UNITED STATES   *6 servings*

The Puritans observed how Native Americans lined a hole with heated stones and placed in it a pottery vessel filled with beans, water, and fat to cook. Cooking was forbidden on the Sabbath, so the Puritans placed a crock of beans, along with Boston Brown Bread (recipe follows), in the oven on Saturday night and the heat of the untended embers gently cooked them for Sunday dinner. So pervasive was this practice in Boston that it came to be known as "Beantown."

STEP ONE

2 cups (400 g) dried navy beans

STEP THREE

3 medium tomatoes, puréed
½ cup (120 ml) dark unsulphured
  molasses
½ cup (100 g) raw or packed dark
  brown sugar

2 tablespoons ghee or oil
Pinch of hing (optional)
½ teaspoon salt
¼ teaspoon ground cloves
Pinch of ground mustard

1. Clean the beans. Place in a bowl with at least 5 cups (1.2 l) of water and soak overnight.
2. Preheat the oven to 350°F (180°C). Drain and rinse the beans, and place in a pot with water to cover. Bring to a boil.
3. Pour into a baking dish, making sure that the liquid covers the beans. Stir in the remaining ingredients.
4. Cover and bake for 5 hours, checking every hour or so and replenishing the water so that it continually covers the beans.
5. After 5 hours, remove the lid. Add water to cover the beans once more, then bake, uncovered, until a little liquid remains as a thick sauce and the beans are a rich brown color, 1 to 1½ hours.

VARIATION
Add Miriam's Sofrito (p. 218) in Step 4.

BOSTON BROWN BREAD

UNITED STATES   *1 loaf*

A dense, moist, steamed loaf that can be prepared in a cylindrical mold or in a deep baking dish for a less authentic shape. Those more prone to luxury than the Boston brethren of old eat it with unpuritanical dabs of cream cheese.

STEP TWO

1 cup (130 g) cornmeal
1 cup (125 g) rye flour
1 cup (150 g) whole wheat
  flour

½ teaspoon salt
1½ teaspoons baking powder
½ teaspoon soda

STEP THREE

¾ cup (180 ml) unsulphured
  molasses

1⅓ cups (320 ml) buttermilk or
  sour milk

STEP FOUR

3/4 *cup (95 g) raisins*   *1 tablespoon finely grated orange zest*
1/2 *cup (50 g) chopped walnuts*

1. Preheat the oven to 350°F (180°C). Butter a 1-quart (1 l) mold or casserole.
2. Mix the dry ingredients together.
3. Mix the molasses and buttermilk or sour milk together and pour over the dry ingredients.
4. Add the raisins, nuts, and orange zest. Mix everything together well.
5. Pour into the mold. The container should be no more than 2/3 full. Cover tightly with a lid or with foil.
6. Place the mold in a pan with 1 inch (2.5 cm) of boiling water. Bake for 2 hours, replacing the water from time to time as it evaporates. Allow to cool before carefully unmolding.

 # RED BEANS AND RICE

UNITED STATES   *4 servings*

Red beans and ricely yours,   —HOW LOUIS ARMSTRONG SIGNED HIS LETTERS

Monday is red beans and rice day in New Orleans. Why? It was a universal wash day, and the long, slow simmering of the dish accommodated the women's absence from the kitchen. Also, the starch left in the rice's cooking water could be used to starch the freshly laundered shirts!

STEP ONE

1 *cup (185 g) dried kidney beans*

STEP TWO

6 *cups (1.4 l) water*

STEP THREE

3 *tablespoons ghee or oil*   1 1/2 *cups (175 g) finely chopped*
Pinch of hing (optional)   *celery*
1 *teaspoon dried thyme*   1 *cup (140 g) finely chopped bell*
1 *teaspoon dried oregano*   *peppers*

STEP FOUR

1 *teaspoon white pepper*   1 *teaspoon paprika*

STEP FIVE

Salt   *Cooked rice*

1. Clean the beans. Place in at least 3 cups (700 ml) of water and soak for 4 to 6 hours or overnight.

2. Drain, rinse, and place the beans in a medium saucepan with the water. Bring to a boil, reduce the heat, and simmer until tender.
3. Meanwhile, heat the ghee or oil in a skillet. Add the hing, thyme, and oregano and sauté over low heat until fragrant, about 30 seconds. Stir in the celery and bell peppers and sauté, stirring frequently, until tender, about 10 minutes.
4. Add the sautéed vegetables, white pepper, and paprika to the beans. Simmer until the beans are tender and most of the water is absorbed to form a gravylike consistency, 2¾ to 3 hours.
5. Add salt to taste. Serve over cooked rice.

VARIATION
Replace the paprika with cayenne to taste.

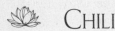 # CHILI

UNITED STATES   *4 servings*

A bowl of blessedness!   —WILL ROGERS, DESCRIBING TEXAS CHILI

Chili powder is derived from spice combinations of the ancient Aztecs as interpreted by a German food producer in New Braunfels, Texas, in 1902! This is a particularly useful blend to make at home if you want to avoid garlic, which all commercial chili powders contain. Add plenty of black pepper or red chilies if you like your "bowl of red" red-hot. Serve with rice to provide balance for Vata and Pitta or with tortillas to keep Kapha home on the range. Vatas can garnish with a dollop of sour cream.

STEP ONE

1 cup (185 g) dried Anasazi, pinto, black, or kidney beans

STEP THREE

2 tablespoons ghee or oil | *1 bell pepper, cut into chunks*
1 teaspoon dried oregano | *2 cups (460 g) chopped tomatoes*
1 stalk celery, thinly sliced | *1 bay leaf*

STEP FOUR

1 teaspoon ground coriander | *¾ teaspoon paprika*
½ teaspoon ground cinnamon | *¼ teaspoon ground cloves*

STEP FIVE

2 tablespoons ghee or oil | *Salt*
Pinch of hing (optional) | *Black pepper*
2 teaspoons ground | *Pinch of sugar*
  cumin | *Chopped fresh cilantro*

1. Clean the beans. Place in about 3 cups (700 ml) of water and soak overnight.
2. Drain, rinse, and place the beans in a pot with 6 cups (1.4 l) of water. Bring to a boil, reduce the heat, and simmer until tender, 2 to 2½ hours. Drain.
3. Meanwhile, heat the ghee or oil in a large skillet. Add the oregano, celery, and bell pepper and sauté for 2 to 3 minutes, stirring frequently. Add the tomatoes and the bay leaf. Cover and simmer over low heat until a thick sauce has formed, stirring occasionally.
4. Stir in the beans, coriander, cinnamon, paprika, and cloves.
5. Heat the second amount of ghee or oil in a small skillet. Add the hing and cumin and sauté over low heat until fragrant, 30 to 60 seconds. Add to the beans. Season to taste with salt, pepper, and a pinch of sugar. Garnish with chopped cilantro.

VARIATIONS

Stir in chopped sautéed seitan or firm tofu during the last 10 minutes of cooking.

Dried Tomato Chili: Omit the fresh tomatoes. Drain some of the water out of the beans after Step 2, leaving enough to barely cover the beans. Continue with Step 3, adding the vegetables to cook with the beans at the point where you would ordinarily throw in the fresh tomatoes. Add a handful of coarsely chopped dried tomatoes and simmer until all the vegetables are tender. Proceed to the spices in Steps 4 and 5.

LENTIL BURGERS WITH HERBED CHÈVRE SAUCE

10 to 12 burgers

The best of the burgers. Serve on burger rolls with all the trimmings. Try one of the mock mayonnaises as a topping or Vata-balancing Herbed Chèvre Sauce (recipe follows).

STEP ONE

1 cup lentils

3 cups (720 ml) vegetable stock or water

STEP TWO

2 tablespoons ghee or oil
Pinch of hing (optional)
1 carrot, grated

1 stalk celery, sliced
½ cup (70 g) minced bell peppers

STEP THREE

½ cup (75 g) bulgar
1 teaspoon salt
  (*less if using salted stock*)

Black pepper

STEP FOUR

Dry bread crumbs or *breading mixture (p. 210)*

STEP FIVE

Ghee or oil

1. Bring the lentils and stock or water to a boil in a medium saucepan. Reduce the heat and simmer, uncovered, for 30 minutes.
2. Meanwhile, melt the ghee or oil in a small skillet. Add the hing, carrot, celery, and bell peppers, and sauté over low heat, stirring frequently, until they start to become tender.
3. Stir the bulgar and sautéed vegetables into the simmering lentils. Cover and simmer over very low heat until the water is completely absorbed and the lentils and bulgar are tender. Be careful the mixture doesn't burn. Season to taste with salt and pepper. Allow the mixture to cool thoroughly to become firm.
4. Place bread crumbs or breading mixture in a shallow bowl. Shape the cooled mixture into burgers and gently dredge in the breading to coat on both sides.
5. *To fry:* Melt a liberal coating of ghee or oil on a griddle or large skillet. The idea is to thoroughly moisten the breading without saturating the burgers. Fry over low heat on both sides until the breading is nicely browned and the burgers are heated through. Replenish the ghee or oil as necessary to coat the breading.
   To bake: Preheat the oven to 350°F (180°C). Liberally coat a baking sheet with melted ghee or oil. The idea is to thoroughly moisten the breading without saturating the burgers. Place burgers on the baking sheet. Carefully flip each one so that the top side is moistened with oil. Bake until the breading is nicely browned, about 30 minutes.

VARIATION

Lentil Loaf: Add 1 large chopped tomato and 1 cup (60 g) *fresh* bread crumbs to the mixture in Step 3. Press the mixture into an oiled loaf pan and bake in a 350°F (180°C) oven for 40 minutes.

 # HERBED CHÈVRE SAUCE

About 1 cup (240 ml)

Cream cheese, ricotta, or even Tofu Mayonnaise can replace the chèvre. This mixture also makes a lovely spread or dip if you don't thin it to sauce consistency.

1 cup (230 g) creamy chèvre, such as Montrachet	¼ teaspoon salt
½ green bell pepper, finely chopped	⅛ teaspoon curry powder or Maharishi Ayur-Veda churna
1 teaspoon each: dried tarragon, basil, and dill or 1 tablespoon each chopped fresh herbs	Generous sprinkling of black pepper Stock or water

Combine all the ingredients in a food processor or beat together thoroughly. Thin to the desired consistency with stock or water.

TOSTADA WITH REFRIED BEANS (TOSTADA CON FRIJOLES REFRITOS)

MEXICO   *4 to 6 tostadas*

Food

One eats
The moon in a tortilla
Eat frijoles
And you eat earth
Eat chilie
And you eat sun and fire
Drink water
And you drink sky
                 —VICTOR VALLE

Tostadas are highly flexible affairs based on ingredients used by the ancient inhabitants of Mexico: crispy pan-fried tortillas topped with Refried Beans and piled high with toppings. For a road-less-traveled tostada, you could substitute chapatis for tortillas, sautéed chopped spinach or chard for the salad greens, and Avocado-Pecan Chutney (page 000) for the guacamole. Though the combination given here is a tad conventional, it looks and tastes unusually vibrant when prepared with homemade refritos and salsa.

STEP ONE
Sesame or other mild-flavored oil
4 to 6 corn tortillas

STEP TWO
Refried Beans (recipe follows, p. 202)   *Sour cream*
Sprouts or shredded lettuce   *Salsa Cruda (p. 507)*
Guacamole (pp. 279–80) or   *Shredded Monterey Jack cheese or*
  avocado slices   *crumbled feta or panir*

1. Heat ¼ inch (6 mm) oil in a skillet over medium-high heat. Cook each tortilla on both sides until crisp. Drain on paper towels.
2. Gently spread the Refried Beans on the tortillas. Top with a layer of sprouts or shredded lettuce, spoonfuls of Guacamole, sour cream and Salsa Cruda. Sprinkle with cheese.

REFRIED BEANS (FRIJOLES REFRITOS)

2 cups

Serve with rice, or in enchiladas, tacos, and other Mexican tortilla-based dishes. The proportions of beans, oil, and spices are highly flexible. You can also use black, Anasazi, or kidney beans. Refried beans seem to be capable of absorbing staggering amounts of ghee or oil. They give the beans good flavor and a silky texture, and you can add more than I've suggested. However, you can also use half the suggested amounts—or even no oil—and still be all right. You can also purée the beans in a food processor with just enough water to make a smooth paste before frying.

¼ to ⅓ cup (60 to 80 ml) melted ghee   3 cups (470 g) cooked pinto beans
*   or oil   Salt*
Pinch of hing (optional)   Black pepper
2 teaspoons ground cumin

Melt the ghee or oil in a skillet. Add the hing and cumin and sauté over low heat until fragrant, about 30 seconds. Add the beans and stir, mashing with a fork or potato masher while stirring. Sprinkle with salt and pepper and continue mashing and stirring for 5 to 7 minutes.

VARIATION
Fold in a handful of chopped cilantro just before serving.

DOSA (DAL AND RICE PANCAKES)

INDIA   *About 12 dosas*

Marvelous, addictive fare from south India. Dosas are leavened by leaving the batter to ferment for a day or two. Ordinarily, Ayurveda does not recommend fermented foods, but this ancient recipe seems to be an exception to the rule. Blending the batter is traditionally accomplished with a large stone mortar, a pestle, and a person with a lot of time on their very strong hands. Some now use an ingenious electric contraption that holds the batter in a rapidly rotating bowl while a heavy, cone-shaped stone dangling from a chain serves as the pestle. However, armed with a blender and large nonstick skillet or well-seasoned cast-iron skillet, you are set up in the same manner as millions of south Indians preparing breakfast for their families. Traditional accompaniments are Coconut Chutney and Sambar. See the Masala Dosa variation for a great lunchtime main dish.

STEP ONE
1 cup (200 g) split hulled urad dal   1½ cups (300 g) basmati rice

STEP TWO

Water

Pinch of hing (optional)

½ teaspoon ground fenugreek (optional)

1 teaspoon salt

STEP FOUR

Ghee or mild-flavored oil

1. Clean the dal and rice separately. Place in separate bowls and cover with 3 times as much fresh water. Soak for 4 to 6 hours or overnight.
2. Drain. Combine in a blender or food processor with enough water to make a thick pancake batter. The batter should be as smooth as possible. Blend in the hing, fenugreek, and salt.
3. Cover and allow the batter to stand, unrefrigerated, until tiny bubbles form on the surface and the mixture smells sour. In hot weather this can happen overnight, while in colder climes it can take as long as 36 hours. I usually plan on a 24-hour wait.
4. Pour a little ghee or mild-flavored oil into a large skillet over medium-high heat, as for pancakes. Nonstick skillets make for easy work, but a well-seasoned cast-iron skillet produces a crisper result. Pour a little batter onto the skillet. *Unlike pancake batter, dosa batter will not spread of its own accord.* Starting from the middle of the batter, swirl the back of a large spoon in a spiral motion to spread the batter out as thin as possible. If you can't get it very thin, never fear—you have made an *ootapam*, a perfectly respectable thick dosa-like pancake that can be served with pride.
5. Cook like a pancake, turning over when bubbles form on the surface and the underside is a deep golden brown. It takes about 5 minutes to cook the first side, and 2 to 3 minutes for the second side. The first dosa may not come out well, but the rest will.

VARIATIONS

Add a handful of chopped cilantro to the batter before cooking.

Sada Dosa: Add cumin seeds and black pepper to the batter.

Masala Dosa: Place a few spoonfuls of Eggplant-Potato Curry (p. 95), Peas and Potato Curry (pp. 115–16), or other nonjuicy curried vegetables on each dosa. Fold like a crêpe.

OFFERING AND SERVING FOOD

Atithi Devo Bhave—Honor the Guest as God.   —*TAITTIRIYA UPANISHAD*

In many cultures it is considered a spiritual responsibility and privilege to provide hospitality—particularly food—to others with the love and reverence one would show to God. Offering and serving food is a high calling. It is a blessing to have abundant food, and a blessing to to be able to share it. An ancient Indian custom still practiced in some areas is, before eating, to look outside the house and invite any hungry person that might be present to share the meal. In Jewish tradition it is a *mitzvah*, a blessing, to have guests at one's table. Serving a meal to others provides a wonderful opportunity to shower them with love, hospitality, and creativity. One can nourish others through loving service as well as through food itself.

 # DOSA BLINI WITH RATATOUILLE CAVIAR

About 30 blini

A rainbow coalition of ideas that makes for an exciting combination of flavors and gives an example of how dosas can be incorporated into dishes with Western-style sensibilities. If fresh basil and oregano are not available for the ratatouille, add a teaspoon each of dried basil and oregano to the oil in Step 3.

STEP ONE

1 cup (200 g) *basmati rice*   ⅔ cup *split hulled urad dal*

STEP FOUR

1 teaspoon salt
½ cup (120 ml) *chopped fresh basil*
   or parsley

STEP FIVE

3 tablespoons olive oil   4 cups (280 g) *peeled and chopped*
Pinch of hing (optional)   *eggplant*
1 stalk celery or fennel, chopped   ½ teaspoon salt
1 cup (140 g) *chopped red bell*
   peppers

STEP SIX

2 cups (210 g) *chopped zucchini*   ½ cup (120 ml) *minced fresh basil*
½ cup (40 g) *chopped*   ¼ cup (60 ml) *minced fresh oregano*
   dried tomatoes   1 teaspoon fresh or dried thyme
⅓ cup (80 ml) *minced flat-leaf*   1 teaspoon sugar
   parsley   Black pepper

STEP SEVEN

Sour cream

Dosa Blini:

1. Clean the dal and rice separately. Place in separate bowls and cover with 3 times as much fresh water. Soak for 4 to 6 hours or overnight.
2. Drain. Combine in a blender or food processor with enough water to make a thick pancake batter. The batter should be as smooth as possible.
3. Cover and allow the batter to stand, unrefrigerated, until tiny bubbles form on the surface and the mixture smells sour. In hot weather this can happen overnight, while in colder climes it can take as long as 36 hours. I usually plan on a 24-hour wait.
4. Gently stir the salt and basil or parsley into the prepared dosa batter. Make "blini" by dropping dosa batter from a soup spoon onto a heated oiled griddle to form 2-inch (5 cm) pancakes. Cook on each side until golden and crispy. Set aside.

Ratatouille Caviar:

5. Heat the oil in a large skillet. Add the hing and sauté over low heat for 30 seconds, until fragrant. Add the celery or fennel, bell peppers, and eggplant. Sprinkle with salt, cover, and sauté until almost tender, about 7 minutes.
6. Add the zucchini and dried tomatoes. Cover and sauté a few more minutes, until all the vegetables are tender. Stir in the parsley, basil, oregano, and thyme. Add the sugar, adjust the salt, and add black pepper to taste.
7. To assemble, place the dosa blinis on a serving platter. Top each blini with the vegetable mixture and a spoonful of sour cream. Serve immediately.

How vast is heaven? lo it will fit
In any space you give to it . . .
So broad—it takes in all things true;
So narrow—it can hold but you.

—John Richard Moreland

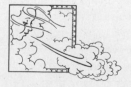

Tofu, Panir, and Seitan

*In bestowing care and nourishment it is important that the right
people be taken care of and that we should attend to our own
nourishment in the right way. If we wish to know what anyone
is like, we have only to observe on whom he bestows his care and
what sides of his own nature he cultivates and nourishes. Nature
nourishes all creatures.*

—I Ching, *The Book of Changes*

Tofu, curd made from soybean milk, and seitan, the protein portion of wheat, hail
from China and have graced dishes throughout East and Southeast Asia for centuries. Both are available in natural foods stores, Asian markets, and often in
supermarkets. Panir, a fresh cheese, is a delicacy from the Middle East and north India.
Rarely available in stores, it is mercifully quick and easy to make. Texturally, tofu,
panir, and seitan are great mimickers that can be used to substitute for meat and, in the
case of tofu and panir, for eggs as well. Tofu is widely employed as a dairy substitute
because it can mimic sour cream and stand in for cottage cheese and cream cheese in
recipes. All have mild flavors that harmonize beautifully with any ingredients with
which they are combined, absorb the flavors of sauces and liquidy dishes, and take on
different attributes when exposed to different cooking methods.

Tofu, panir, and seitan are balancing for Vata, and seitan is also balancing for Pitta.
Some Ayurvedic diners may find all three a bit heavy for their tastes, while others
appreciate their heft and substance and consider them life-savers. They certainly call out
for a strong digestive fire, Agni, to take them in hand. Spices that aid digestion are also
in order, as are sauces and liquid ingredients. While seitan can theoretically be served
anytime—in practice it might prove heavy for the evening—tofu and panir are curds
and thus best suited to the midday meal only.

Seitan, or wheat protein, always has a firm texture, while tofu and panir can have
either a firm texture that can be sliced or a soft, creamy texture.

206

- ❖ Cube firm pieces for Tempura, Pakora, and Kebabs.
- ❖ Stir-fry or deep-fry firm cubes to add to sautéed vegetable dishes, stews, grain dishes, and pastas.
- ❖ Fry, bake, or grill firm slices for sandwiches and cutlets. For additional flavor, marinate the pieces in a flavorful Citrus Vinaigrette before cooking.
- ❖ Mince or crumble and sauté for use in burgers, loaves, stuffings, etc.
- ❖ Crumble or purée soft tofu or panir and use like cottage cheese or ricotta in dishes such as Ravioli, Asparagus Torte, creamy filling for fruit tarts, and Unbaked Cheesecake.
- ❖ Substitute Tofu Mayonnaise and Panir Mayonnaise for Béchamel Sauce, sour cream, and cream cheese. The mock mayonnaises contain a little oil, which gives them a rich, creamy texture that plain purées of tofu and panir do not have.
- ❖ Purée tofu or panir into salad dressings and sauces that contain oil.
- ❖ Add small amounts of puréed tofu to batters for baked goods.

TOFU

Mama de	Made of soybeans	or	Practicing diligence
Shikaku de	Square, cleanly cut	or	Being proper and honest
Yawaraka de.	And soft.	or	And having a kind heart.

—INGEN, 17TH-CENTURY CHINESE CH'AN (ZEN) MASTER, WRITING IN JAPANESE

Tofu, also called *doufu* and *bean curd*, originated in China, where it became especially popular in vegetarian Buddhist monasteries. First used in tenth-century Japan as a food offered in temple worship, tofu soon graced the tables of shoguns, ruling lords, and their samurai, or military elite. Such reverence for tofu is well deserved, but only when it has been treated with reverential care; the slapdash preparation tofu often receives in the West has given it the reputation of being boring and bland.

- ❖ Tofu is usually available in three forms: *firm*, considered Chinese style; *soft*, considered Japanese style; and *silken*, also Japanese style and having a smooth, custardlike texture. Store firm or soft tofu in the refrigerator immersed in water and change the water daily. Kept this way, it will last for several days, sometimes up to to a week, but that's pushing it. If it smells sour, discard it. Silken tofu can be stored unrefrigerated for long periods of time in the market. It is not a fresh product and is therefore less desirable.

 ## DENSE, CHEWY TOFU

This method imparts a particularly chewy texture to tofu that is ideal for preparing cutlets and fried cubes. It also absorbs marinades and other liquids particularly well. When preparing for cutlets, allow ½ pound (230 g) tofu per person.

1. Cut firm tofu into thick slices. Drain thoroughly, pat dry with a towel, and wrap in cellophane or foil. Freeze.
2. The night before you wish to use it, unwrap the tofu and thaw overnight in a colander. It is important that the excess water drains off or it will be reabsorbed by the tofu.
3. Take each slice between your hands and gently squeeze out the remaining water. Pat dry with paper towels. Proceed with your recipe.

 ## SEITAN

4 to 6 servings

Nothing is really work unless you'd rather be doing something else.
—SIR JAMES BARRIE, *Peter Pan*

When wheat flour is mixed with water, its protein molecules form a tangled web of strands. Kneading the dough causes the molecule strands to disentangle and line up. When the bran and starch are rinsed out, what remains is the dense, chewy protein structure called seitan or wheat gluten. This wonderful product deserves more widespread popularity. Seitan can be prepared in the same amount of time as homemade bread. A mixer or food processor with a kneading attachment makes the process faster and less labor intensive.

STEP ONE

6 cups (900 g) whole wheat   2¼ cups (550 ml) water
   flour   (approximately)

STEP FIVE

Water or vegetable stock   2 tablespoons oil

1. Sift the flour and mix in enough water to form a soft dough.
2. Knead on a floured board for 20 to 30 minutes. Do not cut the time short. The dough should feel very smooth and elastic. If using a food processor or mixer, double the time you would usually knead bread dough.
3. Cover the dough with cold water and soak for 1 hour.
4. Now for the fun! Place the dough in a colander under running lukewarm water (the temperature is for the sake of your hands). Work the dough by breaking off pieces, holding under the tap, and squeezing and pinching to release the starch. The water will become milky as the starch is washed away. Continue working and rinsing until the water becomes almost clear—the process will take about 10 minutes. The remaining dough will feel rubbery and spongy.
5. Gather into a ball. Place in water or vegetable stock to cover and add the oil. Bring to a boil, cover, and simmer for 2 hours. Drain. Store seitan immersed in water in the refrigerator for up to a week. Change the water daily.

Sautéed Tofu, Panir, or Seitan

Many people who want to serve tofu, panir, or seitan mixed with vegetables make the mistake of throwing everything into the skillet at the same time. The result is flavorless, insipid-looking, broken-up bits of tofu or seitan forlornly detracting from the vegetables. The story can have a much happier ending. Tofu, panir, and seitan absolutely *must* be sautéed separately from the other ingredients in the dish. They will maintain their shape, brown very nicely, and create a happy marriage with the other ingredients when added a minute or two before serving. Trust me—the extra step is more than worth the trouble.

A nonstick pan is the best tool for the job. You can use less oil, and the lovely browning stays on the food rather than switching allegiance to the pan. To brown tofu more thoroughly, sprinkle on liquid seasoning while cooking. (If not adding liquid seasoning to tofu, it will appear crusty without browning much.)

STEP ONE

Tofu, panir, or seitan

STEP TWO

Ghee or oil *Minced fresh ginger* (optional)
Pinch of hing (optional) *Liquid seasoning* (optional)

1. Slice or cube the tofu, panir, or seitan. Wipe dry with paper towels (very important).
2. Heat the ghee or oil over medium-high heat in a nonstick skillet or wok. Add the hing, ginger, and tofu or seitan. If desired, sprinkle with liquid seasoning. Cook, stirring only occasionally, until nicely browned all over.

No man can be a competent physician who does not have a complete knowledge of cookery.
                                              —Queen Anne's Chef

 # Cutlets with Cranberry Sauce

8 pieces

These marinated, breaded cutlets can be either baked or fried. Serve with Cranberry Sauce (recipe follows), chutney, salsa, or Nut Gravy, or tuck into a sandwich.

STEP ONE

Eight 2 × 2-inch (5 × 5 cm) *1 teaspoon paprika*
cutlets Dense, Chewy Tofu *½ teaspoon salt (if stock is*
(pp. 207–208), firm panir, or *unsalted))*
seitan (2½ pounds/1.1 kg) *½ cup (120 ml) vegetable stock*

STEP THREE

Fine dry bread crumbs

STEP FOUR

Oil

1. Place the cutlets in a shallow pan. Mix the paprika and salt into the stock and pour over them. Squeeze the cutlets gently to help absorb the marinade. Allow to marinate for 1 hour.
2. Drain the cutlets and gently squeeze out any excess marinade so that they are damp but not dripping wet.
3. Place the bread crumbs or breading mixture in a shallow bowl. Gently dredge each cutlet until thoroughly coated.
4. *To bake:* Preheat the oven to 350°F (180°C). Generously oil a baking sheet. Place the cutlets on the sheet, press gently, then turn over so that the breading is lightly coated with oil. Bake until golden brown, about 30 minutes.
5. *To fry:* Fry on both sides over a medium heat in ¼ inch (6 mm) of oil until the breading is golden. Drain on paper towels.

VARIATION

For a thicker, crispier coating, dip the pieces first in yogurt, buttermilk, or Tempura Batter (pp. 47–48), then dredge in the breading mixture until thoroughly coated.

BREADING WITHOUT BREAD CRUMBS

Instead of coating burgers and other foods with bread crumbs, you can utilize any of the following:

Amaranth
Cornmeal
Farina or semolina
Teff
Coarsely ground whole wheat flour, such as graham flour
Wheat germ mixed with other ingredients (alone it can have a bitter flavor)

 # CRANBERRY SAUCE

3½ cups (840 g)

STEP ONE

1½ cups (310 g) sugar
1½ cups (360 ml) water or
  part orange juice

1 teaspoon finely grated
  orange zest

1 pound (455 g) cranberries (4 cups)

1. Combine the sugar, water or orange juice, and orange zest in a saucepan. Boil for 5 minutes.
2. Add the cranberries and return to a simmer until the skins pop and the berries are tender, 5 to 7 minutes.
3. Chill thoroughly so that the sauce jells slightly.

SCRAMBLED TOFU OR PANIR FOR BRUNCH

 Easy, Vata-balancing, and a satisfying dish that can be served in the same manner as scrambled eggs. Three cups (660 g) mashed tofu or panir (720 ml) will serve 4 people. Sauté in a little ghee or oil with some liquid seasoning until it is thoroughly heated through. To impart a creamy texture, stir in dabs of cream cheese and/or grated cheese and/or sour cream and cook until blended. A more Kapha-balancing addition is puréed cooked cauliflower, which is very tasty in this dish (really!). From there the possibilities are endless. A few to try:

❖ Sautéed vegetables, such as chopped bell peppers, artichoke hearts, or arugula
❖ Chopped green herbs, such as basil, cilantro, sage, or epazote
❖ Maharishi Ayur-Veda churnas or curry spices
❖ A dollop of Salsa Cruda (p. 507)
❖ Cilantro or Mint Chutney (pp. 520–21)

TOFU OR PANIR QUICHE WITH BROCCOLI

One 9-inch (23 cm) quiche—6 servings

After a good dinner one can forgive anybody, even one's own relations.
—OSCAR WILDE

Here is a dish bound to create generous feelings. You can be forgiven for substituting asparagus tips, artichoke hearts, cauliflower, or other vegetables for the broccoli. Serve either hot or at room temperature. For a cheeseless option see the following recipe.

Partially Baked Crust (p. 409)

2½ cups drained crumbled tofu (550 g) or panir (500 g)

STEP THREE

½ cup (115 g) cream cheese,
  at room temperature
1½ cups (150 g) grated Swiss
  or Gruyère cheese

¼ cup (30 g) fine dry bread
  crumbs

STEP FOUR

2 cups (180 g) chopped broccoli
  florets

Salt
Pepper

STEP FIVE

2 tablespoons grated Parmesan cheese (optional)

1. Preheat the oven to 350°F (180°C). Place the crust in the freezer until ready to use.
2. Mash the tofu or panir with a fork so there are no large chunks. However, do not purée it or try to make it completely smooth.
3. Beat the cream cheese until soft and smooth. Mix into the tofu or panir. Add the grated cheese and the bread crumbs.
4. Steam the broccoli until just barely tender, 1 to 2 minutes. Drain well and add to the mixture. Season to taste with salt and pepper.
5. Spoon the filling into the pie shell. Spread evenly and smooth the top. Sprinkle on the Parmesan.
6. Bake until the top of the quiche and the crust are golden brown, about 30 minutes. Allow to stand at room temperature for 10 minutes for the filling to set.

VARIATIONS
  Replace the cream cheese with ricotta.
  Add Miriam's Sofrito (p. 218) or green herbs in Step 3.

 # SAVORY TOFU OR PANIR TART

One 9-inch (23 cm) quiche—6 servings

A tart with a colorful confetti of chopped vegetables.

STEP ONE

½ recipe Pastry Crust (pp. 406–407)

STEP TWO

1 tablespoon ghee or oil
Pinch of hing (optional)
1 tablespoon minced fresh
  ginger
1 cup (110 g) finely chopped
  fennel or celery

½ cup (70 g) finely chopped bell
  peppers (red gives the dish the
  best color)
½ cup (45 g) grated carrots
½ teaspoon salt

STEP THREE

1 cup crumbled tofu (220 g)
  or *panir (210 g)*
1 tablespoon melted ghee or oil

1 teaspoon lemon juice
½ teaspoon salt

STEP FOUR

2 cups crumbled firm tofu
  (440 g), *drained thoroughly,*
  or medium-soft panir (420 g)
⅓ cup (40 g) dry bread crumbs

2 tablespoons minced fresh parsley or
  dill
Salt
Pepper

1. Preheat the oven to 350°F (180°C). Place the crust in the freezer until ready to use.
2. Heat the ghee or oil in a skillet. Add the hing and ginger and sauté over low heat for 1 minute. Add the fennel or celery, bell peppers, carrots, and salt. Cover and cook, stirring occasionally, until tender, about 10 minutes.
3. Meanwhile, combine the tofu or panir with the ghee or oil, lemon juice, and salt in a food processor until completely smooth.
4. Gently toss the puréed mixture with the second amount of crumbled tofu or panir and the bread crumbs, parsley or dill, and sautéed vegetables. Season to taste with salt and pepper.
5. Spoon the filling into the pie shell. Spread evenly and smooth the top. Bake until the crust is lightly browned and the filling is set, about 1 hour. Allow to stand at room temperature for 15 minutes before serving.

A NEW YEAR'S WELL-BEGUN-IS-HALF-DONE LUNCH

Creamy Broccoli Soup (pp. 235–36)
Savory Tofu or Panir Tart
Tossed green salad
Holiday Pudding with Caramel Sauce (pp. 450–51)

TOFU OR SEITAN WITH BEAN THREAD NOODLES AND VEGETABLES

VIETNAM   *4 to 6 servings*

A ginger-scented dish with an unusual blend of textures. Preparation is in three steps: soaking the noodles, frying the tofu or seitan, and sautéing the vegetables. The final assembly takes very little time. A shot of liquid seasoning gives the flavor a boost.

STEP ONE

One 3-ounce package (85 g) bean thread noodles

1 pound (500 g) firm tofu or
    seitan
Oil for frying

STEP TWO

Pinch of hing (optional)
Liquid seasoning (optional)

STEP THREE

3 teaspoons mild-flavored oil
Pinch of hing (optional)
2 tablespoons minced fresh
    ginger
1 cup (115 g) green beans
    cut into small pieces

1 cup carrots (90 g) quartered lengthwise
    and thinly sliced
2 cups (210 g) coarsely chopped
    cabbage
½ bell pepper, coarsely chopped

STEP FOUR

Chopped fresh cilantro
Salt

White pepper

1. Soak the noodles in very hot water until they are soft, about 20 minutes. Drain well and set aside. (Do not do this far in advance or they will stick together.)
2. Slice the tofu or seitan into ¾-inch (2 cm) cubes. Wipe dry with paper towels. Heat the oil in a nonstick skillet or wok. Add the hing and the tofu or seitan and cook over medium-high heat, stirring only occasionally, until lightly browned and crusted. If desired, sprinkle with liquid seasoning during the cooking to brown the tofu. Set aside.
3. Heat the oil in a large wok or skillet over medium-low heat. Add the hing and ginger and sauté for 1 minute. Add the vegetables. Sauté, stirring frequently, until tender.
4. Gently mix in the tofu or seitan, the noodles, and the cilantro. Add salt and pepper to taste.

 # TOFU AND VEGETABLES IN COCONUT MILK

VIETNAM   4 to 6 servings

Traditionally prepared with tofu, this recipe works just as well with seitan. Coconut milk adds a cooling note for Pitta. For a more Thai-oriented flavor, stir in chopped cilantro and fresh basil before serving—Thai basil if you can find it.

STEP ONE

1 pound (500 g) tofu, drained
2 tablespoons mild-flavored oil

Pinch of hing (optional)
Liquid seasoning (optional)

STEP TWO

3 tablespoons mild-flavored oil
Pinch of hing (optional)
2 tablespoons minced fresh ginger
1 cup (100 g) cauliflower cut into
 small pieces

1 cup (100 g) green beans cut into
 1½-inch (4 cm) pieces
½ bell pepper, coarsely chopped
1 cup (105 g) coarsely
 chopped cabbage

STEP THREE

1½ cups (360 ml) Coconut Milk
 (p. 494)
Liquid seasoning or salt

White pepper

1. Slice the tofu into ¾-inch (2 cm) cubes. Wipe dry with paper towels. Heat the oil in a nonstick skillet or wok. Add the hing and tofu and cook over medium-high heat, stirring occasionally, until lightly browned and crusted. If desired, sprinkle with liquid seasoning during the cooking to brown the tofu. Set aside.
2. Heat the second amount of oil in a wok or large skillet. Add the hing and ginger and sauté over medium heat for 1 minute. Add the vegetables. Sauté, stirring constantly, for 5 minutes.
3. Add the coconut milk and a sprinkling of liquid seasoning. Bring to a boil. Cover, reduce the heat, and simmer until the vegetables are tender. Gently stir in tofu. Add liquid seasoning or salt and white pepper to taste.

 # SHEPHERD'S PIE WITH SEITAN

ENGLAND   *4 to 6 servings*

Nourishing comfort food. The presence of potatoes with the seitan makes it a luncheon, not evening, dish. Note that the mashed potatoes must be prepared in advance. Grind the seitan in a food processor or just chop it to bits.

STEP TWO

3 tablespoons ghee, butter, or oil
Pinch of hing (optional)
1 tablespoon minced fresh
 ginger
1 cut (110 g) finely chopped
 fennel or celery

1 cup (140 g) finely chopped bell
 peppers
1 cup (90 g) carrots, quartered
 lengthwise and thinly sliced

STEP THREE

2½ cups (325 g) ground seitan
½ cup (65 g) peas
½ cup (120 g) minced fresh
 parsley

1 tablespoon minced fresh sage
 or ½ teaspoon dried
Salt
Black pepper

STEP FOUR

2½ cups (575 g) Mashed Potatoes
(pp. 123–24)

2 tablespoons grated Parmesan cheese
(optional)

1. Preheat the oven to 350°F (180°C). Oil an 8-inch (22 cm) square baking dish.
2. Heat the ghee, butter, or oil in a large skillet. Add the hing and ginger and sauté over low heat for 1 minute. Add the fennel or celery, bell peppers, and carrots. Cover and sauté, stirring occasionally, until tender.
3. Stir in the seitan, peas, parsley, and sage. Season to taste with salt and pepper.
4. Spoon the mixture into the baking dish and spread evenly. Spread the mashed potatoes evenly over the seitan. Sprinkle with Parmesan if desired.
5. Bake until the top is lightly browned in a few spots, 20 to 30 minutes.

VARIATIONS

Add dried rosemary, basil, and thyme in Step 2.
Add other vegetables, such as zucchini and parsnips, in Step 2.
Replace the seitan with sautéed chopped firm tofu.

Our remedies oft in ourselves do lie,
Which we ascribe to heaven.

—WILLIAM SHAKESPEARE

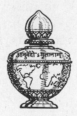

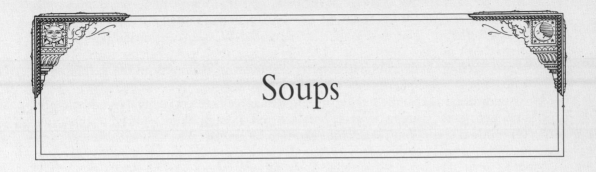

Soups

Only the pure in heart can make a good soup.

—LUDWIG VAN BEETHOVEN

Soup is a very important Ayurvedic food. Maharishi Ayur-Veda recommends making a supper out of soup, as it is both light and nourishing. Its liquid nature makes soup more easily digestible than drier, heavier foods, and many people eat it every evening. After first perfecting one's character as prescribed by the great composer, the second challenge in Ayurvedic vegetarian soup making is coaxing enough flavor out of the ingredients; many beautiful-looking soups prove disappointingly bland. A mistake made by many well-intended cooks is to throw all their good ingredients into a pot of water and boil them up. Good soup? Unfortunately not. Most vegetarian cookbooks rise to the challenge by calling for copious amounts of onions in every recipe. However, aside from Ayurvedic recommendations concerning onions, their flavor is so assertive it can drown out the subtler influences of other ingredients.

❖ Always use fresh, high-quality ingredients. Enlisting the soup pot as a dumping ground for over-the-hill vegetables never works to magically resurrect them.
❖ Peas, greens (such as watercress and arugula) in *small* amounts, and tomatoes (skinned, seeded, and puréed for best texture) add excellent flavor when simmered in soup liquid *without* prior sautéing.
❖ Broccoli, Brussels sprouts, and cauliflower tend to overwhelm soups with their sulphurous flavors, so perhaps you'll want to honor these vegetables in other dishes rather than disgrace them in soup. Also, cabbage can give off a sour flavor if it is cooked much longer than 30 minutes, so time your soup-simmering accordingly.
❖ Liquid seasonings are helpful time-savers for adding flavor. Broth powders made of dried, powdered vegetables and herbs are fine to use in Ayurvedic cooking. They can be found in bulk in natural foods stores. Look for broth powders that

don't contain onions. Flavor alert: Use a light hand with these seasonings—just enough to round out the taste—or all your soups will taste somewhat the same.

❖ Green herbs are almost essential for flavoring Western vegetarian soups. Sauté *dried* herbs in ghee, butter, or oil before adding the stock. Adding them without prior sautéing tends to impart a bitter flavor or no flavor. With the exception of rosemary, stir *fresh* herbs into soup just before serving.

❖ As with dried herbs, the flavors of most vegetables are greatly enhanced by a preliminary gentle sautéing in ghee, butter, or oil. In soup you can achieve this using very little oil; you don't want your broth to be greasy.

 # MIRIAM'S SOFRITO

Here is my Ayurvedic version of the all-purpose, flavor-bestowing *sofrito* or *soffrito* of Latin countries, and the *holy trinity* of New Orleans cooking. It is an excellent soup base as well as a good starting point for creating various stews, gumbos, and other savory dishes. Grated carrots, minced fresh parsley, and chopped tomatoes (added after the vegetables have cooked for a few minutes) also add lovely flavor.

1 tablespoon ghee, butter, or oil
Pinch of hing (optional)
¾ cup (90 g) finely chopped fennel or celery (fennel is preferable)

¾ cup (100 g) finely chopped bell peppers (any color)
1 tablespoon minced fresh ginger

Heat the oil in a small skillet. Add the hing, fennel or celery, bell peppers, and ginger. Cover and cook over very low heat, stirring occasionally, until tender. Add to dishes at the *beginning* of cooking to further cook and blend with the other flavors.

SOUP STOCKS

Soup stocks are a classic method of providing subtle undercurrents that give flavor a head start. When time is of the essence, a shot of liquid seasoning or broth powder in water can provide enough oomph to build on. On the other hand, homemade stocks are fresher tasting and fresher, period, than instant flavorers. Make one when you have the time.

❖ Many people collect the edible vegetable scraps left from preparing the daily meals, such as parsley stems, potato peels, and so forth. They prepare soup stock by simmering them in water until tender and then straining them out. About 2½ cups (600 ml) of scraps flavor 1 quart (1 l) of water. In my experience, unless you are careful to use truly edible scraps, these stocks taste like what they are made from: garbage. Use only your most palatable scraps, and expect the soup ingredients to provide most of the flavor. Also, use vegetable peels only from unsprayed produce.

❖ Diluted fresh vegetable juices make good soup stocks. Try carrot, tomato, or mixed green vegetable juices, mixed at a ratio of 3 to 5 parts water to 1 part juice.

TO THICKEN A THIN STOCK:

❖ Replace part of the broth with cooked vegetable purée.

❖ Add fresh bread crumbs during the last minute or two of cooking. Good-looking they're not, but they taste wonderful.

❖ Cook barley or rice in the soup; their natural starches help thicken the stock, and the grains also absorb the stock and expand.

❖ Beat in a roux during the last few minutes of cooking.

I live on good soup, not fine words.   —MOLIÈRE

 # VEGETABLE STOCK

1 quart (1 l) strained

½ *cup (65 g) peas*	*1 carrot, sliced*
1 stalk celery with leaves, sliced	½ *bell pepper, chopped (any color)*
¼ *cup (60 ml) minced parsley*	*4¼ cups (1 l) water*

Bring all the ingredients to a boil. Cover, reduce the heat, and simmer until the vegetables are tender, about 20 minutes. Either strain out the vegetables or purée them into the stock.

VARIATION

Vegetable Purée Stock: For 1 quart (1 l) of stock, simmer 1½ cups (360 ml) finely cut or grated vegetables, such as peas, carrots, potatoes, turnips, or green beans, in 3½ cups (840 ml) water until the vegetables are tender, about 20 minutes. Purée in a blender in 3 small batches, holding the lid firmly closed with a folded towel. Strain if desired.

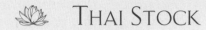

THAI STOCK

THAILAND   *7 cups (1.7 l) unstrained, 6 cups (1.4 l) strained*

This makes good use of the copious cilantro stems that usually get discarded.

6 cups (1.4 l) water
2 cups (230 g) grated daikon
1 cup (90 g) grated carrot

1 cup (240 ml) chopped fresh cilantro
*   stems and leaves*
3 tablespoons minced fresh ginger

Bring all the ingredients to a boil. Cover, reduce the heat, and simmer for 20 minutes. Strain.

CREATING DELICIOUS VEGETABLE SOUPS

Vegetables soups can be served all year long and incorporate whatever vegetables are in season. They are very accommodating to additions.

❖ Grains can be added at the beginning of cooking. Remember that they will swell. One tablespoon of grain per cup of soup stock is sufficient. Allow enough time for the grains to cook, and in the case of grains with lengthy cooking times, cook them first until at least halfway done. In Europe small amounts of semolina and oats are added to soups. These soups are quite thin and bear no resemblance to porridge. Try adding 1 to 2 tablespoons—you'll be pleasantly surprised. Attila the Hun's troops subsisted on oat soup, and what was good enough for Attila. . . .

❖ Add beans, allowing enough time for them to cook. Soak overnight when necessary, and remember that they will expand to 2 to 2½ times their uncooked volume. You can also partially precook them before adding, especially in the case of soups containing acid ingredients, such as tomatoes, which toughen beans.

❖ For added richness, replace part of the stock with nondairy milk—especially coconut milk—or with crème fraîche. Add toward the end of the cooking.

❖ Add pasta or Asian bean thread or rice noodles. Dried pasta can take on a slimy texture when cooked in soup stock. Try the Persian method of toasting noodles in a 350°F (180°C) oven, stirring frequently, or sautéing slowly in ghee or oil for a few minutes until golden before adding them to soup.

VEGETABLE SOUP WITH LEMON PISTOU

About 7 cups (1.7 l)

A recipe is only a theme, which an intelligent cook can play each time with a variation.   —MADAME BENOIT

A good basic vegetable soup for lunch or dinner that can be varied in hundreds of ways.

STEP ONE

2 tablespoons ghee or oil
Pinch of hing (optional)
¼ cup (60 ml) minced fresh
    parsley

¼ teaspoon dried rosemary
½ teaspoon dried basil
1 bay leaf

STEP TWO

1 tomato, chopped
    (optional)

4 to 5 cups (940–1200 ml) thinly
    sliced mixed vegetables

STEP THREE

6 cups (1.4 l) stock or water
Salt

Black pepper

1. Melt the ghee or oil in a soup pot. Add the hing and herbs and sauté over low heat for 1 minute.
2. Add the tomato and mixed vegetables. Sauté over low heat for another 5 to 10 minutes.
3. Add the stock or water to the vegetables. Bring to a boil. Cover, reduce the heat, and simmer for 45 to 60 minutes. Season to taste with salt and pepper. Remove the bay leaf before serving. Pass Lemon Pistou (recipe follows) at the table.

 # LEMON PISTOU

FRANCE   *⅔ cup (260 g)*

A variation on a soup garnish from southern France. Its flavors are different but equal with or without cheese. Replace some of the parsley with fresh oregano for a different flavor.

1 cup (240 ml) minced fresh
    parsley
1 cup (240 ml) minced fresh basil
1 tablespoon lemon zest (optional)

4 to 5 tablespoons olive oil
Up to ½ cup (50 g) grated Parmesan
    cheese (optional)
Salt

Use the lesser amount of olive oil when not including the Parmesan. Blend everything together—a food processor works well. If not using cheese, add salt to taste.

Broccoli-Potato Soup

UNITED STATES   *10 cups (2.4 liters)*

An east Texas–style, Kapha-balancing lunchtime soup from a recipe idea by Chris Soth. Use a flavorful stock for best results. You can also stir in an herb pesto, Lemon Pistou, or minced green herbs after cooking.

STEP ONE

¼ cup (55 g) ghee
Pinch of hing (optional)
½ green bell pepper, coarsely chopped

½ cup (120 ml) coarsely chopped fresh parsley
4 cups (400 g) coarsely chopped broccoli

STEP TWO

3 medium potatoes, peeled and cut into chunks

5 cups (1.2 l) vegetable stock

STEP THREE

Salt
Black pepper

Sour cream (optional)

1. Melt the ghee in a soup pot over a low heat. Add the hing, bell pepper, parsley, and broccoli, and sauté for 7 to 10 minutes, stirring frequently.
2. Add the potatoes and stock. Bring to a boil. Cover, reduce the heat, and simmer until the vegetables are tender, about 30 minutes.
3. Blend the soup in 3 batches in the blender, holding the lid tightly shut with a folded towel. Season to taste with salt and pepper. Serve with a dollop of sour cream if desired.

VARIATION

Broccoli Vichysoisse: For adding a Pitta-balancing influence, replace 2 cups (500 ml) stock with coconut milk. For more balance to Vata, stir in ½ cup (120 ml) crème fraîche or sour cream. Cool to room temperature. Strain and garnish with fresh minced tarragon.

Minestrone

ITALY   *9 cups (1.9 l)*

M. F. K. Fisher aptly advises, "There is no point in doing much else, the night you make Minestrone, because nobody will eat anything else, anyway. Save your tarts for a leaner hungrier night." *Minestra, minestrina, minestrone*—all simply mean "soup" and are closely related to the words *minister* and *administer*, cloaked with meanings of beneficent service. Note that the beans must be soaked and cooked in advance. Pass Lemon Pistou at the table for more flavor.

STEP ONE

¼ cup (50 g) dried garbanzo
   beans (chickpeas)

¼ cup (45 g) dried kidney beans

STEP THREE

8 cups (2.4 l) Vegetable
   Stock (p. 219)
2 cups (460 g) chopped
   tomatoes (optional)

1 bay leaf

STEP FOUR

2 tablespoons olive oil
Pinch of hing (optional)
½ teaspoon dried basil

½ teaspoon dried thyme
¼ teaspoon fresh or dried
   rosemary

STEP FIVE

½ cup (50 g) shredded cabbage or
   spinach
½ cup (60 g) sliced green beans

1 carrot, sliced
1 zucchini, quartered
   lengthwise and thinly sliced
½ bell pepper, chopped

STEP SEVEN

½ cup (65 g) peas
1 cup (110 g) small uncooked
   pasta shapes, such as macaroni
   or fusilli

Salt
Black pepper

1. Clean the beans. Place in a bowl with at least 3 cups (700 ml) of water and soak overnight.
2. Drain the beans. Place in a saucepan with 1 quart (1 l) fresh water. Bring to a boil, reduce the heat, and simmer for 1 hour. Drain again.
3. Place the stock, tomatoes, and bay leaf in a soup pot and bring to a boil. Add the beans and reduce to a simmer.
4. Heat the olive oil in a wok or large skillet. Add the hing, basil, thyme, and rosemary and sauté over low heat for 1 minute.
5. Add all the vegetables listed for Step 5. Sauté for another 5 minutes.
6. Add the vegetable mixture to the stock. Cover the soup and simmer for 1½ hours.
7. Add the peas and pasta. Simmer for 10 to 15 minutes more. Season to taste with salt and pepper.

In the Persian tradition, sharing a bowl of soup with someone is a bond of friendship. So important is soup in Persia that the Farsi word for cook is *ashe-paz*, "soup-maker," and a kitchen, *ashe-paz khaneh*, is literally "a room where soup is cooked."

 ## BARLEY SOUP

About 6 cups (1.4 l)

A hearty European peasant soup for which a flavorful stock is essential. Add a sprinkling of vegetable broth powder or liquid seasoning for best results. I use both.

STEP ONE

2 tablespoons ghee or butter	*½ teaspoon dried basil*
¼ cup (60 ml) minced fresh parsley	*Pinch of hing* (optional)
	½ medium bell pepper, chopped
¼ teaspoon fresh or dried rosemary	*1 stalk celery with leaves, sliced*
	1 carrot, grated

STEP TWO

5 cups (1.2 l) vegetable stock	*1 bay leaf*
¼ cup (40 g) barley	*Salt*
1 turnip, cut into small pieces	*Black pepper*

1. Melt the ghee or butter in a soup pot. Add the parsley, rosemary, basil, hing, bell pepper, celery, and carrot and sauté over low heat for 10 minutes.
2. Add the stock to the vegetables. Add the barley, turnip, and bay leaf. Bring to a boil. Cover, reduce the heat, and simmer until the barley is very tender, 1½ to 2 hours. Season to taste with salt and pepper.

 ## SHCHI (CABBAGE SOUP)

RUSSIA/EASTERN EUROPE   *About 7 cups (1.7 l)*

[Shchi is] quite drinkable . . . though it contained some sour element, which perhaps is necessary for Russian palates. Proper accompaniment should be a jug of sour cream to be stirred into it. —LEWIS CARROLL, *Journal of a Tour in Russia*

At one time Shchi was a staple meal in Russia. Additional ingredients depended on desire, availability, and the prosperity of the household. (So what else is new?) I've given a recipe for the simplest *vegetariansky* version, and some of the things you can add are listed in the Variations.

A flavorful stock is essential to this good, simple soup. Serve Shchi with rye or pumpernickel bread.

STEP ONE

3 tablespoons ghee or butter
Pinch of hing (optional)

2½ to 3 cups (260 to 315 g) shredded
green cabbage

STEP TWO

5 cups (1.2 l) vegetable stock
Chopped fresh dill
Salt

Black pepper
Sour cream

1. Melt the ghee or butter in a soup pot. Add the hing and cabbage and sauté over low heat for 5 to 7 minutes, stirring frequently.
2. Add the stock and bring to a boil. Cover, reduce the heat, and simmer until the cabbage is tender, about 30 minutes. Season to taste with dill, salt, and pepper. Pass a bowl of sour cream at the table.

VARIATIONS

You can add many other vegetables, particularly greens such as sorrel, or root vegetables such as carrots, beets, potatoes, and turnips.

One traditional addition is a handful of short, flat noodles, thrown in for the last 10 to 15 minutes of simmering.

Add a handful of toasted kasha, white rice, or cooked barley in Step 2.

Add cooked white beans before serving.

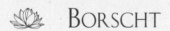 # BORSCHT

UKRAINE/RUSSIA   *About 7 cups (1.7 l)*

Borscht, the center of everything.   —UKRAINIAN SAYING

Borscht can be either simple or complex—Ukrainian-style borscht can contain upward of twenty different ingredients. In the United States, Borscht is strongly associated with Jewish cooking. However, as the old Hebrew proverb goes, "In matters of taste and smell, don't argue," and millions of non-Jewish Russians and eastern Europeans inarguably claim Borscht as part of their own culinary heritage.

STEP ONE

5 cups (1.2 l) water or vegetable
  stock
¼ cup (60 ml) lemon juice
1 tablespoon sugar
1 bay leaf

2½ cups (600 g) grated beets
1 stalk celery, sliced
1 tomato, chopped
1 large potato, cubed
1 cup (100 g) shredded cabbage

STEP TWO

Salt
Black pepper
Sour cream

Minced fresh parsley or dill
  (optional)

1. Combine all the ingredients in a soup pot. Simmer, covered, until all the vegetables
   are tender, 40 to 60 minutes.
2. Season to taste with salt and pepper. Remove the bay leaf before serving. Serve
   with a spoonful of sour cream in each bowl. Garnish with a sprinkling of parsley
   or dill.

VARIATIONS

Beet Borscht: Omit the cabbage, potato, and pepper and add ½ cup (45 g) more
grated beets. Serve the finished soup either hot or at room temperature with sour cream.
For a wild magenta color, blend sour cream into cold borscht.

Spicy Borscht: Add 1 teaspoon toasted cumin seeds, ⅛ teaspoon ground cloves, and
½ teaspoon ground cinnamon toward the end of cooking.

> *I believe it is one of the best soups in the world. It can be hot, cold, thick, thin,
> rich, meager—and still be good. It can be easy or intricate to make.*
>
> —M. F. K. FISHER, ON BORSCHT

POTAGE ST. GERMAIN

FRANCE   *About 6 cups (1.4 l)*

This delightful summertime puréed soup of peas and other vegetables can be served
either hot or at room temperature, omitting the ghee for the room temperature version.

STEP ONE

3 cups (390 g) peas
2 tablespoons ghee
2½ cups (600 ml) vegetable stock
  or water
¼ cup (30 g) thinly sliced radishes

2 cups (180 g) packed shredded
  lettuce
1 celery stalk with leaves, sliced
¼ cup (60 ml) minced fresh parsley

STEP THREE	
1 teaspoon crumbled dried mint or 2 tablespoons minced fresh	Salt White pepper
½ cup (120 ml) crème fraîche or sour cream	

1. Bring all the ingredients for Step 1 to a boil in a medium saucepan. Cover, reduce the heat, and simmer until the vegetables are tender, about 15 minutes.
2. Purée the soup in a blender until smooth. Do this in 2 or 3 batches, holding the lid tightly shut with a folded towel. Return to the pot.
3. Add the mint and crème fraîche or sour cream. Heat to serving temperature. Season to taste with salt and white pepper.

PUMPKIN SOUP

1 quart (1 l)

Pumpkin soup can be prepared from any winter squash. Butternut and kabocha squashes have particularly attractive colors.

2⅔ cups (615 g) puréed cooked pumpkin	2 tablespoons ghee or butter
2 cups (500 ml) nondairy milk	1½ tablespoons raw or brown sugar
¼ teaspoon ground ginger	Salt

Combine the pumpkin, nondairy milk, and ginger in a blender. Pour into a medium saucepan. Add the ghee or butter and the sugar and bring to a boil. Add salt to taste.

VARIATION
    Curried Pumpkin Soup: Omit the ginger. Add ¾ to 1 teaspoon curry powder.

TORTILLA SOUP (SOPA DE TORTILLA)

MEXICO   *7 cups (1.7 l)*

A hearty one-dish lunch idea from Georgina Wilson. In Mexico the first step is to pat out fresh tortillas by hand and set them on the roof to dry in the tropical sun. For those preparing the soup on a freezing January day in Iowa, I've included two options: drying fresh tortillas in the oven or using purchased tortilla chips, which reduce the total preparation time considerably.

STEP ONE

8 ounces (230 g) tortilla chips or   Oil for deep-frying
  8 fresh corn tortillas,   (if using fresh tortillas)
  cut into 1-inch (2.5 cm) strips

STEP TWO

1 tablespoon ghee or   4 cups (1 l) vegetable stock or water
  mild-flavored oil   1 teaspoon epazote (optional)
Pinch of hing (optional)   3 medium potatoes, peeled and diced

STEP THREE

2 tomatoes   ½ cup (120 ml) water

STEP FIVE

1 cup (240 ml) loosely packed   Salt
  chopped fresh cilantro   Black pepper

STEP SIX

¾ cup (180 ml) crème fraîche or sour   Grated Monterey Jack cheese
  cream   Avocado slices

To prepare fresh tortilla strips:
1. Preheat the oven to 350°F (180°C). Spread the tortilla strips on a cookie sheet. Toast in the oven until crisp, about 10 minutes. Heat oil at least 1-inch (2.5 cm) deep in a pot. Have a tray covered with paper towels nearby. Fry the tortilla strips until golden brown. Drain on paper towels.

To prepare the soup:
2. Heat the ghee or oil in a large soup pot over medium heat. Add the hing and sauté until fragrant, about 30 seconds. Add the stock or water, epazote, and diced potatoes.
3. Purée the tomatoes with the water in a blender or food processor. Add to the soup.
4. Bring the soup to a boil. Stir in the tortilla strips or chips. Cover, reduce the heat, and simmer until the potatoes are tender, about 15 minutes.
5. Purée the soup with the cilantro in a blender or food processor. It should have the texture of thin porridge. Thin with stock or water if necessary. Season to taste with salt and pepper.
6. Garnish each bowl of soup with crème fraîche or sour cream, a sprinkling of grated cheese, and avocado slices.

VARIATION
Grill poblano chilies on the stovetop and serve 1 chili on the side of each soup bowl.

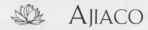

AJIACO

COLOMBIA　　　*8 cups (1.9 l)*

A vegetarian version of the traditional soup. In Colombia it is made with a green herb called *guasca*.

STEP ONE

2 tablespoons ghee, butter, or oil
Pinch of hing (optional)

1 teaspoon cumin seeds
½ cup (120 ml) minced fresh parsley

STEP TWO

3 cups (700 ml) vegetable stock

4 medium potatoes, peeled and diced

STEP THREE

2 ears corn, shucked and cut into 1-inch (2.5 cm) pieces

STEP FOUR

1 cup (240 ml) coarsely chopped
　fresh cilantro
¼ cup (60 ml) water
Salt

Black pepper
Crème fraîche or sour cream
Avocado slices

1. Melt the ghee, butter, or oil in a large soup pot over low heat. Add the hing, cumin seeds, and parsley and sauté for 1 minute, stirring constantly, until the spices are fragrant.
2. Add the vegetable stock and potatoes. Bring to a boil. Cover, reduce the heat, and simmer until the potatoes are tender, about 15 minutes. Lightly mash the potatoes into the stock, leaving some texture.
3. Add the corn pieces. Simmer until tender, about 5 minutes.
4. Purée the cilantro in the water. Stir into the soup. The soup should be thick but not like a porridge. Thin with stock or water if necessary. Season to taste with salt and pepper. Garnish with crème fraîche or sour cream and avocado slices. Serve immediately.

SIZZLING RICE SOUP (GUO BA TANG)

CHINA　　　*4 to 6 servings*

Ayurveda states that good food stimulates all the senses. Here is one dish where the sense of hearing is the most important! The drama of sizzling rice soup is its presentation. The last steps are performed at the table, where a just-fried rice crust is dropped into the soup, eliciting a sizzling noise as the oil meets the stock. The Chinese say it should sound "like the chirping of birds." It's cooking as theater. Note that the rice crust must be prepared at least 4 hours ahead of the soup.

STEP ONE

⅔ cup (140 g) white rice   *1⅔ cups (400 ml) water*

STEP FOUR

1 cup (75 g) mung sprouts   *5 cups (1.2 l) vegetable stock (must*
½ cup (100 g) snow peas   *be very flavorful)*

STEP FIVE

Oil for deep-frying

To prepare the rice crust:
1. Preheat the oven to 250°F (120°C). Bring the rice and water to a boil. Cover, reduce the heat, and simmer for 10 minutes.
2. Spread out in a thin layer—about 2 grains deep—on a buttered pan. Bake for 1 hour.
3. Allow to stand and dry for a few hours, preferably in the sun.

To prepare the soup:
4. Shortly before serving, simmer the vegetables in the stock for 5 minutes.
5. Break the rice crust into pieces. Heat the oil for deep-frying and have a platter covered with paper towels nearby.
6. Place the soup in a tureen ready for serving and have another bowl ready to receive the rice crust.

To assemble:
7. Drop the rice crust into the oil. Call the diners to the table.
8. Deep-fry the rice crust until just a hint of browning appears. Drain on the paper towels for a second and then transfer to the bowl.
9. Immediately bring the rice crust and the soup to the table. With one swoop, drop the rice crust into the soup and savor the sizzle.

The legend goes that Emperor Chien Lung, while traveling in the countryside, repaired to an inn and imperially commanded a bowl of soup for his repast. Mealtime was over, and only a bit of crusted rice remained in the bottom of the pot. The resourceful innkeeper quickly prepared a simple broth and set it before the emperor, then fried up the rice crust and dropped it in. Chien Lung was delighted, the innkeeper relieved, and a stellar dish was born.

COLD SOUPS

According to Ayurveda, chilled foods inhibit digestion, and it is healthier to keep foods more within body temperature range. Therefore, Ayurvedic "cold" soups are actually room temperature or even lukewarm, as opposed to hot. Besides the following recipes, you can serve Potage St. Germain and Beet Borscht as cold soups. Do not use butter to make cold soups. It can harden, lending an unpleasant texture and lumpy appearance.

AVOCADO SOUP

IVORY COAST   *1 quart (1 l)*

A rich, cold soup from a land that seasonally overflows with purplish-skinned avocados.

2 cups (440 g) mashed ripe avocado   1 cup (240 ml) nondairy milk
   (about 2 large avocados)   Seasoned salt
¼ cup (60 ml) lime juice   White pepper
1½ cups (360 ml) cooled vegetable   Chopped fresh cilantro (optional)
   stock

Combine the avocado, lime juice, and stock in a blender. Add the nondairy milk and blend again. Season to taste with seasoned salt, white pepper, and chopped cilantro.

 # CUCUMBER-BEET SOUP

A little over 1 quart (1 l)

Very refreshing, with a complex, subtle mélange of flavors. If using fresh herbs, you may want to add more than the suggested amount, or garnish the soup with a chiffonade of dill and mint.

STEP ONE

1 cup (95 g) grated peeled beets

STEP TWO

2 cups (380 g) grated peeled   Salt
   cucumbers

STEP THREE

3 cups (700 ml) buttermilk   1 tablespoon minced fresh
½ cup (120 ml) sour cream   or ½ teaspoon finely crumbled
2 teaspoons sugar   dried mint
½ tablespoon minced fresh   Salt
   ginger   White pepper
1 tablespoon minced fresh
   or ½ teaspoon dried dill

1. Steam the beets until tender. Drain well, pressing out the excess water.
2. While the beets are cooking, toss the cucumbers with a sprinkling of salt and set in a colander to drain for 10 minutes. Squeeze out the juice.

3. Beat the buttermilk and sour cream with a whisk until smooth. Add the beets, cucumbers, sugar, ginger, dill, and mint. Season to taste with salt and white pepper.

4. Purée half of the soup in a blender. Mix with the unblended soup.

 ## Sorrel Soup

NORTHEASTERN EUROPE/RUSSIA   *7 cups (1.7 l)*

Called *schav* by Ashkenazic Jews, sorrel soup is uniquely tart. My mother would nostalgically describe the "sour grass soup" of her New York childhood, but alas, in my California childhood the requisite green was nowhere to be found. Sorrel soup can be served either hot or cold; I confess to preferring its sourness in a cold brew. Be sure to use a flavorful stock. Sorrel leaves should be bunched up and sliced crosswise into thin strips to cook without becoming stringy.

STEP ONE

*2 tablespoons mild-flavored
   oil (or ghee if serving hot)*
Pinch of hing

1 cup (110 g) finely chopped celery
*½ cup (70 g) finely chopped green
   bell peppers*

STEP TWO

1 quart (1 l) vegetable stock
*8 cups (720 g) loosely packed
   shredded sorrel*

*½ cup (120 ml) chopped flat-leaf
   parsley*

STEP THREE

*1 cup (240 ml) crème fraîche or
   sour cream*
Salt

Black pepper
2 teaspoons sugar (optional)

1. Heat the oil in a soup pot. Add the hing and sauté over low heat until fragrant, about 30 seconds. Add the celery and bell peppers. Cover and cook very slowly, stirring occasionally, until almost tender, about 10 minutes.

2. Add the stock, sorrel, and parsley. Bring to a boil. Cover, reduce the heat, and simmer for 30 minutes.

3. Uncover and allow to cool for a few minutes if serving hot, or let cool to room temperature if serving cold. Purée in two batches in a blender with the crème fraîche or sour cream. Return to the pot and season to taste with salt and pepper. If you wish to cut the sourness a little, add the sugar.

VARIATIONS

Replace up to half the sorrel with mild-flavored greens, such as spinach or chard.

For the Russian version, boil, peel, and dice 2 potatoes and add to the finished soup. Garnish with thinly sliced peeled cucumbers, and pass more crème fraîche or sour cream at the table.

FRUIT SOUP (SØTSUPPE)

NORWAY/SCANDINAVIA   *About 1 quart (1 l)*

Fruit soups, originally from Scandinavia, are served as light meals or for dessert. Fruit soups can be varied considerably depending on the types of fruit you employ. You can use one type of fruit alone, or a mixed batch. Here is a general recipe:

STEP ONE

3 cups (700 ml) peeled, sliced mixed fruits (cherries, plums, mangoes, melons, apricots, peaches, seedless grapes, small amounts of berries)	1 cup (240 ml) water ¼ cup (60 ml) lemon juice

STEP THREE

1 teaspoon arrowroot or cornstarch 2 tablespoons water	¼ cup (50 g) sugar (approximate— adjust to the fruits)

STEP FOUR

1 cup (150 g) halved pitted cherries or sliced strawberries	Whipped cream, sour cream, crème fraîche, or yogurt

1. Purée the fruits, water, and lemon juice in a blender or food processor.
2. Place in a medium saucepan, bring to a boil, and then reduce the heat. Simmer until the fruit is tender, 10 to 20 minutes.
3. Mix the arrowroot or cornstarch with the water until smooth. Add to the soup, beating with a whisk to avoid lumps. Stir and simmer for 2 minutes. Stir in the sugar and adjust to taste. Let cool to room temperature.
4. Add the cherries or strawberries just before serving. Serve with spoonfuls of whipped cream, sour cream, crème fraîche, or yogurt.

CREAM SOUPS

Of all items on the menu, soup is that which extracts the most delicate perfection and the strictest attention.   —AUGUSTE ESCOFFIER

Cream soups are traditionally made by combining puréed vegetables with cream and stock and thickening them with a roux. However, Ayurveda does not recommend mixing dairy milk with any taste other than sweet. (See "The Six Tastes," pp. 27–28). Both the salt and the bitter taste in most vegetables are therefore incompatible with milk. Fortunately, there are nontraditional methods of making cream soups that are equally, if not more, delicious and are also kinder to your body.

❖ Prepare cream soups using nondairy milk, such as soy milk, Nut Milk, or diluted coconut milk. You can also blend nuts and coconut into the soup stock with the vegetables and strain out, rather than preparing Nut Milk separately.

❖ Prepare luncheon cream soups with vegetable stock, replacing ½ cup (120 ml) stock in a recipe for 4 to 6 servings with crème fraîche, sour cream, or buttermilk. Whisk the dairy into soup just before serving. Do not boil, or the dairy will curdle. Crème fraîche has the least sour flavor and will not separate when heated.

❖ Sauté vegetables very, very slowly in a covered pot with a large amount of ghee (a technique that goes by the inelegant cooking term *sweating*), then purée with a small amount of vegetable stock or nondairy milk, gradually adding more until the desired texture is achieved. The ghee substitutes for cream, making the soup rich and smooth.

❖ Sweat vegetables as above, or steam them. Purée with cooked rice or a peeled cooked sweet potato or white potato to thicken the soup, adding nondairy milk or vegetable stock until the desired texture is achieved.

❖ *Flour-free and oil-free cream soups:* In addition to the methods described above, omit the flour and/or ghee or oil from a roux-thickened cream soup recipe for 4 to 6 servings, and mix 1½ tablespoons arrowroot or cornstarch into the unheated soup liquid. Add to the soup and heat slowly, stirring constantly, until thickened. Do not boil.

❧ CLASSIC CREAM OF ASPARAGUS SOUP

About 5 cups

Here is a basic recipe for an Ayurvedic take on the classical construction of a cream soup. The variations give you many options for other soups. You may wish to add a sprinkling of broth powder for more flavor; liquid seasoning alters the subtle color.

STEP ONE

1 pound (500 g) asparagus

STEP TWO

3½ cups (840 ml) nondairy milk

STEP THREE

3 tablespoons ghee or butter   *3 tablespoons flour*
Pinch of hing (optional)

STEP FOUR

Salt   *White pepper* (optional)

1. Steam the asparagus until just barely tender. Drain. Slice off the tips and reserve.
2. Purée the stalks with the nondairy milk in a blender. Strain. Discard the pulp.

3. Melt the ghee or butter in a medium saucepan. Add the hing and sauté over low heat until fragrant, about 30 seconds. Add the flour and cook for 1 minute, stirring constantly with a whisk.

4. Slowly add the asparagus purée, stirring constantly. Heat the soup to a simmer, stirring constantly. Add the asparagus tips. Add salt and, if desired, white pepper to taste.

VARIATIONS

Cream of Celery or Fennel Soup: Fennel is Vata and Pitta balancing, and celery balances Pitta and Kapha. Replace the asparagus with 1½ cups (175 g) finely chopped celery or fennel, ½ teaspoon dried thyme, and ½ teaspoon dried basil. Sauté with the hing in Step 3 until tender before adding the flour.

Cream of Spinach or Watercress (or Arugula or Chard) Soup: More Kapha balancing, and chard will balance Pitta as well. Replace the asparagus with 3 cups (285 g) washed, dried, packed spinach or watercress and a pinch of nutmeg. Skip Step 1; blend with the nondairy milk in Step 2. Do not strain (in any sense of the word). If you desire more texture, blend briefly until the leaves are just chopped.

Cream of Cauliflower Soup: More Kapha balancing. Replace the asparagus with 1⅔ cups (175 g) finely chopped cauliflower. Sauté in ghee until tender in Step 3 before adding the flour. Add ¼ teaspoon paprika, or add curry powder or Maharishi Ayur-Veda churnas to the finished soup.

Cream of Corn Soup: A more Kapha-balanced soup. Omit the asparagus and steps up to Step 3. Add 2 cups (300 g) corn kernels and the nondairy milk in Step 4. Simmer for 3 to 4 minutes until the corn is tender. Stir in 2 tablespoons minced flat-leaf parsley or cilantro.

 # CREAMY BROCCOLI SOUP

7 cups (1.7 l)

This intensely flavored soup, thickened and flavored with vegetables alone, makes good use of broccoli stalks. I save up stalks that would otherwise be discarded over a week, then prepare a big pot of soup. It's important to peel the stalks before cooking; otherwise, they will jam up your sieve when you strain the purée. Broccoli is balancing to Kapha, and the ghee adds balance for Vata and Pitta.

STEP ONE

⅓ cup (75 g) ghee	1 green bell pepper, sliced
Pinch of hing (optional)	1 cup (110 g) sliced fennel or celery
6 cups (660 g) chopped broccoli	½ teaspoon salt

STEP TWO

4 cups (940 ml) vegetable stock

STEP FOUR

Vegetable stock (if needed)   Salt
1 to 2 teaspoons sugar   Black pepper

STEP FIVE

1½ cups (130 g) tiny broccoli   ¼ cup (60 ml) minced fresh
  florets (optional)   parsley
2 teaspoons ghee or butter
  (optional)

1. Melt the ghee in a large soup pot. Add the hing, broccoli, bell pepper, fennel or celery, and salt. Stir, cover, and cook over very low heat until the vegetables are completely tender, 30 to 40 minutes. Stir occasionally.
2. Purée the vegetables very thoroughly with the stock in a blender or food processor. The smoother the mixture is, the easier the next step will be.
3. Place a large sieve over the soup pot. Strain the mixture through it, stirring and pressing with the back of a large spoon. Scrape the underside of the sieve periodically. Do not skip this step! It is essential for a creamy texture. In the end, there should remain a small amount of fibrous material that pulls away from the sieve. Discard it.
4. Heat the soup to serving temperature. Thin with more stock if necessary. Season to taste with the sugar, salt, and pepper.
5. For added texture, if desired, sauté the broccoli florets in the ghee or butter over low heat, stirring frequently, until tender. Stir into the finished soup with the minced parsley.

VARIATIONS

For a very smooth and creamy—and scrumptious—soup, increase the ghee in Step 1 to 1 cup (230 g).

Replace the vegetable stock with nondairy milk.

CREAMY GINGERED CARROT SOUP
WITH OR WITHOUT WILD RICE

7 cups (1.7 l)

Subtle accents of ginger and orange make this Vata-balancing soup unique. Wild rice adds a Kapha-balancing influence, plus color, texture, and flavor that complement the suave mixture and make it worthy of the grandest occasions.

STEP ONE (OPTIONAL)

1½ cups (360 ml) water   *⅓ cup (60 g) wild rice*

STEP TWO

⅓ cup (75 g) ghee or butter   *6 cups (720 g) sliced carrots*
Pinch of hing (optional)   *1½ cups (175 g) thinly sliced*
2 tablespoons minced fresh   *celery*
  ginger   *½ teaspoon salt*

STEP THREE

4 cups (950 ml) vegetable stock   *½ cup (120 ml) orange juice*

STEP FIVE

Vegetable stock (if needed)   *Salt*
1 to 2 teaspoons sugar   *White pepper*

1. *To prepare the optional wild rice:* Bring the water to a boil. Stir in the wild rice. Cover, reduce the heat, and simmer until the water is absorbed and the rice is tender, 50 to 60 minutes.
2. Melt the ghee or butter in a large soup pot. Add the hing, ginger, carrots, celery, and salt. Stir, cover, and cook over a very low heat until the vegetables are very tender, 30 to 40 minutes.
3. Purée the vegetables, stock, and orange juice very thoroughly in a blender or food processor. The smoother the mixture is, the easier the next step will be.
4. Place a large sieve over the soup pot. Strain the mixture through it, stirring and pressing with the back of a large spoon. Scrape the underside of the sieve periodically. Do not skip this step! It is essential for a creamy mixture. In the end, there should remain a small amount of fibrous material that pulls away from the sieve. Discard it.
5. Heat the soup to serving temperature. Thin with more stock if necessary. Season to taste with the sugar, salt, and white pepper.

VARIATION

For a very smooth and creamy texture, use up to 1 cup (230 g) of ghee or butter in Step 2.

CREAMY CAULIFLOWER SOUP WITH ALMONDS

7 cups (1.7 l)

You can use toasted cashews, pecans, or other nuts instead of almonds. You can also omit the nuts entirely and still have a tasty soup.

STEP ONE

¼ cup (60 ml) ghee
Pinch of hing (optional)

6 cups (630 g) coarsely chopped
*   cauliflower*
½ teaspoon salt

STEP TWO

1 medium sweet potato or white potato

STEP THREE

1½ cups (210 g) blanched almonds,
*   toasted*

5 cups (1.2 l) vegetable stock

STEP SIX

Vegetable stock, if needed
Salt

White pepper

1. Melt the ghee in a large soup pot. Add the hing, cauliflower, and salt. Stir, cover, and cook over very low heat until the cauliflower is tender, 30 to 40 minutes. Stir occasionally.
2. While the cauliflower is cooking, boil the potato in water to cover until tender. Drain and peel when cool enough to handle.
3. Blend the almonds thoroughly into the stock. For a completely smooth soup, strain through a sieve lined with a clean muslin cloth. Squeeze all the liquid out of the almond meal.
4. Purée the cauliflower and potato thoroughly with the almond milk in a blender or food processor. The smoother the mixture is, the easier the next step will be.
5. Place a large sieve over the soup pot. Strain the mixture through it, stirring and pressing with the back of a large spoon. Scrape the underside of the sieve periodically. Do not skip this step! It is essential for a creamy texture. In the end, there should remain a small amount of fibrous material that pulls away from the sieve. Discard it.
6. Heat the soup to serving temperature. Thin with more stock if necessary. Season to taste with salt and white pepper.

VARIATIONS

Replace the cauliflower with broccoli or other vegetables.
Garnish with Sweet Red Pepper Purée (p. 513).
Replace the potato with ⅓ cup (70 g) rice, simmered in the stock until tender, about 20 minutes.

Corn Chowder

4 to 6 servings

The day has the color and sound of winter. Thoughts turn to chowder.
Chowder breathes reassurance. It steams consolation.

—Clementine Paddleford

Chowder was originally a stew from Brittany that often featured crème fraîche and was cooked in a pot called a *chaudière*. The translation on America's eastern seaboard is usually made with milk and, in the Ayurvedic translation, with either nondairy milk or the original Breton ingredient.

STEP ONE

1 potato

STEP TWO

1 tablespoon ghee or butter
Pinch of *hing* (optional)
1 carrot, thinly sliced
1 stalk celery, sliced
½ teaspoon dried thyme

½ teaspoon dried basil
⅛ teaspoon dried or fresh
  rosemary
2 tablespoons minced fresh
  parsley

STEP THREE

2 large tomatoes, chopped

STEP FOUR

3 tablespoons ghee or butter
¼ cup (35 g) flour

3½ cups (840 ml) nondairy milk

STEP FIVE

2½ cups (375 g) corn kernels
½ teaspoon paprika

Salt
Black pepper

1. Boil the potato until tender. Drain. When cool enough to handle, peel and cut into chunks.
2. While the potato cooks, melt the ghee or butter in a skillet. Add the hing, carrot, celery, and herbs and sauté over low heat for 5 minutes, stirring frequently.
3. Add the tomatoes and cook until the vegetables are tender, 5 minutes or more.
4. Melt the second amount of ghee or butter in a medium saucepan. Add the flour and cook for 1 minute over low heat, stirring constantly with a whisk. Slowly add the nondairy milk. Beat with the whisk to remove any lumps.
5. Add the sautéed vegetables, potato, corn, and paprika. Bring to a simmer, stirring constantly. Simmer until the corn is tender and the soup is thickened, 3 to 4 minutes. Season to taste with salt and pepper.

VARIATION

Replace the nondairy milk with 3 cups (700 ml) vegetable stock or water. Stir ½ cup (120 ml) crème fraîche into the finished soup.

 # VELVET VEGETABLE SOUP

A little over 6 cups (1.4 l)

Different vegetables and herbs completely change the flavor of this soup. It is the cooking method—a royally slow simmering in ghee—that creates the soup's unforgettable flavor and texture.

STEP ONE

1 cup (230 g) ghee	*4 carrots, sliced*
Pinch of hing (optional)	*1 bell pepper, coarsely chopped*
4 stalks celery, sliced	*2 cups (260 g) peas*

STEP TWO

2 teaspoons dried tarragon or 1½ tablespoons fresh

STEP THREE

4 cups (1 l) vegetable stock	*1 to 2 teaspoons sugar*
1 tablespoon lemon juice	

STEP FIVE

Vegetable stock,	*Salt*
* if needed*	*White pepper*

1. Melt the ghee in a heavy soup pot. Add the hing and sauté over low heat until fragrant, about 30 seconds. Add the vegetables. Stir, cover, and cook over very low heat, stirring occasionally, until the vegetables are very tender, about 45 minutes.
2. Add the tarragon and cook for a few minutes more.
3. Purée the vegetables with the stock, lemon juice, and sugar in a blender or food processor. The smoother the mixture is, the easier the next step will be.
4. Place a large sieve over the soup pot. Strain the mixture through it, stirring and pressing with the back of a large spoon. Scrape the underside of the sieve periodically. Do not skip this step! It is essential for a creamy texture. In the end, there should remain a small amount of fibrous material that pulls away from the sieve. Discard it.
5. Heat to serving temperature. Thin with more stock if necessary. Season to taste with salt and white pepper.

VARIATIONS

Use any vegetables that will cook to a soft texture: zucchini, green beans, tomatoes, turnips, etc.

Instead of tarragon, substitute any combination of green herbs: basil, thyme, rosemary, parsley, etc.

Add curry powder or Maharishi Ayur-Veda churna in Step 5.

 # CREAMY ZUCCHINI-CASHEW SOUP

7 cups (1.7 l)

Of soop and Love the first is best.   —THOMAS FULLER

A cream soup made with cashew milk and thickened with puréed rice (a technique Julia Child developed to substitute for a roux). You can use other nuts to vary the flavor and other types of summer squash. The soup also works with winter squash.

STEP ONE

¼ cup (55 g) ghee or butter   *1 cup (110 g) thinly sliced celery*
Pinch of hing (optional)   *½ green bell pepper, sliced*
6 cups (700 g) sliced zucchini   *½ teaspoon salt*

STEP TWO

⅓ cup (70 g) long-grain white rice   *2 cups (480 ml) vegetable stock*

STEP THREE

1½ cups (200 g) cashews, toasted   *2 cups (480 ml) vegetable stock*

STEP SIX

Salt   *Black pepper*

1. Melt the ghee or butter in a large soup pot. Add the hing, zucchini, celery, bell pepper, and salt. Stir, cover, and cook over very low heat until the vegetables are tender, about 30 minutes.
2. While the vegetables are cooking, simmer the rice in the stock in a covered saucepan until tender, about 15 minutes. Set aside.
3. Purée the cashews in the second amount of stock in a blender or food processor. For a completely smooth soup, strain through a sieve lined with a piece of muslin cloth. Squeeze all the liquid out of the cloth.
4. Combine the rice and stock mixture, the vegetables, and the cashew and stock mixture in a blender. Purée very thoroughly. The smoother the mixture is, the easier the next step will be.
5. Place a large sieve over the soup pot. Strain the mixture through it, stirring and pressing with the back of a large spoon. Scrape the underside of the sieve periodically. Do not skip this step! It is essential for a creamy texture. In the end, there should remain a small amount of fibrous material that pulls away from the sieve. Discard it.

6. Heat the soup to serving temperature. Thin with more stock if necessary. Season to taste with salt and pepper.

VARIATION

Add a little curry powder or Maharishi Ayur-Veda churna or chopped fresh green herbs in Step 6.

BEAN SOUPS

It is best to serve bean soups in general for the midday meal rather than in the evening. However, dal soups made with moong or toor dal are light and digestible anytime. Crock-Pots are ideal for making long-cooking bean soups. First, prepare your soup on the stove, and when all is boiling merrily, transfer to a Crock-Pot for a long, leisurely simmering.

 ## BLACK BEAN SOUP

About 5 cups (1.2 l)

Black bean soup is popular in the United States—but it is even more popular in the Caribbean and Central America. Note that the beans must be soaked overnight.

STEP ONE

1 cup (185 g) dried black beans

STEP TWO

5 cups (1.2 l) unsalted vegetable stock or water   *1 bay leaf*

STEP THREE

2 tablespoons ghee or butter   *¼ cup (60 ml) minced fresh parsley*
Pinch of hing (optional)   *½ bell pepper, chopped*
1 stalk celery, sliced

STEP FOUR

1 tomato, chopped   *1 teaspoon raw or brown sugar*

STEP SIX

Salt   *Lemon or lime juice*
Black pepper   *Lemon or lime wedges*

1. Clean the beans. Place in at least 3 cups (700 ml) of water and soak overnight. Drain.
2. Place the beans in a large pot with the stock or water and bay leaf. Bring to a boil, cover, and reduce the heat to a simmer.

3. Melt the ghee or oil in a skillet. Add the hing, celery, parsley, and bell pepper. Sauté for 5 to 10 minutes over low heat, stirring frequently.
4. Add the chopped tomato and sugar. Sauté for 2 minutes more.
5. Add the vegetables to the beans and simmer until the beans are very tender, about 2½ hours or more.
6. Remove the bay leaf. Purée the soup in a blender in 2 or 3 batches, holding the lid tightly shut with a folded towel. Season to taste with salt, pepper, and a sprinkling of lemon or lime juice. Garnish with lemon or lime wedges.

VARIATION

Refrito Soup: A one-pot meal of soup given a treatment like a tostada. Use black beans or pinto or Anasazi beans. Add 1 tablespoon ground cumin with the hing in Step 3. Purée the finished soup in a blender and garnish with chopped cilantro, avocado slices, Salsa Cruda (p. 507), tortilla chips, sour cream, and shredded Monterey Jack cheese.

 # FASÓULADA

GREECE   *About 7 cups (1.7 l)*

Fassóulatha essosetin Elatha. Fasóulada saved Greece.   —GREEK SAYING

Nontraditional dried limas give this soup a creamy texture. Note that the beans must be soaked overnight.

STEP ONE
1 cup (190 g) dried navy beans or other white beans

STEP TWO

2 tablespoons olive oil	*1 stalk celery with leaves, sliced*
Pinch of hing (optional)	*½ teaspoon dried basil*
1 carrot, sliced	*¼ cup (60 ml) minced fresh parsley*

STEP THREE
2 tomatoes, chopped

STEP FOUR
5 cups (1.2 l) unsalted vegetable stock or water

STEP FIVE

2 tablespoons	*Salt*
lemon juice	*Black pepper*

1. Clean the beans. Place in at least 3 cups (700 ml) of water and soak overnight. Drain.

2. Heat the olive oil in a soup pot and sauté the hing, carrot, celery, basil, and parsley over low heat for 5 to 10 minutes, stirring frequently.
3. Add the tomatoes and sauté for 2 to 3 minutes more.
4. Add the stock or water and the beans. Simmer, covered, until the beans are very tender, 2½ to 3 hours.
5. Add the lemon juice and season to taste with salt and pepper.

 # PERSIAN NEW YEAR'S SOUP WITH TOASTED NOODLES (ASH-E RESHTEH)

IRAN   *10 cups (2.4 l)*

Here are two soups from the Persian tradition. This one is a complex, soul-satisfying meal-in-itself, and the toasted noodles ensure good fortune in the coming year. It is also served to family and friends when a baby cuts his or her first tooth. Note that the beans should be soaked overnight.

STEP ONE

¼ cup (45 g) dried kidney beans
¼ cup (45 g) dried navy beans

¼ cup (50 g) dried garbanzo beans
   (chickpeas)

STEP TWO

½ cup (100 g) mung
   beans or split moong dal

6 cups (1.4 l) water

STEP THREE

2 tablespoons ghee or butter
Pinch of hing (optional)
2 celery stalks, thinly sliced

1 bell pepper, chopped
1 medium tomato, puréed

STEP FOUR

1 quart (1 l) vegetable stock
1 beet, peeled and diced

STEP FIVE

4 ounces (105 g) long pasta, such as linguine or fettuccine

STEP SIX

2 cups (190 g) chopped spinach
   leaves
½ cup (120 ml) chopped fresh
   cilantro
½ cup (120 ml) chopped
   fresh dill or 1 tablespoon dried

⅓ cup (80 ml) chopped fresh mint or
   1 tablespoon dried
½ teaspoon turmeric
1 tablespoon sugar

STEP SEVEN

*½ cup (120 ml) sour cream
 or buttermilk
Salt*

*White or black pepper
Sour cream for garnishing*

1. Clean the kidney, navy, and garbanzo beans. Place in at least 3 cups (700 ml) of water and soak overnight.
2. Drain the soaked beans. Clean the mung beans. Place all of them in a heavy soup pot with the water and bring to a boil. Partially cover, reduce the heat, and simmer until almost tender, 1½ to 2 hours.
3. Meanwhile, melt the ghee or butter in a skillet over low heat. Add the hing, celery, and bell pepper. Sauté for 5 minutes, stirring frequently. Add the puréed tomato and continue to cook for 2 to 3 minutes.
4. After the beans have cooked in Step 2, add the sautéed mixture, vegetable stock, and beet. Partially cover and cook until the beans are completely tender, about 45 minutes.
5. Meanwhile, preheat the oven to 350°F (180°C). Break the pasta into fourths. Scatter on a baking sheet and toast in the oven until lightly browned. Stir every few minutes and be very alert not to burn. Add to the soup.
6. Add the spinach, cilantro, dill, mint, turmeric, and sugar. Simmer until the pasta is tender.
7. Stir in the sour cream or buttermilk. Add salt and pepper to taste. Serve immediately. Pass a bowl of sour cream at the table.

 # PERSIAN BEAN AND BARLEY SOUP (SOUP-E JOW)

IRAN   *8 cups (1.9 l)*

In the olden days of Persia, when someone had a special desire in their hearts, they would place a soup pot at the side of the road. Those passing by would drop in coins for purchasing soup ingredients, to add support for the desire. The more people who contributed, the more powerful the force behind the desire. To this day, Iranians invite their friends over on a day they plan to make a wish. The guests bring soup ingredients, and all prepare and make the soup together to collectively support the desire.

Note that the beans must be soaked overnight.

STEP ONE

*¼ cup (45 g) dried kidney
 beans*

*¼ cup (50 g) dried garbanzo
 beans (chickpeas)*

STEP TWO

*¼ cup (50 g) lentils,
 mung beans, or split moong dal*

1 quart (1 l) water

STEP THREE

2 tablespoons ghee or butter
Pinch of hing (optional)
2 stalks celery, minced

1 bell pepper, minced
1 carrot, minced

STEP FOUR

5 cups (1.2 l) vegetable stock
⅔ cup (140 g) pearl barley

2 tablespoons rice

STEP FIVE

½ cup (120 ml) minced fresh
  parsley
½ cup (120 ml) chopped fresh
  cilantro
½ cup (120 ml) chopped fresh
  dill or 1 tablespoon dried

¾ cup (180 ml) sour cream
  or buttermilk
2 teaspoons sugar
Salt
White or black pepper

1. Clean the kidney and garbanzo beans. Place in at least 2 cups (500 ml) of water and soak overnight.
2. Drain the soaked beans. Place in a heavy soup pot with the lentils or mung beans and the water. Bring to a boil. Partially cover, reduce the heat, and simmer for 1½ hours.
3. Meanwhile, melt the ghee or butter in a skillet. Add the hing, celery, bell pepper, and carrot. Sauté over low heat, stirring frequently, until tender, about 5 minutes. Add to the beans after they have cooked in Step 2.
4. Bring the vegetable stock to a boil. Add the stock, barley, and rice to the beans. Partially cover and simmer until the beans and barley are completely tender, about 1 hour.
5. Stir in the parsley, cilantro, and dill. Stir in the sour cream or buttermilk. Add the sugar and season to taste with salt and pepper.
6. Purée half of the soup in a blender or food processor. Return to the pot. Heat to serving temperature but do not boil.

Dal Soups

Dal soup is served daily throughout much of India and is also daily fare in many Ayurvedic homes around the world. Served with rice and vegetables, it is an excellent choice for a light Ayurvedic meal; add a chutney and Indian unleavened breads, and you have a feast.

Creating Delicious Ayurvedic Dal Soups

❖ Add sliced vegetables in the last 15 to 30 minutes of cooking. Carrots, green beans, sweet potatoes, and chopped tomatoes are nice additions. Chopped spinach can be added 1 to 2 minutes before serving.

❖ Spices are always added to dal a few minutes before serving; they lose their flavors or turn bitter with long simmering. However, fresh cilantro should be added just before serving; it loses its flavor and attractive green color when cooked even for a minute. A pinch of sugar added with the salt rounds out the flavors.

❖ Garnish dal soup with crème fraîche or coconut milk, a sprinkling of lemon or lime juice, plain Pakoras (pp. 291–92), or plain Vadas (pp. 295–96).

Dal Soup with Barley: Steve's favorite evening soup. Barley is a Kapha-balancing addition. After 1 hour of cooking, add ⅓ cup (70 g) barley to any of the dal soups. Continue to simmer until the dal and barley are tender, then add the seasonings.

DAILY DAL

About 6 cups (1.4 l)

This is more or less the way I prepare dal every day. I vary the types of pulses, though, tending to stick with yellow split moong dal. I usually add a sprinkling of broth powder and/or liquid seasoning.

STEP ONE

1 cup (200 g) dal   *6 cups (1.4 l) water*

STEP TWO

2 tablespoons ghee   *2 teaspoons cumin seeds*
Pinch of hing (optional)   *¾ teaspoon mustard seeds*
2 tablespoons minced fresh ginger

STEP THREE

¾ teaspoon turmeric   *¾ cup (180 ml) loosely packed*
2 teaspoons sugar   *chopped fresh cilantro*
Salt

1. Clean the dal. Place in a pot with the water and bring to a boil. Reduce the heat and simmer until the dal is tender, 2 to 4 hours, depending on the type of dal.
2. Melt the ghee in a small skillet over low heat. Add the hing, ginger, cumin seeds, and mustard seeds. Sauté, stirring frequently, until the spices become fragrant and the mustard seeds dance, 1 to 2 minutes. Add to the simmering dal.
3. Stir in the turmeric, sugar, and salt to taste. Simmer for 1 to 2 minutes for the flavors to blend. Just before serving, stir in the cilantro.

DAL I

INDIA   *About 6 cups (1.4 l)*

STEP ONE

1 cup (200 g) dal, lentils,   6 cups (1.4 l) water
  or split peas

STEP TWO

1 tablespoon ghee, butter, or oil   ½ teaspoon ground coriander
Pinch of hing (optional)   ⅛ teaspoon ground cloves
½ teaspoon black mustard seeds   ¾ teaspoon ground turmeric
1 teaspoon cumin seeds

STEP THREE

Salt   Chopped fresh cilantro (optional)

1. Clean the dal. Place in a pot with the water and bring to a boil. Reduce the heat and simmer until the dal is tender, 2 to 4 hours, depending on the type of dal.
2. Heat the ghee, butter, or oil in a small pot. Add the spices in order and sauté over low heat until the mustard seeds dance, 1 to 2 minutes. Remove from the heat.
3. Pour a little soup into the spices and stand back while it sputters. When the sputtering subsides, pour the mixture back into the soup and stir well. Beat with a whisk to break up the pulses. Add salt to taste. Stir in a handful of chopped cilantro if desired.

 # DAL II

About 6 cups (1.4 l)

Coconut and lime juice are characteristic ingredients of Gujarati cooking.

STEP ONE

1 cup (200 g) yellow split peas,   6 cups (1.4 l) water
  masoor, split moong, or toor dal

STEP TWO

2 tablespoons grated unsweetened coconut, toasted

STEP THREE

2 tablespoons ghee, butter, or oil   2 tablespoons minced fresh ginger
Pinch of hing (optional)   1 teaspoon cumin seeds

	STEP FOUR
½ *teaspoon ground coriander*	*Salt*
¼ *teaspoon ground cinnamon*	*Chopped fresh cilantro* (optional)
1 *teaspoon ground turmeric*	

	STEP FIVE
Freshly squeezed lime juice	*Melted ghee*

1. Clean the dal. Place in a pot with the water and bring to a boil. Reduce the heat and simmer until the dal is tender, 2 to 4 hours, depending on the type of dal.
2. Add the toasted coconut.
3. Heat the ghee, butter, or oil in a small saucepan. Add the hing, ginger, and cumin seeds, and sauté for 1 minute.
4. Pour a little soup into the spices and stand back while it sputters. When the sputtering subsides, pour the mixture back into the soup and stir well. Add the remaining spices. Beat with a whisk to break up the pulses. Add salt to taste. Stir in a handful of chopped cilantro if desired.
5. To serve, pour into individual bowls. Top each bowl with a sprinkling of lime juice and a teaspoonful of melted ghee.

 # SAMBAR

INDIA   *About 6 cups*

Sambar is served on a daily basis throughout much of south India, often with dosas served with coconut chutney. The recipe has been tested with homemade sambar powder containing black pepper instead of chilies. If using commercial powders (which contain garlic and chilies), *add to taste*. Also, toor dal can take a long time to cook. I make the soup in a Crock-Pot and just forget about it all morning while it does its own thing.

	STEP ONE
1 *cup (200 g) toor dal*	6 *cups (1.4 l) water*

	STEP TWO
2 *tablespoons mild-flavored oil*	1 *teaspoon cumin seeds*
½ *teaspoon urad dal* (optional)	½ *teaspoon black mustard seeds*
Pinch of hing (optional)	

	STEP THREE
2 *medium tomatoes, chopped*	1 *tablespoon sambar powder*
1 *teaspoon black pepper*	(*recipe follows, p. 250*)
½ *teaspoon turmeric*	2 *teaspoons sugar*

STEP FOUR

2 teaspoons tamarind paste mixed
*   with ¼ cup (60 ml) hot water,*
*   or tamarind water (p. 571)*

Salt
¾ cup (180 ml) chopped fresh cilantro

1. Wash the toor dal thoroughly. Place in the water and bring to a boil. Cover, reduce the heat, and simmer until the dal is tender, about 4 hours.
2. Heat the oil in a small skillet. Add the urad dal and sauté over low heat, stirring frequently, until the dal starts to darken. Add the hing, cumin seeds, and mustard seeds and sauté until the mustard seeds "dance."
3. Add the tomatoes, pepper, turmeric, Sambar Powder, and sugar. Cook, stirring constantly, until the tomatoes are mushy.
4. Add the spice mixture to the dal. Add the tamarind mixture. Add salt to taste. Simmer 5 to 10 minutes for the flavors to blend. Stir in the cilantro just before serving.

VARIATIONS

If you don't like hot food, reduce the black pepper. If you do, replace the pepper with crumbled dried red chilies, added with the spices in Step 2.

Add cubed potatoes, sliced green beans, or sautéed eggplant cubes for the last 20 minutes of cooking.

 # SAMBAR POWDER

About 5 tablespoons

For best flavor, grind whole spices to a powder just before preparing the recipe.

STEP ONE

1 tablespoon ground coriander
2½ teaspoons ground cumin
1½ teaspoons ground black pepper

1½ teaspoons ground fenugreek
1 teaspoon ground mustard seeds

STEP TWO

¼ teaspoon hing (optional)

1 tablespoon turmeric

1. Place the ground coriander, cumin, pepper, fenugreek, and mustard seeds in a dry skillet. Toast over low heat, stirring constantly, until the spices become fragrant and are smoking.
2. Add the hing and toast for 30 seconds more, stirring constantly. Stir in the turmeric and remove from the heat. Store in an airtight container.

> *Certainly it is heaven upon earth to have a man's minde move in*
> *charitie, rest in Providence, and turn upon the poles of truth.*
>
> —SIR FRANCIS BACON, *Essays of Truth*

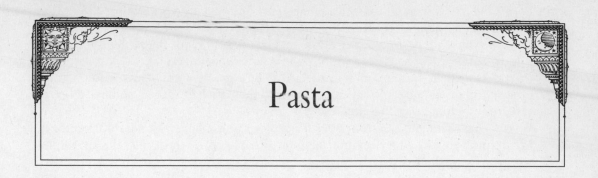

Pasta

Life is a combination of magic and pasta. —FEDERICO FELLINI

By the time Marco Polo observed noodle making in twelfth-century China, it had already been well established in India, China, and the Middle East. It also existed in Italy. Travelers in bygone days describe mile upon mile of craggy Italian coastline festooned with racks of pasta drying in the sea breezes and warm Mediterranean sunshine. Pasta is excellent fare for balancing Vata and Pitta, and there are nonwheat pastas that balance Kapha. It can be prepared both warm and cool, making it adaptable for all seasons. Served without cheese, pasta dishes make a lovely evening meal.

> Until recently, no one made dried pasta better than the Italians. The government strictly controls the ingredients used in commercially produced pasta: The flour must be durum (semolina), which gives pasta a superior texture and golden color. However, farmers in the United States are growing exceptional durum wheat for making pasta—so much so that there is a demand for it in Italy! You can now find quality American pasta made from organically grown durum wheat.

❖ *Whole wheat pasta* has a rough, firm texture and strong, wheaty flavor. It can be used for both Asian and Italian dishes. Some people find its character too assertive; Japanese whole wheat *somen* and *udon* noodles are smoother and milder tasting.

❖ *Soy pasta* is made from a combination of soy and whole wheat flours. It has a smoother texture than whole wheat pasta.

- ❖ *Quinoa pasta* is made from a combination of quinoa and whole wheat flours that provides more balance for Kapha.
- ❖ *Corn pasta* is made from corn flour and has a subtle cornmeal flavor. It is an option both for Kapha types and for people with wheat allergies. Corn pasta tends to stick together during cooking, so boil it in copious amounts of water with a tablespoon of oil and stir frequently. Small shapes, such as macaroni, have a better texture than long, thin noodles.
- ❖ *Brown rice pasta* is made from brown rice flour and a binder of vegetable gum. In my opinion, it is a gooey textural disaster. People with wheat allergies or Kapha constitutions who are desperately seeking pasta might try it, but they'd be better off with corn pasta.

Asian Pasta

In China long noodles are symbolic of long life and are served on New Year's, birthdays, and other auspicious celebrations. Asian noodles come only in long, thin shapes—none of the twists and turns of Italian varieties.

- ❖ *Chinese noodles* are made with white flour and water. Some contain eggs and others don't. You can find fresh Chinese noodles in supermarkets in a refrigerated case.
- ❖ *Japanese noodles: Somen* and *udon* are whole wheat noodles. *Jijenjo* are made from a combination of wheat flour and *jijenjo*, wild mountain yam flour. *Kuzu noodles,* used in traditional Zen temple cuisine, are made from kuzu root powder and potato starch. *Soba,* buckwheat noodles, are noisily slurped up in bowls of broth by millions of Japanese at fast food lunch counters. They are also the object of mastery of perhaps fifty chefs, who elevate soba preparation to an art form.
- ❖ *Rice sticks,* dried noodles made from rice flour and water, and *bean thread noodles* or *saifun*, made from mung bean flour, are used throughout Southeast Asia. You can purchase them from Asian markets. Rice sticks and bean thread noodles come in bundles that are brittle and unyielding. Breaking off the amount you need involves kitchen shears or a sharp knife and a major wrestling match. Soak in cold water for 20 minutes. Drain, then drop into boiling water and simmer for 2 to 3 minutes, until tender.

Puffed Bean Thread Noodles: Puffed bean threads are light and crunchy. They can serve as a bed for stir-fried vegetables or can decorate the top of a vegetable dish or a casserole. Cut the desired amount of bean thread noodles from the bundle. Deep-fry until they are puffed and rise to the top of the oil, about 5 seconds. Drain on paper towels.

Homemade vs. Commercial vs. Fresh vs. Dried Pasta

In Italy, fresh pasta, in the northern style, is made with flour and eggs. Dried pasta from the south is made from flour and water. *Fresh pasta* has a texture that is, well, just different from *dried pasta*. Comparison is an apples-and-oranges proposition. Fresh is preferable in Ayurvedic cooking, but freshly made eggless pasta means homemade. Homemade pasta may not always be a viable time option, and the finely milled semolina that makes the best Italian-style pasta is largely unavailable to home cooks. You could make large amounts and dry your own, or just eat good-quality store-bought pasta and enjoy. Store fresh pasta in the refrigerator for a day or two and in the freezer for a week or two. Store dried pasta in airtight containers in a dry area.

Four Noble Truths of Creating Delicious Fresh Pasta

1. It is important to knead the dough very well—for at least 10 minutes by hand. It should be quite dry. If you press your finger into the dough and it comes out with sticky bits clinging to it, the dough is too wet.
2. Roll out and cut pasta into the shape you desire just after kneading it. The traditional and most effective rolling pin is long and thin, like a broomstick. You can obtain a similar one in Indian markets, where they are sold for rolling out Chapatis.
3. Allow freshly made pasta to rest and dry a little before cooking; 10 minutes spread on a dry towel is sufficient. However, if you are making ravioli or another type of filled pasta, stuff and seal it immediately after rolling out.
4. If you wish to dry pasta for later use, allow it to rest on a towel until completely dry. To avoid breaking long noodles such as spaghetti or fettuccine, Italians form small amounts of pasta into nest shapes while still fresh and dry them in that form. When thoroughly dry (it usually takes 24 hours or more), store the pasta in airtight containers away from moisture.

To Cook Pasta (Fresh or Dried)

1. For 1 pound (500 g) of pasta, bring 6 quarts (6 l) of water to a boil. A teaspoon of oil added to the water will help keep the pasta from sticking together and the water from boiling over.
2. When the water is boiling rapidly, drop in 1 pound (500 g) of fresh pasta or ½

pound (230 g) dried pasta for 4 people. Push the strands into the water as they soften, if necessary.

3. The cooking time will vary according to the size and thickness of the pasta. Pastas containing whole grain flours take a little longer to cook than those made with white flour. The noodles should be at the point that Italians call *al dente*—tender but offering a little resistance to the teeth. Timing is everything—texture is what pasta has going for it. Immediately drain in a colander.

Cascare come il cacio sui maccherone. To fall like the cheese on macaroni.
—OLD ITALIAN SAYING, WHEN SOMEONE OR SOMETHING ARRIVES
JUST AT THE PROPITIOUS MOMENT OR IS ESPECIALLY WELCOME

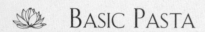 # BASIC PASTA

1 pound (500 g)

If you have access to powder-fine semolina—not the grainy product used as a breakfast cereal and sometimes incorrectly sold specifically for pasta—by all means use it.

2 cups (280 g) unbleached white flour   ½ to ⅔ cup (120 to 160 ml) water

1. Sift the flour. Add the water and mix to form a soft, nonsticky dough.
2. Turn out on a floured board. Knead until completely smooth, about 10 minutes.
3. Wrap the dough in a lightly dampened dish cloth and allow to rest for 10 to 30 minutes.
4. Divide the dough into 4 parts for easier handling. Roll out very thin on a well-floured board. Fold the dough over loosely 2 or 3 times and cut noodles to the width you desire.

VARIATIONS

Soy or Chickpea Pasta: Replace 1 cup (140 g) white flour with 1 cup (120 g) soy flour or besan (chickpea flour). Use 6 to 8 tablespoons (90 to 120 ml) water.

Udon: For Japanese whole wheat noodles, prepare Basic Pasta with sifted whole wheat flour. Cut into noodles ¾-inch (2 cm) wide.

Soba: Popular in Japan, buckwheat noodles are also eaten in parts of Italy. Replace 1 cup (140 g) white flour with buckwheat flour (130 g).

Vegetable: Use vegetable juice instead of water to give the pasta different colors and flavors. Try beet juice or carrot juice.

Pasta Verde (Green Pasta): Purée 1 cup (240 ml) spinach leaves in a blender with ½ cup (120 ml) water. Strain out the spinach and use the green water to prepare Basic, Soy or Chickpea, or Udon pasta dough.

SPAGHETTI WITH CARROT-PEPPER SAUCE AND WHEAT BALLS

4 servings

Says M. F. K. Fisher, "Spaghetti, one of the most misunderstood simple foods in the world, can be one of the best if properly treated." Her idea of proper treatment is a tossing of Parmesan and butter—which is wonderful—but here is a dish that upgrades the childhood favorite of many to an Ayurvedic vegetarian status: a flavorful alternative to tomato sauce and walnut-laced wheat balls. Proper treatment, indeed.

½ pound (230 g) dried spaghetti
Carrot-Pepper Sauce
  (recipe follows)

Wheat Balls (recipe follows, p. 256)

Cook and drain the spaghetti. Mound on a plate. Spoon on the sauce and top with Wheat Balls.

CARROT-PEPPER SAUCE

3 cups (720 ml)

The flavor mimics a sweeter version of tomato sauce, and the color almost makes it to "red sauce."

STEP ONE

¼ cup (60 ml) olive oil
Pinch of hing (optional)
2 teaspoons dried basil
1 teaspoon dried thyme
½ teaspoon chopped fresh
  or dried rosemary

3 cups (270 g) sliced carrots
2 cups (280 g) chopped red bell
  peppers
1 cup (110 g) chopped fennel or
  celery
Liquid seasoning or salt

STEP TWO

1 cup (240 ml) vegetable stock
  or water

Black pepper

1. Heat the olive oil in a large skillet. Add the hing and herbs and sauté over a low heat for 30 seconds, until fragrant. Add the carrots, peppers, and fennel or celery. Sprinkle with liquid seasoning or salt, cover, and sauté over low heat, stirring occasionally, until the vegetables are very tender.
2. Purée in a food processor with the stock or water. Season with pepper and adjust the salt.

WHEAT BALLS

About 25

You can also shape the mixture into patties and serve as burgers, sans spaghetti.

STEP ONE

1½ cups (205g) *walnut pieces*

STEP TWO

1 cup (240 ml) *water*   1 carrot, grated
½ cup (85 g) *bulgar*   ½ cup (120 ml) *minced fresh parsley*
1 stalk celery,
  finely chopped

STEP FOUR

¼ cup (30 g) *fine dry bread*   2 tablespoons flour
  crumbs   Liquid seasoning or salt
1 teaspoon paprika   Black pepper

STEP SIX

Fine dry bread crumbs

STEP SEVEN

Oil

1. Preheat the oven to 350°F (180°C). Place the walnuts in an ungreased baking pan and toast until lightly browned, 20 to 30 minutes. Shake the pan every 5 minutes.
2. While the walnuts are toasting, bring the water to a boil. Add the bulgar, celery, carrot, and parsley. Cover, reduce the heat, and simmer until the water is absorbed and the bulgar is tender, about 15 minutes.
3. Grind the walnuts to a powder in a blender or food processor. Place in a mixing bowl.
4. Add the bulgar mixture to the walnut powder. Add the bread crumbs, paprika, and flour. Add liquid seasoning or salt and pepper to taste. Allow the mixture to cool.
5. Squeeze and roll the mixture into balls 1 inch to 1½ inch (2.5 to 3.5 cm) in diameter.
6. Place a thick layer of bread crumbs in a shallow bowl. Roll the balls in it to coat.
7. *To pan-brown:* Heat ½ inch (1.5 cm) oil in a heavy skillet over medium-low heat. Fry the balls in uncrowded batches, turning on all sides, until browned. Drain on paper towels.
   To bake: Preheat the oven to 350°F (180°C). Place the balls on a very well-oiled baking sheet. Roll them around gently to lightly coat the crumbs with oil. Bake until the crumbs are nicely browned, about 30 minutes.

Spaghetti can be eaten successfully if you inhale it like a vacuum cleaner.

—SOPHIA LOREN

In a custom dating from the olden days in Persia, Iranians eat long noodles before starting something new: a project, a business, and especially a new year. Long, thin strands of pasta represent the different paths and choices in life, with all their attendant possibilities. Eating them disentangles the complex, intertwined situations life offers and puts them in order. The right choices will then be made, and good fortune will smile on the endeavor.

 # LEMON-SCENTED FETTUCCINE WITH ARTICHOKE HEARTS

4 servings

To adhere to the Ayurvedic recommendation of not mixing salt into fresh milk, the Alfredo-type sauce is prepared with crème fraîche or thick coconut milk. For color contrast, use half Pasta Verde and half regular pasta for a green-and-white mixture Italians call *paglia e fieno*, "straw and hay." The lemon flavor acts as an undertone; if you want it to be more assertive, add another tablespoon of lemon juice. A cheese-free version is given in the first variation.

STEP ONE

3 large cooked artichoke hearts　　　*1½ teaspoons lemon juice*
1 teaspoon finely grated lemon zest　　*Salt*

STEP TWO

1 pound (500 g) fresh fettuccine or ½ pound (230 g) dried

STEP THREE

¾ cup (165 g) ghee or butter　　　*½ cup (120 ml) crème fraîche or*
Pinch of hing (optional)　　　　　　*thick coconut milk*

STEP FOUR

¾ cup (75 g) grated Parmesan cheese　　*Black pepper*
¼ cup (60 ml) minced fresh parsley

1. Slice the artichoke hearts and toss with the lemon zest, lemon juice, and a sprinkling of salt. Set aside.
2. Cook the fettuccine until al dente. Drain.
3. Melt the ghee or butter in a saucepan. Add the hing and sauté for 30 seconds, until fragrant. Add the crème fraîche or coconut milk and bring to a boil.

4. Toss the fettuccine with the cream mixture, artichokes, Parmesan, and parsley. Add a sprinkling of pepper and adjust the salt. Serve immediately.

VARIATIONS

Omit the Parmesan. Return the drained pasta to the pot and add the cream mixture. Sauté 2½ to 3 cups (600 to 720 ml) vegetables, such as cubed eggplant, green beans, or sliced fennel, and substitute for the artichoke hearts.

HOMAGE TO VIVALDI: THE THREE AYURVEDIC SEASONS OF PASTA

An epicure eats with his brain as well as his mouth. —CHARLES LAMB

Pasta tossed with sautéed vegetables, besides being delicious, is about as fast as Ayurvedic fast food can be. Great for dinner and a lovely lunchtime meal with cheese and nuts added, pasta with vegetables is my first and last resort when mealtime calls and cook time is in short supply. Here are three seasonal vegetable combinations. They all contain tri-doshic elements: asparagus in spring, French beans in summer, and fennel in winter, so you can create each mixture with the types of oils, pastas, and additions that are most balancing for you.

ADDITIONS TO TOSS WITH PASTA WITH SAUTÉED VEGETABLES:

Toasted nuts and seeds
Sautéed tofu, panir, or seitan cubes
Pesto
Sweet Red Pepper Purée (p. 513)
Grated Parmesan cheese
Dabs of cream cheese or chèvre, added to the vegetables while cooking
Thick Coconut Milk (p. 494), added to the vegetables while cooking
Maharishi Ayur-Veda churnas

 # SPRING PASTA FOR KAPHA

4 servings

Slicing snap pea pods brings out a different personality in the vegetable than leaving them whole.

STEP ONE

*½ pound (230 g) dried fettuccine
or linguine or 1 pound (500 g) fresh*

STEP TWO

*⅓ cup (80 ml) sunflower oil
Pinch of hing (optional)
2 cups (240 g) snap peas,
  stringed and cut into thirds
4 cups (350 g) coarsely chopped
  arugula*

*2½ cups (375 g) asparagus, trimmed and
  cut into 2-inch (5 cm) pieces
Liquid seasoning or salt
Black pepper*

1. Cook the pasta until al dente. Drain.
2. Heat the oil in a large wok or skillet. Add the hing and sauté over medium heat for 30 seconds, until fragrant. Add the vegetables. Sprinkle with liquid seasoning or salt and pepper to taste, cover, and cook for 3 to 5 minutes, until tender, stirring a few times. Toss with the pasta. Adjust the seasoning.

 ## SUMMER PASTA FOR PITTA

4 servings

From the wonderful summertime bounty of fresh vegetables and herbs, here is a combination that nourishes and balances Pitta and would be equally balancing for Kapha. Because of the oil, it could also be considered within range for Vata. The mint should be minced to smithereens, as the leaves can be a bit coarse.

STEP ONE

*½ pound (230 g) dried
pasta shapes, such as penne,
small shells, or orecchiette*

STEP TWO

*¼ cup (60 ml) olive oil
Pinch of hing (optional)
2 cups (200 g) French or
  green beans, trimmed and
  halved crosswise*

*3 cups (320 g) zucchini or other summer
  squash, quartered lengthwise
  and sliced
Liquid seasoning or salt*

STEP THREE

*2 tablespoons olive oil
Pinch of hing (optional)
¾ cup (90 g) dry bread crumbs
¾ cup (180 ml) finely chopped fresh
  basil*

*½ cup (120 ml) finely chopped
  flat-leaf parsley
¼ cup (60 ml) minced fresh mint
Black pepper*

1. Cook the pasta until al dente. Drain.
2. Heat the ghee or oil with the hing in a skillet over low heat. Add the French or green beans, cover, and sauté for 2 to 3 minutes. Add the zucchini or summer squash, sprinkle with liquid seasoning or salt, cover, and cook until tender, stirring occasionally.
3. Heat the second amount of oil in a skillet. Add the hing and sauté for 30 seconds, until fragrant. Add the bread crumbs and sauté, stirring constantly, until golden brown and crisp. Add the basil, parsley, mint, and a sprinkling of black pepper, and stir. Toss with the pasta and vegetables. Adjust the seasoning.

 # WINTER PASTA FOR VATA

4 servings

A julienne of carrots and fennel tossed with Ginger Gremolata. Whole wheat pasta offers a nice color contrast to the fennel. If fennel is not in season, substitute slivered celery or even julienned green beans. (Don't worry about the fennel tops—I just like to utilize them if the fennel bulb has been gracious enough to provide them.) You can toast fennel seeds in the toaster oven, which works perfectly when you watch them like a hawk. They go from lightly toasted to burned in seconds.

STEP ONE

*1 pound (500 g) fresh
    linguine, fettuccine, or spaghetti or
½ pound (230 g) dried*

STEP TWO

⅓ cup (80 ml) olive oil	*Up to 4 tablespoons chopped fennel tops*
Pinch of hing (optional)	*(if on the fennel bulb)*
2 cups (180 g) carrots, cut into	*Liquid seasoning or salt*
2-inch (5 cm) lengths and finely	
julienned	
3 cups (330 g) fennel stalks, cut into	
2-inch (5 cm) lengths and	
slivered lengthwise	

STEP THREE

1 tablespoon fennel seeds	*½ cup (50 g) slivered pecans, lightly*
2 tablespoons lemon juice	*toasted*
Ginger Gremolata (recipe	*Black pepper*
follows)	

1. Cook the pasta until al dente. Drain
2. Heat the oil in a large skillet over low heat. Add the hing and sauté for 30 seconds,

until fragrant. Add the carrots, fennel, and fennel tops and sprinkle with liquid seasoning or salt. Stir, cover, and cook until tender, stirring occasionally.
3. Toss the vegetables, fennel seeds, lemon juice, Ginger Gremolata, pecans, and a sprinkling of black pepper with the pasta. Adjust the seasoning.

GINGER GREMOLATA

Gremolata is a flavorful garnish for soups and stews as well as for pasta. Everything should be very finely minced—a whirl in a food processor is a good final step.

1 tablespoon minced fresh ginger
1 tablespoon finely grated
  lemon zest

1 cup (240 ml) minced flat-leaf
  parsley

Mix all the ingredients together.

HALUSKY KAPUSTA

POLAND/SLOVAKIA   *4 servings*

Mary Dicasali Hospodar, my Italian mother-in-law, prepares it like this for her Slovak relatives who insist on its cultural purity. When making it for herself, she can't resist adding red bell peppers and sometimes finishing it with cheese.

STEP ONE

½ cup (115 g) ghee or butter

STEP TWO

Pinch of hing (optional)
7 cups (730 g) finely chopped cabbage

1 teaspoon salt
½ teaspoon black pepper

STEP THREE

½ pound (230 g) dried wide,
  flat noodles, or shapes such as
  farfalle or conchiglie, or 1 pound
  (500 g) fresh noodles

1. Melt the ghee or butter in a large skillet. Cook over medium heat until golden brown.
2. Add the hing, cabbage, salt, and pepper. Cover, reduce the heat, and cook, stirring frequently, until some of the cabbage browns. Be careful not to burn it.

3. While the cabbage is cooking, cook the noodles according to package directions. Drain.
4. Toss the noodles and cabbage together. Adjust the seasonings.

VARIATIONS

Sauté chopped bell pepper, fennel, or carrots with the cabbage in Step 2.
Add a sprinkling of poppy seeds before serving.
Stir in sour cream before serving.

 ## CURRIED PASTA WITH APRICOTS AND PINE NUTS

6 to 8 servings

Sometimes an unlikely occurrence triggers the imagination. Once in Switzerland, while exiting a restaurant, my glance momentarily fell on an abandoned plate of pasta in a golden sauce. What immediately came to mind was a curry sauce with a Middle Eastern slant of dried apricots and pine nuts.

STEP ONE

¼ cup (55 g) ghee or butter	*1 cup (240 ml) crème fraîche or*
4 teaspoons mild curry powder	*sour cream*

STEP TWO

1½ pounds (680 g) fresh linguine or fettuccine or 12 ounces (350 g) dried

STEP THREE

¼ cup (35 g) pine nuts, toasted	*2 tablespoons lemon juice*
⅓ cup (40 g) finely sliced dried	*Salt*
apricots, soaked if necessary	*White pepper*

1. Melt the ghee or butter in a saucepan with the curry powder. Stir in the crème fraîche or sour cream and remove from the heat.
2. Cook the pasta until al dente. Drain.
3. Toss the pasta, cream sauce, pine nuts, and apricots together in a serving bowl. Add the lemon juice and toss again. Add salt and pepper to taste. Serve immediately.

VARIATION

Add a little finely grated orange zest to the sauce.
❂ Replace the crème fraîche or sour cream with thick coconut milk.

CAPELLINI WITH PEPPERS

ITALY   *6 to 8 servings*

Mary Zamarra's formula for a colorful dish. Roast the peppers in advance. You can replace one or two peppers with yellow ones to make the pasta even more colorful.

STEP ONE

2 red bell peppers, cut into strips	*Olive oil*
2 green bell peppers, cut into strips	*Salt*

STEP TWO

12 ounces (350 g) dried capellini

STEP THREE

3 tablespoons ghee or butter
3 tablespoons olive oil
Pinch of hing (optional)
8 oil-packed sun-dried tomatoes, drained and finely chopped

¼ cup (60 ml) torn fresh basil
¼ cup (60 ml) minced fresh flat-leaf parsley

STEP FOUR

¼ cup (25 g) grated Parmesan cheese (optional)

Salt
Black pepper

1. Preheat the oven to 350°F (180°C). Scatter the bell peppers on a baking sheet. Drizzle with olive oil, sprinkle lightly with salt, and toss to coat. Bake, stirring once or twice, until tender, 20 to 30 minutes.
2. While the peppers are roasting, cook the pasta until al dente. Drain.
3. Melt the ghee or butter with the olive oil. Add the hing and sauté until fragrant, about 30 seconds. Add the tomatoes, roasted peppers, basil, and parsley.
4. Toss the vegetables and Parmesan with the pasta in a serving bowl. Season to taste with salt and pepper. Serve immediately.

VARIATION

When adding the vegetables in Step 3, toss in crumbled feta cheese or panir.

ALTERNATIVE MACARONI AND CHEESE

4 servings

*I like all simple things . . . but the one I can eat day in and day out, not only
without disgust but with the eagerness of an appetite unimpaired by excess is
Macaroni.* —SOMERSET MAUGHAM

In 1789 an agent was dispatched to Naples on a diplomatic mission for Thomas Jefferson. His assignment? To learn the secrets of making "maccarony" and to obtain the necessary equipment for the job. When the agent returned bearing a spaghetti-making device, the founding father summarily ordered pasta slathered with butter and cheese to be served forth at a formal dinner. And lo, the formal debut of macaroni and cheese on North American shores came to pass. Let us now fast-forward past any lingering images of packaged mac 'n' cheese dinners to a lunchtime dish you can prepare with fresh cheese. Rigatoni, penne, and other small pasta shapes can stand in for macaroni.

STEP ONE

*3 cups (720 ml) drained cooked
  macaroni*

*1½ cups (325 g) coarsely crumbled
  soft cheese, such as panir, feta,
  chèvre, or chopped fresh mozzarella*

STEP TWO

½ cup (120 ml) sour cream
*½ cup (120 ml) nondairy milk,
  vegetable stock, or water*

2 tablespoons ghee or butter
Salt
White pepper

STEP THREE

*¼ cup (30 g) fine dry
  bread crumbs*
2 teaspoons melted ghee or butter

*2 tablespoons grated Parmesan
  cheese* (optional)

1. Preheat the oven to 350°F (180°C). Generously butter a baking dish. Toss the macaroni and cheese in the baking dish.
2. Blend the sour cream, nondairy milk, stock or water, and ghee or butter in a blender until smooth. Pour over the pasta. Sprinkle with salt and pepper and toss lightly. Smooth the top.
3. Toss the bread crumbs with the melted ghee or butter until thoroughly moistened. Mix in the Parmesan, if desired. Sprinkle evenly over the macaroni mixture.
4. Bake until the bread crumbs are nicely browned and the mixture is bubbly, about 30 minutes.

VARIATIONS

Add chopped spinach, asparagus tips, peas, or other vegetables. Lightly cook longer-cooking vegetables before adding.

Replace the liquid with Béchamel Sauce (p. 498) or one of its variations.

PIZZOCCHERI

ITALY   *4 to 6 servings*

Pizzoccheri is the name given to wide, short buckwheat pasta from Valtellina in the Italian Alps. Here is the dish traditionally prepared with it.

STEP ONE

1 cup (165 g) thickly sliced new potatoes

STEP TWO

3 tablespoons ghee or butter
Pinch of hing (optional)
2 teaspoons chopped fresh sage
  or ½ teaspoon dried

4 cups (360 g) coarsely chopped greens,
  such as chard, Savoy cabbage,
  collard, or kale

STEP FOUR

½ pound (230 g) dried
  buckwheat (soba or pizzoccheri)
  noodles or 1 pound (½ kg)
  fresh (p. 254)

STEP FIVE

1½ cups (150 g) diced fontina cheese
⅓ cup (35 g) grated Parmesan cheese

Salt
Black pepper

1. Steam the potatoes until tender. Drain and set aside.
2. Melt the ghee or butter in a skillet. Add the hing and sauté over low heat until fragrant, about 30 seconds. Add the sage and greens, cover, and cook, stirring occasionally, until tender but not well cooked. Set aside.
3. Preheat the oven to 400°F (200°C). Butter a casserole dish.
4. Cook the pasta until al dente. Drain thoroughly.
5. Toss the pasta with the greens, potatoes, and cheeses. Season to taste with salt and pepper.
6. Place in the casserole dish and smooth the top. Cover. Bake until the cheeses have melted, 10 to 15 minutes. Serve immediately.

GREEN AND WHITE LASAGNA (LASAGNA VERDE BIANCA)

10 to 12 servings

> *He who looks at magnitude*
> *Is often mistaken.*
> *A grain of pepper conquers*
> *Lasagna with its strength.*
> —IACOPONE DA TODI, 13TH CENTURY

Green lasagnas are often prepared with spinach; this version utilizes an emerald green parsley sauce and artichoke hearts. Don't expect to be able to slice this lasagna into perfect, firm squares. See the variations for a fresh cheese version.

STEP ONE

2 tablespoons olive oil	2 cups (220 g) thinly sliced celery or fennel
Pinch of hing (optional)	2 cups (180 g) chopped broccoli

STEP TWO

¼ cup (32 g) arrowroot or cornstarch	3 pounds (6 cups/1.4 kg) ricotta cheese
¼ teaspoon freshly grated nutmeg	

STEP THREE

2½ cups (415 g) sliced cooked artichoke hearts	Salt
	White pepper

STEP FOUR

½ cup (115 g) ghee or butter	½ cup (70 g) unbleached white flour
Pinch of hing (optional)	

STEP FIVE

4 cups (940 ml) nondairy milk

STEP SIX

¼ teaspoon freshly grated nutmeg	Salt
3 cups (720 ml) minced fresh parsley (about 2 bunches)	White pepper

STEP SEVEN

1 pound (500 g) fresh pasta dough or 12 ounces (345 g) dried lasagna noodles

STEP NINE

6 cups (600 g) grated Swiss, mozzarella, or Monterey Jack cheese	¾ cup (75 g) grated Parmesan cheese

To prepare the filling:

1. Heat the olive oil and hing in a large skillet over low heat. Add the celery and broccoli and sauté, stirring frequently, until tender.
2. Beat the arrowroot or cornstarch and nutmeg into the ricotta.
3. Mix the sautéed vegetables and the artichoke hearts into the ricotta. Season to taste with salt and pepper. Set aside.

To prepare the sauce:

4. Melt the ghee or butter in a saucepan over low heat. Add the hing and sauté for about 30 seconds, until fragrant. Add the flour and stir with a whisk for 1 minute to make a roux.
5. Slowly add the nondairy milk. Beat with a whisk to remove any lumps, then heat slowly, stirring almost constantly, until thickened. Do not boil.
6. Remove the sauce from the heat. Stir in the nutmeg and parsley. Season to taste with salt and white pepper. Set aside.
7. *If using fresh pasta,* roll out 3 very thin sheets of dough to fit the lasagna pan. Do not cook. *If using dried noodles,* cook according to package directions. Lasagna noodles tend to stick together—cook in plenty of water and stir occasionally to separate. Drain the noodles in a colander. Run cold water over them until cool enough to handle and gently separate any that are stuck together.

To assemble:

8. Preheat the oven to 350°F (180°C). Oil a lasagna pan with olive oil.
9. Place a little sauce in the bottom of the pan. Place 1 sheet of dough or ⅓ of the noodles, slightly overlapping each other, to cover the bottom of the pan. Cover with ½ of the filling. Spread evenly. Spread ⅓ of the sauce over the filling. Sprinkle on ⅓ of the grated Swiss, mozzarella, or Jack cheese, then ⅓ of the Parmesan.
10. Place another layer of dough or noodles over the cheeses. Repeat with another layer of each ingredient in the same order as in Step 9.
11. Place the remaining dough or noodles over the second layer. Top with the remaining sauce, then with the remaining grated Swiss, then with the last of the grated Parmesan.
12. Cover the lasagna with foil. Bake for 45 minutes. Allow to stand at room temperature for 20 minutes to firm up before serving.

VARIATIONS

You can replace the hard cheeses with crumbled panir or more ricotta. Add 1 tablespoon arrowroot or cornstarch for each cup of soft cheese. The lasagna will be less firm.

Replace part of the ricotta with a creamy chèvre or with crumbled panir.

✪ Replace the ricotta with crumbled tofu.

✪ If desired, replace the cheeses with enough fine dry bread crumbs to sprinkle a layer over the sauce. For the top layer, moisten the bread crumbs with olive oil so that they brown nicely. Do not cover the lasagna while baking.

All the Colors of the Rainbow Celebration Menu

Antipasti
Green and White Lasagna (Lasagna Verde Bianca)
Broccoli with Peppers and Cashews (pp. 70–71)
Focaccia Rossa (with Sun-Dried Tomatoes and Peppers) (p. 344)
Mango, Kiwi, and Raspberry Salad with Ginger-Honey Dressing (p. 316)

Pierogen

JEWISH/RUSSIA/EASTERN EUROPE   *About 25*

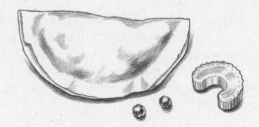

You can use sweet potatoes or winter squash instead of potatoes. Serve these half-moon-shaped treats with plenty of sour cream.

STEP ONE

1 recipe any pasta dough

STEP TWO

2 cups (460 g) Mashed Potatoes (pp. 123–24) or Potato Filling (p. 294)

STEP FOUR *(for fried version only)*

Oil for frying

1. Roll out the pasta dough on a floured board. Cut into 3-inch (7.5 cm) circles with the rim of a glass or a cookie cutter.
2. Place a spoonful of filling on half of each circle. Make a paste of flour and water to moisten the edges, fold the dough over, and seal *very* thoroughly—it is easy for them to fall apart during cooking.
3. Allow the pierogen to dry in the sun for 2 to 3 hours on a floured board.
4. *To boil:* Drop the pierogen into 3 quarts (3 l) of rapidly boiling water. Reduce the heat and boil gently for 6 to 8 minutes. Drain very gently by removing each pierogen with a slotted spoon and tenderly placing in a colander.
   To fry: Heat ½ inch (1.5 cm) oil in a large skillet. Fry in uncrowded batches on both sides over medium-low heat until golden brown. Drain on paper towels.

CELERIAC-FILLED RAVIOLI

ITALY   *20 large ravioli*

There are various machines to roll out and cut ravioli dough; the hand-operated crank type does a very good job. If you do not have one, a rolling pin and a sharp knife or pie edge trimmer will do fine. Either way, you'll need a clean, small paintbrush like the ones in watercolor kits to seal the edges most easily. Seal the edges thoroughly and handle the ravioli gently to ensure a successful conclusion. The delicate flavor of the filling would be overwhelmed by a heavy sauce; melted ghee or Sauce Noisette work very well.

STEP ONE

1 tablespoon olive oil
Pinch of hing (optional)
1 stalk celery, finely chopped
2 cups (190 g) grated celeriac

¼ cup (60 ml) minced celery leaves or
  parsley
Salt

STEP TWO

⅔ cup (160 g) ricotta cheese
⅓ cup (75 g) cream cheese
¼ cup (30 g) ground pistachios or
  blanched almonds

Salt
Black pepper

STEP THREE

1 pound (500 g) fresh pasta dough

1. To make the filling, heat the oil in a large skillet. Add the hing and sauté over low heat for 30 seconds, until fragrant. Add the celery, celeriac, and celery leaves or parsley. Sprinkle with salt, cover, and sauté, stirring occasionally, until the vegetables are tender, about 10 minutes. Allow to cool to room temperature.
2. Place the vegetable mixture in a food processor with the ricotta, cream cheese, and nuts. Process until almost but not completely smooth. Season to taste with salt and pepper. Set aside.
3. Divide the pasta dough into 2 pieces. Roll out each piece on a well-floured board into a 9 × 11-inch (23 × 28 cm) rectangle.
4. Place little spoonfuls of filling on 1 sheet of dough 1 inch (2.5 cm) apart, in rows with 4 across and 5 down, with a ¾-inch (2 cm) edge around the outside.
5. Make a thin flour and water paste. Using a clean paintbrush, brush lines of paste between each row and around the outside edge.
6. Place the second rectangle of dough on top. Gently press down to seal between the rows and around the edges. With a sharp knife or a pie edge trimmer, carefully cut down and across the rows to form the ravioli. Make sure each ravioli is thoroughly sealed. Trim excess dough from the edges if necessary.
7. Place on a floured tray and allow to dry, preferably in the sun, for 2 to 3 hours.
8. Cook in 2 batches. Drop 1 batch at a time into 3 quarts (3 l) of boiling water.

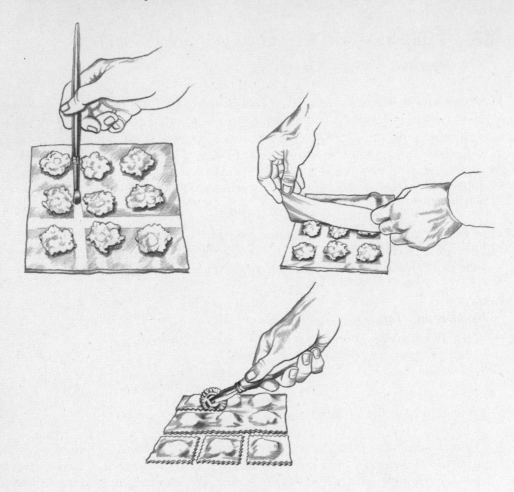

Reduce the heat and gently simmer for 8 to 10 minutes. Remove with a slotted spoon and transfer very gently to a colander.

VARIATIONS

Add ¼ cup (25 g) grated Parmesan cheese to the filling.

Pumpkin Ravioli (Ravioli di Popone): Replace the celeriac with puréed cooked pumpkin or kabocha squash, or replace the entire filling with 1¾ cups (400 g) seasoned pumpkin or squash purée.

Spinach Ravioli (Ravioli di Spinaci): Replace the celery and celeriac with 1 cup (200 g) chopped cooked spinach. Drain very thoroughly before mixing with the cheeses.

Fox's Noodles (Kitsune Udon)

JAPAN 4 servings

Foxes are said to like tofu; hence, the name of this dish.

STEP ONE
½ pound (230 g) fresh Udon Noodles (p. 254) or ¼ pound (115 g) dried

STEP TWO
1 quart (1 l) vegetable stock (p. 219)   *Twenty 1-inch (2.5 cm) cubes firm tofu,*
2 teaspoons sugar   *sautéed*

1. Cook the noodles according to the directions on pages 253–54. Drain.
2. Bring the stock and sugar to a boil. Divide the noodles among 4 bowls. Cover with the stock. Place 5 pieces of tofu on top of the noodles in each bowl.

VARIATION

Noodles and Tempura (Tempura Udon): Replace the tofu with pieces of vegetable tempura (pp. 47–48).

Gnocchi

In parts of Italy little girls and boys are affectionately called *gnoccha* and *gnoccho*. The term *gnocchi* (NYO-kee), meaning "knobs" or "lumps," encompasses a variety of delicious Italian dumpling-type dishes. Serve gnocchi as a light main dish.

 # Gnocchi alla Romana

ITALY 4 to 6 servings

A gently flavored and textured semolina gnocchi.

STEP ONE
1½ cups (360 ml) nondairy milk   *⅔ cup (120 g) semolina*
1½ cups (360 ml) vegetable stock or water

STEP TWO
¼ teaspoon ground nutmeg   *½ teaspoon salt*

STEP SIX
¼ cup (60 ml) melted ghee or   *2 tablespoons grated Parmesan*
butter   *cheese* (optional)

STEP SEVEN

Minced fresh parsley   *Black pepper*

1. Bring the water or stock and milk to a boil. Slowly pour in the semolina with one hand, stirring the mixture constantly with the other.
2. Cook over low heat, stirring constantly, until the mixture is thick and pulls away slightly from the sides of the pan. This will take just a few minutes. Beat in the nutmeg and salt.
3. Spread the mixture about ⅛ inch to ¼ inch (3 to 6 mm) thick on a buttered baking sheet. Chill to harden.
4. Preheat the oven to 400°F (200°C). Butter a baking dish.
5. Gently peel the semolina off the pan and place on a cutting board. Cut out circles with the rim of a glass. Cut each circle in half to form a half moon.
6. Arrange the half moons in a baking dish, slightly overlapping. Brush with melted ghee or butter and pour the remaining ghee or butter over them. Sprinkle evenly with the Parmesan.
7. Bake until the edges of the gnocchi and the cheese are golden brown, 20 to 30 minutes. Sprinkle with parsley and pepper. Serve immediately.

VARIATIONS

Serve with Tomato Sauce (pp. 505–506) or pesto (pp. 509–12).
Use Monterey Jack or mozzarella cheese instead of Parmesan.

 # Spinach Gnocchi (Gnocchi di Spinaci)

ITALY   *6 servings*

Prepared with homemade ricotta, these Tuscan delights have an incomparably delicate flavor and texture. Gentle handling throughout the whole process is the key to success.

STEP ONE

6 cups (570 g) coarsely chopped spinach leaves

STEP TWO

2 cups (500 g) ricotta cheese or soft panir   *6 tablespoons flour*
¼ cup (25 g) grated Parmesan cheese   *1 teaspoon salt*
2 tablespoons arrowroot or cornstarch   *½ teaspoon freshly grated nutmeg*

STEP THREE

Flour

STEP SEVEN
¼ cup (60 ml) melted ghee or butter   *2 tablespoons grated Parmesan cheese*

1. Steam the spinach just until wilted. Drain well, squeezing out the water. Chop fine.
2. Gently mix the spinach with all the ingredients for Step 2.
3. Sprinkle flour on a cutting board. Roll the gnocchi mixture into balls the size of large marbles. Gently roll in the flour to form egg shapes.
4. Bring a large pot of water to a boil. Have a watch, a colander, and a slotted spoon ready at the starting gate.
5. Gently drop the gnocchi into the water. Look at your watch to time the cooking at exactly 2 minutes. Gently jostle the pot to keep the gnocchi from sticking to the bottom. After a minute or so they will rise to the top.
6. After 2 minutes, gently remove the gnocchi with a slotted spoon to the colander. Do not drop them; they are quite fragile. From the colander, place them side by side in a buttered baking dish.
7. Preheat the broiler. Pour the melted ghee or butter over the gnocchi. Sprinkle on the Parmesan. Place under the broiler for a minute to lightly brown the cheese. Serve immediately.

VARIATIONS
Use watercress or arugula instead of spinach.
Add a few basil leaves to the spinach.
Top the gnocchi with shredded Jack or mozzarella cheese instead of Parmesan.
Top with sour cream instead of, or in addition to, the hard cheese. Do not broil if using sour cream only.

POLENTA GNOCCHI (GNOCCHI DI POLENTA)

ITALY   *4 servings*

Serve with a salad or some sautéed vegetables and focaccia for a lovely lunch.

STEP ONE
2 cups (480 ml) vegetable   *½ teaspoon salt*
stock or water   *½ cup (75 g) polenta*

STEP TWO
2 tablespoons flour

STEP FOUR
3 quarts (3 l) water   *1 tablespoon salt*

2 tablespoons ghee or butter
Pinch of hing (optional)
2 tablespoons chopped fresh sage

STEP SIX

2 tablespoons grated Parmesan
cheese (optional)

1. Bring the stock or water and salt to a boil. Stirring constantly, add the polenta in a steady stream. Reduce the heat and simmer, stirring constantly, until very thick.
2. Beat in the flour. Let cool until hardened, 45 to 60 minutes.
3. Preheat the oven to 350°F (180°C). Butter a 9-inch (23 cm) baking pan.
4. Bring the water and salt to a boil over high heat. Meanwhile, with moistened hands roll spoonfuls of the polenta into ¾-inch (2 cm) round marbles. Make sure they have no cracks.
5. Drop the gnocchi into the water all at once. Watch carefully, and after a minute or two they will all rise to the surface. The moment the last gnocchi has risen, count 20 seconds, then gently remove them with a slotted spoon to a colander.
6. Melt the ghee or butter in a small skillet. Add the hing and sauté over low heat until fragrant, about 30 seconds. Gently place the gnocchi in the baking pan. Sprinkle the sage over them, then pour the melted ghee or butter on top. Sprinkle with Parmesan if desired.
7. Bake for 20 minutes. Serve immediately.

VARIATIONS

Omit the sage or replace with dried basil leaves.
Serve with a tomato sauce or a pesto.

POTATO GNOCCHI (GNOCCHI DI PATATE)

ITALY   *4 servings*

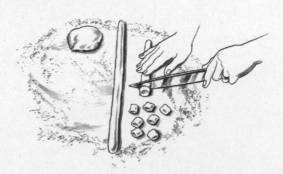

Potato gnocchi's purpose in life is to be a neutrally flavored foil for a flavorful sauce. They are traditionally slathered with tomato sauce and grated Parmesan. You can also sauce them with pesto or Salsa di Noci. A caution: use only thin-skinned "boiling" potatoes, eschewing new potatoes and baking potatoes, or you won't be able to look anyone in the eye with the results in hand.

STEP ONE

1½ cups (340 g) cooked, peeled, and thoroughly mashed boiling potatoes (about 4)

1½ cups (210 g) unbleached white flour

STEP TWO

3 quarts (3 l) water

1 tablespoon salt

STEP FOUR

Sauce, as described above

1. Make sure the potatoes are free of lumps—pass through a food mill if you have one. Add 1¼ cups (175 g) of the flour and mix together well. Continue to add flour until you have a soft dough that has some slight stickiness to it.
2. Bring the water and salt to a boil in a wide casserole or soup pot. Meanwhile, using your hands, roll out pieces of the dough on a lightly floured board to form long, rounded ropes ¾-inch (2 cm) thick. Slice off ¾-inch (2 cm) pieces with a sharp knife.
3. When the water comes to a full boil, stand by with a serving bowl, a slotted spoon, and a watch or clock. Drop half of the gnocchi into the water. Do not settle in with a copy of *War and Peace*; watch with baited breath until they rise, which they will do in a minute or so. If there are a few laggards, give them a gentle nudge with your spoon. The moment all are floating, wait 10 seconds, then gently remove them to the bowl. Repeat with the second batch.
4. Toss the gnocchi with plenty of your chosen sauce.

In the heaven-world there is no fear; thou are not there, O Death, and no one is afraid on account of old age. Leaving behind both hunger and thirst, and out of reach of sorrow, all rejoice in the world of heaven.

—KATHA UPANISHAD

Appetizers, Finger Foods, and Savories

For us winds do blow,

The earth resteth, heav'n moveth, fountains flow;

Nothing we see but means our good,

As our delight or as our treasure;

The whole is either our cupboard of food

Or cabinet of pleasure.

—George Herbert

Ayurveda generally recommends having ample time to digest one meal before consuming the next. Therefore, small dishes such as these might more often be served as part of a meal rather than as a preprandial or between-meal snack. Almost every culture has a tradition of small savory tidbits. Partake of *hors d'oeuvres* in France, *zakuski* in Russia, *meze* in Greece, or *mazza* in the Middle East, a Scandinavian *smörgåsbord*, Spanish *tapas*, or Chinese *dim sum*—presumably not all on the same day.

Antipasto and Mezethakia or Mazza

Antipasto, "before the meal," is the first course of an Italian meal. Though many dishes can be served as a first course, a true antipasto often comprises a lovely composed salad featuring several or many cooked and lightly dressed vegetables and beans served at room temperature. It is a warmer weather option that is adaptable as a salad course or as a lunch unto itself. Spread a bed of greens on a serving platter or individual plates and decoratively arrange a variety of any or all of the foods suggested below. Serve with crusty Italian-style bread.

Vegetables such as cucumbers, beets, fennel, green beans, carrots, eggplant, zucchini, and artichoke hearts, dressed with olive oil and lemon juice
Greek-Style Marinated Vegetables (pp. 304–305)

Bean salads (p. 311)
Sesame Radish Salad (p. 311)
Whole cooked artichokes
Roasted Peppers (pp. 116–17)
Oil-packed dried tomatoes
Spoonfuls of ricotta and other soft cheeses

Mezethakia, "opens the appetite" in Greek, becomes *mazza* in Arabic—tidbits that are eaten to allay hunger in the hours before the customarily late dinner. Some restaurants in Greece and the Middle East feature tables with hundreds of little dishes for patrons to choose from. A typical repast includes bowls of plain yogurt, minced fresh herbs, and pita bread, plus a variety of other dishes. Fill small dishes and bowls with a variety of the suggested foods.

Toasted salted almonds, pine nuts, sunflower seeds, pistachios (Greeks also
    serve watermelon seeds), sometimes served with honey for dipping
Greek-Style Marinated Vegetables (pp. 304–305)
Bean salads (p. 311)
Cakik (p. 305)
Roasted Peppers (pp. 116–17)
Fresh figs
Dolmáthes (pp. 297–98)
Melon cubes
Puréed vegetables, drizzled with olive oil
Baba Ghanouj (recipe follows)
Cashew-Coconut Hummus (pp. 280–81)
Borani (recipe follows, pp. 278–79)

BABA GHANOUJ (EGGPLANT DIP)

MIDDLE EAST   *3 cups (720 ml)*

Baba ghanouj means something like "pampered father," for this rich, tangy eggplant purée was originally created by a devoted daughter to please her toothless progenitor. Traditionally served with pita bread, Baba Ghanouj can also be used as a filling for Falafel and other pita sandwiches. Use a heavier hand (or should I say, a heavier thumb and forefinger) with the hing than usual.

STEP ONE

2 large eggplants

STEP THREE

½ cup (120 ml) olive oil   ½ cup (70 g) sesame seeds
Large pinch of hing

STEP FOUR

1 tablespoon minced fresh ginger   ½ cup (120 ml) lemon juice

STEP FIVE

Liquid seasoning or salt   Black pepper

1. To grill the eggplants, either either place in the broiler, or spear each one whole with a large fork and hold over the flame on a gas burner. Turn repeatedly until the skin is charred and blackened and the eggplants are tender.
2. As soon as they are cool enough to handle, peel the eggplants. Using a fork or potato masher, mash them to make a rough paste.
3. Place the olive oil, hing, and sesame seeds in a small skillet. Sauté over low heat, stirring frequently, until the sesame seeds are golden brown. Remove from the heat immediately. Allow to cool for a few minutes.
4. Place the sesame seed mixture, ginger, and lemon juice in a blender and blend on high speed until smooth.
5. Beat into the mashed eggplants. Season to taste with liquid seasoning or salt and pepper. Serve at room temperature with toasted pita triangles.

VARIATIONS

For a pungent flavor, sauté crumbled red chilies or powdered cayenne in the oil.

Baba Ghanouj à la Less Work: Homemade tahini has a more interesting texture, but there are times when less work is more. Replace the ingredients in Steps 3 and 4 with ½ cup (130 g) prepared tahini.

Faites simple—Keep it simple.   —ESCOFFIER'S CREDO

 # BORANI (SPINACH-YOGURT DIP)

IRAN   2½ cups (600 ml)

In the first millennia A.D. there lived a Persian queen named Poorandolet. She was immensely fond of yogurt, so a special dish containing her favorite ingredient was created and christened "poorani" in her honor. The name evolved into *borani* and has come to connote a variety of vegetables mixed with yogurt. You'll find variations on spinach purée mixed with yogurt from Greece to Afghanistan. Serve with pita wedges.

STEP ONE

1 pound (500 g) spinach

STEP TWO

¼ cup (60 ml) lemon juice *½ teaspoon ground cumin, toasted*
2 tablespoons olive oil *Salt*
1 cup (240 ml) yogurt

1. Wash the spinach thoroughly and remove the stalks. Steam the leaves just until wilted, about 1 minute. Drain well and let cool to room temperature.
2. Purée the spinach with the remaining ingredients in a blender or food processor. Adjust the salt.

VARIATION
✪ Replace the yogurt with Tofu or Cashew Mayonnaise (pp. 503–504).

To eat is a necessity, but to eat intelligently is an art. —LA ROCHEFOUCALD

 # GUACAMOLE (AVOCADO DIP)

MEXICO *About 2 cups (480 ml)*

Guacamole is Aztec fare, enthusiastically perpetuated by its inheritors throughout the world family. There are many ways to prepare it, some distinctly better than others, as the delicate flavor of the avocado is often drowned out by the noisy carousing of masses of onions and chilies. Prepare no more than an hour in advance; avocado flesh turns brown when exposed to air, and its subtle flavor also alters dismally quickly.

1 tablespoon oil *Liquid seasoning or salt*
Pinch of hing *Black pepper*
1 teaspoon cumin seeds *⅓ cup (80 ml) finely chopped fresh*
2 cups (450 g) mashed avocado   *cilantro*
  (about 2 large) *¼ cup (20 g) chopped dried*
2 tablespoons lemon or lime juice   *tomatoes soaked in hot water*
1 tablespoon minced fresh ginger   *to soften if necessary* (optional)

1. Heat the oil in a small skillet. Add the hing and cumin seeds and sauté over low heat until fragrant, about 1 minute.
2. Mix the avocado with the hing, lemon or lime juice, and ginger. Season to taste with liquid seasoning or salt, pepper, and chopped cilantro. Stir in the dried tomatoes. Serve at room temperature with tostaditas or corn chips.

VARIATIONS
   Add ¼ cup sour cream or Cashew, Panir, or Tofu Mayonnaise.
   Replace the fresh ginger with chopped crystallized ginger.

 # CASHEW-COCONUT HUMMUS (GARBANZO PURÉE)

MIDDLE EAST   *2 cups (480 ml)*

A version that marches to the beat of a different drummer from the usual garlic-laden, tahini-based Middle Eastern *hummus bi tehina*. Note that you must soak the garbanzos overnight.

STEP ONE

1 cup (190 g) dried garbanzo beans
   (chickpeas)

STEP THREE

¼ cup (60 ml) olive oil	*⅓ cup (50 g) chopped bell peppers*
Pinch of hing (optional)	*2 tablespoons minced fresh ginger*
2 teaspoons cumin seeds	

STEP FOUR

3 tablespoons lemon juice	*¾ cup (180 ml) coconut milk*
¾ cup (105 g) cashews, toasted	

STEP FIVE

½ cup (120 ml) minced fresh parsley	*Liquid seasoning or salt*
3 tablespoons fresh dill	*Black pepper*
1 teaspoon raw sugar	

1. Clean the garbanzos. Place in a bowl with at least 3 cups (720 ml) of water and soak overnight.
2. Drain, then place in a pot with at least 6 cups (1.4 l) of water. Bring to a boil, reduce heat, and simmer until very tender, about 2½ hours. Drain well.
3. Heat the oil in a skillet. Add the hing, cumin seeds, and bell peppers. Sauté over low heat for a few minutes, until the peppers are tender. Stir in the ginger and remove from the heat.
4. Purée the pepper mixture in a food processor or blender with the lemon juice, cashews, and coconut milk until smooth. (A blender makes the smoothest purée, if you can stand to clean it up in addition to a food processor for the next step.)
5. Purée with the garbanzos in a food processor. Blend in the parsley, dill, and raw sugar, and season with liquid seasoning or salt and pepper to taste. Serve at room temperature with pita wedges.

VARIATIONS
Add 2 to 3 tablespoons chopped dried tomatoes.
Add cayenne or chopped fresh chilies.

 # DIP WITH THREE FENNELS AND THREE PEPPERS

2 cups (480 ml)

Here is a basic way to build a creamy dip using sautéed vegetables and seasonings to flavor and color it. For the best texture, peel the bell pepper with a vegetable peeler before chopping. You can substitute sour cream for the thinned cream cheese, use different vegetables, grill the vegetables for a smoky flavor, or replace the vegetables with mashed avocado.

STEP ONE

2 tablespoons olive oil
Pinch of hing (optional)
1 cup (110 g) finely chopped fennel
1 cup (140 g) finely chopped red
    bell peppers

Liquid seasoning or salt
1 teaspoon sugar

STEP TWO

1 tablespoon fennel seeds

STEP THREE

2 cups (two 8-ounce packages/
    450 g) cream cheese
1 tablespoon water
2 tablespoons finely chopped fennel
    tops (if not enough on the fennel
    bulb, make up the difference
    with parsley)

2 tablespoons minced fresh parsley
½ teaspoon paprika
White pepper

1. Heat the oil in a skillet. Add the hing and sauté over low heat for 30 seconds, until fragrant. Add the fennel and bell peppers, sprinkle with liquid seasoning or salt and with the sugar. Cover and sauté until very tender and slightly browned.
2. Lightly toast the fennel seeds in a dry pan. Crush to a coarse powder with a rolling pin.
3. Whirl all the ingredients except the liquid seasoning or salt and the pepper in a food processor, stopping before completely smooth. Add plenty of pepper and adjust the liquid seasoning or salt.

VARIATIONS
Replace the cream cheese and water with Panir, Tofu, or Avocado Mayonnaise (pp. 503–504).

Replace the seasonings with ¼ teaspoon curry powder or Maharishi Ayur-Veda churna.

Add finely chopped dried tomatoes or Dried Tomato Paste (p. 506).

Replace the seasonings with a pesto.

 # MOUSSE D'AVOCAT (AVOCADO MOUSSE)

WEST AFRICA   *About 10 servings*

STEP ONE

1½ cups (360 ml) vegetable stock   *1 tablespoon agar agar flakes**

STEP TWO

3 cups (650 g) mashed avocado   *2 cups (480 ml) sour cream*
(about 3 large)   *Liquid seasoning*
¼ cup (60 ml) lemon juice   *Seasoned salt*
1 tablespoon sugar

STEP FOUR

Lettuce leaves or mesclun

1. Bring the stock to a boil. Reduce the heat, stir in the agar agar flakes, and simmer for about 5 minutes, stirring constantly, until the agar agar is dissolved.
2. Combine the broth with the mashed avocado, lemon juice, sugar, and sour cream in a blender until completely smooth. Season to taste with liquid seasoning and seasoned salt.
3. Pour into a 1½-quart (1.5 l) ring mold. Chill to set.
4. Cover a platter with lettuce leaves or mesclun. To unmold, dip the mold into hot water for 1 second, then invert on the platter and shake gently.

VARIATIONS

✪ Replace the sour cream with tofu.

Frozen Mousse: Allow to set in a pan, not a mold. Freeze in an ice cream maker, or in the same manner as Fruit Ice (pp. 480–81). Serve in scoops on a bed of mesclun.

---

*This measurement is for agar agar flakes of which 1 tablespoon flakes thickens 1 quart (1 l) liquid. If your brand requires more to thicken 1 quart (1 l), increase the measurement to 4 teaspoons.

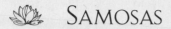

SAMOSAS

INDIA   *24 to 30 pastries*

In this aesthetically pleasing dish, flaky, fluted pastry encloses a delicately spiced vegetable filling. Mint Chutney (p. 520) is the traditional accompaniment.

STEP ONE

2 cups (280 g) unbleached white
   flour
¼ cup (60 ml) melted ghee or butter

½ cup (120 ml) water
   (approximately)

STEP THREE

3 tablespoons ghee or butter
Pinch of hing (optional)
1½ teaspoons ground cumin

2½ cups peeled, coarsely chopped
   potatoes (355 g) or chopped
   cauliflower (265 g)

STEP FOUR

⅔ cup (90 g) peas
1 teaspoon turmeric
1 teaspoon ground coriander

¼ teaspoon ground fenugreek
½ teaspoon sugar
Salt

STEP NINE

Oil for deep-frying

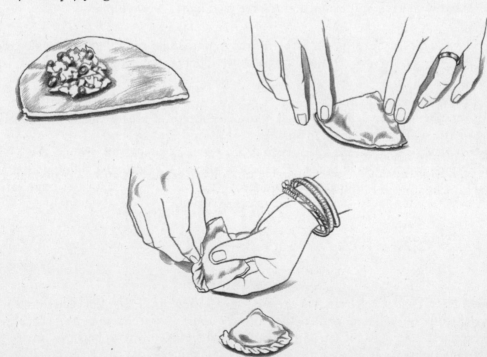

To prepare the dough:
1. Sift the flour. Add the melted ghee or butter and mix in enough water to form a soft, nonsticky dough.
2. Turn out on a floured board. Knead lightly just a few times, cover, and set aside to rest while preparing the filling.

To prepare the filling:
3. Melt the ghee or butter in a skillet. Add the hing and cumin and sauté over low heat until fragrant, about 1 minute. Add the potatoes or cauliflower and sauté, stirring frequently, until they begin to soften, 10 to 15 minutes.
4. Add the peas, spices, and sugar. Continue to sauté until the potatoes and peas are tender. Add salt to taste and cook for another 30 seconds.
5. Remove from the heat and mash to a rough—not completely smooth—consistency. Let cool to room temperature.

To assemble:
6. Divide the dough into 12 to 15 pieces and roll into 1-inch (2.5 cm) balls.
7. On a floured board, roll out each ball into a 3½-inch (9 cm) round. Cut each round in half.
8. Place a spoonful of filling on a half round. Fold the dough in half to form a triangle. Make a thin paste of flour and water and moisten the edges with it. Pinch closed. Be sure they are thoroughly sealed. For a beautiful touch, starting at one end along the curved edge, pinch a little of the dough between the thumb and forefinger and twist over. Continue pinching and twisting along the edge to form a fluted pattern. Repeat with each half round and reserve on a lightly floured plate.

To cook:
9. Heat the oil for deep-frying. Deep-fry the samosas just until they are a pale golden color—do not brown. Drain on paper towels. Serve immediately.

VARIATIONS

Add cayenne to the filling.

An inauthentic but delicious touch is to place a dab of cream cheese on top of the filling before sealing the dough in Step 8.

Sambousic: These cheese-filled pastries are eaten as snacks all around the Middle East. Prepare samosas as in the above recipe, replacing the vegetable filling with a mixture of 3 cups (600 g) crumbled semisoft cheese, such as panir, feta, or fresh mozzarella, and 1 tablespoon minced fresh dill or 1 teaspoon dried.

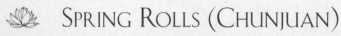

SPRING ROLLS (CHUNJUAN)

CHINA   *12 to 14 rolls*

Chinese New Year is celebrated at the advent of spring, and these delicacies are shared among friends and relatives gathered for the occasion. Hence the name *spring rolls*. Serve with Sweet-and-Sour Sauce (p. 514). Ready-made spring roll wrappers are often available in supermarkets and Asian markets. (Some contain eggs, so check the label.)

STEP ONE

1 tablespoon mild-flavored oil

Pinch of hing (optional)

1 tablespoon minced fresh ginger

3 cups (720 ml) shredded or minced
 vegetables (use at least 3 of the
 following: carrot, turnip, celery,
 bell pepper, bok choy, cabbage,
 spinach, whole mung sprouts)

STEP TWO

½ teaspoon sugar

Finely chopped fresh cilantro

Liquid seasoning or salt

White pepper

A few drops toasted sesame oil

STEP THREE

Prepared spring roll wrappers or
 Basic Pasta or Soy or Chickpea
 Pasta Dough (p. 254)

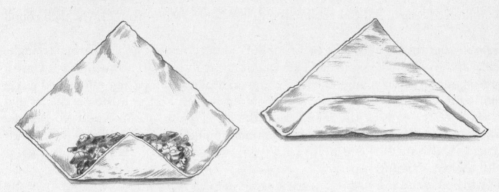

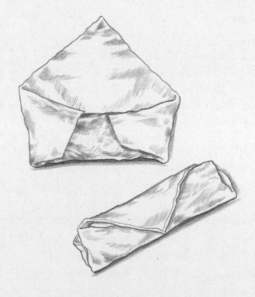

STEP FOUR
Flour

STEP FIVE

Oil for deep-frying

To prepare the filling:
1. Heat the oil in a small wok or skillet. Add the hing and ginger and sauté over low heat for 1 minute, stirring frequently. Add the vegetables. Cook over medium-high heat, stirring constantly, until they are crisp-tender.
2. Add the sugar. Remove from the heat and season to taste with cilantro, liquid seasoning or salt, white pepper, and a few drops of toasted sesame oil. Let cool to room temperature.

To prepare the wrappers:
3. If using pasta dough, roll out very thin on a floured board in as close to a rectangular shape as you can manage. Using a sharp knife or a pizza cutter, cut the dough into 6 × 6-inch (15 × 15 cm) squares.

To assemble and cook:
4. Place a wrapper on the table in a diamond shape with one point toward you. Place a large spoonful of the filling on half a wrapper. Make a thin paste of flour and water and lightly moisten the edges with it. Fold up the left and right points of the diamond over the ends of the filling. Fold the lower point of the diamond over the filling and, holding the 2 ends shut, continue rolling to form a tube with the ends tucked in. Moisten the end point with flour and water paste and seal shut. Repeat with the remaining wrappers.
5. Heat the oil for deep-frying. Deep-fry the rolls until light golden brown, turning gently once or twice. Drain on paper towels. Serve immediately.

VARIATION
Replace some of the filling with sautéed crumbled tofu or seitan.

 # RICE PAPER SPRING ROLLS (CHA GIO)
SOUTHEAST ASIA   *12 to 14 rolls*

I first tasted these crispy spring rolls when Klaus, a family friend, stepped off the plane from Vietnam with his bride. After a week with my family, she spent a day in the kitchen preparing a Vietnamese meal for us. My young senses had never before been so sorely tried by The Great Unknown. (I'm sure that Uyen had spent a sorely trying week attempting to down my mother's best efforts.) I made a meal of her light, crispy spring rolls—the closest to anything I had ever experienced before.

In Southeast Asia spring rolls are prepared with translucent-white, crispy rice flour wrappers instead of the Chinese wheat flour variety. Their presentation, cut into pieces and wrapped in lettuce leaves with basil and cucumber, is also quite different from that of their Chinese cousins. Serve plain or with Sweet-and-Sour Sauce (p. 514) or Sambal (pp. 515–16). Rice paper or rice noodle sheets can be found in Asian markets. You may want to use two or even three skillets to accomplish the leisurely cooking process in one fell swoop rather than in batches.

STEP ONE

1 tablespoon mild-flavored oil,
   such as sesame or sunflower
Pinch of hing (optional)

1 cup (220 g) chopped firm tofu
Liquid seasoning or salt

STEP TWO

1 tablespoon mild-flavored oil
1 tablespoon minced fresh ginger
2 stalks celery, finely chopped
1 cup (100 g) chopped chard or spinach

¼ cup (60 ml) finely chopped fresh
   mint
3 tablespoons finely chopped fresh
   cilantro

STEP THREE

½ cup (40 g) mung bean thread noodles, broken into small pieces

STEP FOUR

Rice paper

STEP FIVE

Oil for frying

STEP SIX

Tender lettuce leaves, such as bibb
   or green leaf

Fresh basil leaves
1 cucumber, peeled and sliced

1. Heat 1 tablespoon oil in a skillet. Add the hing and sauté over medium heat for 30 seconds, until fragrant. Add the tofu, sprinkle with liquid seasoning or salt, and sauté, stirring frequently, until lightly browned. Set aside.
2. Heat another tablespoon of oil in the skillet. Add the ginger and celery and sauté until crisp-tender. Stir in the chard or spinach and stir until wilted. Stir in the mint and cilantro.
3. Simmer the bean thread noodles in water until tender, about 10 minutes. Drain and mix together with the tofu and sautéed vegetables. Adjust the seasoning.
4. Cut the rice paper into 6 × 6-inch (15 × 15 cm) rectangles. Brush both surfaces of 1 or 2 pieces with water. In 1 minute they should become quite flexible. Do not let them sit; they will get soggy. Fill and fold as described in Step 4 of the preceding recipe for Spring Rolls.
5. Heat the oil ½ inch (1.5 cm) deep in a large skillet over low heat. Place as many spring rolls in the skillet as possible without crowding. Fry slowly, turning once or twice. It will take about 6 minutes of slow frying on each side to cook them. The wrappers will not brown very much; a crisp texture is a better indication of doneness. Drain on paper towels.

6. Slice each spring roll into 3 or 4 pieces. Place each piece in a lettuce leaf, along with 1 or 2 basil leaves and a few cucumber slices. Roll up in the lettuce leaf.

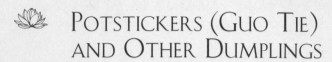

POTSTICKERS (GUO TIE) AND OTHER DUMPLINGS

CHINA   *About 25*

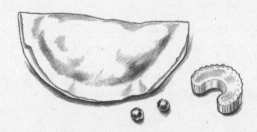

The culinary saving grace for a small band of *mei-gwo ren* (American persons) on the loose in Taichung, Taiwan, was a little vegetarian hole-in-the-wall featuring an enclosed fire pit with a built-in cauldron of boiling soup and a stack of bamboo steamers that rose to a towering height. After some unnecessary gesticulation on our part, Mama or Papa would throw exactly the right amount of noodles into the cauldron and hand each of us a steamer filled with dumplings, a pair of chopsticks, and, almost instantaneously, a bowl of fresh noodle soup. We then sat at the only table, inevitably sharing it with a child doing homework, to savor our fast food feast. Potstickers, the famous element of dim sum, are cooked by the dual method of frying followed by steaming. They can also be boiled or steamed.

STEP ONE

1 tablespoon mild-flavored oil
Pinch of *hing* (optional)
1 tablespoon minced fresh ginger
2 cups (480 ml) shredded or minced
   vegetables (*use at least 3 of the
   following: carrot, turnip, celery,
   bell pepper, bok choy, cabbage,
   spinach, whole mung sprouts*)

1 cup (220 g) well-drained,
   crumbled firm tofu

STEP TWO

½ teaspoon sugar
Liquid seasoning or salt
White pepper

A drizzle of toasted sesame oil
Finely chopped fresh cilantro

STEP THREE

Prepared spring roll wrappers, or Basic Pasta or Soy or Chickpea Pasta Dough
   (p. 254), prepared with boiling water

Flour

2 tablespoons mild-flavored oil

To prepare the filling:
1. Heat the oil in a small wok or skillet. Add the hing and ginger and sauté over low heat for 1 minute, stirring frequently. Add the vegetables and cook over medium-high heat, stirring constantly, until crisp-tender. Stir in the tofu and cook for 1 minute.
2. Add the sugar. Remove from the heat and season to taste with liquid seasoning or salt, white pepper, toasted sesame oil, and cilantro. Let cool to room temperature.

To prepare the wrappers:
3. If using pasta dough, roll out very thin on a floured board. Cut out 3-inch (7.5 cm) rounds with a cookie cutter or the rim of a glass.

To assemble and cook:
4. Place a spoonful of filling on half of a wrapper. Make a thin paste of flour and water and lightly moisten the edges with it. Fold the dough in half. Pinch closed and seal thoroughly, as in the diagram. Repeat with the remaining wrappers and reserve on a floured platter.
5. Place the oil in a wide skillet over medium heat. Add about ⅓ of the potstickers; do not crowd them. Cook until they are nicely browned on one side. Do not stir during the frying. Check one by lifting with a spatula.
6. Add ½ inch (1.5 cm) of water to the skillet. Bring to a boil. Cover, reduce the heat, and steam for a few minutes, until the wrappers are slightly translucent and shiny, like al dente pasta. Try one potsticker to check that the dough is cooked. (potstickers do tend to be a *little* gummy; if that is the case, you haven't failed.) Serve immediately.

VARIATIONS
Boiled Dumplings (Shui Jiao Guo Tie):
1. Prepare potstickers but do not cook. Bring 6 quarts (6 l) of water to a boil in a large soup pot. Leave on high heat.
2. Gently drop in the dumplings. When the water boils again, add 2 cups of cold water to break the boil.
3. Bring to a boil again, reduce the heat to medium, and boil until tender, 5 to 6 minutes.
4. Quickly and gently lift each dumpling out of the water with a slotted spoon and transfer to a serving plate. Do not try to pour them into a colander; they will break.

Steamed Dumplings (Zheng Jiao Guo Tie):
1. Prepare potstickers but do not cook. Place the dumplings in a steaming basket over boiling water. (Chinese bamboo steamers are especially suited for the purpose.) If

you do not have a steaming basket, you can improvise by placing the dumplings on a heatproof plate and setting the plate on an inverted flat-bottomed heatproof bowl in a large pot. Fill the pot with water to just below the plate and bring to a boil.
2. Cover and steam over medium heat until the wrappers are done, about 15 minutes.

WONTONS (HUN TUN)

Wontons were originally a Mongolian delicacy, first served in China during the reign of the Mongol conqueror Kublai Khan. They are made in the same manner as other dumplings but are shaped differently. Ready-made "wonton wrappers" are often available in supermarkets and Asian markets. (Some contain eggs, so check the label.)

Otherwise, trim dough into 3-inch (7.5 cm) squares. Place filling on half of each square. Moisten the edges with a flour and water paste. Fold over and seal thoroughly. Bend the outside edges of the square toward you, as in the diagram. Seal the edges that meet.

WONTON SOUP (HUNTUN TANG)

Cook as for Boiled Dumplings (previous page). For Wonton Soup, drain very gently by removing a few at a time with a slotted spoon. Divide the wontons among 5 or 6 individual bowls. Pour a hot, flavorful vegetable stock over them. Serve immediately.

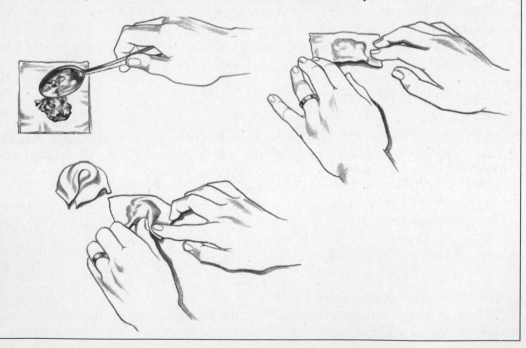

PAKORAS
(SPICED CHICKPEA BATTER FRITTERS)

INDIA   *4 servings*

On a rainy night an ancient bus with canvas shades flapping inadequately over open windows rattled through the western Ghat mountains of India, bearing a young Indian couple, my husband, Steve, and me. Two hours of mutually endured torture sealed a friendship. They gave us their address in a small village hundreds of miles away with an invitation to visit any Sunday. Miles and months later, another bus bumped and rattled through a Kerala jungle and deposited us in their tiny village. We were greeted with surprise, delight, and after a quiet exit by the wife to the kitchen, with a tray of sizzling potato pakoras—manna from heaven. Pakoras are made by dipping vegetables or panir in a spicy chickpea flour batter and deep-frying them. The batter can also be fried by itself in spoonfuls. Serve with a chutney for dipping.

STEP ONE

1½ cups (180 g) besan (chickpea
    flour)
¼ teaspoon baking powder
1¼ teaspoons salt
1 teaspoon turmeric

1½ teaspoons cumin seeds
1 tablespoon minced fresh ginger
Pinch of hing (optional)
1 to 1⅓ cups (240 to 320 ml) water

STEP TWO

Oil for deep-frying
Fillings: 4 cups (940 ml) thinly
    sliced vegetables, such as
    eggplant, potatoes, summer or
    winter squash, and spinach
    leaves, or bananas, or cubed
    panir

1. *To prepare the batter:* Combine the besan, baking powder, salt, and spices. Add the water and mix in a blender or food processor to make a thick batter—use 1 cup (240 ml) of water for plain pakoras and 1⅓ cups (320 ml) for filled pakoras.
2. Heat oil for deep-frying. To make *plain pakoras,* drop spoonfuls of batter into the oil and deep-fry until golden brown, turning once or twice. To make *filled pakoras,* dip each piece of filling in the batter separately to coat it thoroughly, then deep-fry until golden brown, turning once or twice.
3. Drain on paper towels. Serve immediately.

VARIATIONS
    Blend fresh or dried chilies into the batter.
    For an inauthentic but delicious variation, dip cubes of fresh mozzarella or cream cheese in the batter and deep-fry.

Add shredded cabbage or spinach to the batter and fry in spoonfuls as for plain pakoras.

Prasad Pakoras: Place a generous dab of cream cheese between 2 thin slices of zucchini and press to hold. Dip in pakora batter and deep-fry.

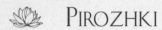

PIROZHKI

RUSSIA   *20 pirozhki*

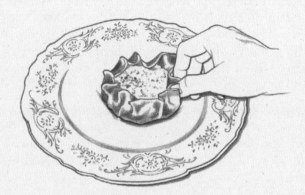

When I was a child, for a wondrous treat my mother would take me to the Russian Miniature Bakery in San Francisco to feast on freshly made pirozhki. Here is a group-sized amount of these rich, filling pastries. The crust completely encloses the filling in some pirozhki; in this recipe it forms a decorative cradle for the filling. Note that the crust is prepared in advance and can even be made the night before.

STEP ONE

*1¼ cups (175 g) unbleached white
    flour*
1¼ cups (155 g) rye flour

1 teaspoon salt
⅔ cup (145 g) butter

STEP TWO

⅔ cup (160 ml) sour cream

STEP FIVE

*Kasha or Potato Filling (recipes
    follow)*

Sesame or poppy seeds

To prepare the crust:

1. Sift the flours and salt into a bowl. Add the butter and work with your fingers or a pastry cutter until the mixture resembles coarse meal.
2. Add the sour cream. Mix until the ingredients just hold together in a ball. For best

results, wrap in waxed paper and refrigerate for 1 to 6 hours, or prepare the night before and refrigerate. Allow to stand at room temperature for 20 to 30 minutes to soften before rolling out.

To assemble and cook:

3. Preheat the oven to 375°F (190°C). Butter a baking sheet.
4. Roll the dough out ⅛-inch (3 mm) thick on a floured board. Cut out 4½-inch (11 cm) rounds.
5. Place a large spoonful of filling in the middle of each round. Sprinkle with sesame or poppy seeds. Bring up the dough, making little pinches in it to encase, but not completely enclose, the filling (see diagram).
6. Place the pirozhki on the baking sheet and bake until the crust is lightly browned, 30 to 40 minutes. Carefully remove with a spatula. Serve hot.

KASHA FILLING

2 cups (480 ml)

Also good for stuffing Golubsti (pp. 77–78).

STEP ONE

2 tablespoons ghee or oil	1 stalk fennel or celery, thinly sliced
Pinch of hing (optional)	½ bell pepper, chopped

STEP TWO

⅔ cup (110 g) kasha	Liquid seasoning or salt
1⅓ cups (320 ml) vegetable stock or water	Black pepper
½ cup (120 ml) sour cream	

1. Heat the ghee or oil in a saucepan. Add the hing, fennel or celery, and bell pepper and sauté over low heat, stirring frequently, until tender.
2. Add the kasha and the stock or water. Bring to a boil. Cover, reduce the heat, and simmer for 10 minutes. Turn off the heat and allow to stand, without lifting the lid, until all the water has been absorbed, about 10 minutes. Stir in the sour cream. Season to taste with liquid seasoning or salt and pepper.

VARIATION

✪ Omit the sour cream or replace in Step 2 with tofu or Tofu Mayonnaise (p. 503).

POTATO FILLING

2 cups (480 g)

2 large potatoes

2 tablespoons ghee or oil
Pinch of hing (optional)
1 cup (250 ml) shredded vegetables,
  such as carrot, zucchini, celery,
  bell pepper (for Pirozhki, use
  mixed carrot and cabbage)

¼ cup (60 ml) minced fresh parsley

1 teaspoon caraway seeds
⅓ cup (80 ml) sour cream or
  ricotta cheese
1½ cups (150 g) shredded
  Monterey Jack or other mild
  cheese (optional)

Seasoned salt
Black pepper

1. Place the potatoes in a pot and add water to cover. Bring to a boil, reduce the heat, and simmer until tender.
2. Meanwhile, heat the ghee or oil in a skillet. Add the hing, vegetables, and parsley and sauté over low heat, stirring frequently, until the vegetables are tender.
3. Drain the potatoes. When cool enough to handle, peel and mash them thoroughly. Beat in the vegetables, caraway seeds, sour cream or ricotta, and shredded cheese. Season to taste with seasoned salt and pepper.

VARIATION

❂ Omit the sour cream and cheese or replace in Step 3 with tofu or Tofu Mayonnaise (p. 503).

CRISPY TOFU WITH CASHEW SAUCE (TAHU GORENG)

INDONESIA   *6 to 8 hors d'oeuvre–size servings*

An unusual hors d'oeuvre and a delightful method of preparing tofu. The tofu can be served in other contexts, such as a side dish, or on a salad platter with another sauce, such as Sweet-and-Sour Sauce, a mock mayonnaise, or Taratoor Sauce. You can obtain rice flour from Asian markets and gourmet foods stores.

STEP ONE

1 pound (500 g) firm tofu

STEP TWO

¼ cup (35 g) rice flour   *1 teaspoon salt*
2 tablespoons arrowroot or
* cornstarch*

STEP FOUR

Oil for frying

STEP FIVE

Lettuce leaves   *Sambal (pp. 515–16)*
1 medium cucumber
¼ cup (60 ml) coarsely chopped
* fresh cilantro*

1. Drain the tofu thoroughly in a colander. Pat dry with paper towels. Cut into 1½ × 1 × 1–inch (3.5 × 2.5 × 2.5 cm) pieces.
2. Mix the rice flour, arrowroot or cornstarch, and salt together in a shallow bowl.
3. Dredge the tofu pieces gently in the flour mixture. Shake off the excess.
4. Heat oil ½ inch (1.5 cm) deep in a large skillet over medium heat. Have a platter covered with paper towels nearby. In 2 batches, carefully fry the tofu until golden brown, turning once or twice during the frying. Drain on paper towels.
5. To serve, line a platter with lettuce leaves. Peel the cucumber and slice thinly cross-wise and then into thin julienne strips. Arrange the tofu and cucumber decoratively on the platter and sprinkle the cilantro over them. Serve a bowl of sauce on the side for dipping.

VARIATION

For a golden-colored coating, add a pinch of turmeric to the flour mixture in Step 2.

 # VADA (SPICED LENTIL FRITTERS)

INDIA   *About 30 vadas*

My Indian college roommate frequently made these crispy little balls of puréed legumes for her friends. Her name was Pingala, and we dubbed them "Ping-Pong balls" in her honor. Vadas can also be added to curries like dumplings, and they are served in a cool yogurt sauce in Dahi Vada (recipe follows). Serve with a bowl of chutney for dipping. Note that the legumes must be soaked overnight.

STEP ONE

1 cup (190 g) lentils, yellow split peas, or dal

STEP TWO

2 tablespoons minced fresh ginger   *½ teaspoon turmeric*
1 teaspoon ground coriander   *Pinch of hing* (optional)
2½ teaspoons toasted cumin seeds   *1 teaspoon salt*

STEP THREE

Besan (chickpea flour) or wheat flour

STEP FOUR

¼ teaspoon baking powder (optional)

STEP FIVE

Oil for deep-frying

1. Clean the legumes. Place in a bowl with at least 3 cups (720 ml) of water and soak overnight. Drain.
2. Purée in a blender with just enough water to facilitate grinding. Blend in the ginger, spices, and salt.
3. Place in a bowl and beat in just enough flour to thicken the mixture so that it can be dropped in teaspoonfuls.
4. Test the batter by dropping a little into a bowl of water. If it does not float, add the baking powder to the batter.
5. Heat oil for deep-frying over medium heat. Have a platter covered with paper towels nearby. Fry one vada first to make sure it cooks thoroughly; it must not cook too fast. Drop teaspoonfuls of the mixture carefully into the hot oil and deep-fry until they are golden, turning once or twice, about 3 minutes. Drain on paper towels. Serve hot or at room temperature.

VARIATIONS

Add cayenne or chilies to the batter.

Spinach Vada: Add ¾ cup (70 g) finely chopped spinach to the prepared batter. Prepare the vadas from yellow split peas for an attractive color contrast to the green spinach.

Dahi Vada (4 to 6 servings):
A flavorful, cooling, and nourishing summer side dish.

1. Prepare Vadas as directed. Mix 2 tablespoons salt into 3 cups (720 ml) cold water in a bowl. Drop the vadas into the water in batches. Allow to soak for 2 minutes, then drain. Gently squeeze the water out of each vada. This soaking and draining process removes all the oil from the deep-frying.

2. Gently place the vadas in a serving bowl. Beat 3 cups (720 ml) yogurt with a whisk to make slightly more liquid. Pour over the the vadas and stir gently.

DOLMÁTHES (STUFFED GRAPE LEAVES)

GREECE   *40 dolmáthes*

Pick grape leaves when young, tender, and about 6 inches (15 cm) wide. You can also use large spinach leaves, chard, or tender young cabbage leaves. I serve them on a tray, alternating dolmáthes with lemon slices, rind side up, for color contrast.

STEP ONE

2 tablespoons olive oil   *3 tablespoons pine nuts*
Pinch of hing (optional)

STEP TWO

¾ cup (150 g) uncooked white rice,   *3 tablespoons currants*
* preferably basmati*   *Few threads saffron*
1½ cups (360 ml) vegetable stock   *1½ teaspoons crumbled dried mint*
* or water*

STEP THREE

Salt   *Black pepper*

STEP FOUR

50 grape leaves

STEP SIX

2 tablespoons olive oil

STEP EIGHT

Lemon wedges

To prepare the filling:
1. Heat the olive oil in a small saucepan over low heat. Add the hing and sauté until fragrant, about 30 seconds. Add the pine nuts slowly and sauté until golden.
2. Add the rice and sauté for 1 minute. Pour in the stock or water. Add the currants, saffron, and mint. Increase the heat and bring to a boil. Cover, reduce the heat, and simmer until the water is absorbed, about 20 minutes.
3. Season to taste with salt and pepper and set aside to cool a little while preparing the wrappers.

To prepare the wrappers:
4. Bring about 1 quart (1 l) of water to a boil. Blanch the grape leaves by dropping all of them into the boiling water for no more than 30 seconds. Drain. Gently separate the leaves and lay them flat, stem side up. Cover the bottom of a wide, heavy pot with 10 of the leaves to protect the dolmáthes from burning while cooking.

To assemble and cook:
5. Place a spoonful of the filling on the base of a leaf. Fold over the sides to cover the filling, and roll up tightly to make a small, compact package (see diagram). Continue the procedure with the remaining leaves.

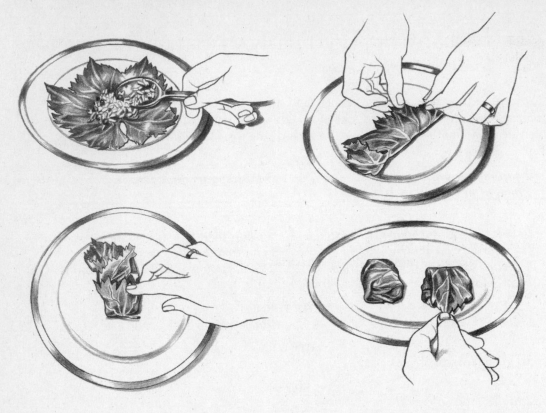

6. Place the dolmáthes close together in the pot. If necessary, make a second row on top of the first. Pour water about ¼ inch (5 mm) deep in the pot. Drizzle the olive oil over the dolmáthes.

7. Bring the water to a boil, cover, and reduce the heat to very low. Simmer gently until the dolmáthes are tender, about 30 minutes.

8. Gently remove from the pot and allow to cool to room temperature. Serve with lemon wedges to squeeze over them.

Earth's crammed with heaven.   —ELIZABETH BARRETT BROWNING

Salads and Salad Dressings

Oh herbaceous treat!
'Twould tempt the dying anchorite to eat;
Back to the world he'd turn his fleeting soul,
And plunge his fingers in the salad bowl;
Serenely full the epicure would say,
"Fate cannot harm me—I have dined today."

—SYDNEY SMITH

THE RAW AND THE COOKED: THE ROLE OF SALADS IN AYURVEDA

According to Ayurvedic principles, a majority of warm, cooked foods are most suitable for human physiologies, with "rabbit food" indeed consigned for the most part to our four-footed neighbors on the earth. Raw vegetables are cold, rough, and require very strong digestive fire, Agni, to digest. They can be a source of toxic impurities, or ama, when eaten in large amounts or at the wrong time of day. This does not mean they should necessarily be entirely eliminated, just that raw vegetable salads play a more minor role in Ayurvedic meals than other dishes—certainly more so than in the West, where a raw salad can comprise a full meal. Salads containing raw vegetables appear in smaller amounts in Ayurvedic meals, served more as a condiment or small side dish. Another Ayurvedic option is to prepare salads based on cooked ingredients, such as grilled vegetables, cooked and cooled beans, pasta, and grains. Don't prepare too far in advance, however; when cooked vegetables stand for more than 6 hours, they become heavy and ama producing, along the lines of leftovers.

❖ In general, serve salads during hot weather, when their cooler temperatures can help balance Pitta. Chilled ingredients extinguish the digestive fire, Agni; room temperature is a wiser choice.

299

❖ Serve salads at the noontime meal, when the digestive fire is most powerful, with spices and seasonings that help digestion. Black pepper, ginger, and cumin are Agni-kindling spices, and lemon juice both kindles Agni and helps cut ama.

❖ People with primarily Vata constitutions would be wise to eat raw vegetable salads in smaller amounts and the least frequently of all the mind-body types. Use Vata-balancing vegetables, such as cucumber, and cooked beets and asparagus. (If you can stand to lightly cook the cucumber, it will help matters.) Serve with plenty of unctuous salad dressing. Fat-free, salt-free dressings are not generally Vata types' best friends. The sweet, sour, and salty tastes and unctuous ingredients such as oil, avocados, and sour cream can help add balance for Vata. Pasta and some grain salads are more workable for managing Vata.

❖ Salads' cooler temperatures are helpful in balancing Pitta. Keep the salt and sour elements reduced in the dressing, and use a bit less oil than Vata types need. Croutons can add more sweet taste (sweet in the Ayurvedic sense) for Vata and Pitta, and pasta and Pitta-balancing grains are good choices.

❖ A wide range of vegetables and beans help balance Kapha, although salads' cooler temperatures are not as balancing. Reduce the sweet, sour, and salt tastes in the dressing, and favor small amounts of Kapha-friendly oils, such as sunflower and corn. Kapha-balancing grains and soba (buckwheat) noodles are good salad ingredients.

 # WILTED GREEK SALAD WITH CARAMELIZED WALNUTS (HORIÁTIKI)

4 servings

Greeks cherish their *horta*, wild greens, and people forage for seasonal greens to use in what is referred to as "rural salad." Feel free to incorporate other tasty leaves, such as lamb's lettuce and not-so-Greek radicchio and arugula in the mixture.

STEP ONE

2 pounds (1 kg) spinach

STEP TWO

Olive oil   *Pinch of hing (optional)*

STEP THREE

2 tablespoons lemon juice   *1 cup (200 g) crumbled feta or*
Salt   *panir*
Pepper   *Caramelized Walnuts (recipe follows)*

1. Remove the stems of the spinach and rinse well. The spinach leaves must be very, very dry for this recipe, or they will leave a watery broth in the pot. Pat them dry with paper towels within an inch of their lives. Tear into large pieces and dry again if necessary.

2. Heat the oil in a large wok or pot. Add the hing and sauté over medium heat until fragrant, about 30 seconds. Add the spinach and toss for 30 to 60 seconds, until wilted.

3. Remove immediately to a bowl. Toss with the lemon juice and a sprinkling of salt and pepper. Arrange on plates and sprinkle with the crumbled cheese and Caramelized Walnuts.

CARAMELIZED WALNUTS

½ cup (60 g)

These sweet-salty nuts make great nibblers as well as a topping for salads. You can add more spice flavoring by sprinkling on a little curry powder or Maharishi Ayur-Veda churna during the last few seconds of cooking.

½ teaspoon ghee or oil
Tiny pinch of hing (optional)
¼ teaspoon ground cumin
½ cup (50 g) coarsely chopped
   walnuts

1 tablespoon turbinado or
   white sugar
Seasoned salt

Heat the oil in a small skillet over low heat. Add the hing and cumin and sauté for 30 seconds, until fragrant. Add the nuts and sauté for about 2 minutes, until lightly toasted. Sprinkle with the sugar and a little seasoned salt. Sauté, stirring constantly, for 1 to 2 minutes, until the sugar is melted and coats the walnuts. Remove from the heat immediately and place the nuts on a plate to cool—the sugar will burn if you continue to cook it. Let cool thoroughly before using.

Dining is and always was a great artistic opportunity.   —FRANK LLOYD WRIGHT

 ## NEW WORLD CHOPPED SALAD

4 servings

A confetti of foods from the lands found by Columbus, with spices from the lands he was searching for. For a summer lunchtime main dish, add cooked, cooled beans—black or aduki beans add lovely color contrast.

STEP ONE

3 tablespoons sunflower or other
   mild-flavored oil
Pinch of hing (optional)
1 tablespoon minced fresh ginger
1½ teaspoons cumin seeds

¾ teaspoon brown mustard seeds
½ cup (70 g) chopped red bell
   peppers
Kernels from 1 large ear yellow corn

STEP TWO

1 cup (140 g) finely cubed jicama
½ cup (70 g) finely cubed
　cucumbers
1 medium avocado, finely cubed
2 to 3 garden radishes, finely cubed
⅓ cup (45 g) pepitas (pumpkin seeds)

1 cup (240 ml) chopped fresh
　cilantro
¼ cup (60 ml) lime juice
Salt
Black pepper

1. Heat the oil in a skillet over medium-low heat. Add the hing, ginger, cumin seeds, and mustard seeds and sauté until fragrant, about 1 minute. Add the bell peppers and corn, cover, and cook for 3 to 4 minutes, until crisp-tender, stirring once or twice.
2. Toss with the remaining ingredients, seasoning to taste with salt and plenty of pepper.

VARIATIONS

For more bite, do not sauté the ginger, add chopped jalapeños, or do both.
Add chopped fresh epazote or oregano.

 # Thai Eggplant Salad (Yum Mekeyau)

THAILAND　　4 servings

Vongduan Silapasorn graciously contributed the ideas for the following two recipes. Thai salads, called *yum* or *yam*, are often based on cooked ingredients. They make delicious appetizers, and you can serve the following two salads together for a light summer repast.

STEP ONE

2 large or 3 medium eggplants

STEP THREE

1 tablespoon mild-flavored oil
Pinch of hing (optional)
1 tablespoon minced fresh ginger

1½ cups (330 g) coarsely chopped
　firm tofu
Liquid seasoning

STEP FOUR

Lettuce leaves
½ cup (120 ml) chopped fresh
　cilantro

2 tablespoons lime juice
3 tablespoons liquid seasoning
1 teaspoon sugar

1. Prick the eggplants with a knife in several places. Place in the broiler on foil or in a baking pan to catch drips. Broil, turning every 5 minutes, until tender when pierced with a knife. The whole cooking process should take 10 to 15 minutes.

2. When cool enough to handle, peel and coarsely chop. Let cool.
3. Heat the oil in a nonstick wok or small skillet. Add the hing, ginger, and tofu. Sprinkle with liquid seasoning and sauté over medium-high heat until the tofu is browned. Let cool.
4. Arrange the lettuce leaves on a plate. Arrange the eggplant over the lettuce. Cover with the tofu. Sprinkle the cilantro on top. Mix the lime juice, liquid seasoning, and sugar together and pour over the salad. Serve at room temperature.

VARIATION
Sprinkle toasted cashews over the salad.

 # Bean Thread Noodle Salad (Yum Woonsén)

THAILAND   *4 to 6 servings*

Bean thread noodles are available in Asian markets and sometimes in the ethnic foods sections of supermarkets. You can substitute rice noodles. Use kitchen shears to cut them into pieces.

STEP ONE

*2 cups (140 g) bean thread noodles
   cut into 1½-inch (4 cm) lengths*

STEP TWO

1 tablespoon mild-flavored oil
Pinch of hing (optional)
1 tablespoon minced fresh ginger

*⅔ cup (145 g) coarsely chopped
   firm tofu*
Liquid seasoning or salt

STEP THREE

3 tablespoons liquid seasoning
2 tablespoons lime juice
1½ teaspoons sugar
1 teaspoon black pepper
*2 cups (270 g) quartered, thinly
   sliced peeled cucumbers*
*2 medium tomatoes, cut into
   thin wedges*

*½ cup (120 ml) chopped fresh
   cilantro*
*1 cup (240 ml) chopped fresh
   mint leaves*
Lettuce leaves

1. Place the bean thread noodles in a bowl and cover with boiling water. Allow to soak until soft, about 20 minutes. Drain thoroughly.
2. Meanwhile, heat the oil in a nonstick skillet or wok. Add the hing, ginger, and tofu. Sprinkle with liquid seasoning or salt and sauté over medium-high heat until the tofu is browned. Let cool.

3. Mix the liquid seasoning, lime juice, sugar, and pepper together. Gently toss with the noodles, tofu, cucumbers, tomatoes, cilantro, and mint. Arrange the salad on a bed of lettuce leaves.

VARIATIONS

Replace the black pepper with finely chopped fresh chilies to taste.
If you don't like heat, omit the black pepper.

PANZANELLA (BREAD SALAD)

ITALY   *4 to 6 servings*

Use the best olive oil you can get your hands on for this flavorful, robust salad. Any crusty unsliced loaf will do but, if there is a Vata type in the house, whole wheat sourdough bread is particularly delicious.

4 cups (200 g) crusty country-style or French bread torn into bite-sized pieces
1 cup (230 g) tomatoes, cut into large chunks
1 cup cucumber (140 g) peeled, quartered, and cut into chunks
1 cup (240 ml) torn basil leaves
½ cup (65 g) thinly sliced fennel or celery

½ cup (70 g) thinly sliced red bell pepper
⅓ cup (80 ml) minced flat-leaf parsley
¼ cup (25 g) grated Parmesan cheese (optional)
½ cup (120 ml) Citrus Vinaigrette (p. 318)

Toss all the ingredients together. The bread should be fairly saturated with the dressing. If it seems too dry after a thorough tossing, sprinkle with a very small amount of water and toss again.

GREEK-STYLE MARINATED VEGETABLES (LÁHANA MARINÁTA)

GREECE   *4 to 6 servings*

Dried herbs are incorporated into the marinade here; however, you can omit them and sprinkle the finished dish with a chiffonade of fresh herbs.

½ cup (120 ml) olive oil
1½ cups (360 ml) vegetable stock
or water
1 cup (240 ml) unsweetened apple
juice or white grape juice
⅓ cup (80 ml) lemon juice

1 bay leaf
1 teaspoon salt
1 teaspoon dried dill
½ teaspoon dried oregano
½ teaspoon dried basil
A few peppercorns

STEP TWO

4 to 6 cups (1 to 1.2 l) cut-up
vegetables

1. Combine all the ingredients for Step 1 in a large nonreactive pot. Bring to a boil, then reduce the heat.
2. Add the vegetables. Simmer, covered, for just a few minutes, until not quite done. They will continue to cook off the heat.
3. Remove from the heat. Allow the vegetables to cool to room temperature in the marinade.
4. Drain, reserving the marinade. At this point you can serve as is. However, for best results, return the marinade to the pot and boil until it is reduced to ¼ its original volume. Let cool to room temperature and spoon over the vegetables.

 # CAKIK (CUCUMBERS WITH YOGURT, DILL, AND MINT)

ARMENIA　　*4 servings*

Traditional Armenian fare for *Khoutum Kisher*, the night before Easter, accompanied by Bulgar with Vermicelli (pp. 158–59) and sautéed spinach. You can also serve it as a *mazza*, as it is found in several Middle Eastern countries.

1 cup (240 ml) yogurt
1 to 2 tablespoons chopped fresh
dill or ¾ teaspoon dried
1 to 2 tablespoons minced fresh
mint or 1 teaspoon crumbled
dried

1 cucumber, peeled and
thinly sliced
Salt
White pepper

Whisk the yogurt gently with the dill and mint. Gently toss with the cucumber slices. Season to taste with salt and white pepper.

YOGURT IN AYURVEDIC SALADS

A good instrument of pleasure.   —Pliny, describing yogurt

Yogurt must be treated carefully to be fully nourishing. Yogurt that is too sour or too old or served too cold and at the wrong time of day can block the microcirculatory channels (shrotas). Eat salads with yogurt at room temperature and at lunchtime rather than at the evening meal.

 # CUCUMBER RAITA (KHIRA RAITA)

INDIA   *4 to 6 servings*

A basic recipe that can be used for many different vegetables, as indicated in the Variations. Small, crisp pickling cucumbers work well. To drain grated cukes, place in a sieve for a few minutes and press with the back of a spoon to release excess moisture that will dilute the yogurt.

2 cups (480 ml) yogurt	Chopped fresh cilantro
1 teaspoon ground cumin, toasted	Salt
1 cup (190 g) coarsely grated and	Black pepper
drained peeled cucumber	Pinch of sugar

Whisk the yogurt with the cumin until the yogurt is free of lumps. Mix in the cucumber and season to taste with chopped cilantro, salt, pepper, and a pinch of sugar.

VARIATIONS

Cucumber-Tomato Raita (Khira Tamatar Raita): Add 1 medium chopped tomato and ¼ cup (35 g) finely chopped toasted cashews or almonds.

Avocado Raita: Avocados are not well known in India. However, they make a great raita. Replace the cucumber with 1 cubed avocado. Add chopped tomato if desired.

Potato (Alu) or Pumpkin (Kaddu) Raita: Replace the cucumber with 1 cup (140 g) cubed cooked potato or pumpkin.

Bless, O Lord, the plants, the vegetation, and the herbs of the field that they may grow and increase to fullness and bear much fruit. And may the fruit of the land remind us of the spiritual fruit we should bear.

—Coptic Orthodox liturgy

EGGPLANT RAITA (BAIGAN RAITA)

INDIA   *4 to 6 servings*

STEP ONE

4 to 5 tablespoons (60 to 75 ml)
   mild-flavored oil
Pinch of hing (optional)
¼ teaspoon black mustard seeds

1 teaspoon ground cumin
1 medium eggplant, peeled and
   diced

STEP TWO

2 cups (480 ml) yogurt
Salt

Black pepper
Pinch of sugar

1. Heat the oil in a skillet or wok. Add the hing, mustard seeds, and cumin and sauté over low heat until the mustard seeds "dance." Add the eggplant and sauté until tender, letting it brown a little. Let cool.
2. Whisk the yogurt until it is free of lumps. Mix in the eggplant. Season to taste with salt, pepper, and a pinch of sugar.

 # MIXED VEGETABLE RAITA (SABJI-KI RAITA)

INDIA   *4 to 6 servings*

A more complex raita with a lively mélange of flavors, colors, and textures. The small amount of curry powder adds a nice undertone, but you can omit it if you want a more authentically Indian dish.

STEP ONE

2 cups (480 ml) yogurt

1 teaspoon sugar

STEP TWO

2 tablespoons mild-flavored oil
Pinch of hing (optional)
1 teaspoon cumin seeds

1 teaspoon black mustard seeds
¼ teaspoon curry powder or
   Maharishi Ayur-Veda churna

STEP THREE

1 cup (190 g) grated peeled
   cucumbers
½ cup (45 g) grated carrots
1 small tomato, coarsely chopped
1 tablespoon minced fresh ginger
½ cup (120 ml) finely chopped
   fresh cilantro

¼ cup (40 g) chopped cashews,
   toasted
Salt
Black pepper

1. Whisk the yogurt with the sugar until it is free of lumps.
2. Heat the oil in a small skillet. Add the spices in order and sauté over low heat until the mustard seeds "dance."
3. Mix the spice mixture into the yogurt. Stir in the vegetables, ginger, cilantro, and cashews. Add salt and pepper to taste.

THE VAIDYA'S SALAD

4 small servings

I am convinced that digestion is the great secret of life.   —SYDNEY SMITH

Here is a delicious, satisfying grated salad that was developed by a traditional Ayurvedic doctor, a vaidya, to serve in very small amounts at lunch. The proportions of the ingredients are flexible; this is a basic guideline.

1 cup (90 g) finely grated carrots
1 cup (240 ml) sprouts
¾ cup (70 g) finely grated beets
¼ cup (30 g) finely grated daikon radish

3 tablespoons minced fresh basil
3 tablespoons minced fresh parsley
2 to 3 teaspoons minced fresh ginger
1 tablespoon lemon juice

Toss all the ingredients together.

CÉLERI RÉMOULADE WITH GINGER-MUSTARD SEED DRESSING

FRANCE   *2½ cups (580 g)*

An East-West version of the classic French celeriac salad. The rich, creamy dressing is also luscious on other salads.

STEP ONE

5 cups (425 g) coarsely grated or finely julienned celeriac

STEP TWO

2 teaspoons sesame or other mild-flavored oil
Pinch of hing (optional)

¾ teaspoon brown mustard seeds
2 tablespoons minced fresh ginger

STEP THREE

*¼ cup (60 ml) sesame or other
    mild-flavored oil*
⅓ cup (45 g) raw sunflower seeds
3 tablespoons lemon juice

¼ cup (60 ml) water
1 tablespoon honey
Liquid seasoning or salt
Black pepper

1. Bring 6 cups (1.5 l) water to a boil. Drop in the celeriac and blanch for 30 seconds. Drain in a strainer, running cold water over it to stop the cooking. Let cool to room temperature.
2. Heat the oil in a small skillet. Add the hing and mustard seeds and sauté over low heat until the mustard seeds "dance." Remove from the heat. Add the ginger and stir a few times to take the raw edge off, but do not cook.
3. Blend in the second amount of oil and the sunflower seeds, lemon juice, water, and honey until smooth, 2 to 3 minutes. Pour over the celeriac, toss, and season to taste with liquid seasoning or salt and pepper.

The art of eating is no slight art, the pleasure no slight pleasure. —MONTAIGNE

 # FENNEL COLE SLAW WITH PECAN DRESSING

6 to 8 servings

The fennel, carrots, pecans, oil dressing, and sweet and sour flavors help balance the Vata-increasing nature of uncooked cabbage; and the general sweetness, the cilantro, and the cool temperature of the dish add some balance for Pitta. If fennel is out of season, increase the carrots and cabbage.

*1½ cups (160 g) finely shredded
    cabbage*
*1½ cups (175 g) finely shredded
    fennel*
1½ cups (135 g) grated carrots
*⅓ cup (55 g) chopped crystallized
    ginger*

1 tablespoon fennel seeds, toasted
*¾ cup (180 ml) finely chopped
    fresh cilantro*
Pecan Dressing (recipe follows)
Black pepper

Mix all the ingredients except the pepper together. Toss with the dressing and a sprinkling of black pepper. Adjust the seasoning.

PECAN DRESSING

About ⅔ cup (160 ml)

*½ cup (120 ml) sesame or other
    mild-flavored oil*
½ cup (50 g) pecans

3 tablespoons lemon juice
2 tablespoons honey
Liquid seasoning or salt

Combine the oil, pecans, lemon juice, and honey in a blender until smooth. Season to taste with liquid seasoning or salt.

VARIATIONS

Add whole seedless grapes or pineapple cubes to the salad.

Replace the pecans in the dressing with sunflower seeds for balancing Kapha, with sour cream for balancing Vata, or with thick coconut milk to balance Pitta.

 ## CARROT-DATE SALAD

4 to 6 servings

A sweet, Vata-balancing condiment salad with Indian and North African flavors.

STEP ONE

*2 tablespoons sesame or other mild-
    flavored oil*
Pinch of hing (optional)

½ teaspoon brown mustard seeds
1½ teaspoons cumin seeds
3 cups (270 g) grated carrots

STEP TWO

½ cup (145 g) chopped dates
¼ cup (30 g) lightly toasted pistachios
*2 tablespoons finely chopped
    crystallized ginger*
2 tablespoons lemon juice

¼ cup (60 ml) orange juice
1 tablespoon finely grated orange zest
½ teaspoon ground cinnamon
¼ teaspoon salt

1. Heat the oil in a large skillet. Add the hing and mustard seeds and sauté over low heat until the mustard seeds "dance." Add the carrots and toss for 30 to 60 seconds, just to take the raw edge off them. Remove immediately to a bowl.
2. Add all the remaining ingredients and toss thoroughly. Serve at room temperature.

Sesame Radish Salad

MEXICO   *4 servings*

Very young radishes are balancing for all three doshas. Cooked with a little oil, they are Vata balancing. I first saw a version of this condiment salad prepared with garden radishes by a Mexican woman and have since only encountered Chinese versions made from daikon. In any case, it would work well as a Middle Eastern *mazza* or tossed with yogurt for an Indian-style raita! You can also use it to dress tossed green salads.

STEP ONE

2 tablespoons sesame or other mild-flavored oil
Pinch of hing (optional)

½ teaspoon brown mustard seeds
1 tablespoon sesame seeds

STEP TWO

2 cups (230 g) grated daikon or garden radishes
2 tablespoons lemon juice
Liquid seasoning or salt

Black pepper
Toasted sesame oil
2 tablespoons minced fresh cilantro

1. Heat the oil in a small skillet. Add the hing, mustard seeds, and sesame seeds. Sauté until the sesame seeds are golden brown.
2. Pour the hot oil-seed mixture immediately over the radishes. Add the lemon juice and season to taste with liquid seasoning or salt and pepper. Let cool to room temperature, then stir in a few drops of toasted sesame oil and the cilantro.

Bean Salads

Both fresh and dried beans marry well with a vinaigrette-type dressing. Serve dressed cannellini beans, fava beans, or garbanzos in an antipasto or as a *mazza*, and of course, there is always the ubiquitous three-bean mixture in every salad bar on God's green earth. Use very good olive oil or walnut or hazelnut oil for exciting flavor. You can mix a variety of beans, but keep kidney beans separate; they give off a color that turns other beans an unappetizing gray.

WILD RICE SALAD WITH DRIED CRANBERRIES

4 servings

A Kapha-balancing dish. You can also prepare it with bulgar, substitute dried cherries for the cranberries, and have something to keep Vata and Pitta happy.

STEP ONE

3 cups (720 ml) water
½ teaspoon salt

¾ cup (135 g) wild rice
½ cup (70 g) dried cranberries

STEP TWO

1 tablespoon oil
Pinch of hing (optional)

*1 cup (115 g) French or green
beans cut in 2-inch (5 cm) lengths*

STEP THREE

*½ cup (70 g) finely chopped red
bell peppers*
½ cup (75 g) chopped cucumbers
*½ cup (120 ml) finely chopped
fresh basil*
*¼ cup (60 ml) finely chopped flat-
leaf parsley*

½ cup (60 g) pistachios
¼ cup (60 ml) oil
¼ cup (60 ml) lemon juice
Liquid seasoning or salt
Black pepper

1. Bring the water and salt to a boil. Stir in the wild rice. Cover and simmer for 30 minutes. Stir in the cranberries, re-cover, and simmer until the water is absorbed and the rice is tender. Allow to cool to room temperature.
2. Meanwhile, heat the oil in a large skillet. Add the hing and sauté over low heat for 30 seconds. Stir in the French or green beans, cover, and cook until the beans are crisp-tender. Allow to cool to room temperature.
3. Gently toss the wild rice, beans, bell peppers, cucumbers, basil, parsley, and pistachios together. Pour the oil and lemon juice over them and toss. Season to taste with liquid seasoning or salt and pepper.

BULGAR AND TOASTED NOODLES WITH FOUR FRESH HERBS

4 to 6 servings

A Vata- and Pitta-balancing salad with a Persian slant. You can change everything around by using quinoa and pumpkin seeds for a more Kapha-balancing mixture.

STEP ONE

3 tablespoons olive oil
Pinch of hing
2 tablespoons minced fresh ginger
2 teaspoons cumin seeds
½ cup (40 g) vermicelli, broken
   into 1-inch (2.5 cm) pieces

¾ cup (130 g) bulgar
1½ cups (360 ml) vegetable stock
   or water
½ teaspoon salt

STEP TWO

1 cup (240 ml) finely chopped fresh
   mint
1 cup (240 ml) finely chopped fresh
   cilantro
½ cup (120 ml) finely chopped flat-
   leaf parsley
¼ cup (60 ml) finely chopped dill
½ cup (60 g) coarsely chopped
   garden radishes
½ cup (75 g) coarsely chopped
   cucumbers

1 cup (140 g) blanched almonds,
   toasted
¼ cup (60 ml) olive oil
⅓ cup (80 ml) lemon juice
1 teaspoon ground allspice
1 teaspoon ground cinnamon
Liquid seasoning or salt
Black pepper

1. Heat the oil in a skillet. Add the hing, ginger, cumin seeds, and vermicelli. Sauté, stirring constantly, over low heat until the vermicelli is nicely browned. Add the bulgar, stock or water, and salt. Bring to a boil, cover, reduce the heat, and cook until the stock or water is absorbed and the bulgar is tender. Let cool to room temperature.
2. Toss the herbs, radishes, cucumbers, and almonds with the bulgar mixture. Mix the oil, lemon juice, allspice, and cinnamon together and mix into the salad. Season to taste with liquid seasoning or salt and pepper.

 # PASTA SALAD WITH PINE NUTS AND DRIED TOMATOES

4 to 6 servings

Use oil-packed tomatoes, or reconstitute dried tomatoes by boiling in water until tender.

STEP ONE

½ cup (120 ml) olive oil
Pinch of hing (optional)

⅓ cup (45 g) pine nuts

STEP TWO

1 cup (80 g) coarsely chopped dried
  tomatoes

3 tablespoons lemon juice
2 teaspoons sugar

STEP THREE

½ pound (230 kg) dried pasta or 1
  pound (500 g) fresh

STEP FOUR

1 cup (200 g) crumbled feta cheese
½ cup (120 ml) minced fresh flat-
  leaf parsley
½ cup (120 ml) chopped fresh basil
  or dill

Lemon juice (optional)
Liquid seasoning or salt
Black pepper

1. Heat the olive oil in a medium skillet. Add the hing and pine nuts and cook over
   low heat until the nuts are golden brown. Remove from the heat.
2. Stir in the tomatoes while the oil is still hot. Let cool, then stir in the lemon juice
   and the sugar.
3. Cook the pasta until al dente. Drain and let cool.
4. Toss the dressing, feta cheese, and herbs with the pasta. Add more lemon juice if
   necessary. Season to taste with liquid seasoning or salt and pepper.

 # Bon Bon Chi with Asparagus (Cold Sesame Noodle Salad)

CHINA   6 servings

A vegetarian version that is mostly balancing for Vata. Since asparagus is tri-doshic,
you could replace the sesame seeds with almonds to better balance Pitta, or replace the
sesame with sunflower seeds and use soba noodles for Kapha.

STEP ONE

2 tablespoons sesame or other mild-
  flavored oil
Pinch of hing (optional)

2 cups (420 g) tofu, cut into
  ½-inch (1.3 cm) cubes
Liquid seasoning

STEP TWO

1 pound (500 g) asparagus,
  trimmed and cut into 2-inch
  (5 cm) lengths

Salt

STEP THREE

⅓ pound (150 g) vermicelli　　　*Salt*
Sesame Dressing (recipe follows)　*Black pepper*

STEP FOUR

2 cups (140 g) julienned cucumbers　*Chopped fresh cilantro*

1. Heat the oil in a skillet over medium-high heat. Add a pinch of hing and the tofu. Sprinkle with liquid seasoning and sauté, stirring frequently, until the tofu is golden brown.
2. Add the asparagus, sprinkle with salt, cover, and cook for 3 to 4 minutes, until crisp-tender. Remove from the heat immediately.
3. Cook the pasta until al dente. Do not, do *not* overcook. Drain and run cold water over it to stop the cooking. Toss with half of the Sesame Dressing. Season to taste with salt and pepper.
4. Spread the noodles on a platter. Spread the tofu-asparagus mixture over them. Sprinkle with the cucumbers. Drizzle with the remaining dressing and sprinkle a generous amount of chopped cilantro on top.

SESAME DRESSING

A little over ½ cup (120 ml)

STEP ONE

⅓ cup (80 ml) sesame or other　　*½ cup (70 g) coarsely chopped bell*
*　mild-flavored oil*　　　　　　　*　peppers*
Pinch of hing (optional)　　　　　*2 tablespoons coarsely chopped fresh*
⅓ cup (45 g) sesame seeds　　　　*　ginger*

STEP TWO

3 tablespoons lemon juice　　　*Toasted sesame oil*
1 tablespoon raw sugar　　　　*Liquid seasoning*
⅓ cup (80 ml) water　　　　　 *Black pepper*

1. Heat the oil in a small saucepan or skillet. Add the hing and sesame seeds and sauté over low heat until the sesame seeds just begin to turn golden. Add the bell peppers and continue to sauté until the sesame seeds are well browned. Add the ginger and stir once or twice to coat with the hot oil before removing from the heat. Allow to cool for a few minutes.
2. Combine the sesame mixture with the lemon juice, sugar, water, and a drizzle of toasted sesame oil in a blender until it is as smooth as possible. Add more water if necessary. Season to taste with liquid seasoning and pepper.

VARIATION

For a spicier dressing, do not sauté the ginger. Or you can add dried red chilies to the oil or do both.

PRASAD FRUIT SALAD (PHAL CHAT PRASADAM)

INDIA   *4 servings*

Prasad or *prasadam* is food that has been prepared for and offered to the gods. After offering, it is eaten as blessed food. Bananas, dates, and coconuts are common ingredients in south Indian *prasad*.

STEP ONE

3 medium bananas, peeled and sliced   ⅓ cup (25 g) grated fresh or dried
⅔ cup (120 g) sliced pitted dates   unsweetened coconut

STEP TWO

2 tablespoons lemon juice   ¼ teaspoon crushed cardamom
2 tablespoons honey   seeds

1. Mix the bananas, dates, and coconut together.
2. Combine the lemon juice, honey, and cardamom. Toss lightly with the fruit.

MANGO, KIWI, AND RASPBERRY SALAD WITH GINGER-HONEY DRESSING

4 to 6 servings

Here is a lovely summer lunchtime mélange of colors with predominantly sweet flavors, subtly accented by sour-astringent lime juice and pungent ginger. Use absolutely ripe fruit and serve at room temperature.

2 large mangoes   *Ginger-Honey Dressing*
4 kiwis   *(recipe follows)*
2 cups (200 g) raspberries

Peel and cube the mangoes. Peel, quarter, and slice the kiwis. Gently toss all the fruit together with the dressing.

GINGER-HONEY DRESSING

⅓ cup (80 ml)

2 tablespoons chopped crystallized   2 tablespoons lime juice
   ginger   3 tablespoons honey

Combine all the ingredients in a blender until smooth.

SALAD DRESSINGS

In the eighteenth century, London was graced by one Marquis d'Albignac, an escapee from the French Revolution. Faced for the first time with having to work, he proceeded to earn a comfortable livelihood by running from house to house each evening concocting the salad dressing! Begging the pardon of Citizen d'Albignac, a few today (or then, for that matter) would confine themselves to this singular talent, for salad dressings are simple to prepare. Like all Ayurvedic foods, dressings are best freshly made. Instead of employing vinegar, which is fermented, the following recipes contain lemon juice—one of the great health-giving ingredients of Ayurvedic cooking—to add the requisite tart note.

Additions

Citrus juice
Small amounts of sweeteners, such as honey or raw sugar
Curry powder and Maharishi Ayur-Veda churnas
Vegetable juices
Pesto
Dried Tomato Paste (p. 506)
Nut Butter (p. 546) and Tahini (p. 512)
Dried green herbs
Mustard powder or prepared mustard
Fennel, poppy, caraway, or toasted sesame or cumin seeds
Minced fresh greens and herbs, such as watercress, spinach, parsley, cilantro, basil
    (you can purée these into the dressing as well)

Additions to Be Puréed in a Blender or Food Processor

Sautéed or grilled bell peppers and other cooked vegetables
Tofu
Soft cheeses, such as cottage cheese and panir
Sesame, sunflower, or pumpkin seeds and nuts
Avocado
Cooked beans

Oil-free salad dressings: Replace oil with vegetable juice, yogurt, puréed tomato, or with tofu, cottage cheese, or panir that has been puréed and thinned with a liquid.

✿ *Dairy-free salad dressings:* Replace dairy products in creamy dressings with puréed tofu. Add a little oil to achieve the proper texture. You can also replace dairy products with mashed avocado or a vegetable purée.

Besides the recipes below, see:

Taratoor Sauce (pp. 512–13)
Guacamole (pp. 279–80)
Creamy Horseradish Sauce (p. 502)

 # CITRUS VINAIGRETTE

⅓ cup (80 ml)

Citrus vinaigrette can also be used as a marinade.

¼ cup (60 ml) oil
2 tablespoons lemon juice

¼ to ½ teaspoon salt
Black pepper

Mix all the ingredients together.

 # YOGURT, BUTTERMILK, AND OTHER CREAMY DRESSINGS

½ cup (120 ml)

Many ingredients can be added to these basic proportions for a creamy dressing. For "ranch" dressing, use buttermilk, sour cream, or crème fraîche.

⅓ cup (80 ml) yogurt, buttermilk,
*   or sour cream*
2 tablespoons oil

2 tablespoons lemon juice
1 teaspoon dried herbs
1 teaspoon honey or sugar (optional)

Mix all the ingredients together.

 # CREAMY SALAD DRESSING

½ cup (120 ml)

A basic creamy dressing based on fresh cheese.

⅓ cup (75 g) cottage cheese, soft
*   panir, crumbled tofu, cream*
*   cheese, or creamy chèvre*
¼ cup (60 ml) oil

3 tablespoons lemon juice
Salt
Black pepper

Purée all the ingredients in a blender until smooth. If too thick, add a little water or vegetable stock.

VARIATION
French Dressing: To make a light, fresh facsimile of creamy French dressing, add ½ tomato and purée. Add green herbs such as dill and basil.

 ## Avocado Dressing

½ cup (120 ml)

½ avocado
3 tablespoons oil
2 tablespoons lemon juice

Salt
Black pepper

Blend all the ingredients together.

 ## Tarragon-Pistachio Goddess Dressing

About 1 cup (240 ml)

Green bean or snap pea purée adds subtle green color, though you could substitute mashed avocado or leave it out altogether and still end up with something delightful. Double the recipe and you have a lovely dip or a tasty dressing for baked potatoes.

STEP ONE

1 tablespoon oil
Pinch of hing (optional)

¾ cup (60 g) finely chopped green beans or snap peas

STEP TWO

1 cup (225 g) sour cream
2 tablespoons finely chopped fresh tarragon
2 tablespoons finely chopped flat-leaf parsley

3 tablespoons finely chopped pistachios, lightly toasted
Seasoned salt
Black pepper

1. Heat the oil in a small skillet. Add the hing and sauté for 30 seconds over low heat, until fragrant. Add the green beans or snap peas, sprinkle with salt, and sauté until tender, stirring frequently.
2. Place in a food processor or blender with just enough of the sour cream to blend to a smooth purée. Mix the purée into the remaining sour cream and stir in the tarragon, parsley, and pistachios. Season to taste with salt and black pepper.

LEMONS AND LIMES IN AYURVEDA

Huge lemons, cut into slices, would sink like setting suns into the dusky sea, softly illuminating it with their radiating membranes, and its clear, smooth surface aquiver from the rising bitter essence.   —RAINIER MARIA RILKE

Lemons are considered a particularly healing and health-giving food in Ayurveda because they stimulate the digestive fire, Agni, and they are both cleansing and nourishing.

❖ Limes present us with a problematical definition: the *Bearss* and *Persian* limes of the United States are actually hybrid lemons coaxed to a green color. What we call *Key* limes, now very rare in this country, are commonly known—and commonly available—to much of the world.

❖ Try, try to find a source of tree-ripened lemons. *Meyer* lemons, a bit milder than ordinary market varieties, are sometimes available from farmers' markets. Standard supermarket lemons often have a very unhappy childhood before you adopt them and take them home. They are picked while still green, then stored for 3 to 6 months. Before being sent out in the marketplace, they are exposed to a gas that turns them yellow but doesn't ripen them. Then they are dipped in fungicide and occasionally waxed to boot. Lemons and limes do not ripen further after they are picked.

❖ Water taken with a little lemon juice, with or without the addition of honey, helps remove the clogging deposits caused by improperly digested food, ama, and can be taken frequently throughout the day.

❖ The use of lemon juice in the kitchen extends beyond cooking to a role as cleanser and freshener. Small amounts of lemon juice and salt mixed into water can be used to wash kitchen surfaces. Use lemon juice and salt full-strength as a natural cleanser.

BROCCOLI AND OTHER PURÉED VEGETABLE DRESSINGS

1 cup (240 ml)

A wonderful way to make use of broccoli stalks. You can substitute other vegetables, such as summer squash, green beans, or bell peppers.

⅓ cup (80 ml) olive oil
Pinch of hing (optional)
1 cup (120 g) chopped peeled
  broccoli stalks

¼ green bell pepper, coarsely
  chopped
1 teaspoon dried basil
½ teaspoon dried thyme

2 tablespoons lemon juice
3 tablespoons vegetable stock or
  water

Liquid seasoning or salt
Black pepper

1. Heat the oil in a small saucepan or skillet. Add the hing and sauté until fragrant, about 30 seconds. Add the broccoli, bell pepper, basil, and thyme. Cover and sauté over low heat until tender, stirring occasionally.
2. Purée the vegetable mixture with the lemon juice and stock or water in a blender until smooth. Season to taste with liquid seasoning or salt and pepper.

VARIATIONS
Endless. Change the herbs, or omit herbs and add curry powder.
Add sour cream or yogurt.

 # TAHINI DRESSING

⅓ cup (80 ml)

3 tablespoons Tahini (p. 512)
2 tablespoons oil (more if the
  Tahini is thick)
1 tablespoon lemon juice

1 tablespoon minced fresh ginger
Liquid seasoning or salt
Black pepper

Mix all the ingredients together and season to taste.

Heaven is for those who think of it. —JOSEPH JOUBERT

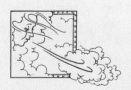

Yeasted Breads and Pizza

What is the bread (which Moses gave the children of Israel to eat)? It is the word which the Lord ordained, and this Divine Ordinance imparts both light and sweetness to the soul which has eyes to see.

—PHILO JUDAEUS

Material bread they already possessed, for the children of Israel are thought to have been the first to harness yeast organisms to lighten and expand flat griddle cakes of ground grain and water, the bread of the entire ancient world. The words lord and lady in Old English are *hlaford*, "keeper of the bread," and *hlaefdigge*, "kneader of the dough." In other words, a basic family unit was defined as the maker and possessor of bread. Furthermore, the words *companion* and *company*, which encompass an expanded range of human relationships, are derived from *companio*, Latin for "one who shares bread."

YEASTED BREAD AND AYURVEDA

Yeast is not a highly favored substance in Ayurvedic cooking. It can contribute to yeast-based diseases when impurities from improperly digested food, ama, are present in the body because yeast feeds on ama. At the same time, people who have been raised on yeasted breads eat them as a staple food, without which they feel uncomfortable. Ayurveda is about comfort. Comfort is good. Comfort helps create the biochemical component of bliss, ojas. So what to do? Take measures to reduce or avoid creating ama in general—a capital idea anyway. You might elect to incorporate unleavened flatbreads into your diet for some meals and eat leavened breads at others. There are also ways to prepare and eat yeasted breads that maximize their good effects and help minimize their less desirable attributes:

❖ Freshly baked bread is the best for health as well as for flavor.

❖ Eat bread that is well cooked. Translation: Toast bread slices before eating.

❖ Ayurveda recommends leaning more toward whole grain breads for maximum nutrition. However, they can be tricky to prepare without producing whole grain bricks, so according to my preference, I have included some unbleached white flour in the recipes. If you have access to spelt flour, you can substitute it successfully for unbleached white flour. For those committed to baking 100 percent whole grain breads at home, consult *The Laurels Kitchen Bread Book* by Laurel Robertson, Carol Flinders, and Bronwen Godfrey (Random House, 1985). The authors maintain that whole grain bread must be handled differently from that containing any amount of refined wheat flour, and they have done exhaustive research and testing. However, I caution you to not use honey to sweeten your loaves, as they often do.

❖ Many breads contain both milk and salt, an incompatible combination. Milk also does not combine well with the taste (in the Ayurvedic sense) of yeast. Water makes a chewier loaf than milk and is used in "lean" breads—loaves prepared without milk or fat—such as country-style crusty loaves and baguettes. Buttermilk, sour milk, and yogurt give bread a more tender texture and do not have to be boiled before being used with yeast. I mix them half and half with water or juice to avoid any potential for gluey texture.

Breadmaking, I have found, is a very personal thing, and what one cook does another cannot or will not do because it does not feel right. . . . Good bread will forever send out its own mysterious and magical goodness, to all the senses, and quite aside from all the cookbooks, perhaps the best way to learn how to make it is to ask an old, wise, and above all, good woman.

—M. F. K. FISHER, *An Alphabet for Gourmets*

BASIC BREAD INGREDIENTS

❖ *Leavening* occurs when gas bubbles produced by the yeast are trapped by the gluten—stringy protein structure—in the flour. The only flour containing significant amounts of gluten is wheat flour. All other types make for heartier, heavier loaves and must be combined with wheat flour to produce a lightweight result. *Hard winter wheat* and *hard spring wheat* flours contain the most gluten. "Pastry" flours are milled from *soft summer wheat*, which is low in gluten and better for cakes and pastries. "All-purpose" flour is usually a blend. *Kamut* and *spelt*, or *dinkel wheat*, ancient varieties of hard wheat with a broader nutritional profile than modern, hybrid wheat varieties, have high gluten contents and are excellent bread flours. They create lighter breads without the addition of unbleached white flour.

The following are some of the low-gluten flours that are best added in small amounts—no more than 1 cup (about 130 g) per loaf of bread.

> Amaranth
> Barley
> Buckwheat
> Millet
> Quinoa
> Rice
> Rye
> Triticale
> ¼ cup (30 g) soy, besan (chickpea), and other bean flours per loaf

---

❖ *Sweetenings* help nourish yeasts. A small amount of sweetening—1 tablespoon per loaf—enhances the flavor of nonsweet loaves. Too much sugar causes the yeast to first stage a feeding frenzy, then later burn out. For breads containing more than 2 tablespoons sugar per cup of flour, increase the amount of yeast.

❖ *Salt* makes the gluten structure strong and keeps the yeast's growth orderly and even. Without salt, bread will not rise quite as high. If not including salt, it is wise to include more sweetening to give the yeast something to chew on.

❖ *Oil* makes breads tender and keeps them that way longer. Small amounts of oil—as little as 3 percent of the total weight of the loaf—actually increase the loaf's volume by 20 percent. Ghee adds subtle, sumptuous flavor and texture. You may also want to use olive or unrefined sesame oil in some loaves for their unique flavors.

LET THERE BE BREAD! THE TEN COMMANDMENTS

The following directions are for bread made with conventional—not quick-rising—yeast and produced without a bread-making machine. Quick-rising yeasts and bread-making machines come with their own sets of injunctions.

I. *Thou shalt be patient and allow the process to happen.* Yeasts are living, growing organisms, and one simply sets up the most supportive conditions for them to accomplish their work—which they do in their own good time.

II. *Let thy bowls be of nonreactive materials, such as glass or pottery, so that the yeast can grow and multiply.* Dissolve yeast in lukewarm water, between 110° and 115°F (43° and 46°C). A whisk works well to incorporate the yeast into the water. Allow to stand for 5 minutes, then mix again to ensure complete dissolution.

III. *Thou shalt keep thy ingredients neither too hot nor too cold, but just right.* Dry ingredients should be at room temperature. Remember to take flour and other ingredients out of the refrigerator or freezer in advance. Liquids should be approximately 110°F (43°C). However, buttermilk curdles when too hot; remove from the heat immediately if it starts to separate.

IV. *Mix thy dough to the proper texture.* Mix in the sweetening, oil, salt, and liquid. Mix in enough flour to make a soft dough. You may have to work in the last 2 to 3 cups with your hands if not using an electric mixer with a dough hook. A conventional food processor cannot handle the amount of dough needed for two loaves, so it is best to do the initial mixing by hand and divide the dough into batches for kneading. A soft dough makes the lightest bread. However, the dough should hold its shape; a moist batter is not the aim here. It is something you simply have to feel—there are no exact measurements to ensure perfection. Don't worry; it's an easy feeling to get.

V. *Let there be nurturing conditions for thy bread to rise.* Do not oil the bowl you intend to use for rising; it can cause an uneven texture in your bread. For rising, always cover the bowl with a dampened clean cloth, which allows the bread to breathe but keeps it from drying out. Place the bowl in a warm, draft-free place between 70° and 80°F (21° and 27°C). Too much heat kills the yeasts. Too little offers them cold comfort and they won't do their job. Do not disturb rising bread—yeasts, like many of us, like quiet and privacy. At this point, most cookbooks advise allowing the dough to rise "until doubled in bulk." However, doughs containing any amount of whole grain flour almost never balloon up that much. The better test is to plunge two fingers into the center after the amount of time specified in the directions has elapsed (usually 1½ to 2 hours).
   ❖ If the holes you've made just stay there, your dough has risen enough.
   ❖ If their sides start to cave in or if the dough clings to your fingers, it needs to rise more.
   ❖ If the dough has the smell of alcohol on its breath and starts to shrink, it has sat too long. The only thing you can do is shorten the third rising and cross those fingers that just gave you the bad news about the dough.

VI. *Honor the gluten in thy dough and keep it holey:* Kneading develops the gluten.
   ❖ Use a minimum amount of flour on your work surface. Scrape up the dough with a pastry cutter, knife, or spatula until it stops sticking, which it will do after about 5 minutes of kneading.
   ❖ Knead bread until it feels silky smooth, springy, and elastic. About 10 minutes by hand is usually enough for two loaves' worth of dough containing unbleached white flour. Laurel Robertson and company recommend 20 to 30 minutes for doughs made solely with whole grain flours.
   ❖ Using a dough hook on an electric mixer slightly shortens the time it takes to hand-knead dough; it all depends on the speed and enthusiasm of your mixer. Check after 6 to 8 minutes for doughs containing unbleached white flour after 10 to 15 minutes for completely whole grain loaves.

❖ Kneading in a food processor is accomplished in about 80 seconds. Unless you own a giant-sized, industrial-strength processor, you will have to knead a two-loaf amount of dough in 2 or 3 batches.

VII. *Punch thy dough and form into loaves with circumspection.* Literally punch down the dough with your fists. For best results, allow it to stand for about 10 minutes before forming into loaves. Everyone has a favorite method of forming loaves. You have two basic options:

❖ *Free-form loaves*, which bake on a baking sheet. These can be round, oval, braided, or made into fancy shapes like people, animals, trees, etc. If trying your hand at bread sculpture, remember that your shapes become less distinct as they rise.

Coat baking sheets with oil or ghee; the loaves won't touch the entire surface of the pan, and butter will burn on the uncovered spots. You can also scatter a liberal amount of cornmeal on an unoiled baking sheet, a technique often used for pumpernickel and rye breads.

An option that produces a crisp bottom crust is to use an unglazed clay surface, such as tiles or a "pizza stone." I've also had good luck with well-seasoned cast-iron griddles and skillets for producing crisp bottom crusts.

❖ *Loaf pans.* For best results, use small or medium-sized pans—not extra-large. Coat the pans with butter for the least amount of sticking. Try to keep manipulation of the dough to a minimum when forming loaves; cracks and fissures prove very stubborn when you try to pinch them closed. If the San Andreas Fault appears and won't go away, put it on the bottom of the loaf and hope it disappears during the baking. It usually doesn't.

VIII. *Thou shalt proof thy loaves.* The final rising, called *proofing*, is vital to the final result. Cover the loaves loosely but thoroughly with a damp cloth so they won't dry out—or you can invert a large pot over them. Don't put them in the oven to rise, as you have to heat the oven at some point during their rising time. Allow to rise for the time given, usually 30 to 45 minutes, then very gently remove the covering and lightly press with your fingertips to leave a very shallow impression. If the impression bounces back very slowly, the loaves are ready to bake.

IX. *Bake thy loaves in a thoroughly preheated oven.* If you warm up the oven with the loaves in it, the yeasts go into high gear in the initial warmth before dying out as the temperature approaches the range for baking, leaving behind an unevenly textured loaf as their legacy. The best bread-baking ovens are made of porous earthen material, such as brick. If you feel serious about your loaves, you can make a temporary bread-baking oven by lining your oven with ceramic tiles or bricks before you turn it on.

❖ If you desire a hard crust, place a pan of boiling water on the bottom rack to create steam.

X. *Know when thy bread is done, and yield not unto the temptation to eat it all the minute it comes out of thy oven.* Bread is done when the top crust is nicely browned and it has a hollow sound when you thump the bottom of the loaf after gently removing it from the pan. Remove bread from the pan to cool on a rack. Bread fresh from the oven will crumble when you try to slice it. If at all possible, wait!

BREAD CRUMBS

❖ *Fresh bread crumbs* are a delicious binder and thickener for loaves, burgers, soups, and stews. Pulverize fresh bread in a blender or food processor. Measure by packing lightly into a measuring cup.

❖ *Dry bread crumbs* are good for coating burgers and other fried foods and for making stuffings. Finely pulverize very dry bread or crackers in a blender or food processor, or place in a sturdy bag and crush with a rolling pin. To dry out bread, bake thin slices in a 300°F (150°C) oven for about 15 minutes, until dry but not browned.

❖ *Buttered bread crumbs:* If you top a casserole with dry crumbs, they emerge looking sandy and unappetizing. Moistening dry bread crumbs with oil helps them brown nicely. Use 2 to 3 tablespoons melted ghee, butter, or oil for ½ cup (50 g) dry fine bread crumbs.

❖ *Savory bread crumbs:* Add small amounts of hing, sesame or sunflower seeds, and dried herbs, such as basil, thyme, oregano, sage, and rosemary.

 ## BASIC BREAD

2 loaves

Our daily bread depends on Heaven; Heaven knows how each man gets his living.
          —WILLIAM SCARBOROUGH, *Chinese Proverbs*

STEP ONE

4½ teaspoons (2 packages) yeast   *1 cup (240 ml) lukewarm water*

STEP TWO

¼ cup (50 g) sugar   *¼ cup (60 ml) melted ghee, butter,*
1 cup (240 ml) lukewarm   *or oil*
   buttermilk   *3 cups (450 g) whole wheat flour*
2 teaspoons salt   *3 to 3½ cups (420 to 490 g)*
                      unbleached white flour

1. Mix the yeast with the water. Allow to stand for 5 minutes. Mix again.
2. Stir in the sugar, buttermilk, salt, oil, and whole wheat flour. Work in enough unbleached white flour to form a soft dough.

3. Turn out on a floured board. Knead until the dough is smooth and elastic, about 10 minutes.

4. Place in a large bowl and cover with a damp cloth. Let the dough rise in a warm place until it tests done, 1½ to 2 hours.

5. Punch down the dough and allow it to rest for 10 minutes. Form 2 loaves and place in buttered 9 × 5 × 3–inch (23 × 13 × 7.5 cm) loaf pans.

6. Redampen the cloth, cover the loaves, and allow them to rise in a warm place—not the oven—until proofed, 30 to 45 minutes.

7. Meanwhile, preheat the oven to 375°F (190°C). Bake the loaves for about 45 minutes.

VARIATIONS

White Bread: Substitute unbleached white flour for the whole wheat flour.

Raisin Bread: Add 1 cup (125 g) raisins in Step 2 or to any bread recipe you fancy having raisins in.

Rye Bread: Substitute for all the flour, 2 cups (280 g) unbleached white flour, 2 cups (250 g) rye flour, and 2 to 2½ cups (300 to 375 g) whole wheat flour. Add 2 tablespoons caraway seeds in Step 2.

Pistachio, Fig, and Anise Bread: Add 1 cup (115 g) coarsely chopped pistachios, 1½ cups (240 g) coarsely chopped figs, and 2 tablespoons anise seeds in Step 2. Add ¼ cup (50 g) more sugar.

Dried Tomato Bread: Add 1 cup (80 g) coarsely chopped dried tomatoes (either well-drained oil-packed or reconstituted dried) in Step 2.

Fennel or Cumin Bread: Sauté 2 tablespoons fennel or cumin seeds in the oil in Step 2 for 1 minute.

Sesame Bread: Toast ⅔ cup (90 g) sesame seeds in a dry skillet over low heat, stirring constantly until they are golden brown. Grind to a powder in a blender. For more intense sesame flavor, add a few drops of toasted sesame oil. Add in Step 2. Press whole sesame seeds into the tops of the loaves after they are formed in Step 5.

Nut or Seed Bread: Add 1 cup (135 g) whole seeds, such as sunflower or pumpkin, or 1 cup (240 ml) coarsely chopped nuts to the dough in Step 2.

 # Swedish Rye Bread (Skräddkakor)

SWEDEN   *2 loaves*

A fragrant, full-flavored bread.

STEP ONE

4½ teaspoons (2 packages) yeast   2 cups (480 ml) lukewarm water

STEP TWO

¼ cup (60 ml) dark
  unsulphured molasses
2 tablespoons finely
  grated orange zest
2 teaspoons salt
2 tablespoons ghee,
  butter, or oil
1 tablespoon caraway seeds

1 tablespoon anise or
  fennel seeds
2 cups (300 g) whole
  wheat flour
2 cups (250 g) rye flour
2 to 2½ cups (280 to 350 g)
  unbleached white flour

1. Mix the yeast with the water. Allow to stand for 5 minutes. Mix again.
2. Mix in the molasses, orange zest, salt, oil, seeds, and whole wheat and rye flours. Work in enough unbleached white flour to form a soft dough.
3. Turn out on a floured board. Knead until the dough is smooth and elastic, about 10 minutes.
4. Place in a large bowl and cover with a damp cloth. Let the dough rise in a warm place until it tests done, 1½ to 2 hours.
5. Punch down the dough and allow it to rest for 10 minutes. Form 2 round loaves. Place on an oiled baking sheet at least 2 inches (5 cm) apart. Make 3 diagonal cuts with a sharp knife ½-inch (1.3 cm) deep on the top of each loaf.
6. Redampen the cloth, cover the loaves, and allow them to rise in a warm place—not the oven—until proofed, 30 to 45 minutes.
7. Meanwhile, preheat the oven to 375°F (190°C). Bake the loaves for about 45 minutes.

If thine enemy be hungry give him bread to eat.   —PROVERBS 25.21

 # OATMEAL AND OTHER COOKED CEREAL BREADS

2 loaves

Here is a generic recipe for producing a variety of scrumptious breads, each with its own unique personality. You can use any cooked cereal or any grain that has a mushy, cooked-cereal-like texture without distinct individual grains, such as bulgar, buckwheat, amaranth, teff, or broken wild rice pieces. Oatmeal and bulgar are my favorites. You may have to slightly alter the amount of flour, depending on the differing amounts of moisture in different cooked grains.

STEP ONE

4½ teaspoons (2 packages) yeast   ¼ cup (60 ml) lukewarm water

STEP TWO

2 cups (480 ml) lukewarm cooked
  cereal or mushy grains
½ cup (120 ml) lukewarm
  buttermilk
⅓ cup (70 g) raw or packed
  brown sugar

¼ cup (60 ml) melted ghee, butter,
  or oil
2 teaspoons salt
2½ cups (375 g) whole wheat flour
2½ to 3 cups (350 to 420 g)
  unbleached white flour

1. Mix the yeast with the water. Allow to stand for 5 minutes. Mix again.
2. Mix in the cooked cereal or grain, buttermilk, sugar, oil, salt, and whole wheat flour. Work in enough unbleached white flour to form a soft dough.
3. Turn out on a floured board. Knead until the dough is smooth and elastic, about 10 minutes.
4. Place in a large bowl and cover with a damp cloth. Let the dough rise in a warm place until it tests done, 1½ to 2 hours.
5. Punch down the dough and allow it to rest for 10 minutes. Form 2 loaves and place in buttered 9 × 5 × 3–inch (23 × 13 × 7.5 cm) loaf pans.
6. Redampen the cloth, cover the loaves, and allow them to rise in a warm place—not the oven—until proofed, 30 to 45 minutes.
7. Meanwhile, preheat the oven to 375°F (190°C). Bake the loaves for about 45 minutes.

 # WHEAT BERRY AND
OTHER WHOLE GRAIN BREADS

2 loaves

Wheat berries and other firm, whole grains add a delightful texture to breads. Use firm, distinct grains, such as whole grain wild rice, rye berries, whole oats, and triticale.

STEP ONE

4½ teaspoons (2 packages) yeast

1¼ cups (300 ml) lukewarm water

STEP TWO

¼ cup (60 ml) unsulphured
  molasses
1 cup (240 ml) lukewarm buttermilk
2 teaspoons salt
¼ cup (60 ml) melted ghee, butter,
  or oil

2 cups (480 ml) lukewarm cooked
  wheat berries or other whole grains
½ cup (60 g) wheat germ
3 cups (450 g) whole wheat flour
3 to 3½ cups (420 to 490 g)
  unbleached white flour

1. Mix the yeast with the water. Allow to stand for 5 minutes. Mix again.

2. Add the molasses, buttermilk, salt, oil, wheat berries, wheat germ, and whole wheat flour. Work in enough unbleached white flour to form a soft dough.
3. Turn out on a floured board. Knead until the dough is smooth and elastic, about 10 minutes.
4. Place in a large bowl and cover with a damp cloth. Let the dough rise in a warm place until it tests done, 1½ to 2 hours.
5. Punch down the dough and allow it to rest for 10 minutes. Form 2 loaves and place in buttered 9 × 5 × 3–inch (23 × 13 × 7.5 cm) loaf pans.
6. Redampen the cloth, cover the loaves, and allow them to rise in a warm place—not the oven—until proofed, 30 to 45 minutes.
7. Meanwhile, preheat the oven to 375°F (190°C). Bake the loaves for about 45 minutes.

 # POLENTA RAISIN BREAD

SWITZERLAND   *2 loaves*

Here is my attempt to replicate the most delicious bread I've ever eaten: a rustic loaf containing coarsely cracked cornmeal made in a small Swiss village. Perhaps the glory was in eating it still warm from the oven when it was delivered at 6 A.M. Maybe it was the crystalline air or the view of a mountain across the lake so massive and powerful it overwhelmed the senses . . . anyway, the bread was really good.

STEP ONE

4½ teaspoons (2 packages) yeast   *¼ cup (60 ml) lukewarm water*

STEP TWO

½ cup (120 ml) lukewarm buttermilk   *¼ cup (60 ml) melted ghee or butter*
½ cup (100 g) raw or packed brown sugar   *2 teaspoons salt*
2 cups (480 ml) cooked Polenta (pp. 164–65), cooled to lukewarm   *1 cup (125 g) raisins*
      ½ cup (60 g) toasted wheat germ
      5 to 6 cups (700 to 840 g) unbleached white flour

1. Mix the yeast with the water. Allow to stand for 5 minutes. Mix again.
2. Mix in the buttermilk, sugar, Polenta, melted ghee or butter, salt, raisins, and wheat germ. Beat and work in enough flour to form a soft dough.
3. Turn out on a floured board. Knead until the dough is smooth and elastic, about 10 minutes.
4. Place in a large bowl and cover with a damp cloth. Let the dough rise in a warm place until it tests done, 1½ to 2 hours.
5. Punch down the dough and allow it to rest for 10 minutes. Form 2 round free-form loaves. Scatter a little cornmeal on an oiled baking sheet and place the loaves on it at least 2 inches (5 cm) apart.

6. Redampen the cloth, cover the loaves, and allow them to rise in a warm place—not the oven—until proofed, 30 to 45 minutes.
7. Meanwhile, preheat the oven to 375°F (190°C). Bake the loaves for about 45 minutes.

The eating of bread is under the providence of God; he is an ignorant man that disputeth it.   —Ptah-Hotep, 3350 b.c.

 # Granola Bread

2 loaves

A sweet bread with a bit of crunch.

STEP ONE

4½ teaspoons (2 packages) yeast   1¼ cups (300 ml) lukewarm water

STEP TWO

½ cup (100 g) raw or packed   2 teaspoons salt
    brown sugar   3 cups (375 g) Granola (p. 155)
¾ cup (180 ml) lukewarm   3 cups (450 g) whole wheat flour
    buttermilk   3 to 3½ cups (420 to 490 g)
¼ cup (60 ml) melted ghee or   unbleached white flour
    butter

1. Mix the yeast with the water. Allow to stand for 5 minutes. Mix again.
2. Mix in the sugar, buttermilk, melted ghee or butter, salt, Granola, and whole wheat flour. Work in enough unbleached white flour to form a soft dough.
3. Turn out on a floured board. Knead until the dough is smooth and elastic, about 10 minutes.
4. Place in a large bowl and cover with a damp cloth. Let the dough rise in a warm place until it tests done, 1½ to 2 hours.
5. Punch down the dough and allow it to rest for 10 minutes. Form 2 loaves and place in buttered 9 × 5 × 3–inch (23 × 13 × 7.5 cm) loaf pans.
6. Redampen the cloth, cover the loaves, and allow them to rise in a warm place—not the oven—until proofed, 30 to 45 minutes.
7. Meanwhile, preheat the oven to 375°F (190°C). Bake the loaves for about 45 minutes.

VARIATION
    Add 1 cup raisins (125 g) or chopped dates (285 g) after the first rising.

I am going to bake bread tomorrow. So you may imagine me with my sleeves
rolled up, mixing flour, milk, saleratus [leavening], etc. with a deal of grace. I
advise you if you don't know how to make the staff of life to learn with dispatch.
—EMILY DICKINSON

 # HERB BREAD

2 loaves

There are many green herbs that make delicious bread; one luscious bread contains only
rosemary leaves. Dried herbs briefly sautéed in oil add the most flavor, with the exception of rosemary, thyme, and sage, which have powerful flavors whether fresh or dried.
Minced fresh herbs, such as parsley and cilantro, give a pretty appearance but don't do
much for the taste buds. The following recipe combines both fresh and dried herbs for
the best of both sensory experiences.

STEP ONE

¼ *cup (60 ml) olive oil*
Pinch of hing (optional)
2 teaspoons dried basil

1 teaspoon rosemary
2 teaspoons dill seeds
2 tablespoons minced fresh parsley

STEP TWO

4½ *teaspoons (2 packages) yeast*
1 cup (240 ml) lukewarm
   vegetable stock or water

STEP THREE

3 tablespoons raw or brown sugar
1 cup (240 ml) lukewarm
   buttermilk
2 teaspoons salt

3 cups (450 g) whole wheat flour
3 to 3½ cups (420 to 490 g)
   unbleached white flour

1. Heat the olive oil in a small skillet. Add the hing and herbs and sauté over low heat,
   stirring constantly, until fragrant. Allow to cool to lukewarm.
2. Mix the yeast with the stock or water. Allow to stand for 5 minutes. Mix again.
3. Add the herb mixture, sugar, buttermilk, salt, and whole wheat flour. Work in
   enough unbleached white flour to form a soft dough.
4. Turn out on a floured board. Knead until the dough is smooth and elastic, about 10
   minutes.
5. Place in a large bowl and cover with a damp cloth. Let the dough rise in a warm
   place until it tests done, 1½ to 2 hours.
6. Punch down the dough and allow it to rest for 10 minutes. Form 2 loaves and place
   in buttered 9 × 5 × 3–inch (23 × 13 × 7.5 cm) loaf pans.

7. Redampen the cloth, cover the loaves, and allow them to rise in a warm place—not the oven—until proofed, 30 to 45 minutes.

8. Meanwhile, preheat the oven to 375°F (190°C). Bake the loaves for about 45 minutes.

VARIATIONS

Replace the herbs with 1 tablespoon each chopped fresh rosemary and fresh sage leaves.

Replace 1 cup (150 g) of whole wheat flour with 1 cup (125 g) rye flour.

Add sliced dried tomatoes in Step 3.

For an earthier, crustier bread, make free-form loaves. Spritz with water before baking and place a pan of boiling water on the lower rack of the oven to provide steam.

 # PUMPERNICKEL BREAD

2 loaves

From the Middle Ages onward, the bakers of western Europe labored under regulations so strict they could produce loaves containing only the most basic ingredients. Their colleagues to the east led much less fettered professional lives. Free to respond to new ingredients, old customs, and their own inner callings, they created great holiday loaves bursting with fruits and nuts, as well as an everyday receptacle of a-little-bit-of-this-and-that: pumpernickel. This version was obviously created after the discovery of the New World because of its inclusion of cornmeal.

STEP ONE

¾ cup (180 ml) water　　　*¾ cup (95 g) cornmeal*

STEP TWO

4½ teaspoons (2 packages) yeast　　　*½ cup (120 ml) lukewarm water*

STEP THREE

¼ cup (60 ml) dark unsulphured　　*2 tablespoons caraway seeds*
*　molasses*　　　　　　　　　　　*2 cups (250 g) rye flour*
2 tablespoons oil　　　　　　　　*4 to 4½ cups (600 to 675 g)*
2 teaspoons salt　　　　　　　　　*　whole wheat flour*

1. Bring the water to a boil. Stir in the cornmeal and cook for 1 minute, stirring constantly, until thick.

2. Mix the yeast with the lukewarm water. Allow to stand for 5 minutes. Mix again.

3. Mix in the cooked cornmeal, the molasses, water, oil, salt, caraway seeds, and rye flour. Work in enough whole wheat flour to form a soft dough.

4. Turn out on a floured board. Knead until the dough is smooth and elastic, about 20 minutes.

5. Place in a large bowl and cover with a damp cloth. Let the dough rise in a warm place until it tests done, about 2 hours.

6. Punch down the dough and allow it to rest for 10 minutes. Form 2 free-form oval loaves. Make 3 shallow diagonal cuts with a sharp knife on the top of each loaf.
7. Oil a baking sheet and scatter cornmeal on it. Place the loaves on the cornmeal at least 2 inches (5 cm) apart.
8. Redampen the cloth, cover the loaves, and allow them to rise in a warm place—not the oven—until proofed, 45 to 60 minutes.
9. Meanwhile, preheat the oven to 375°F (190°C). Bake the loaves about 45 minutes.

VARIATION

For a darker loaf, mix 1 tablespoon herbal coffee substitute powder (preferably Raja's Cup) into the water in Step 1.

> *And the best bread was of my mother's own making—the best in all the land!*
> —HENRY JAMES

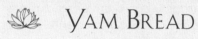
YAM BREAD

UNITED STATES   *2 loaves*

Sam McIlhenny introduced me to a sweet, golden loaf from Louisiana that can be prepared from any type of puréed cooked winter squash. The beautiful golden color shows up best when you use turbinado or white sugar.

STEP ONE

4½ teaspoons (2 packages) yeast   *¼ cup (60 ml) lukewarm water*

STEP TWO

2 cups (460 g) puréed cooked yams or winter squash   *1 tablespoon ground cinnamon*
⅔ cup (140 g) sugar   *½ cup (65 g) raisins*
¼ cup (60 ml) melted ghee or butter   *½ cup (50 g) chopped walnuts*
2 teaspoons salt   *6½ to 7 cups (900 to 980 g) unbleached white flour*

1. Mix the yeast with the water. Allow to stand for 5 minutes. Mix again.
2. Beat in the yams or squash, sugar, ghee or butter, salt, and cinnamon. Mix in the raisins and nuts. Beat and work in enough of the flour to form a soft dough.
3. Turn out on a floured board. Knead until the dough is smooth and elastic, about 10 minutes.
4. Place in a large bowl and cover with a damp cloth. Let the dough rise in a warm place until it tests done, 1½ to 2 hours.
5. Punch down the dough and allow it to rest for 10 minutes. Form 2 loaves and place in buttered 9 × 5 × 3–inch (23 × 13 × 7.5 cm) loaf pans.

6. Redampen the cloth, cover the loaves, and allow them to rise in a warm place—not the oven—until proofed, 30 to 45 minutes.

7. Meanwhile, preheat the oven to 375°F (190°C). Bake the loaves for about 45 minutes.

VARIATION

For a loaf that is not sweet, reduce the sugar to ¼ cup (50 g) and omit the raisins.

Open thine eyes, and thou shalt be satisfied with bread.   —PROVERBS 20.13

DINNER ROLLS

Dinner-type rolls can be made from any bread dough. One bread recipe yields enough rolls to feed an army, so unless you have one handy, cut the recipe in half to yield 12 to 16 rolls. To ensure that rolls are well cooked, which Ayurveda recommends, split and toast baked rolls before eating.

1. Prepare bread dough as directed. Instead of shaping into loaves, form rolls in the shapes described below, or any other shape you desire. If you wish, press seeds firmly into the tops.

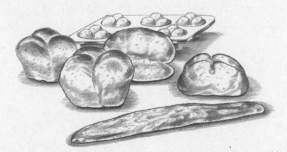

2. Place on an oiled baking sheet. Allow the rolls to proof for 30 to 45 minutes, as described in your selected bread recipe.

3. Bake in a 375°F (190°C) oven for 20 to 25 minutes.

Roll Shapes

❖ *Burger Rolls:* Roll the dough into 1½-inch (3.5 cm) balls. Flatten the balls on the bottom but leave the tops rounded. Press sesame seeds into the tops if desired.

❖ *Parkerhouse Rolls:* Roll the dough into 1-inch (2.5 cm) balls. Flatten them and fold in half.

❖ *Cloverleaf Rolls:* Roll the dough into tiny balls. Place 3 balls in each cup of a buttered muffin pan to form cloverleafs.

❖ *Petit Pains (French-Style Rolls):* Focaccia dough makes nice rolls—and no need to halve the recipe. Roll the dough into 1½-inch (3.5 cm) balls. Place on an oiled baking sheet and flatten the bottoms. With a sharp knife, slash crosscuts about ¼-inch (6 mm) deep in the top of each roll. For a hard crust, place the rolls on the upper oven shelf and a pan of boiling water on the lower shelf.

❖ *Bread Sticks:* Roll out long, thin ropes of dough. If desired, roll in poppy, caraway, or other seeds. Bake 10 to 15 minutes.

❖ *Fan Tans:* Roll out 5 thin 4 × 5-inch (10 × 13 cm) rectangles. Stack them on top of each other, brushing each rectangle with melted ghee or butter before laying down the next one. Fold in half from the wide end to form a 2 × 5-inch (5 × 13 cm) rectangle. Cut out 3 rolls. Place, "fan" side up, in buttered muffin cups. Repeat until you have used up all the dough.

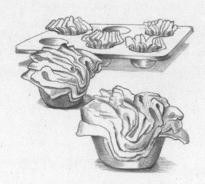

Sage Dressing

UNITED STATES   *4 to 6 servings*

Sage is sacred to many Native American tribes. It is sprinkled on the ground or burned like incense to purify the environment, as well as added to foods for its unparalleled flavor. How fitting that sage graces this classic Thanksgiving dish. Whole grain breads give it extra flavor and texture. Serve with gravy if desired.

STEP ONE

4 cups (200 g) cubed bread

STEP TWO

⅓ cup (75 g) ghee or butter
Pinch of hing (optional)
1¼ teaspoons dried thyme
½ teaspoon dried sage or
  2 teaspoons chopped fresh

½ teaspoon rosemary
1 carrot, grated
3 cups (330 g) thinly sliced fennel
  or celery

¼ cup (60 ml) minced fresh
  parsley
Vegetable Stock (p. 219)

Liquid seasoning
Seasoned salt
Black pepper

STEP FOUR

Cabbage or lettuce leaves

1. Spread the bread cubes on a baking sheet. Toast in a 350°F (180°C) oven until very dry. Let cool.
2. Meanwhile, melt the ghee or butter in a large skillet. Add the hing and herbs and sauté for about 30 seconds over low heat. Add the carrot and fennel or celery and sauté until tender, stirring frequently. Remove from the heat.
3. Toss the bread cubes and parsley with the vegetables. Add just enough stock to moisten. Season to taste with liquid seasoning, seasoned salt, and pepper.
4. Preheat the oven to 325°F (160°C). Butter a 2-quart (2 l) casserole dish and line it with cabbage or lettuce leaves to keep the dressing from drying out and forming a crust.
5. Place the dressing over the leaves. Do not pack down. Cover and bake for 1 hour.

CROUTONS

Homemade croutons make excellent garnishes for soups and salads. Cube bread in ½-inch to 1-inch (1.3 to 2.5 cm) pieces. Scatter the cubes on a baking sheet and toast in a 325°F (160°C) oven until very dry, about 15 minutes.

❖ *Herb Croutons:* Heat ⅓ cup (80 ml) olive oil in a skillet with a pinch of hing (optional). Add and sauté until fragrant, about 30 seconds:

½ teaspoon dried thyme
½ teaspoon dried basil
¼ teaspoon crumbled dried sage
¼ teaspoon dried rosemary

Add the croutons and stir for a minute to coat.

Pandolce (Sweet Bread)

ITALY   *2 loaves*

A holiday specialty of Genoa, fragrant with anise and studded with colorful fruits and nuts. Though it is traditionally prepared with glacéed citron and candied fruit, I have substituted dried fruits, which many people prefer. When using hard, unsulphured dried fruit, soak it in boiling water to soften before adding.

STEP ONE

4½ teaspoons (2 packages) yeast   ¼ cup (60 ml) lukewarm water

STEP TWO

2 tablespoons anise seeds   1 teaspoon salt
1 cup (240 ml) lukewarm   1 cup (125 g) raisins
  orange juice   ½ cup (60 g) sliced dried apricots
1 cup (240 ml) lukewarm   ½ cup (80 g) coarsely chopped
  buttermilk   crystallized ginger
½ cup (120 ml) melted ghee or   ½ cup (65 g) dried cherries (or other
  butter   dried fruit)
⅔ cup (140 g) sugar   ½ cup (70 g) shelled pistachios
2 tablespoons finely grated orange ⅓ cup (45 g) pine nuts
  zest   7 to 7½ cups (980 g to 1.1 kg)
1 tablespoon finely grated lemon   unbleached white flour
  zest

1. Mix the yeast with the water. Allow to stand for 5 minutes. Mix again.
2. Beat in the ingredients in order, working in enough flour to form a soft dough.
3. Turn out on a floured board. Knead until the dough is smooth and elastic, about 10 minutes.
4. Place in a large bowl and cover with a damp cloth. Let the dough rise in a warm place until it tests done, about 1½ hours.
5. Punch down the dough and allow it to rest for 10 minutes. Form 2 round loaves and place on a buttered baking sheet at least 2 inches (5 cm) apart.
6. Redampen the cloth, cover the loaves, and allow them to rise in a warm place—not the oven—until proofed, 30 to 40 minutes.
7. Meanwhile, preheat the oven to 350°F (180°C). Bake the loaves for 50 to 60 minutes.

WEIHNACHTSTRIEZEL (CHRISTMAS BRAID)

GERMANY   *1 long loaf*

A talented German chef—named, would you believe, Klaus Chef—lent me his baker father's personal handwritten recipe book. Unfortunately, Mr. Chef, Sr., penned his notes for the most part in elegant, beautiful, and utterly unreadable old German script. However, a precious few recipes—all gems—were written in a modern hand. Here is one of them.

STEP ONE

3½ teaspoons (1½ packages) yeast

1 cup (240 ml) lukewarm water

STEP TWO

⅔ cup (140 g) sugar
1 cup (240 ml) lukewarm buttermilk

¼ cup (60 ml) melted ghee or butter
1 teaspoon salt

STEP THREE

2 tablespoons finely grated orange zest
1 cup (125 g) raisins
¾ cup (100 g) slivered blanched almonds

6 to 6½ cups (840 to 910 g) unbleached white flour

1. Mix the yeast with the water. Allow to stand for 5 minutes. Mix again.
2. Beat in the sugar, buttermilk, melted ghee or butter, and salt.
3. Stir in the orange zest, raisins, and almonds. Beat and work in enough of the flour to form a soft dough.
4. Turn out on a floured board. Knead until the dough is smooth and elastic, about 10 minutes.
5. Place in a large bowl and cover with a damp cloth. Let the dough rise in a warm place until it tests done, about 1½ hours.
6. Punch down the dough and allow it to rest for 10 minutes. Divide into 3 parts. Roll each piece into a long, even, fat rope. Place on an oiled baking sheet. Pinch the ends together securely on one end. Gently braid the ropes and pinch the other end together. Tuck both ends under for a smooth appearance.
7. Redampen the cloth, cover the loaf, and allow it to rise in a warm place—not the oven—until proofed, 30 to 45 minutes.
8. Meanwhile, preheat the oven to 350°F (180°C). Bake the loaf for about 1 hour.

CINNAMON ROLLS

1 dozen

When preparing rolls for breakfast, to avoid the 1½-hour rising time, you can make the dough the night before and let it rise overnight in the refrigerator.

STEP ONE

2¼ teaspoons (1 package) yeast	½ cup (120 ml) lukewarm water

STEP TWO

¼ cup (60 ml) melted ghee or butter	½ teaspoon salt
⅓ cup (70 g) raw or packed brown sugar	3 to 3½ cups (420 to 490 g) unbleached white flour
½ cup (120 ml) lukewarm buttermilk	

STEP SIX

3 tablespoons melted ghee or butter	¼ cup (50 g) sugar
	1 tablespoon ground cinnamon

STEP TEN: OPTIONAL GLAZE

½ cup (60 g) confectioner's sugar	A few drops of water
1 teaspoon finely grated orange zest	

1. Mix the yeast with the water. Allow to stand for 5 minutes. Mix again.
2. Beat in the melted ghee or butter, sugar, buttermilk, and salt. Work in enough flour to form a soft dough.
3. Turn out on a floured board. Knead until the dough is smooth and elastic, about 10 minutes.
4. Place in a large bowl and cover with a damp cloth. Let the dough rise in a warm place until it tests done, about 1½ hours.
5. Punch down the dough and allow it to rest for 10 minutes. Roll out on a floured board in a 9 × 14-inch (23 × 36 cm) rectangle.
6. Brush the dough with the melted ghee or butter. Mix the sugar and cinnamon together and sprinkle evenly over the surface of the dough.
7. Roll up the dough tightly from a long side to make a long, thin tube. Slice off 1-inch (2.5 cm) rolls. Place on an oiled baking sheet, cut side up.
8. Cover the rolls with a damp cloth and allow them to rise in a warm place—not the oven—until proofed, 30 to 45 minutes.
9. Meanwhile, preheat the oven to 375°F (190°C). Bake the rolls until golden brown, 20 to 25 minutes.
10. Allow to cool for 10 minutes. If desired, mix all the ingredients for the glaze together and drizzle over the rolls.

YAM-PECAN STICKY BUNS

1 dozen

Yams and dry winter squash, such as kabocha, work beautifully to make these golden-colored buns. You can also make sticky buns using uncooked Cinnamon Rolls (previous recipe), starting at Step 8.

STEP ONE

2¼ teaspoons (1 package) yeast	*½ cup (120 ml) lukewarm water*

STEP TWO

1 cup (230 g) puréed cooked yams or winter squash	*3 tablespoons melted ghee or butter*
½ teaspoon salt	*3 to 3½ cups (420 to 500 g) unbleached white flour*
⅓ cup (70 g) sugar	

STEP SIX

3 tablespoons melted ghee or butter	*1 tablespoon cinnamon*
	¼ cup (50 g) sugar

STEP EIGHT

¾ cup (150 g) raw or packed brown sugar	*½ cup (50 g) finely chopped pecans*
6 tablespoons (90 ml) melted ghee or butter	

1. Mix the yeast with the water. Allow to stand for 5 minutes. Mix again.
2. Beat in the yams or squash, salt, sugar, and melted ghee or butter. Beat and work in enough flour to form a soft dough. Add more flour if necessary.
3. Turn out on a floured board. Knead until the dough is smooth and elastic, about 10 minutes.
4. Place in a large bowl and cover with a damp cloth. Let the dough rise in a warm place until it tests done, about 1½ hours.
5. Punch down the dough and allow it to rest for 10 minutes. Roll out on a floured board to form a 9 × 14-inch (23 × 36 cm) rectangle.
6. Brush the dough with the melted ghee or butter. Mix the sugar and cinnamon together and sprinkle evenly over the surface of the dough.
7. Roll up the dough lengthwise to form a long rope. Slice into 12 equal pieces to form the buns.
8. Mix the brown sugar and ghee or butter together. Spread over the bottom of a 10-inch (26 cm) cast-iron skillet. Sprinkle the pecans evenly over the bottom. Arrange the buns in the skillet about equal distance from each other.
9. Redampen the cloth, cover the buns, and allow them to rise in a warm place—not the oven—until proofed, 30 to 45 minutes.

10. Meanwhile, preheat the oven to 350°F (180°C). Bake the buns until golden brown, about 30 minutes. Do not bake a moment past the time they are done.
11. Invert a large plate over the skillet. Reverse the skillet and plate so that the rolls will come out in a single cake, covered with syrup and nuts.

VARIATION
Add raisins to the dough.

A SUNDAY BRUNCH FOR THE BOOK DISCUSSION GROUP

Tomatoes Stuffed with Vegetable Hash (pp. 138–39)
Scrambled Panir (p. 211)
Yam-Pecan Sticky Buns
Spice Nectar (p. 486)

 # FOCACCIA

ITALY   *One 11 × 15-inch (28 × 38 cm) flatbread*

The smell of good bread baking, like the sound of lightly falling water, is indescribable in its evocation of innocence and delight.   —M. F. K. FISHER

Focus is Latin for "hearth," and this wonderful, earthy bread was known in ancient Rome as *panis focacius*, "hearth bread." It was possibly the forerunner of pizza: a flat loaf sprinkled with toppings and baked on the hearth amongst the ashes.

Unglazed tiles or a pizza stone is ideal for replicating a hearth. However, a cookie sheet does just fine, and I often divide the dough and bake it in oiled cast-iron skillets. I like focaccia to have the thickness of a slightly-too-thick pan pizza crust—it fits my fantasy of the hearth bread of the ancients. However, your focaccia fantasy may be of something more thick and breadlike. If so, shape it more thickly and bake in a smaller pan. The flavorings and toppings that follow the recipe can be combined with each other ad infinitum. Serve focaccia with olive oil for dipping; Lemon-Pepper Oil is a particularly lovely anointment.

	STEP ONE
2¼ teaspoons (1 package) yeast	*1 cup (240 ml) lukewarm water*
	STEP TWO
¼ cup (60 ml) olive oil	*2⅓ cups (325 g) unbleached*
1 teaspoon salt	*white flour*
⅔ cup (100 g) whole wheat flour	

STEP FIVE

Cornmeal

1. Mix the yeast with the water. Allow to stand for 5 minutes. Mix again.
2. Mix in the olive oil, salt, and flours to form a soft dough.
3. Turn out on a floured board. Knead until the dough is smooth and elastic, about 10 minutes.
4. Place in a bowl and cover with a damp cloth. Let the dough rise in a warm place until it tests done, about 1¼ hours.
5. Punch the dough down. Scatter cornmeal on an oiled 11×15-inch (28 × 38 cm) cookie sheet or a baker's peel. Stretch out the dough until it resembles a too-thick pizza crust. Avoid having any thin, translucent spots, which will bake to a cracker-like hardness. If using any toppings, sprinkle them over the dough now.
6. Allow the dough to rest for 20 minutes. Meanwhile, preheat the oven to 425°F (220°C).
7. If baking on tiles, transfer the loaf to the heated tiles. Bake until the focaccia is lightly browned in a few places on top and lightly browned on the bottom, about 20 minutes. For the best flavor, serve warm from the oven.

VARIATIONS

Herbed Focaccia (Focaccia con Erbe): Brush the dough with 1 to 2 tablespoons olive oil in Step 5. Sprinkle lightly with chopped rosemary or sage leaves, fresh thyme, or dried green herbs, such as basil.

Salt-Crusted Focaccia (Focaccia Incrostata di Sale): Brush the dough with 1 to 2 tablespoons olive oil in Step 5. Sprinkle lightly with coarse (kosher) salt and/or cracked black pepper.

Focaccia with Fennel (Focaccia con Finocchio): Add 1 tablespoon fennel seeds to the dough in Step 2. While the dough is rising, heat 2 tablespoons olive oil in a skillet. Add a pinch of hing and sauté over low heat until fragrant, about 30 seconds. Add 2 cups (220 g) very thinly sliced fennel and sprinkle lightly with salt and pepper. Cover and sauté, stirring occasionally, until just barely tender, 5 to 10 minutes. Let cool to lukewarm. Spread over the dough after stretching out in Step 6, making sure the olive oil is distributed evenly. If desired, sprinkle with 2 tablespoons grated Parmesan. Allow the dough to rest for 20 minutes before baking.

Focaccia Rossa (Red Focaccia with Peppers and Dried Tomatoes): Add ½ cup (40 g) chopped sun-dried tomatoes to the dough in Step 2. Prepare as for Focaccia with Fennel, above, substituting 2 cups (280 g) very thinly sliced red bell peppers for the fennel. For an even rosier focaccia, replace part of the water in the dough with tomato juice.

PIZZA

One legend of the origins of pizza as we know it today is found in the *Aeneid*, where Virgil tells of a group of Trojans who, after the fall of Troy, consulted with an oracle before sailing in search of a new home. The oracle predicted that they would settle in a land where they would eat their dishes. A violent storm sank their ships off the coast of Naples, and they straggled to shore and fixed a meal for themselves as best they could. Their pewter dishes and utensils at the bottom of the watery deep, the refugees proceeded to eat their food atop makeshift flatbreads they baked on a stone, and then they hungrily consumed the breads as well. The people realized that they had "eaten their dishes" and took it as a sign to settle on that land.

Five-Star Pizza

☆ For a crisp crust, shape the dough by hand, and bake the pizza for a short time on the floor or the lowest rack of a very hot oven.

☆ For serious pizzophiles, the best medium for baking pizza crust is unglazed clay—either a pizza stone or unglazed tiles. You'll need a *baker's peel*, a large wood spatula, for maneuvering your pizza in and out of the oven.

☆ A wide variety of vegetables that do not ordinarily find their way onto pizzas, such as winter squash, can be successfully incorporated by cooking them first. When using tomato sauce or Carrot-Pepper Sauce, you can cook vegetables in the sauce.

☆ Tomato sauce is not absolutely necessary on pizza. Try a pesto or Tofu or Panir Mayonnaise, a flavored vegetable purée, or no sauce at all. A layer of panir, ricotta, chèvre, or even cream cheese makes a delicious base for pizza instead of sauce.

☆ You can make marvelous pizza with fresh cheeses like fresh mozzarella, feta, panir, and other soft cheeses, or omit the use of cheese entirely.

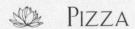 PIZZA

ITALY   *2 medium or 1 large pizza*

The following is a recipe for a conventional pizza setup, with options for fresh cheese and a sauce that is not based on tomatoes.

STEP ONE

2¼ teaspoons yeast (1 package)   *1 cup (240 ml) lukewarm water*

STEP TWO

¼ cup (60 ml) olive oil   *⅔ cup (100 g) whole wheat flour*
1 teaspoon salt
2⅓ cups (325 g) unbleached white flour

STEP SIX

Thick tomato sauce or
  Carrot-Pepper Sauce (p. 255)
2 cups (480 ml) or more lightly
  sautéed sliced vegetables: bell
  pepper, zucchini, eggplant, etc.
2 to 2½ cups (200 to 250 g)
  chopped fresh mozzarella, crumbled
  panir or feta, or grated firm mozzarella

Dried basil
Dried oregano
Grated Parmesan cheese (optional)
Olive oil

To prepare the crust:

1. Mix the yeast with the water and let stand for 5 minutes. Mix again.
2. Add the oil, salt, and the flours. Mix, turn out on a floured board, and knead the dough for 5 to 10 minutes.
3. Place in a glass or ceramic bowl, cover with a dampened dish towel, and let the dough rise in a warm place for 1½ hours or until it tests done.

To assemble:

4. Preheat the oven to 475°F (240°C). Place unglazed tiles in the oven before heating it, or oil an 11 × 15-inch (28 × 39 cm) baking sheet or 12-inch (30 cm) pizza pan with olive oil and set aside.
5. Punch down the dough. For two pizzas, divide in half. Spread and pinch *with your hands* to the desired size on a baker's peel that has been liberally dusted with cornmeal or on the prepared pan. Pinch a ridge around the edges of the dough to hold the topping.
6. Spread the sauce over the dough. Spread the vegetables over the sauce. Sprinkle on the cheese and a little basil, oregano, and grated Parmesan. Drizzle a little olive oil on top.
7. Bake on the lowest rack in the oven until the crust is done, about 15 minutes.

VARIATIONS

Those feeling less bold can bake the pizza for 30 minutes at 350°F (180°C).

✪ Omit the cheese.

CALZONE

Calzone, "trousers," are the Neapolitan equivalent of *empanadas* and Cornish pasties: half-moon-shaped pastries of pizza dough enclosing a filling. Use pizza fillings that are not juicy (fresh tomatoes and tomato sauce do not work well), such as sautéed vegetables, thick pesto, sautéed ground seitan, fresh or grated cheeses, and dried tomato paste. The fillings for Artichoke-Filo Pie, Spinach-Cheese Pie, and Asparagus Torte all make excellent fillings for Calzone. To make 6 large Calzone:

1. Prepare the dough for Pizza. When it is ready to form into a crust, divide into 6 pieces. Stretch and roll out each piece into a 7-inch (18 cm) round.
2. Divide your chosen filling equally among the 6 rounds. Prepare a thin paste of flour and water and dab around the edges of each round. Fold in half over the filling to form a half round and pinch the edges shut.
3. Place on oiled baking sheets. Bake at 450°F (230°C) until the crusts are browned and crispy, about 20 minutes.

 # LACHMANJUNS (SPICED PITA "PIZZAS")

ARMENIA/SYRIA/LEBANON   *12 individual pizzas*

I spent my seventeenth summer with my best friend, Dana Gilbert, in a suburb of Boston. We were dispatched on an errand to the Armenian district to pick up some lachmanjuns (more or less pronounced *lama-junes*) for her father's Syrian wife—a grand adventure for two California girls with newly acquired driver's licenses. Here is a vegetarian version. Grind the seitan in a food processor.

STEP ONE

2¼ teaspoons (1 package) yeast   *1 cup (240 ml) lukewarm water*

STEP TWO

2 tablespoons mild-flavored oil   *1½ cups (225 g) whole wheat flour*
1 teaspoon sugar   *1½ cups (210 g) unbleached*
1 teaspoon salt   *white flour*

STEP FIVE

3 tablespoons mild-flavored oil   *¾ cup (100 g) finely chopped bell*
Pinch of hing (optional)   *peppers*
1 teaspoon cumin seeds   *¼ cup (60 ml) minced fresh parsley*
2 tablespoons minced fresh ginger
¾ cup (90 g) finely chopped fennel
*   or celery*

STEP SIX

1 medium tomato

STEP SEVEN

2 cups (260 g) coarsely ground
  seitan
⅓ cup (45 g) pine nuts
⅔ cup (160 ml) yogurt
½ teaspoon ground allspice

¼ teaspoon ground cinnamon
¼ teaspoon ground nutmeg
1 teaspoon paprika
Salt
Black pepper

STEP ELEVEN

Olive oil

To prepare the crust:

1. Mix the yeast with the water. Allow to stand for 5 minutes. Mix again.
2. Add the oil, sugar, and salt. Beat in the flours to form a soft dough.
3. Turn out on a floured board. Knead the dough until smooth and elastic, about 10 minutes.
4. Place in a bowl. Cover with a damp dish towel and let the dough rise in a warm place until it tests done, about 1½ hours.

To prepare the filling:

5. While the dough is rising, heat the oil in a large skillet. Add the hing, cumin, seeds, and ginger, and sauté over low heat until fragrant, about 1 minute. Add the fennel or celery, bell peppers, and parsley. Cover and cook, stirring occasionally, until the vegetables are almost tender, 7 to 8 minutes.
6. Add the tomato and cook until the tomato is mushy, 2 to 3 minutes.
7. Stir in the seitan, pine nuts, yogurt, and spices. Season to taste with salt and pepper. Cook for 1 minute for the flavors to blend. Set aside.

To assemble and bake:

8. Preheat the oven to 400°F (200°C). Oil 2 baking sheets.
9. Punch down the dough. Divide into 12 pieces and roll into smooth balls.
10. Roll out each ball on a floured board to form a 4½-inch (11 cm) round. Place on the baking sheets. Top each round with the filling and spread evenly, leaving a ¼-inch (6 mm) edge of dough uncovered.
11. Brush the edges of the dough with olive oil. Bake until the dough is lightly browned but not crisp at the edges, about 20 minutes. Serve hot or at room temperature.

In heaven I hope to bake my own bread and clean my own linen.

—HENRY DAVID THOREAU

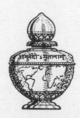

Unleavened and Quick Breads, Biscuits, Muffins, and Pancakes

This is the bread which cometh down from heaven, that a man may eat thereof, and not die.

—John 6.50

Indian Flatbreads

Indian flatbreads are ancient, purely Ayurvedic food: They are made with whole grain flour, contain no leavening, and are baked fresh for every meal. Flatbreads can be served any time of day, and while they are more balancing for Vata and Pitta, Kapha types can enjoy them as well. As with much simple cooking, a number of subtleties are involved in the process. Indian cooks sail through them on automatic pilot with speed and grace. Little wonder, considering that, like their ancestors through the millennia, they have been doing so since they could hold a rolling pin. For those of us enrolling in Indian Breads 101 later in life—without a handy grandmother to guide us—the process can feel awkward at first. However, practice makes perfect, and even imperfect results that are freshly and lovingly prepared are sublime.

❖ The best flour is *ata*, or *chapati flour*, available in Indian markets. It is a fine grind of soft whole wheat and makes a soft, pliable dough that is easy to work with. There is no comparable flour in the West; even whole wheat pastry flour is too coarse. If you can't obtain ata, use a mixture of equal parts unbleached white flour and whole wheat pastry flour. Don't try making these breads with conventional whole wheat flour—you'll be frustrated and disappointed.

❖ Although not absolutely necessary, the right tools make the job much easier. These are inexpensive and available in Indian markets. A small, thin, curved *chapati rolling pin* is the most helpful; it is much easier to maneuver than conventional Western types. Flatbreads are cooked individually on a *tava*, a small, round, slightly concave griddle, often with a long handle.

To keep the body in good health is a duty, for otherwise we shall not be able to trim the lamp of wisdom or keep our mind strong and clear.   —BUDDHA

 # BASIC DOUGH FOR INDIAN FLATBREADS

INDIA

The simplest, most basic dough is composed of flour and water alone. The additions of salt and ghee or oil make a tastier, more tender bread.

½ teaspoon salt
2 cups (260 g) ata (chapati flour),
or a mixture of equal parts
whole wheat pastry and
unbleached white flours

2 teaspoons melted ghee or oil
Approximately ½ cup (120 ml)
water

1. Mix the salt into the flour. Add the ghee or oil and enough water to make a soft, nonsticky dough.
2. Turn out on a floured board and knead vigorously for 5 to 10 minutes. Alternatively, knead in a food processor for 1 minute.
3. Cover with a damp cloth or inverted bowl to keep the dough from drying out, and allow it to rest for 10 to 30 minutes.

VARIATIONS

For a flaky, rich dough, use a total of 2 to 4 tablespoons melted ghee or butter in Step 1.

For a golden dough, add a little turmeric in Step 1.

For a more tender dough, substitute ¼ cup (60 ml) buttermilk or yogurt for ¼ cup (60 ml) water in Step 1.

 # CHAPATIS

INDIA   *About 16*

The basic bread of India. In wheat-growing Sonora, Mexico, they are served as "wheat tortillas." Keep finished chapatis under a cloth while the rest are cooking to keep them warm and to absorb the steam that would otherwise make them flabby. If desired, brush with ghee before serving.

STEP ONE

Basic Dough for Indian Flatbreads

1. Pinch off pieces of the dough and roll into 1½-inch (3.5 cm) balls.
2. Roll out each ball on a floured board into 4- to 5-inch (10 to 13 cm) round. Try to make each as round as possible. Indian mothers chide their children's first attempts by exclaiming, "You make chapatis that look like a map of India!" The tapered rolling pin designed for chapatis can be manipulated more easily to achieve circular perfection. But don't worry, maps of Iowa taste just as good as those of India— which taste just as good as perfect rounds.
3. *Griddle and Flame Method:* The best method of cooking chapatis is to partially cook them on a griddle, then finish them by placing directly on a heat source, which causes them to puff up like a balloon. Traditionally, they are thrown onto hot coals, which you can certainly do. However, the flame of a gas stove burner works fine. With an electric stove, you'll need some sort of apparatus, like an angel food cake cutting tool, to hold the chapati above the coils. Yamuna Devi in *Lord Krishna's Cuisine* suggests bending a wire coat hanger into a U shape that can be used to hold chapatis over both gas and electric stoves.
   ❖ Place an ungreased tava, skillet, or griddle over high heat. When hot, gently slap a chapati flat onto it and cook just until it looks dry, about 20 seconds. Flip with a spatula and cook the other side for 20 seconds.
   ❖ Remove from the griddle and place directly onto the heat source: glowing charcoals, a gas burner on medium heat, or a rack over a glowing electric burner. After a second or two, flip over and cook the other side for a second or two. If the chapati is fairly round, it should puff up. If less perfectly shaped, it will probably puff in a few places. A finished chapati should look perfectly dry, with a few dark marks on it from the heat source.

Griddle Method: Blessed are the meek, for they shall cook their chapatis without throwing them onto the fiery flames. Cook on each side in an ungreased skillet, tava, or griddle over medium-high heat until they look dry and have a few dark spots on their surfaces, about 30 seconds for each side.

VARIATIONS

Large Individual Chapatis (makes 4 to 6): Roll out 4 to 6 very large chapatis instead of the 1½-inch (3.5 cm) balls. Cook by the griddle method, above. If you have a tava or a flat griddle and a gas stove, tilt the griddle and quickly push an edge of the chapati over the flame for a second to puff up, then pull it back. Continue with all edges. Fold in quarters. Serve 1 per person.

Amaranth Chapatis: Eaten in the Himalayan regions. Substitute 1 cup (130 g) amaranth flour for 1 cup ata or whole wheat pastry flour.

Flavored Chapatis: Add to the flour 2 teaspoons cumin, fennel, or kalonji seeds.

Spinach Chapatis (Palak Chapati): For a bright green, delicately flavored bread, purée 1 cup (90 g) packed chopped spinach leaves in a blender with the water for Basic Dough for Indian Flat Breads. Do not strain out the leaves.

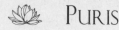

PURIS

INDIA   *About 14*

Puris, light, deep-dried breads that puff up like balloons are served at celebratory occasions and festivals. Perfect puris can be achieved by rolling them out very round and by pressing them with a spatula as described below.

STEP ONE

Basic Dough for Indian Flatbreads
   (p. 350)

STEP TWO

Oil or ghee for deep-frying

1. Roll the dough into 1½-inch (3.5 cm) balls. Roll out into 3-inch to 4-inch (8 to 10 cm) rounds.
2. Heat oil or ghee for deep-frying in a flat-bottomed pot. (Do not try this in a wok—it is the wrong shape.) Have a platter covered with paper towels nearby.
3. Drop the puris, one at a time, into hot oil or ghee. Gently press each one flat to the bottom of the pot with the flat part of a spatula and hold for 1 second, then release. This helps distribute the air evenly throughout the puri so that it will puff evenly. The puri should then rise to the top.
4. Fry until golden on one side, then flip and fry on the other side for a few seconds. Drain on paper towels. The puris should be very tender, and they will lose their "puff." Keep prepared puris warm under a towel until all are cooked. Serve immediately.

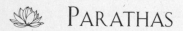

PARATHAS

INDIA   *6 to 8*

For parathas, the dough is folded and rolled out twice, then pan-fried to make a crisp, flaky bread.

STEP ONE

Basic Dough for Indian Flatbreads
   (p. 350)

STEP THREE

Melted ghee

1. Form the dough into six to eight 2-inch (5 cm) balls.
2. Roll out each ball on a floured board into a 7-inch to 8-inch (18 to 20 cm) round.

3. Brush each paratha with ghee. Fold in half. Brush with ghee and fold in half again, forming a somewhat triangular shape. Gently roll out the folded parantha as thin as a chapati or puri.
4. Heat a griddle or skillet over medium heat. Coat with 1 to 2 tablespoons ghee. Add a paratha and cook until browned and crispy on one side. Drizzle with a spoonful of ghee and flip over with a spatula. Drizzle the cooked side with more ghee and cook until lightly browned and crispy all over. Serve immediately.

Stuffed Parathas: Prepare parathas as described in the above recipe, sprinkling a little of the vegetables and pinches of spice and salt on each surface before folding:

Vegetables (choose one):

²/₃ *cup (60 g) finely grated carrots
  or daikon radish*
²/₃ *cup (70 g) finely chopped
  cauliflower or cabbage*

*1 cup (95 g) finely chopped spinach
  or watercress*

Spices (choose one):

*Ground cumin
Garam masala (pp. 565–66)*

*Maharishi Ayur-Veda churna
Salt*

Stuffed Chapatis: Roll out chapatis. Place a spoonful of filling for Samosas (pp. 283–84) on half of each round. Moisten the edges of the dough with yogurt or water, fold the dough in half, and seal the edges thoroughly. Fry on each side in ¼-inch (8 mm) ghee or oil until golden brown and crisp. Drain on paper towels and serve at once with a chutney.

 # TORTILLAS

MEXICO   *1 dozen*

The word *tortilla* is a linguistic mishmash concocted when Spanish *conquistadores* applied their word for flatbread, *torta*, to Aztec corn griddle breads, *tlaxcalli*. Well known today as the basis for tacos, tostadas, and similar Mexican dishes, corn griddle breads are also served in north India, where they are known as *makki ki roti*.

The traditional dough used throughout Central America is *masa*, freshly ground hominy. Sometimes you can find it in Hispanic markets. *Masa harina*, flour made from dry hominy, is more widely available. In the southwestern United States, *blue cornmeal* is often employed to make tortillas. It is moister than masa harina, so less water must be used.

If you have not grown up patting out these breads by hand and cooking them on a heated stone, the dough can prove difficult to work with because it doesn't contain gluten to hold it together. Don't tell the Mexican food police, but you can mix masa harina with an equal amount of ata (chapati flour) or unbleached white flour to produce a nicely flavored and textured half chapati/half tortilla that will not cause you to want to throw the dough on the floor and stomp on it.

A *tortilla press*, which forms the breads by flattening pieces of dough, is a useful tool. The equipment suggested for making Indian flatbreads on pages 349–50 is also helpful for making tortillas.

1½ cups (200 g) masa harina   *½ teaspoon salt* (optional)
½ cup (120 ml) or more hot water

1. Mix the ingredients in a bowl, starting with ½ cup (120 ml) water and adding more, 1 tablespoon at a time, to form a soft, nonsticky dough.
2. Knead on a floured board until smooth, 5 to 10 minutes. Alternatively, knead in a food processor for 1 minute.
3. Cover with a damp cloth or an inverted bowl and allow the dough to rest for 30 minutes.
4. Pinch off a piece of dough and roll into a ball the size of a Ping-Pong ball. Roll out into a thin circle between 2 pieces of waxed paper or plastic wrap.
5. Heat an ungreased heavy skillet over medium-high heat. Gently peel off the waxed paper or plastic wrap, slap the tortilla onto the skillet, and cook until it looks dry and has dark marks in a few spots, 20 to 25 seconds. Flip over and cook on the other side. If there are cracks around the edges, the dough is too stiff. Add more water and divide the dough into 11 more pieces. Roll into balls and continue to roll out and cook tortillas. Stack one on top of the other and cover with a cloth until all are cooked. Serve warm.

VARIATIONS

Add sprinklings of spice to the dough, such as hing, powdered cumin, cracked black pepper, or Maharishi Ayur-Veda churnas.

Tostaditas: The original tortilla chips, thoroughly delicious because they are home-made. Roll out tortillas 2 to 3 inches (5 to 8 cm) in diameter on a floured board. Cut into quarters or eighths to form chips. Allow to dry for 30 minutes. Deep-fry until golden and crispy. Drain on paper towels.

PUPUSAS
(STUFFED CORNMEAL GRIDDLE BREADS)
WITH CURTIDO (SPICED CABBAGE SALAD)

EL SALVADOR   *8 pupusas*

Ceci, the El Salvadoran chef at the Maharishi Ayur-Veda Health Center in Los Angeles, mentioned that she would be preparing a special dish for dinner. At the appointed hour the kitchen was filled with her relatives, all laughing, singing to Spanish songs on the radio, and patting out pupusas. They served them hot off the griddle with spoonfuls of tomato sauce and Curtido (recipe follows), a spicy cole slaw, on the side. A choice of three fillings is given. You could serve the pupusas with a pesto, salsa, or chutney instead of the authentic accompaniments given below.

STEP ONE

2⅓ cups (300 g) masa harina
½ teaspoon salt

Approximately 1⅓ cups (320 ml) water

STEP TWO

Cheese Filling:

1½ cups (250 g) crumbled fresh cheese, such as queso ranchero, panir, farmer's cheese, or grated Monterey Jack cheese

1½ tablespoons minced fresh loroco, basil, or parsley
Salt (optional)

Bean Filling:

2 tablespoons ghee or mild-flavored oil
Pinch of hing (optional)

1½ cups (330 g) mashed well-cooked pinto or kidney beans
Salt

Chicharron "Sausage" Filling:

1 tablespoon ghee or mild-flavored oil
Pinch of hing (optional)
2 teaspoons minced fresh ginger
⅓ cup (40 g) finely chopped fennel or celery

⅓ cup (45 g) finely chopped bell peppers
1 small Roma tomato, chopped
1⅓ cups (175 g) ground seitan
¼ teaspoon black pepper
Salt

To prepare the dough:

1. Combine the masa harina and salt with enough water to form a soft dough. Knead on a masa harina–floured surface until smooth, 5 to 10 minutes. Cover with a damp dish towel and set aside.

To prepare the filling:

2. *For the cheese filling:* Mix the cheese and herbs together. Add salt to taste if needed.
   For the bean filling: Heat the oil in a small skillet. Add the hing and sauté over low heat until fragrant, about 30 seconds. Add the beans and sauté, stirring constantly, for a few minutes, until smooth. Add salt to taste.
   For the chicharron filling: Heat the oil in a skillet. Add the hing and ginger and sauté until fragrant, about 30 seconds. Add the fennel or celery and bell peppers and sauté, stirring frequently, until tender. Stir in the chopped tomato and cook until it becomes mushy, 2 to 3 minutes. Stir in the seitan, pepper, and salt to taste. Cook for 1 minute to blend the flavors.

To assemble and cook:

3. Keep your hands moistened to prevent sticking when working with masa dough. Rinse them frequently. Always keep the dough under a damp towel when not working with it. Divide the dough into 8 pieces and roll each into a smooth ball.

4. Gently make an indentation into a ball to form a small bowl. Place some of the filling into the hollow. Carefully coax the sides of the bowl to enclose the filling, and roll the dough back into a smooth ball. Repeat with all the balls, keeping them under the damp cloth when not forming them.

5. Pat out each ball by slapping between your hands to form a 5-inch (13 cm) circle. Alternatively, you can roll them out on a masa harina–coated board, but it doesn't work as well and isn't half as much fun.

6. Generously coat a griddle or large skillet with ghee or oil and place over medium heat. Cook the pupusas until nicely browned on each side, about 5 minutes for the first side. They will puff up slightly. Serve with tomato sauce and Curtido (following recipe).

 # CURTIDO (SPICED CABBAGE SALAD)

EL SALVADOR   *4 servings*

Here is an East-West version spiced with black pepper and fresh ginger. You can substitute crumbled dried red chilies to heat things up, or reduce the amount of black pepper to cool things down.

1½ cups (160 g) finely shredded cabbage	*1 tablespoon minced fresh ginger*
⅓ cup (30 g) grated carrots	*3 tablespoons lemon juice*
⅓ cup (40 g) grated daikon radish or garden radishes	*3 tablespoons water*
	¼ teaspoon black pepper
	Salt

Mix all the ingredients together, adding salt to taste.

SOCCA (CHICKPEA FLOUR CRACKERS)

FRANCE/ITALY   *About 24 crackers*

Socca's ancestor is dried pieces of *pulmentum*, a staple of the Roman legions. It is now enjoyed by legions as street food on the French and Italian Rivieras. If you replace the olive oil with ghee or mild-flavored oil and throw a sprinkling of kalonji or cumin seeds into the batter, you'll have something that could pass as street food in Bombay. Besan is available in Indian markets.

STEP TWO

1½ cups (360 ml) water   *½ teaspoon salt*
1½ cups (180 g) besan (chickpea flour)

STEP FOUR

1 tablespoon olive oil

STEP FIVE

Olive oil for frying

1. Preheat the oven to 350°F (180°C). Butter a 9 × 13-inch (23 × 33 cm) baking pan.
2. Combine the water, besan, and salt in a blender or food processor until smooth.
3. Pour the batter into a saucepan and cook over low heat, stirring constantly with a whisk, until it is thickened but still pourable. If lumps form, blend again until smooth.
4. Pour the batter into the baking pan and spread evenly. Sprinkle the olive oil over it and gently spread evenly over the batter with the back of a spoon. Bake until golden brown and somewhat cracked, about 30 minutes. Let cool to room temperature.
5. Heat the olive oil ⅛-inch (3 mm) deep in a skillet. Have a platter covered with paper towels nearby.
6. Cut the socca into 2-inch (5 cm) squares. Fry on both sides until golden brown. Drain.

WHEAT GERM STICKS

2 dozen

STEP TWO

1 cup (140 g) unbleached white flour   *½ cup (40 g) grated dried*
1 cup (150 g) whole wheat flour   *unsweetened coconut*
1 cup (120 g) wheat germ   *1 teaspoon salt*
¼ cup (35 g) sesame seeds   *¼ cup (50 g) raw or packed*
                                brown sugar

STEP THREE

½ cup (120 ml) ghee or oil   *1 cup (240 ml) yogurt*

1. Preheat the oven to 350°F (180°C). Butter a baking sheet.
2. Mix the dry ingredients together.
3. Add the ghee or oil and the yogurt. Mix to form a soft dough.
4. Roll out on a floured board ½-inch (1.3 cm) thick. Slice into sticks ½-inch (1.3 cm) wide and about 4 inches (10 cm) long.
5. Place the sticks on the baking sheet. Bake until golden, 30 to 35 minutes.

VARIATION
   ✹ Replace the yogurt with nondairy milk, stock, or water.

QUICK BREADS

In general, quick breads emphasize the sweet taste and are balancing for Vata and Pitta. In some cases they also feature the sour taste of citrus ingredients, making them especially balancing for Vata. They are less balancing for Kapha, but quick breads contain less oil than cakes, and some feature Kapha-balancing ingredients such as cornmeal, cranberries, and apples. Eggless quick bread batters are usually quite thick, so don't worry if you're expecting a soupier mixture.

   ❖ Quick breads fall apart when sliced fresh from the oven. Give them plenty of time to cool.
   ❖ To make quick breads even quicker, prepare in a food processor. Be careful not to overmix. Stir in by hand only the ingredients you don't want chopped up, such as nuts and raisins.
   ❖ Quick breads are done when they shrink slightly from the sides of the pan, the top is lightly browned, and a toothpick inserted into the middle comes out dry.

QUICK BREAD MUFFINS AND CUPCAKES

Place quick bread batter in buttered muffin cups and bake in a 375°F (190°C) oven for 25 to 30 minutes. Test for doneness using a toothpick.

APPLESAUCE BREAD

One 9 × 5 × 3–inch (23 × 13 × 7.5 cm) loaf

STEP TWO

¼ cup (55 g) ghee or butter
1⅓ cups (280 g) raw or packed
  brown sugar

STEP THREE

1¼ cups (210 g) unbleached
  white flour
¾ cup (115 g) whole wheat flour
2 tablespoons arrowroot or
  cornstarch

1 tablespoon baking powder
½ teaspoon salt
1½ teaspoons ground cinnamon
¼ teaspoon ground cloves

STEP FOUR

1½ cups (335 g) puréed steamed
  apples or unsweetened
  applesauce

½ cup (65 g) raisins
½ cup (60 g) chopped nuts

1. Preheat the oven to 350°F (180°C). Butter and lightly flour 9 × 5 × 3–inch (23 × 13 × 7.5 cm) loaf pan.
2. Cream the ghee or butter and the sugar.
3. Mix the dry ingredients together and add to the creamed mixture.
4. Add the apples and mix just until all the ingredients are blended. Stir in the raisins and nuts.
5. Spoon the mixture into the loaf pan and spread evenly. Bake about 1 hour.

VARIATION

  Persimmon Bread: Replace the apples with 1½ cups (360 g) puréed peeled persimmon pulp(!) from fully ripe hachiya persimmons. Replace the baking powder with 1 teaspoon baking power and 1 teaspoon baking soda.

BANANA-APRICOT BREAD

One 9 × 5 × 3–inch (23 × 13 × 7.5 cm) loaf

Soak hard unsulphured apricots in hot water to soften and drain well before using.

STEP TWO

¼ cup (55 g) ghee or butter
1½ (310 g) cups raw or packed
  brown sugar

STEP THREE

1½ cups (210 g) *unbleached*
    white flour
¾ cup (115 g) *whole wheat flour*
2 tablespoons *arrowroot or*
    cornstarch

2 teaspoons *baking powder*
½ teaspoon *baking soda*
½ teaspoon *salt*
1½ teaspoons *ground cinnamon*

STEP FOUR

2 cups (480 g) *mashed ripe*
bananas

½ cup (60 g) *chopped dried apricots*
¾ cup (90 g) *chopped nuts*

1. Preheat the oven to 350°F (180°C). Butter and lightly flour a 9 × 5 × 3–inch (23 × 13 × 7.5 cm) loaf pan.
2. Cream the ghee or butter and the sugar.
3. Mix the dry ingredients together and add to the creamed mixture.
4. Add the mashed bananas and mix just until blended. Stir in the dried apricots and nuts.
5. Spoon the mixture into the buttered loaf pan and spread evenly. Bake about 1 hour.

 # CORNBREAD

One 9-inch (23 cm) square pan

The Flour of Mayz, mix'd with that of Wheat, makes excellent Bread, sweeter, and more agreeable than that of Wheat alone.   —BENJAMIN FRANKLIN

American colonists first incorporated New World cornmeal into their Old World breads. Try the variations separately, or put them all together in one go-for-broke batter.

STEP TWO

1½ cups (210 g) *unbleached*
    white flour
1½ cups (195 g) *cornmeal*
2 teaspoons *baking powder*
½ teaspoon *baking soda*

2 tablespoons *arrowroot or*
    cornstarch
⅓ cup (70 g) *raw or packed*
    brown sugar
1 teaspoon *salt*

STEP THREE

⅓ cup (80 ml) *melted ghee or oil*
1 cup (240 ml) *buttermilk*

1 cup (240 ml) *water*

1. Preheat the oven to 400°F (200°C). Butter a 9-inch (23 cm) square baking pan. For crusty cornbread, place in the oven to heat.

2. Mix the dry ingredients together.
3. Add the melted ghee or oil, buttermilk, and water. Mix just until blended.
4. Pour into the pan. Bake until golden, 25 to 30 minutes. Unlike other quick breads, cornbread can be eaten as soon as it is baked—hot and crumbly is heavenly.

VARIATIONS

Reduce the sugar to 3 tablespoons and add chopped jalapeño chilies, chopped bell peppers, and/or sliced dried tomatoes to the batter.

Add chopped green herbs, such as sage, cilantro, or dill, to the batter.

Add fresh corn kernels to the batter.

 # CRANBERRY-ORANGE NUT BREAD

One 9 × 5 × 3–inch (23 × 13 × 7.5 cm) loaf

Cranberries are somewhat elusive when you attempt to chop them with a knife, so use a food processor or place them in a blender in 3 batches and blend for 1 or 2 seconds. The necessary amount of liquid seems to vary from batch to batch—probably dependent on the amount of moisture in the cranberries. Mix in all the liquid thoroughly before deciding to add more orange juice if the batter appears to be too dry.

STEP TWO

¼ *cup (55 g) ghee or butter*
1⅓ *(280 g) cups raw or packed*
  dark brown sugar

STEP THREE

1½ *cups (210 g) unbleached*   1½ *teaspoons baking powder*
  white flour   ½ *teaspoon baking soda*
¾ *cup (115 g) whole wheat flour*   ¾ *teaspoon salt*
2 *tablespoons arrowroot or*
  cornstarch

STEP FOUR

1 *tablespoon finely grated*   2½ *cups (280 g) chopped cranberries*
  orange zest   ¾ *cup (75 g) chopped walnuts*
½ *cup (120 ml) orange juice (or more)*

1. Preheat the oven to 350°F (180°C). Butter and lightly flour a 9 × 5 × 3–inch (23 × 13 × 7.5 cm) loaf pan.
2. Cream the butter and sugar.
3. Mix the dry ingredients together and add to the creamed mixture.

4. Add the orange zest, orange juice, and cranberries, and mix just until all the ingredients are blended. Mix in the nuts.
5. Spoon into the loaf pan and spread evenly. Bake for about 1 hour.

 # DATE-PISTACHIO BREAD

One 9 × 5 × 3–inch (23 × 13 × 7.5 cm) loaf

Before you slice dates for baked goods, dust with a little flour to help keep the knife from sticking.

STEP TWO

¼ cup (55 g) ghee or butter
1¼ cups (260 g) raw or packed
  brown sugar

STEP THREE

1½ cups (210 g) unbleached   *½ teaspoon salt*
  white flour   *1½ teaspoons ground cardamom*
¾ cup (115 g) whole wheat flour   *2 teaspoons baking powder*
2 tablespoons arrowroot   *½ teaspoon baking soda*
  or cornstarch

STEP FOUR

½ cup (120 ml) buttermilk   *1 cup (285 g) chopped pitted dates*
½ cup (120 ml) water   *1 cup (115 g) chopped pistachios*

1. Preheat the oven to 350°F (180°C). Butter and lightly flour a 9 × 5 × 3–inch (23 × 13 × 7.5 cm) loaf pan.
2. Cream the butter and sugar.
3. Mix the dry ingredients together and add to the creamed mixture.
4. Add the buttermilk and water, and mix just until all the ingredients are blended. Mix in the dates and nuts.
5. Spoon into the loaf pan and spread evenly. Bake for about 1 hour.

 # PUMPKIN BREAD

One 9 × 5 × 3–inch (23 × 13 × 7.5 cm) loaf

A moist, golden autumn loaf that can be made with any type of winter squash or with sweet potatoes. You may need to add a little more liquid when using a drier squash such as kabocha.

STEP TWO

¼ cup (55 g) ghee or butter
1½ cups (310 g) raw or packed
   brown sugar

STEP THREE

1½ cups (210 g) unbleached
   white flour
¾ cup (115 g) whole wheat flour
2 tablespoons arrowroot or
   cornstarch
¼ teaspoon salt

1½ teaspoons baking powder
1 teaspoon baking soda
1 teaspoon ground cinnamon
¼ teaspoon ground cardamom
¼ teaspoon ground cloves
¼ teaspoon ground ginger

STEP FOUR

2 tablespoons water
1¾ cups (400 g) puréed cooked
   pumpkin or other winter squash

⅓ cup (55 g) chopped crystallized
   ginger (optional)

1. Preheat the oven to 350°F (180°C). Butter and lightly flour a 9- × 5- × 3-inch (23 × 13 × 7.5 cm) loaf pan.
2. Cream the ghee or butter and the sugar.
3. Mix the dry ingredients together and add to the creamed mixture.
4. Add the water and pumpkin and mix just until all the ingredients are blended. Stir in the crystallized ginger.
5. Spoon into the loaf pan and spread evenly. Bake for about 1 hour.

 # SAFFRON-LEMON-ALMOND BREAD

One 9 × 5 × 3–inch (23 × 13 × 7.5 cm) loaf

Saffron was brought to Europe from Asia by the Phoenicians. Murals in the Cretan palace of Knossos show people harvesting saffron crocuses, and the saffron color came to signify royalty in Greece.

STEP TWO

¼ teaspoon loosely packed
   saffron threads

¼ cup (60 ml) hot water

STEP THREE

¼ cup (55 g) ghee or butter
1 cup (210 g) sugar
1 cup (240 ml) sour cream

1 tablespoon finely grated
   lemon zest
¼ cup (60 ml) lemon juice

STEP FOUR

2½ cups (350 g) unbleached
   white flour
2 tablespoons arrowroot or
   cornstarch
2 teaspoons baking powder

½ teaspoon baking soda
1 teaspoon salt
1 cup (140 g) sliced almonds,
   toasted

1. Preheat the oven to 350°F (180°C). Butter and lightly flour a 9 × 5 × 3–inch (23 × 13 × 7.5 cm) loaf pan.
2. Crumble the saffron threads with your fingers into a small cup. Pour the hot water over them, stir, and set aside for a few minutes.
3. Cream the ghee or butter and sugar. Beat in the sour cream, lemon zest, and lemon juice until smooth. Add the saffron water.
4. Mix the flour, arrowroot or cornstarch, baking powder, soda, and salt together and add to the moist ingredients. Mix just until all the ingredients are blended. Mix in the almonds.
5. Spoon the batter into the loaf pan and spread evenly. Bake for about 1 hour.

VARIATION

Even without the saffron, this is a nice tea loaf. I have prepared it with pecans, replaced the sugar with brown sugar, and omitted the saffron.

❀ Zucchini Bread

One 9 × 5 × 3–inch (23 × 13 × 7.5 cm) loaf

STEP TWO

2 cups (210 g) drained grated
   zucchini
¼ cup (55 g) melted ghee or butter

1¼ cups (260 g) raw or
   packed brown sugar

STEP THREE

1¼ cups (175 g) unbleached
   white flour
1 cup (150 g) whole wheat flour
2 tablespoons arrowroot or
   cornstarch
½ teaspoon salt
2 teaspoons baking powder

½ teaspoon baking soda
1 teaspoon ground cinnamon
¼ cup (60 ml) buttermilk
¾ cup raisins (95 g) or chopped
   dates (215 g)
1 cup (95 g) coarsely chopped
   pecans

1. Preheat the oven to 350°F (180°C). Butter and lightly flour a 9 × 5 × 3–inch (23 × 13 × 7.5 cm) loaf pan.

2. Mix the zucchini, ghee or butter, and sugar.
3. Mix the dry ingredients together and add to the zucchini mixture. Add the buttermilk and mix just until all the ingredients are blended. Stir in the raisins or dates and the nuts.
4. Spoon into the baking pan and spread evenly. Bake for about 1 hour.

BISCUITS

❖ For the most tender biscuits, handle the dough as little as possible to keep the gluten from developing.
❖ For the flakiest biscuits, use cold butter and do not blend it thoroughly into the flour but allow it to remain in tiny pieces. Have the dough cold and the oven very hot, and the separation of butter and flour will cause the dough to flake in the same manner as pie crust.
❖ Biscuits become hard if they sit around too long. For best results, serve them forth hot from the oven, and cast old biscuits upon the waters.

Strange to see how a good dinner and feasting reconciles everyone.

—SAMUEL PEPYS

 ## BISCUITS

1 dozen

This recipe produces a full-flavored whole grain biscuit. If your tastes run way down upon the Swanee River to more traditional southern fare, substitute unbleached white flour for the whole wheat flour.

STEP TWO

1¼ cups (175 g) unbleached white flour	2 teaspoons baking powder
¾ cup (115 g) whole wheat flour	1 teaspoon baking soda
½ teaspoon salt	2 teaspoons sugar (optional)

STEP THREE

⅓ cup (75 g) butter

STEP FOUR

⅓ cup (80 ml) buttermilk   ⅓ cup (80 ml) water

1. Preheat the oven to 450°F (230°C). Butter a baking sheet.
2. Mix the dry ingredients together.

3. Add the butter and work in with your fingers or a pastry cutter until the mixture resembles coarse meal.

4. Mix in the buttermilk and water. Knead a few times to make a smooth dough.

5. Roll out ½-inch (1.3 cm) thick on a floured board. Cut out biscuits with the rim of a glass or a cookie cutter.

6. Place on the baking sheet and bake until golden brown, 8 to 10 minutes. Serve hot.

VARIATIONS

Replace ¼ cup (40 g) of the whole wheat flour with ¼ cup (30 g) wheat germ, cornmeal, barley flour, or rye flour.

❁ Replace the buttermilk with nondairy milk mixed with 1 tablespoon lemon juice.

Seeded Biscuits: Add 1½ teaspoons caraway, fennel, or poppy seeds in Step 4.

Drop Biscuits: Drop biscuits look less elegant but are lighter than rolled biscuits. Add ⅓ cup (80 ml) more buttermilk in Step 4. Drop spoonfuls of batter onto the baking sheet.

Skillet Biscuits: Instead of baking, cook over low heat in an ungreased skillet until browned, at least 5 minutes on each side.

Benne Seed Biscuits: In South Carolina *benne* (sesame) seeds were believed to bring good luck. Stir in ⅓ cup (45 g) toasted sesame seeds with the liquids in Step 4, and expect good things to happen.

Herb Biscuits: Add 1½ teaspoons dried herbs (such as basil, thyme, sage, or rosemary) or 2 tablespoons minced fresh herbs in Step 4. Replace the salt with seasoned salt.

Bell Pepper Biscuits: Red peppers look especially beautiful, or you could do a confetti mixture of red, yellow, and green peppers. Sauté ½ cup (70 g) chopped peeled bell peppers in 1 teaspoon ghee or butter over low heat until almost tender, about 5 minutes. For added flavor, add a pinch of hing and 1½ teaspoons cumin or fennel seeds while sautéing. Allow to cool to room temperature. Add to the biscuit dough between Steps 3 and 4.

Feta Cheese Biscuits (Biscotákia Me Feta): Common breakfast fare in Greece. Add ½ cup (100 g) crumbled feta cheese with the butter in Step 3. Replace the liquids with ¾ cup (180 ml) buttermilk. Serve warm.

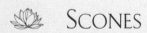

SCONES

BRITISH ISLES   *18 scones*

Here is a rendition of Richard Swinehart's rendition of the classic teatime favorite. He prefers to use all pastry flour, which can be found unbleached. Serve warm with butter.

STEP TWO

3 cups (420 g) unbleached
 white flour
2½ teaspoons baking powder
¾ teaspoon baking soda

¾ teaspoon salt
⅓ cup (70 g) sugar
6 tablespoons (85 g) butter

STEP THREE

½ cup (65 g) currants or raisins
1 teaspoon finely grated orange
 zest (optional)

½ cup (120 ml) buttermilk or
 yogurt
½ cup (120 ml) water

1. Preheat the oven to 400°F (200°C). Butter a baking sheet.
2. Mix the dry ingredients together. Cut the butter into small pieces and work in with your fingers or a pastry cutter until the mixture resembles coarse meal.
3. Add the currants or raisins and orange zest if desired. Add the buttermilk or yogurt and the water and mix to form a soft dough.
4. Roll out ½-inch (1.3 cm) thick and cut out rounds with a cookie cutter or the rim of a glass. Place on the baking sheet.
5. Bake until nicely browned, 15 to 20 minutes.

VARIATIONS

For wedge-shaped scones, divide the dough into 2 balls and roll out into 8-inch (20 cm) rounds. Slice like pies into 6 wedges each, place separately on a baking sheet, and bake.

❂ Replace the buttermilk or yogurt with nondairy milk mixed with ½ tablespoon lemon juice.

 # WELSH CAKES

WALES   *12 individual cakes*

Little buttery skillet cakes that are served in Wales for dessert. I tested the recipe out on two fiery Welsh brothers who were members of my kitchen staff in Switzerland. These two gruff souls suddenly became misty-eyed and dreamy, muttering, "Perfect! Just like Mom's." A higher compliment I have never received.

STEP ONE

½ cup (115 g) unsalted butter

1 cup (210 g) sugar

STEP TWO

2 cups (280 g) unbleached
 white flour
¾ teaspoon baking powder

¼ teaspoon baking soda
½ teaspoon salt
½ teaspoon ground nutmeg

½ cup (65 g) currants or raisins
½ to ⅔ cup (120 to 160 ml)
   buttermilk

1. Cream the butter and sugar thoroughly.
2. Mix the dry ingredients together and sift into the creamed mixture.
3. Add the currants or raisins and enough buttermilk to make a fairly firm dough like biscuit dough.
4. Roll out ⅓-inch (1 cm) thick on a floured board. Cut out rounds with the rim of a glass or a cookie cutter.
5. Cook the cakes over low heat on an ungreased griddle or skillet until golden brown, about 5 minutes on each side.

MUFFINS

Charles Dickens's character Ralph Nickleby, uncle of Nicholas, saw the future and it was "The United Metropolitan Improved Hot Muffin Baking and Punctual Delivery Company." His marketing instinct certainly ran true—muffins can be prepared in a snap, and everybody loves them.

The Seven Pillars of Eggless Muffin Wisdom

   I. Have the oven heated and the muffin tins buttered and ready to go before preparing the batter.
  II. Place the dry ingredients in a bowl, add the wet ones, and stir just until the dry ingredients are moistened, about 15 strokes. It's all right if there are lumps remaining. Mix the batter quickly and with a light touch to avoid developing the gluten in the flour.
 III. Immediately after the batter is mixed, pour into the muffin cups. It's all right to fill the batter up to the brim of the cups in these recipes.
  IV. There is no need to use paper muffin cups—they pull off some of the crust, and if the tin is well buttered or made of nonstick material, the muffins will come out easily.
   V. Place in the hot oven immediately after pouring, and bake just until golden brown.
  VI. Remove muffins from the tin a few minutes after removing from the oven.
 VII. Eggless muffins become leaden and clunky if they sit too long, so it is best to bake them just before serving.

UNIVERSAL MUFFINS

1 dozen

A basic recipe intended to be altered to create your own original muffins.

STEP TWO

1 cup (150 g) whole wheat flour
1 cup (140 g) unbleached
  white flour
1 teaspoon baking powder

¾ teaspoon baking soda
¾ teaspoon salt
⅓ cup (70 g) sugar

STEP THREE

¾ cup (180 ml) buttermilk
¾ cup (180 ml) water

¼ cup (60 ml) melted ghee,
  butter, or oil

1. Preheat the oven to 400°F (200°C). Butter 12 muffin cups.
2. Mix the dry ingredients together.
3. Mix the buttermilk, water, and oil. Pour over the dry ingredients. Beat until just barely mixed, about 15 strokes.
4. Pour the batter into the muffin cups. Bake until nicely browned, about 20 minutes.

VARIATIONS

Date-Nut Muffins: Add ⅔ cup (120 g) chopped dates and ½ cup (50 g) chopped walnuts or pecans in Step 3. (Yields 1 to 2 additional muffins.)

Orange Muffins: Add 1 tablespoon finely grated orange zest and replace the water with orange juice in Step 3.

Spice Muffins: In Step 2, add ½ teaspoon each: ground cinnamon, ground allspice, and ground ginger; ¼ teaspoon each: ground nutmeg and ground cloves.

Banana or Pumpkin Muffins: Add 1 cup (235 g) puréed ripe bananas or puréed cooked pumpkin in Step 3. Reduce the buttermilk (but not the water) to ½ cup.

❖ Replace no more than ½ cup (70 g) wheat flour with nonwheat flours such as barley, buckwheat, cornmeal, or bran.

❖ Replace buttermilk or sour milk with nondairy milk or fruit juice mixed with 2 tablespoons lemon juice.

❖ Add 1 cup (100 g) drained grated carrot, zucchini, apple; reduce the buttermilk to ½ cup (120 ml).

BLUEBERRY, BLACKBERRY, OR CRANBERRY MUFFINS

14 to 16 muffins

All one's muffin desires fulfilled. The batter is just a medium for the berries.

2 cups (280 g) *unbleached*
  white flour
1 teaspoon *baking powder*
¾ teaspoon *baking soda*

STEP TWO

¾ teaspoon *salt*
½ cup (100 g) *raw or packed brown*
  sugar

¾ cup (180 ml) *buttermilk*
¾ cup (180 ml) *water*
¼ cup (60 ml) *melted ghee, butter,*
  or oil

STEP THREE

1¼ cups (175 g) *blueberries or*
  blackberries or 1 cup (115 g)
  chopped cranberries

1. Preheat the oven to 400°F (200°C). Butter 14 to 16 muffin cups.
2. Mix the dry ingredients together.
3. Mix the buttermilk, water, and oil and add to the dry ingredients. Add the berries. Beat until just barely mixed, about 15 strokes.
4. Pour into the muffin cups. Bake until nicely browned, about 20 minutes.

BRAN MUFFINS

1 dozen

1 cup (90 g) *wheat bran*
1 cup (140 g) *unbleached*
  white flour
½ cup (100 g) *raw or packed*
  brown sugar

STEP TWO

1 teaspoon *baking powder*
¾ teaspoon *baking soda*
¾ teaspoon *salt*

¾ cup (180 ml) *buttermilk*
½ cup (120 ml) *water*

STEP THREE

¼ cup (60 ml) *melted ghee,*
  butter, or oil
½ cup (65 g) *raisins*

1. Preheat the oven to 400°F (200°C). Butter 12 muffin cups.
2. Mix all the dry ingredients together.

3. Mix the buttermilk, water, and oil and add to the dry mixture. Add the raisins. Beat until just barely mixed, about 15 strokes.
4. Pour into buttered muffin cups and bake until nicely browned, about 20 minutes.

 # CEREAL OR GRAIN MUFFINS

1 dozen

These muffins have an unusual texture—crunchy on the outside and moist and chewy within. This will vary from batch to batch, depending on the moisture in the cooked grains. The recipe works best with flaked cereals and with grains that are somewhat mushy when cooked. Try rolled oats, broken-up wild rice, or bulgar—divine! Avoid whole grain berries, such as wheat berries and rye berries. Be sure to eat them warm.

STEP TWO

1 cup (235 ml) cooked cereal or grains
1 cup (240 ml) buttermilk

¼ cup (60 ml) melted ghee, butter, or oil

STEP THREE

1½ cups (210 g) unbleached white flour
¾ teaspoon salt
1 teaspoon baking powder

1 teaspoon baking soda
⅓ cup (70 g) raw or packed brown sugar

1. Preheat the oven to 400°F (200°C). Butter 12 muffin cups.
2. Mix the cereal with the buttermilk and oil.
3. Mix the dry ingredients together and add to the wet ingredients. Beat until just barely mixed, about 15 strokes.
4. Pour into muffin cups and bake until nicely browned, about 20 minutes.

VARIATION

Savory Grain or Cereal Muffins: Reduce the sugar to a total of 2 tablespoons. Add any or all of the following: ¼ cup (60 ml) finely chopped fresh herbs, such as cilantro, dill, or flat-leaf parsley; ½ cup (60 g) coarsely chopped nuts; 1 to 2 teaspoons curry powder or Maharishi Ayur-Veda churna; up to ½ cup (40 g) sliced dried tomatoes.

Tell me what you eat, and I will tell you what you are.　　—BRILLAT-SAVARIN

CILANTRO-PUMPKIN SEED CORN MUFFINS

1 dozen

European colonists applied European baking techniques to New World cornmeal to create a whole genre of baked goods such as hushpuppies, corn dodgers, and corn muffins. This recipe features other New World ingredients as well. You could use pine nuts instead of pumpkin seeds and vary the color of cornmeal for different results.

STEP ONE

¼ cup (60 ml) melted ghee, butter, or oil
Pinch of hing (optional)

1½ teaspoons cumin seeds, toasted
½ cup (70 g) pumpkin seeds

STEP TWO

1 cup (130 g) cornmeal
¾ cup (180 ml) buttermilk
¾ cup (180 ml) water

¼ cup (50 g) raw or packed brown sugar

STEP THREE

1 cup (140 g) unbleached white flour
1 teaspoon baking powder

¾ teaspoon baking soda
¾ teaspoon salt
¼ cup (60 ml) minced fresh cilantro

1. Heat the ghee, butter, or oil in a skillet. Add the hing, cumin seeds, and pumpkin seeds and sauté over low heat until the pumpkin seeds puff up a little. Place in a mixing bowl and let cool for a few minutes to room temperature.
2. Preheat the oven to 400°F (200°C). Butter 12 muffin cups.
3. Add the cornmeal, buttermilk, water, and sugar to the cooled oil mixture.
4. Mix the dry ingredients together. Add to the cornmeal mixture. Add the cilantro. Beat until just barely mixed, about 15 strokes.
5. Pour into buttered muffin cups. Bake until nicely browned, about 20 minutes.

VARIATIONS
  Add chopped bell peppers or mild chilies.
  Add up to ½ cup (40 g) sliced dried tomatoes.
  Add ⅔ cup (100 g) fresh corn kernels.

PANCAKES

The Art of tossing a Pancake: This is a Thing very easy to a bold Hand, but which a timorous Person will never be able to do well; for such a one, she is to know that the first Thing to be done is to get rid of her Fear, and then a little Practice will make it quite familiar.

—Mrs. Martha Bradley, a British housewife (circa 1770)

A classic American breakfast, pancakes also make a nice Ayurvedic supper.

Six Habits of Highly Effective Eggless Pancakes

1. For best results, prepare pancake batter, minus the leavening, at least an hour in advance (or the night before) and let it sit in the refrigerator. This allows the flour to swell so the pancakes hold together better. Beat in the baking powder and soda before cooking.
2. Use a heavy skillet or a griddle. A well-seasoned cast-iron or a soapstone surface is ideal, and nonstick cookware also works well.
3. Very little oil is needed to cook pancakes. Ghee or oil work well, but if your cooking surface isn't well seasoned, such as a stainless-steel surface, butter stands the least chance of causing pancakes to stick. (However, it also stands the most chance of burning.)
4. The pan should be hot enough that a drop of water flicked on it sputters and dances. If the water evaporates immediately, the pan is too hot, and if it just sits there, it is too cold.
5. Pour the batter onto the skillet to form small circles. A 3-inch (8 cm) circle is manageable for flipping. When bubbles form all over the surface, the pancake is ready to be turned over. Check to see that it is golden brown and not too pale. Flip with a spatula or by quickly shaking the pan with the "bold Hand" of the *British Housewife*. The second side will cook in half the time. The first batch may stick to the pan a little, but the succeeding batches will not. Add more butter to the pan as necessary.
6. Do not stack the finished pancakes until they are brought to the table—the steam they produce will make them soggy.

 # UNIVERSAL PANCAKES

20 to 24 pancakes

This batter makes great basic pancakes and can also serve as a foil for different additions to take on multiple personalities.

1 cup (150 g) whole wheat flour
1 cup (140 g) unbleached white flour
2 tablespoons arrowroot or cornstarch
½ teaspoon salt

1½ teaspoons baking powder
¼ teaspoon baking soda
2 tablespoons melted ghee, butter, or oil
1 cup (240 ml) buttermilk
1 cup (240 ml) water

1. Blend all the ingredients in a blender or food processor or beat together well. For best results, omit the baking powder and soda and allow to stand in the refrigerator for at least 1 hour. (You can prepare the batter the night before if desired.) Beat in the leavenings just before cooking.
2. Cook according to the directions for pancakes on page 373.

VARIATIONS

Fruit Pancakes: Add 2 cups (480 ml) thinly sliced ripe fruit, drained, or 1½ cups (360 ml) berries just before cooking.

Vegetable Pancakes: For a main dish, add 2 cups (480 ml) minced or shredded vegetables just before cooking. If desired, blend in a blender or food processor for 1 second just to ensure that the vegetables are fine enough. Do not purée. Cook small pancakes and serve with sour cream, a pesto, a mock mayonnaise, or other sauces.

Buckwheat Pancakes: Popular American breakfast food in the nineteenth century that adds a Kapha-balancing ingredient. Replace the whole wheat flour with 1 cup (130 g) buckwheat flour.

Two dozen dainty flapjacks of buckwheat covered with a pitcher of honey and treacle and soaked by a hogshead of butter!
—WASHINGTON IRVING'S IDEA OF A HEAVENLY BREAKFAST

Create a plethora of pancakes by stirring any of the additions listed for muffins on page 369 into the batter just before cooking. The standard American pancake topping is a pat of butter and a healthy drizzle of syrup. Europeans more readily anoint theirs with jam, fresh fruit, and whipped cream. Try some of the following for a change of pace:

A fruit sauce or Dried Fruit Purée (p. 462)
Rice, barley malt, or sorghum syrup
Flavored butters or ghee
Crème Fraîche (p. 535), Hung Yogurt (p. 534), sour cream
Ricotta cheese, mascarpone, Panir Mayonnaise (p. 503)

WILD RICE-PECAN PANCAKES

18 pancakes

Serve with either sweet accompaniments, or as an elegant savory side dish with sour cream, salsa, pesto, or chutney.

STEP ONE

⅓ cup (60 g) wild rice	*1 to 1¼ (240 to 300 ml) cups water*

STEP TWO

¾ cup (110 g) unbleached white flour	*½ teaspoon salt*
	2 teaspoons baking powder
⅓ cup (50 g) whole wheat flour	*1 teaspoon baking soda*
2 tablespoons arrowroot	

STEP THREE

2 tablespoons melted ghee, butter, or oil	*¾ cup (180 ml) water*
	⅓ cup (30 g) finely chopped pecans
¾ cup (180 ml) buttermilk	

1. Bring the wild rice to a boil in 1 cup water. Cover, reduce the heat, and simmer until the water is absorbed and the rice is tender, about 50 minutes. If too chewy, add ¼ cup more water and simmer until tender.
2. Mix the dry ingredients together.
3. Add the oil, buttermilk and water and mix until smooth. Stir in the wild rice and the nuts.
4. Cook small pancakes according to the directions on page 373.

VALENTINE'S DAY BRUNCH

Avocado Soup (p. 231)
Wild Rice–Pecan Pancakes topped with crème fraîche and chopped fresh herbs
Wilted Greek Salad with Caramelized Walnuts (pp. 300–301)
Butter Cookies in heart shapes (pp. 430–31)

 # CRÊPES

FRANCE   *7 to 12 crêpes*

Crêpe, from the word meaning "crisp," is simply the French word for pancake. Today the word is associated with delicate, thin pancakes that are often elegantly wrapped around vegetable or dessert fillings.

2½ cups (600 ml) nondairy milk
1¾ cups (245 g) unbleached
   white flour
½ teaspoon salt

2 tablespoons arrowroot or
   cornstarch
2 tablespoons melted ghee, butter,
   or oil

1. Blend the ingredients in a blender or food processor. Allow the mixture to stand for at least 1 hour. Add more milk if the batter is too thick.
2. Place an 8-inch (22 cm) crêpe pan or skillet on medium-high heat. Lightly coat with butter. Pour a little batter into the center of the pan. Immediately lift the pan and swirl it around to distribute the batter over the bottom in a thin layer. Replace the pan on the heat.
3. After 30 seconds, gently check the bottom of the crêpe (the top will not form bubbles). When golden brown, carefully flip with a spatula and cook until the other side is golden brown.

THE CRÊPE UNIVERSE

❖ *Vegetable-Filled Crêpes:* Vegetable crêpes make light entrées that look very elegant. For a summer luncheon, serve vegetable-filled crêpes with a salad and a cold soup. You can also serve tiny individual crêpes for appetizers. Wrap crêpes around cooked mixtures of thinly sliced vegetables, such as:

> Curried vegetables
> Creamed vegetables
> Ratatouille Caviar (see pp. 204–205)
> Roasted Peppers (pp. 116–17)
> Zucchini in Sour Cream with Fennel and Dill (pp. 131–32)

If desired, add to the filling, or top with:

> Ricotta cheese, sour cream, chèvre, mascarpone, or other creamy cheeses
> Panir
> One of the mock mayonnaises
> A pesto
> Red Pepper Purée (p. 513)

❖ *Crêpe Cake:* Instead of rolling crêpes in the traditional manner, pile them in layers with vegetable fillings, soft cheeses, and anything else you wish to form a cake. Crêpes should be of a uniform size. If they are not, trim the larger crêpes to match the smaller ones. For best results, use firm fillings. Vegetables should be well chopped or thinly sliced—not in large chunks. Use a very sharp knife to slice the cake. Serve cut into wedges like a cake.

❖ *Dessert Crêpes:* Dessert crêpes' patrician appearance belies their essential simplicity. You can, of course, go to great lengths to embellish them; for instance, you can wrap crêpes around ice cream and top with Caramel Sauce, whipped cream, and chopped nuts, as a sort of crêpe ice cream sundae. On the other hand, a more innocent presentation, such as a filling of fresh, ripe berries and a sprinkling of confectioner's sugar over the rolled-up crêpes, is also elegant without being overly time-consuming to prepare. Fill and/or top with:

> Fresh berries, sliced peaches, mangoes, bananas, apricots, or other soft, juicy fruits
> Fruit sauces
> Ice cream
> Ricotta cheese, mascarpone, Hung Yogurt (p. 534), or sour cream
> Whipped cream, crème fraîche, or Tofu Dessert Cream (p. 503)

❖ *Swedish Pancake Cake (Pannkakstårta):* In Sweden this cake would be prepared with lingonberry jam. Prepare crêpes. Spread a layer of jam or thick fruit sauce on each crêpe. Follow with a layer of whipped cream. Cover with another crêpe and repeat the process, stacking evenly to form a many-layered cake. Chill thoroughly. To serve, cut into wedges like a cake. Serve for dessert or for an elegant, not-so-*petit déjeuner*.

BLINTZES

JEWISH   *8 to 10 blintzes*

And what about blintzes? How does one go about describing them? All you can do is wait for the next holiday and throw a garland in the air for those Delancey Street blintzes—those flat squares of dough folded lovingly over cottage cheese or jelly and fried in butter; and eaten as you prefer, plain or with sour cream.
                                                —HARRY GOLDEN, *Only in America*

Although associated with Jewish cooking, blintzes started out as Ukrainian Lenten fare. The round shape of the pancakes symbolized the sun at spring equinox. Jews interpreted the shape of two folded blintzes side-by-side as the tablets on which the Ten Commandments were inscribed by God and originally served them on Shavuot, the holiday commemorating the day Moses received the Commandments on Mount Sinai. Today blintzes are served either as a Vata-balancing main course for breakfast or lunch or as a dessert.

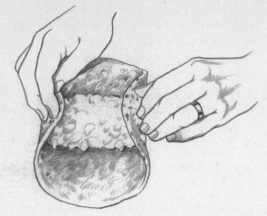

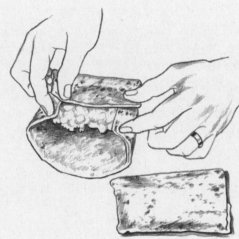

STEP ONE

Crêpe batter (pp. 375–76)

STEP TWO

*1 cup (8 ounces/230 g) cream
  cheese, softened*
*2 cups (400 g) farmer's cheese,
  hoop cheese, Tvorog (pp. 539–40),
  or crumbled firm panir*

⅓ cup (70 g) sugar
*1 tablespoon arrowroot or
  cornstarch*
¾ teaspoon ground cinnamon
¼ teaspoon ground nutmeg

STEP FOUR

Ghee or butter
*Fresh sliced strawberries, blueberries,
  or Fresh Summer Fruit Sauce (p. 456) (optional)*

Sour cream

1. Prepare the crêpes in a 10-inch (26 cm) skillet, *frying on one side only*. The top side
    should be firm and nonsticky. Set aside.

2. To prepare the filling, mix the cheeses, sugar, arrowroot or cornstarch, cinnamon, and nutmeg. Beat until smooth with a mixer or spoon—do not use a food processor.
3. Place a crêpe, cooked side up, on a plate and place a large spoonful of the cheese filling in the center. Gently bring up the 2 opposite edges of the crêpe over the filling, then roll up from an unfolded edge to form a tubelike package that completely encloses the filling. Be careful not to break the crêpe.
4. Coat a skillet with a generous amount of ghee or butter. Cook the blintzes on both sides until golden brown, turning very gently. To serve, top with sour cream or with fruit and sour cream.

 ## JONNYCAKES

UNITED STATES   *1 dozen*

At last—a Kapha-balancing pancake. To Rhode Island Yankees these cornmeal cakes can be Serious Business. In the 1890s the legislature of Rhode Island made the proper spelling of Jonnycake into law. They would have made the correct recipe into law as well if only the South County and Newport County representatives could have agreed. The debate rages on—all in good fun, they say—with "The Society for the Propagation of the Jonnycake Tradition" fanning the flames. If white cap cornmeal, a Rhode Island–grown type of white cornmeal, is available, you can prepare the absolute maybe real thing. However, if you don't, you won't get a citation—yet.

STEP ONE

1 cup (130 g) cornmeal   *1 teaspoon sugar* (optional)
½ teaspoon salt

STEP TWO

1 cup (240 ml) boiling water   *½ cup (120 ml) cold water*

STEP THREE

Ghee or butter for frying (or   *Rice or barley malt syrup or honey*
sunflower oil for Kapha)

1. Mix the cornmeal, salt, and sugar.
2. Make a well in the center. Pour the boiling water into the well. Beat with a whisk until smooth. Beat in the cold water to make a thick, smooth batter.
3. Fry small pancakes in plenty of ghee or butter. Jonnycakes take longer to cook than ordinary pancakes. Make sure they are brown and crusty before flipping or they will fall apart in midair. Keep thinning the batter as necessary with water; the cornmeal will swell. Serve hot with syrup or, for balancing Kapha, lukewarm with honey.

The love of heaven makes one heavenly.

—WILLIAM SHAKESPEARE

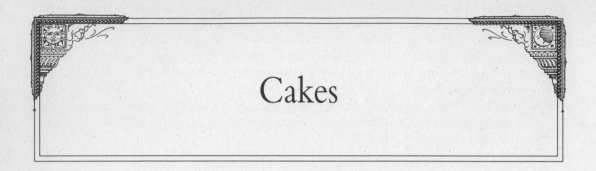

Cakes

A house is not beautiful because of its walls, but because of its cakes.
           —Old Russian proverb

Cakes represent all that is celebratory, rich, and sweet in life. In the western world, the rituals of holidays and rites of passage are punctuated by beautifully decorated cakes such as those cut and shared by a newly joined couple or topped by candles to joyously mark another year of life. Cakes as we know them today are relative newcomers to the world's culinary repertoire. In earlier centuries butter, milk, finely milled flour, and sugar were luxuries—not to mention a chef capable of coaxing a properly baked cake from the unreliable ovens of the day. However, for those of us with reliable ovens and easy access to fine ingredients, all we need is a little confidence and know-how to create a sweet source of universal delight to celebrate any whim or fancy.

Baking and Ayurveda

It is difficult to add any notes of seriousness or caution when discussing festive, joyful cakes, cookies, and pastries. Most of us have them for an occasional treat, not as a staple food. Unless you have a serious imbalance that is triggered by one of the ingredients, and if eating cake once in awhile at a celebration produces bliss, then at that moment it constitutes health food.

Cakes, cookies, and such are basically heavy, sweet, and unctuous, making them ultimately most balancing for Vata. Pitta comes in a close second, although large amounts of oil and fat are less balancing than for Vata dosha. The tastes and qualities of flavorings and other added ingredients influence the overall effect: add more sour flavors, such as lemon or sour cream, and the result will be less balancing for Pitta. Add dry, astringent ingredients such as apples or cranberries, and a note of balance for Kapha has been sounded.

❖ *Flour:* Although Ayurveda recommends eating whole grain flour, a 100 percent whole wheat cake is not an object of desire for most people. I use unbleached white flour in the recipes in the interests of making the cake light and helping hold it together. These factors are more important in layer cakes and less so in moist tea cakes containing ingredients such as dried fruits and nuts, which can be cut and served from the pan.

You can substitute about ½ cup (75 g) whole wheat flour for unbleached white flour without any noticeable change in texture or flavor. If anything, it improves the cake. It is possible to substitute more whole wheat flour, even for the total amount. However, the cake will be heavier, more crumbly, and have a not-so-subtle wheaty flavor. (You may want these qualities in heavier cakes, such as fruitcake.)

Bleached white all-purpose flour can cause uneven rising in eggless cakes unless it is mixed with at least ½ cup (75 g) whole wheat flour. Bleached white pastry or cake flour does not work well in eggless cakes.

❖ *Fats:* The *ne plus ultra* of fats for cake baking is unsalted butter. Although ghee is the most lauded oil in Ayurveda, it can give cakes a dense, oil-saturated texture. However, substituting ghee for up to half the butter doesn't affect the flavor and texture of most cakes very much. (Cake recipes calling for *melted* butter or oil are much more delicious if you substitute ghee.)

If you are wedded to only using ghee in your baking, you can substitute ghee for unmelted butter if you use 20 percent less ghee than the amount of butter specified.

Oil also imparts its own flavor and dense texture to cakes. I don't recommend it. However, if you insist on using it, reduce the liquid in the recipe slightly when substituting oil for unmelted butter.

❖ *Eggs:* Eggless cakes follow somewhat different rules of construction than ordinary cakes. See the section on "Baking Without Eggs," pages 575–76, to understand the general *modus operandi*.

❖ *Sweeteners:* I use raw sugar, the preferred sugar of Ayurveda, for baking. My favorites are *gur*, available in Indian markets, or a mixture of half Sucanat and half turbinado sugar. You can, however, also use white or packed brown sugar with equal success in any of the recipes, so I only specify "sugar." The choice is yours.

❖ *Liquids:* Ayurveda does not recommend combining milk with "mixed tastes," which in the case of baked goods means the salt and bitter taste of the leavening. Serendipitously, buttermilk, which combines perfectly well with other tastes, is the best dairy liquid for eggless cakes anyway. Its acidity interacts with the alkaline qualities of baking powder and soda to facilitate the leavening process. I use a mixture of half buttermilk and half water, as buttermilk on its own can sometimes make a cake gluey.

❖ To substitute yogurt for buttermilk, mix the yogurt and water together thoroughly, as if preparing lassi. If your yogurt is very thick, reduce the amount slightly and increase the water. For instance, instead of ½ cup (120 ml) each of yogurt and water, use ⅓ cup (80 ml) yogurt and ⅔ cup (160 ml) water.

☻ When using nondairy milk, add 2 teaspoons lemon juice per cup of milk.

AYURVEDA AND SWEETS

Honey and very sweet food enlighten the eyes of man.　　—THE TALMUD

There is much ambivalence surrounding sweeteners today: a desire to eat them yet an uneasy feeling that they are unhealthy, plus a widely marketed hope that somehow they are fine as long as they are in fat-free foods! This fosters a guilty "can't live with 'em, can't live without 'em" attitude. In Ayurveda sweeteners are a source of one of the six major tastes. The right type in the right amount at the right time, in harmony with the constitution of the individual eating it, can be nourishing and have wonderful health benefits.

A little sweetness along with the other five creates balance and a feeling of well-being. However, too much of any one taste can create imbalance. All would agree that excessive use of sugar can lead to health problems. As with all foods, moderation is the key.

❖ One quality of the sweet taste is heaviness, which balances the light quality of Vata dosha. However, heavy foods are more difficult to digest than light ones. Some vaidyas recommend eating sweets at the beginning of the meal rather than as a finale. (So the world's kids were right after all!) Agni, the digestive fire, is strongest when you first sit down hungry to a meal and therefore is most prepared to tackle a heavy dessert.

THE NOBLE NINEFOLD PATH OF EGGLESS CAKES

1. Butter baking pans by rubbing a thin film of butter on the bottom and sides of the pan. Ghee and oil don't do the job; cakes will stick to the pan. Alternatively, use nonstick bakeware or line the pans with baker's parchment.
2. Do a very thorough job of creaming the butter and sugar together—it makes the cake lighter. However, when combining the dry and wet ingredients, mix just until blended together, and no more. (Forget about the 400 to 600 strokes that egg batter cakes receive.)

3. Cake batter can be prepared quickly and easily in a food processor. Use the blade attachment to first cream the butter and sugar. Next, add the dry ingredients and process. Last, add the liquids and process just until blended.

4. When you spoon the batter into the cake pans, the pans should be no more than ⅔ full. The batter should be between 1 and 1½ inches (2.5 and 4 cm) deep—no more and no less—for best results.

5. Try not to poke or jiggle cakes or slam the oven door while they are baking—sharp movements can cause a beautifully rising cake to mimic a prickled balloon.

6. A cake is done when:
   - A toothpick or knife inserted in the center comes out clean, without any wet batter clinging to it.
   - The top is lightly browned and the sides shrink away slightly from the pan.
   - When pressed lightly, the cake feels fairly solid underneath—not squishy.

7. Allow the cakes to cool for 15 minutes, then gently run a knife around the edges of a pan to loosen the cake. Invert a plate over the pan and turn the whole thing over to release the cake onto a rack—or directly onto a plate. Now perform the same maneuver, using your serving plate to put it right side up. Invert the second layer onto a rack to cool—it will stick to a plate.

8. If a cake stubbornly refuses to give up its hold on the pan, invert it and place a cold wet dish towel over the bottom of the pan. Now drum on it with some military "Forward march!" beat to encourage it. If that doesn't work, gently coax the cake loose with a knife and spatula. If occasionally a cake breaks in the birthing process, you can always glue it back together again and disguise the breaks with frosting.

9. Allow cakes to cool very thoroughly before frosting. Attempting to frost a cake that is even slightly warm is courting disaster. Believe me, I've done it—and ended up serving my mother's birthday cake in ragged pieces mixed up with gobs of frosting in individual bowls. On another occasion, a top layer unceremoniously slid off the bottom layer and plopped on the floor as the bride-to-be I was "helping" watched in horror. Patience is a necessity—not only a virtue—when icing cakes.

HOW TO BAKE PERFECTLY FLAT LAYERS FOR LAYER CAKES

Here is a trick to make a cake rise perfectly flat instead of having a hump in the middle—a distinct advantage when more than one layer is involved:

1. Preheat the oven to 250°F (120°C). Bake the cake for 10 minutes on the middle rack.

2. Raise the heat to 300°F (150°C) without opening the door or removing the cake from the oven. Bake for another 10 minutes.

3. Now raise the temperature to 350°F (180°C) and bake until the cake is done, about 20 minutes for 8-inch (22 cm) or 9-inch (23 cm) layers.

MULTILAYER CAKE
One 8-inch (22 cm) or 9-inch (23 cm) cake

No matter how hard people have tried to solve the problem—and I've been given hundreds of "foolproof" recipes and solutions to combat it—the fact remains that eggless cakes are generally heavier than those containing eggs. A method that produces an overall lighter result, and the one I've found to work best, was developed by Jim Meredith. I now make all my layer cakes this way. Instead of preparing a traditional two-layer cake, the same amount of batter is used to prepare three or four thin layers, and an almost equal amount of frosting is placed between each layer.

> **1 recipe any layer cake**
>   (*pp. 385–93*)

1. Line three 9-inch (23 cm) or four 8-inch (22 cm) cake pans with kitchen parchment that has been trimmed to fit the bottom of the pan. Butter and lightly flour the paper.
2. You may need to thin the batter so that it spreads more easily. Add a little more buttermilk and water until the batter is almost pourable. The layers here are too thin to develop an uneven texture from such treatment.
3. Spread the batter evenly in the pans, leaving no thin spots where the paper shows through.
4. The layers will bake more quickly than the usual thicker ones. Check the oven 10 minutes earlier than the recipe calls for.
5. Allow the layers to cool in the pan. To remove, invert the pans gently, then peel off the waxed paper.
6. Prepare a double batch of frosting. When the layers have thoroughly cooled, spread the frosting between them—as thick as the cake layers themselves. Whipped cream frostings give an especially light effect.

CUPCAKES

Butter and flour a 12-cup muffin tin or line the tin with paper muffin cups. Fill each cup ⅔ full with cake batter. Bake in a 375°F (190°C) oven about 25 minutes.

White Cake with Buttercream Frosting

Two 8-inch (22 cm) layers

Two classics, very basic, to serve as is, or ready and willing to receive your creative flavoring additions. Buttercream frosting can absorb any of the flavoring additions used in other frostings in this chapter.

	STEP TWO
⅔ *cup (145 g) unsalted butter*	2 *cups (420 g) sugar*
	STEP THREE
3½ *cups (490 g)* **unbleached white flour**	2½ *teaspoons baking powder*
2 *tablespoons arrowroot or cornstarch*	½ *teaspoon baking soda*
	½ *teaspoon salt*
	STEP FOUR
1 *cup (240 ml) buttermilk*	1 *cup (240 ml) water*

1. Preheat the oven to 350°F (180°C). Butter and lightly flour two 8-inch (22 cm) baking pans.
2. Cream the butter and sugar thoroughly.
3. Mix the dry ingredients and sift them over the butter-sugar mixture.
4. Mix the buttermilk with the water. Pour over the dry ingredients and mix just until blended.
5. Spoon into the pans. Bake about 35 minutes.

VARIATIONS

Poppy Seed Cake: Add 2 tablespoons poppy seeds in Step 4. Also try this with Orange Cake or Lemon Cake.

Nut Cake: Add ¾ cup (85 g) finely chopped toasted nuts and 2 teaspoons herbal coffee substitute powder (preferably Raja's Cup) to the batter in Step 4.

Buttercream Frosting

2 cups (240 g)

	STEP ONE
½ *cup (120 g) unsalted butter, at room temperature*	1 *pound (455 g)* **confectioner's sugar, sifted**
	STEP TWO
2 *to 3 tablespoons milk*	

1. Cream the butter and sugar thoroughly.
2. Beat in 2 tablespoons milk. Add the remaining tablespoon if the frosting is too thick. The mixture will harden if it sits—thin with milk to the desired texture if this happens.

VARIATIONS

✿ *Mint Frosting:* Replace the milk with chilled strong mint tea.

Nut Frosting: Pistachios look particularly exquisite. Frost the cake. Set on a baking sheet to catch falling nuts. Gently press handfuls of ground nuts into the cake. Brush away the excess.

Here is a professional cake decorator's technique for preventing crumbs from mixing into the frosting as you work: Make a small amount of very thin Buttercream Frosting. Spread a very thin layer over all cake layers to seal in the crumbs. Allow it to dry completely before applying a second, final layer of thicker frosting, 20 to 30 minutes.

ORANGE CAKE WITH ORANGE-COCONUT CREAM CHEESE FROSTING

Two 8-inch layers

This could also be a lemon or lime cake with lemon- or lime-coconut cream cheese frosting (see Variation).

⅔ cup (145 g) unsalted butter

STEP TWO
2 cups (420 g) sugar

3½ cups (490 g) unbleached white flour
3½ tablespoons arrowroot or cornstarch

STEP THREE
2½ teaspoons baking powder
½ teaspoon baking soda
½ teaspoon salt

1 cup (240 ml) orange juice
1 cup (240 ml) buttermilk

STEP FOUR
2 tablespoons finely grated orange zest

1. Preheat the oven to 350°F (180°C). Butter and lightly flour two 8-inch (22 cm) round cake pans.
2. Cream the butter and sugar.

3. Mix the dry ingredients and sift over the butter-sugar mixture.
4. Mix the orange juice, buttermilk or sour milk, and grated orange zest together. Add to the dry ingredients and mix just until blended.
5. Spoon into the pans and spread evenly. Bake about 35 minutes.

VARIATION

Lemon or Lime Cake: Lemon or lime juice causes the batter to rise very high, so use 9-inch (23 cm) cake pans. Replace the orange zest with 1 tablespoon plus 1 teaspoon finely grated lemon or lime zest. Substitute the following for the total amount of liquid in Step 4: ¾ cup (180 ml) water, ½ cup (120 ml) lemon or lime juice, ¾ cup (180 ml) buttermilk.

ORANGE-COCONUT CREAM CHEESE FROSTING

2 cups (250 g)

You can turn any frosting into a coconut frosting by this method. Cream cheese frosting is quite flexible in its preparation—all's fair that renders the cream cheese spreadable and sweet. Be careful when adding liquid ingredients to thin the cream cheese—it becomes soupy amazingly easily. Allow the cream cheese to stand at room temperature for an hour or more to soften, and add liquid very conservatively, a little at a time, until the desired consistency is achieved. Use "natural" cream cheese without salt and gum additives if possible.

STEP ONE

With Honey:

2 cups (1 pound/500 g) cream cheese, softened
¼ to ½ cup (60 to 120 ml) honey

2 tablespoons finely grated orange zest

With Sugar:

1¾ cups (400 g) softened cream cheese
¼ cup (60 ml) buttermilk, water, or fruit juice

2 tablespoons finely grated orange zest
1 cup (115 g) sifted confectioner's sugar or to taste

STEP TWO

Grated fresh or dried unsweetened coconut, toasted if desired

1. Beat the ingredients together until smooth.
2. Ice the cake and place over a baking sheet to catch falling coconut. Gently press handfuls of grated coconut into the frosting, allowing the excess to fall away.

VARIATION
   Lemon- or Lime-Coconut Cream Cheese Frosting: Substitute lemon or lime zest for the orange.

 ## MOCHA SPICE CAKE WITH COFFEE WHIPPED CREAM AND CREAM CHEESE FROSTING

Two 8-inch (22 cm) layers

Give me the luxuries of life and I will willingly do without the necessities.
                                    —FRANK LLOYD WRIGHT

At one time in Olde Europe, both spices and coffee were rare imports from mysterious countries. Here is an Ayurvedic upgrade on a delicacy originally called "Egyptian cake," a title that was geographically confused but rife with exoticism.

STEP TWO
⅔ cup (145 g) unsalted butter
2 cups (420 g) raw or packed
   brown sugar

STEP THREE

3 cups (420 g) unbleached white flour	*½ teaspoon salt*
½ cup (75 g) whole wheat flour	*2 teaspoons ground cinnamon*
2 tablespoons arrowroot or cornstarch	*½ teaspoon ground cloves*
2½ teaspoons baking powder	*½ teaspoon ground ginger*
½ teaspoon baking soda	*3 tablespoons herbal coffee substitute powder (preferably Raja's Cup)*

STEP FOUR
1 cup (240 ml) buttermilk   *1 cup (240 ml) water*

1. Preheat the oven to 350°F (180°C). Butter and lightly flour two 8-inch (22 cm) round cake pans.
2. Cream the butter and sugar.
3. Mix the dry ingredients and sift over the butter-sugar mixture.
4. Mix the buttermilk with the water. Pour over the dry ingredients and mix just until blended.
5. Spoon into the pans. Bake about 35 minutes.

Coffee Whipped Cream and Cream Cheese Frosting

3 cups (360 g)

This is my favorite frosting. It is light, but the small amount of cream cheese gives more body to the whipped cream. The only way to make the frosting completely smooth—unless Superman is mixing it for you—is to use a food processor or electric mixer. Use "natural" cream cheese without salt and gum additives. You can beat herbal coffee substitute powder into any other type of frosting as well.

STEP ONE

½ cup (120 g) cream cheese, softened

2 tablespoons honey or 3 to 4 tablespoons confectioner's sugar

STEP TWO

1 cup (250 ml) heavy (whipping) cream

2 teaspoons herbal coffee substitute powder (preferably Raja's Cup)

1. Beat the cream cheese and honey or sugar until completely free of lumps. Set aside.
2. Whip the cream until stiff. Beat in the herbal coffee substitute powder and cream cheese just until thoroughly blended.

To Frost or Not to Frost

Frostings are best suited to layer cakes and to drier baked goods that need a rich accompaniment. Moist, rich, fruity cakes are often best left to their own devices—they already "have it all." There are also some cakes with strong flavors that are not served well by conflicting or distracting accompaniments. Here are some alternatives to all-out frostings for cakes that you want to dress in slacks and sweaters rather than in floor-length gowns and tuxedos:

❖ Spoon a fruit sauce, such as Fresh Summer Fruit Sauce (p. 456) or Applesauce (p. 463), over individual cake slices.
❖ Spoon unsweetened crème fraîche, lightly whipped cream, or Hung Yogurt (p. 534) over individual cake slices.
❖ Dried Fruit Purées (p. 462) are naturally sweet alternatives to frostings. Spread a thin layer, as you would butter, on individual cake slices.

✿ COCONUT CAKE WITH APRICOT OR DATE FROSTING

Two 8-inch (22 cm) layers

¼ *cup (55 g) unsalted butter*

STEP TWO

1½ *cups (310 g) sugar*

2½ *cups (350 g) unbleached white flour*
2 *tablespoons arrowroot or cornstarch*

STEP THREE

½ *teaspoon salt*
2½ *teaspoons baking powder*
½ *teaspoon baking soda*

1¾ *cups (140 g) grated fresh or dried unsweetened coconut*
⅔ *cup (160 ml) buttermilk*

STEP FOUR

⅔ *cup (160 ml) water*
1 *teaspoon finely grated lemon zest*

1. Preheat the oven to 350°F (180°C). Butter and lightly flour two 8-inch (22 cm) round cake pans.
2. Cream the butter and sugar thoroughly.
3. Sift the dry ingredients over the butter-sugar mixture.
4. Add the coconut. Mix the buttermilk with the water and lemon zest. Pour over the dry ingredients and mix just until blended.
5. Spoon into the pans. Bake about 35 minutes.

VARIATIONS

Tuck drained crushed pineapple and mango slices between the layers.

Orange-Coconut Cake: Replace the lemon zest with 2 tablespoons finely grated orange zest, and replace the water with orange juice.

APRICOT OR DATE FROSTING

2 cups

Puréed dried fruits offer delicate flavor to frostings. Apricots and dates impart the most attractive colors and blend in most smoothly, but you can experiment with other dried fruits with the awareness that their bright colors may not translate perfectly to this medium and they may not be completely smooth when blended.

¾ cup (110 g) packed chopped
   dried apricots or dates
½ cup (120 ml) water or
   fruit juice

1¾ cups (400 g) softened cream
   cheese or Hung Yogurt
Honey

1. Place the dried fruit and water or fruit juice in a saucepan. Bring to a boil, cover, and simmer over very low heat until the fruit is soft and most of the water is absorbed, about 10 minutes. Let cool to room temperature.
2. Combine with the cream cheese or yogurt in a food processor until smooth. Add honey to taste and to spreading consistency. In the unlikely event that the frosting is becoming too liquid but is not sweet enough, switch to sifted confectioner's sugar.

SOUR CREAM SPICE CAKE WITH GINGERED MOLASSES FROSTING

Two 8-inch (22 cm) layers

½ cup (115 g) unsalted butter
2 cups (420 g) raw or packed
   brown sugar

STEP TWO

1 cup (240 ml) sour cream

STEP THREE
1 cup (240 ml) water

3½ cups (490 g) unbleached
   white flour
3 tablespoons arrowroot or
   cornstarch
1 teaspoon herbal coffee substitute
   powder (preferably Raja's Cup)

STEP FOUR
½ teaspoon salt
1½ teaspoons baking powder
1 teaspoon baking soda
1½ teaspoons ground cinnamon
½ teaspoon each: ground cloves,
   ginger, nutmeg, cardamom

1. Preheat the oven to 350°F (180°C). Butter and lightly flour two 8-inch (22 cm) round cake pans.
2. Cream the butter and sugar thoroughly.
3. Add the sour cream and beat until smooth. Mix in the water.
4. Mix the dry ingredients together and sift over the sour cream mixture. Mix just until blended.
5. Spoon into the pans. Bake about 35 minutes.

GINGERED MOLASSES FROSTING

2 cups

Beat 2 to 3 teaspoons unsulphured molasses into Buttercream Frosting (pp. 385–86). After frosting the cake, sprinkle on a small amount of finely chopped crystallized ginger.

BANANA CAKE WITH PECAN PRALINÉ HUNG YOGURT FROSTING

Two 8-inch (22 cm) layers

	STEP TWO
⅔ cup (145 g) unsalted butter	2 cups (480 g) mashed ripe bananas
2 cups (420 g) sugar	

	STEP THREE
3 cups (420 g) unbleached white flour	2½ teaspoons baking powder
	½ teaspoon baking soda
2 tablespoons arrowroot or cornstarch	½ teaspoon salt

	STEP FOUR
⅓ cup (80 ml) buttermilk	⅓ cup (80 ml) water

1. Preheat the oven to 350°F (180°C). Butter and lightly flour two 8-inch (22 cm) round cake pans.
2. Cream the butter and sugar thoroughly. Beat in the mashed bananas until smooth.
3. Mix the dry ingredients and sift over the banana mixture.
4. Mix the buttermilk with the water. Pour over the dry ingredients and mix just until blended.
5. Spoon into the pans. Bake 35 to 40 minutes.

PECAN PRALINÉ HUNG YOGURT FROSTING

2 cups (250 g)

You can make praliné frosting from any other type of frosting by this method. The secret of preparing praline is to remove the mixture from the heat the moment the sugar melts and spread it on a tray with lightning speed. If you stop right there, allow it to cool, and break it into pieces, you have nut brittle candy. The saucepan will look impossible to clean, but before your Vata goes out of balance with worry, know that a little soaking in hot water easily removes the sugar residue.

STEP ONE

1½ cups (300 g) turbinado, white, or packed light brown sugar

STEP TWO

1½ cups (150 g) coarsely chopped pecans

STEP THREE

2 cups (480 ml) Hung Yogurt (p. 534)   *4 to 6 tablespoons (60 to 90 ml) honey*

1. Butter a 13 × 9-inch (33 × 23 cm) pan. Place the sugar in a saucepan over medium heat. Stir constantly until the sugar melts. Be very careful not to burn it.
2. Stir in the nuts, remove from the heat, and immediately spread in the pan with the back of a wooden spoon. Allow the mixture to harden. Break into pieces and pulverize in a food processor.
3. Mix the yogurt just until blended with honey to taste. You'll have to adjust the sweetening depending on the sourness of the yogurt.
4. Frost the cake. Place on a baking sheet to catch praliné as it falls, then lightly press handfuls of praline onto the cake.

VARIATION

For a thicker consistency, add sifted confectioner's sugar instead of honey to the Hung Yogurt.

TEA CAKES, FRUITED CAKES, AND OTHER SINGLE-LAYER CAKES

Tea cakes are often baked in a single layer and cut into squares right from the pan. Rich and moist, they are sometimes prepared with melted ghee or butter or even with oil to increase their density. Because such cakes are traditionally heavier than layer cakes, the absence of eggs offers little-to-no loss to their texture. These are good cakes to serve to people who are unfamiliar with—and maybe unreceptive to—eggless baked goods.

❖ Sweet quick breads can be baked in 9-inch (23 cm) square cake pans and served as cake. They contain less fat than cake recipes and are therefore a little drier. A rich frosting helps pass them off as their richer brethren.

CARROT CAKE

One 13 × 9-inch (33 × 23 cm) cake

Here is a rich, moist, almost puddinglike version of this classic cake. Prepare with ghee for superlative flavor. This cake is so rich it really does not need frosting. If you wish to gild the lily, very lightly sweetened, unflavored Cream Cheese Frosting (use recipe on p. 387, omitting juice, orange zest, and coconut), Whipped Cream and Cream Cheese Frosting (p. 389), or whipped cream will do the job nicely.

STEP TWO

⅔ cup (160 ml) melted ghee or oil or ¾ cup (180 ml) melted butter
1¼ cups (260 g) raw or packed brown sugar
2 cups (180 g) grated carrots
⅓ cup (25 g) grated fresh or dried unsweetened coconut

1 cup (250 g) drained chopped pineapple
1 cup (100 g) chopped walnuts or pecans
¾ cup (100 g) raisins

STEP THREE

2 cups (280 g) unbleached white flour
¼ cup (40 g) whole wheat flour
2 tablespoons arrowroot or cornstarch
2 teaspoons baking powder

½ teaspoon baking soda
½ teaspoon salt
1 teaspoon ground cinnamon
½ teaspoon ground cardamom
½ teaspoon ground ginger

STEP FOUR

⅓ cup (80 ml) buttermilk   ½ cup (80 ml) water

1. Preheat the oven to 350°F (180°C). Butter and lightly flour a 13 × 9-inch (33 × 23 cm) baking pan.
2. Beat the oil and sugar together until smooth. Beat in the carrots, coconut, pineapple, nuts, and raisins.
3. In a separate bowl, mix together the dry ingredients.
4. Add the dry ingredients, buttermilk and water to the carrot mixture and mix together. The batter will be extremely thick.
5. Spoon into the pan and spread evenly. Bake until lightly browned on top, 40 to 45 minutes. Do not underbake. The cake will be more moist than other cakes.

VARIATION
    Add ¼ cup (40 g) chopped crystallized ginger in Step 4.

ÄPFELTORTE (APPLE TORTE)

GERMANY   *One 9-inch (23 cm) cake*

This cake looks quite professional when served in squares.

STEP ONE

4 cups (480 g) coarsely chopped
   peeled apples
⅓ cup (30 g) raisins

⅓ cup (70 g) sugar
½ teaspoon ground cinnamon

STEP THREE

2¼ cups (315 g) unbleached
   white flour
2 tablespoons arrowroot or
   cornstarch
1½ teaspoons baking powder
¼ teaspoon baking soda
¾ cup (150 g) sugar

½ teaspoon salt
1 teaspoon finely grated lemon zest
⅓ cup (40 g) finely chopped
   pistachios or toasted almonds
   (optional)

STEP FOUR

½ cup (115 g) unsalted butter
3 tablespoons buttermilk

3 tablespoons water

STEP SEVEN

Confectioner's sugar

To prepare the filling:
1. Steam the apples until soft. Drain thoroughly. Mix in the raisins, sugar, and cinnamon.
2. While the apples are steaming, preheat the oven to 325°F (160°C). Butter and lightly flour a 9-inch (23 cm) square cake pan.

To prepare the cake:
3. Mix the dry ingredients together.
4. Cut in the butter and work with your fingers or a pastry cutter until the mixture resembles coarse meal. Add the buttermilk and water to make a crumbly dough. Be careful—it's easy to use too much liquid and end up with a solid mass of dough.
5. Crumble half the dough evenly into the pan. Do not pat down. Spread the apple mixture over the dough. Crumble the remaining dough evenly over the apple mixture to completely cover it.
6. Bake 40 to 45 minutes. Turn the heat off and let the cake sit in the oven for another 10 minutes, until the top is golden brown.
7. Allow to cool thoroughly. Sift a little confectioner's sugar over the top. Cut into squares and remove from the pan to reveal the filling.

APPLESAUCE GINGERBREAD

One 13 × 9-inch (33 × 23 cm) cake

If I had one penny in the world, thou shouldst have it for gingerbread.
—WILLIAM SHAKESPEARE, *Love's Labors Lost*

Applesauce adds moistness, and the crystallized ginger provides a little kick.

¼ cup (55 g) ghee or butter
⅓ cup (80 ml) unsulphured molasses
1 cup (210 g) raw or packed brown sugar

STEP TWO

1 tablespoon finely grated orange zest

2½ cups (350 g) unbleached white flour
2 tablespoons arrowroot or cornstarch
½ teaspoon salt

STEP THREE

2 teaspoons baking powder
½ teaspoon baking soda
1 teaspoon ground ginger
1 teaspoon ground cinnamon

1⅔ cups (360 g) puréed steamed apples or unsweetened applesauce
⅓ cup (55 g) chopped crystallized ginger

STEP FOUR

½ cup (65 g) currants, soaked in warm water for 30 minutes and drained

1. Preheat the oven to 350°F (180°C). Butter and lightly flour a 13 × 9-inch (33 × 23 cm) pan.
2. Cream the ghee or butter with the molasses, sugar, and orange zest.
3. Mix the dry ingredients together and add to the creamed mixture.
4. Add the applesauce and mix just until all the ingredients are blended. Stir in the crystallized ginger and currants.
5. Spoon into the pan and spread evenly. Bake about 1 hour.

CARDAMOM TEA CAKE (KARDEMUMMAKAKA)

SWEDEN   *One 13 × 9-inch (33 × 23 cm) cake*

The dessert is said to be to the dinner what the madrigal is to literature—it is the light poetry of the kitchen.
—GEORGE ELLWANGER

¼ cup (55 g) unsalted butter

2½ cups (350 g) unbleached
  white flour
2 teaspoons baking powder

⅔ cup (160 ml) buttermilk

1 cup (210 g) sugar
¾ cup (110 g) flour

STEP TWO
1¼ cups (260 g) sugar

STEP THREE
½ teaspoon baking soda
1½ teaspoons ground cardamom
½ teaspoon salt

STEP FOUR
⅔ cup (160 ml) water

STEP FIVE
½ cup (115 g) butter

1. Preheat the oven to 350°F (180°C). Butter and lightly flour a 13 × 9-inch (33 × 23 cm) pan.
2. Cream the butter and sugar thoroughly.
3. Mix the dry ingredients and sift over the butter-sugar mixture.
4. Mix the buttermilk with the water. Pour over the dry ingredients and mix just until blended. Spoon into the pan.
5. *To prepare the streusel topping:* Mix the sugar and flour together. Cut the butter into small pieces and work into the dry ingredients with your fingers or a pastry cutter until the mixture resembles coarse meal. Sprinkle evenly over the cake batter.
6. Bake 30 to 40 minutes.

APPLE, RHUBARB, OR BLUEBERRY TEA CAKE

9-inch (23 cm) cake

STEP TWO

½ cup (115 g) unsalted butter
1 cup (210 g) raw or packed light
  brown sugar

STEP THREE

2 cups (280 g) unbleached
   white flour
2 tablespoons arrowroot or
   cornstarch

2 teaspoons baking powder
½ teaspoon baking soda
½ teaspoon salt

STEP FOUR

½ cup (120 ml) sour cream or
   yogurt
½ cup (120 ml) water

1½ cups (180 g) coarsely chopped
   apples, sliced rhubarb (180 g),
   or blueberries (210 g)

STEP FIVE

½ cup (100 g) sugar
½ cup (50 g) chopped pecans

1 tablespoon butter
1 teaspoon ground cinnamon

1. Preheat the oven to 350°F (180°C). Butter and lightly flour a 9-inch (23 cm) square cake pan.
2. Cream the butter and sugar thoroughly.
3. Mix the dry ingredients and sift over the butter-sugar mixture.
4. Add the sour cream or yogurt and water and mix just until blended. Gently fold in the fruit. Spoon into the pan and spread evenly.
5. Mix the sugar, pecans, butter, and cinnamon together. Sprinkle evenly over the cake batter.
6. Bake about 1 hour.

SHORTCAKE—STRAWBERRY, BLUEBERRY, MANGO, PEACH, ETC.

One shortcake with two 9-inch (23 cm) layers

STEP TWO

4 cups (560 g) unbleached white
   flour
1 cup (210 g) sugar

1 tablespoon baking powder
1 teaspoon baking soda
1 teaspoon salt

STEP THREE

1 cup (230 g) unsalted butter

STEP FOUR

⅔ cup (160 ml) buttermilk

⅔ cup (160 ml) water

1 quart/liter berries or *4 cups (860 g) sliced peaches or mangoes*   *Confectioner's sugar*

1 cup (240 ml) heavy (whipping) cream

1. Preheat the oven to 425°F (220°C). Butter and lightly flour two 9-inch (23 cm) round cake pans.
2. Mix the dry ingredients and sift into a bowl.
3. Cut in the butter and work with your fingers or a pastry cutter until the mixture resembles coarse meal.
4. Mix the buttermilk with the water. Pour over the dry ingredients and mix to make a soft dough.
5. Press evenly into the pans. Bake 25 to 30 minutes. Allow to cool thoroughly.
6. If using strawberries, slice half of them, reserving the most beautiful strawberries to be used whole on the top. Sweeten the sliced fruit with a little confectioner's sugar.
7. Whip the cream until it stands in soft peaks.
8. Place one layer of cake on a plate. If the top is very rounded, trim it flat. Spread half the whipped cream over it and cover with half of the sliced fruit. Place the second layer on top. Spread with the remaining whipped cream and top with the remaining fruit in a pretty design.

VARIATIONS

Cover the first layer with blueberries or sliced peaches and cover the second layer with whole strawberries for a double fruit shortcake.

Mix a little chopped crystallized ginger into the fruit.

Mix a little ground cardamom into the whipped cream.

Spread each cooled cake layer with a thin layer of Marzipan (pp. 453–54) before assembling the cake.

 # PINEAPPLE UPSIDE-DOWN CAKE

One 10-inch (26 cm) cake

This exquisite cake is best prepared in a 10-inch (26 cm) all-metal skillet, such as cast iron or stainless steel. Serve warm with whipped cream.

1 small pineapple

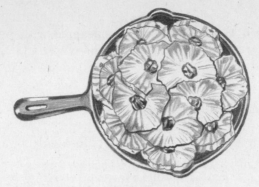

STEP THREE

¼ *cup (55 g) ghee or unsalted butter*

¾ *cup (150 g) packed dark brown sugar*

STEP FOUR

10 *to 12 pecan halves*

STEP FIVE

2 *cups (280 g) unbleached white flour*
2 *teaspoons baking powder*

½ *teaspoon baking soda*
½ *teaspoon salt*
1 *cup (210 g) sugar*

STEP SIX

½ *cup (120 ml) buttermilk*
½ *cup (120 ml) water*

2 *tablespoons melted ghee or unsalted butter*

1. Preheat the oven to 350°F (180°C).

To prepare the topping:

2. Peel the pineapple. Slice thin. Remove the core from each slice with an apple corer or a paring knife.
3. Melt the ghee or butter in a 10-inch (26 cm) all-metal skillet. Add the brown sugar and stir for a minute. Remove from the heat. Spread the mixture as evenly as possible over the bottom of the pan.
4. Arrange five pineapple slices, overlapping, in a circular pattern in the bottom of the skillet. Cut the remaining slices in half and arrange along the sides of the skillet, cut side down. Place a pecan half in the center hole of each pineapple slice.

To prepare the cake:

5. Mix all the dry ingredients and sift into a bowl.
6. Mix the buttermilk with the water. Pour over the dry ingredients. Add the melted ghee or butter and mix just until blended.
7. Gently pour the batter over the pineapple design and spread evenly. Bake 40 to 45 minutes.
8. Allow to cool for 5 minutes. Very gently loosen with a knife. Invert a plate over the top of the skillet. Invert the skillet and plate to release the cake onto the plate. If any pineapple slices slip off in the unmolding, simply put them back in place.

VARIATION

Peach Upside-Down Cake: Replace the pineapple with peach slices and arrange them, overlapping, in a pinwheel formation in the center and along the sides. Omit the pecans.

 # GINGER FRUITCAKE

Two 9 × 5 × 3–inch (23 × 13 × 7.5 cm) loaves

Fruitcake is of Roman origin. Derived from its name, *satura,* are the words *saturate* and also *satire*—from its sour ingredients mixed in with the sweet. This particular version is prepared with natural dried fruits and is dedicated to the hordes and masses that dislike candied fruit peel in fruitcake. Vary the color by using either light or dark brown sugar or different proportions of unbleached white and whole wheat flour.

STEP ONE

¾ cup (95 g) raisins
2½ cups (540 ml) chopped mixed
  dried fruit

½ cup (80 g) chopped crystallized
  ginger
2 cups (480 ml) apple juice

STEP THREE

3¼ cups (490 g) whole wheat or
  part unbleached white flour
2 teaspoons baking powder
1 teaspoon baking soda
1½ teaspoons ground cinnamon

1 teaspoon ground cardamom
1 teaspoon ground cloves
2 cups (420 g) raw or
  packed brown sugar

STEP FOUR

2 cups (480 ml) chopped mixed nuts

STEP FIVE

Pecan halves

1. Soak the raisins, mixed dried fruit, and crystallized ginger overnight in the apple juice.
2. Preheat the oven to 300°F (150°C). Butter and lightly flour two 9 × 5 × 3–inch (23 × 13 × 7.5 cm) loaf pans.
3. Mix the flour, baking powder, soda, and spices and sift into a bowl. Stir in the sugar.
4. Add the apple juice mixture and the nuts. Stir until blended.
5. Spoon into the pans. Decorate the tops with pecan halves. Bake about 1¼ hours.

CHEESECAKES

Cheesecakes were popular fare in ancient Greece. They were offered up to the gods and were the subjects of philosophical writings—perhaps existential musings on the fact that some types of Greek cheesecake didn't contain cheese! Serve cheesecakes at lunch to balance Vata. These recipes are designed to be made in a 9-inch (23 cm) pie pan or springform cake pan—more common equipment in home kitchens than larger springform pans. If you do have a 12-inch (30 cm) springform pan, prepare 1½ recipes and spread the crumb crust on the bottom only, not up the sides.

AT PLAY IN THE CHEESECAKE UNIVERSE

❖ Replace Crumb Crust with Granola Crust or, European style, with Pastry Crust.

❖ Replace the water with fruit juice. Orange juice is particularly nice.

❖ Top a finished cheesecake with:

Toasted nuts
Sliced fresh fruit or cooled fruit sauce
A drizzle of Caramel Sauce (p. 458) or preserves thinned with lemon juice
Crumbled Louisiana Pralines (pp. 452–53)
Candied rose petals or violets

 # BAKED CHEESECAKE

One 9-inch (23 cm) cheesecake

STEP TWO

1½ *tablespoons arrowroot or cornstarch*
½ *cup (120 ml) water*
¼ *cup (120 ml) sour cream*

2 *cups (1 pound/500 g) cream cheese, softened*
¾ *cup (150 g) sugar*
1 *teaspoon finely grated lemon zest*

STEP THREE

9-*inch (23 cm) unbaked Crumb Crust (p. 410)*

STEP FOUR

1¼ *cups (300 ml) sour cream*

1. Preheat the oven to 350°F (180°C).
2. Mix the arrowroot or cornstarch, water, and sour cream in a blender or food processor. Add the cream cheese, sugar, and lemon zest. Blend until smooth.
3. Pour into the crust. Bake until the top is lightly browned in a few places, about 45 minutes. Don't mind any cracks that might appear.
4. Chill until firm. Spread the sour cream evenly over the top.

UNBAKED CHEESECAKE

One 9-inch (23 cm) cheesecake

STEP ONE

½ cup (120 ml) water

1 teaspoon agar agar flakes*

STEP TWO

2 cups (1 pound/500 g) cream
   cheese, softened
¼ cup (60 ml) sour cream

¾ cup (150 g) sugar
1 teaspoon finely grated lemon zest

STEP THREE

9-inch (23 cm) prebaked Crumb
   Crust (p. 410)

1¼ cups (300 ml) sour cream

1. Bring the water to a boil and sprinkle in the agar agar flakes. Stir, reduce the heat, and simmer for 5 minutes to dissolve the flakes.
2. Place the agar agar mixture in a blender with the cream cheese, sour cream, sugar, and lemon zest. Blend until smooth.
3. Pour into the crust. Chill until firm. Spread the sour cream evenly over the top.

 # COFFEE-ALMOND CHEESECAKE

One 9-inch (23 cm) cheesecake

STEP TWO

1½ teaspoons herbal coffee
   substitute powder (preferably
   Raja's Cup)

½ cup (120 ml) boiling water

STEP THREE

1¼ cups (125 g) finely crushed
   graham cracker crumbs
3 tablespoons sugar

¼ cup (35 g) slivered almonds
¼ cup (60 ml) melted ghee or butter

STEP FOUR

2 cups (1 pound/500 g) cream
   cheese, softened
¼ cup (60 ml) sour cream

1½ tablespoons arrowroot or
   cornstarch
¾ cup (150 g) sugar

STEP SIX

1¼ cups (300 ml) sour cream

¼ cup (35 g) blanched almonds,
   toasted

*This measurement is for agar agar flakes of which 1 tablespoon flakes thickens 1 quart (1 l) liquid. If your brand requires more to thicken, increase the measurement to 4 teaspoons.

1. Preheat the oven to 350°F (180°C). Butter a 9-inch (23 cm) pie pan or springform cake pan.
2. Place the herbal coffee substitute powder in a blender. Pour the boiling water over it and set aside.
3. Mix the graham cracker crumbs, sugar, and slivered almonds together. Add the melted ghee or butter and mix together well. Immediately sprinkle into the pan and press evenly over the bottom (and sides if using a pie pan). Set aside.
4. Add the cream cheese, sour cream, arrowroot or cornstarch, and sugar to the blender containing the coffee mixture. Blend until completely smooth.
5. Pour the filling evenly over the crust. Place in the oven and bake until the top is very lightly browned in a few places, about 45 minutes. Don't mind any cracks that might appear. Chill until firm.
6. Spread the sour cream evenly over the top. Decorate with the almonds.

 # LEMON-YOGURT CHEESECAKE FOR JERRY

One 9-inch (23 cm) cheesecake

My father's favorite recipe in the book—a high recommendation! The yogurt produces a light, fluffy cake with a special flavor and texture.

STEP TWO

3 cups (720 ml) yogurt	*½ cup (100 g) sugar*
3 tablespoons arrowroot or cornstarch	*1½ teaspoons finely grated lemon zest*

STEP THREE
9-inch unbaked Crumb Crust (p. 410)

1. Preheat the oven to 350°F (180°C).
2. Combine all the ingredients for the filling in a blender until smooth.
3. Pour into the crust. Bake until the top is lightly browned in a few places, 50 to 60 minutes.
4. Chill until firm. The filling will sink slightly.

COOKING AYURVEDIC FOOD FOR CHILDREN

Obstetrics and Pediatrics are major branches of Ayurvedic medicine. Ayurveda has specific recommendations for facilitating conception, healthy pregnancy and childbirth, and for caring for children's health and happiness—and also caring for the parents, especially the special needs of women who have just given birth.

❖ Knowing your children's doshas can help you better understand their personality traits and physiological needs. In fact, some parents learn pulse diagnosis so that they can determine what foods they need to maintain balance day-to-day. Also remember that childhood is the Kapha time of life, and children with a fair amount of Kapha in their makeup are particularly susceptible to Kapha-based illnesses like colds, flu, and congestion—especially during Kapha season and during damp, Kapha-aggravating weather

❖ Obviously mother's milk is the most perfectly designed first food. When a baby begins to take solids, freshly prepared foods are the most life-supporting. Bottled or frozen baby foods, even from the health food store, have heavy, ama-creating qualities.

❖ Ayurvedic recommendations for the proper preparation of milk on page 487 help give children the maximum benefit from cow's milk and minimize milk's congesting qualities.

❖ Following the seasonal dietary recommendations can help avoid some of the seasonal illnesses that children are so prone to and keep children more comfortable during "cold season," "flu season," and climatic extremes.

Parents who are deeply committed to Ayurveda in their own lives have told me that, while it is easy to follow the principles with babies and young children, once kids reach the age where they interact with other children and attend school, it can become very challenging to keep them on track. Kids are constantly exposed to less-than-balancing foods—at their friends' and relatives' houses, at school, and in a barrage of media enticements. Whether or not a child is willing to eat the way parents want depends on many factors: the child's personality, the relationship with the parents, and the influences the child is exposed to.

Parents who wish to keep their own doshas in balance will best succeed by staying very, very, flexible about keeping kids on an Ayurvedic routine. Tension and stress create ama—for you as well as for your kids! In the interest of promoting a lifetime of good physical and mental health, avoid creating pressure and guilt around food. Just do your best, practice what you preach (and don't preach too much), and be loving, patient, and accepting. Know that the loving attention you put into your food is the most nourishing element of Ayurvedic cooking, that although important, diet is only one part of the Ayurvedic picture, and that your unqualified love is the most Ayurvedic thing you can give to your children.

Who has not found heaven below will fail of it above.

—EMILY DICKINSON

Pies and Pastries

Pie is the food of the heroic. No pie-eating people can ever be permanently vanquished. —*New York Times, 1902*

Bake a good pie and the world will flock to your door—if not your kitchen. Different types of pies require different types of treatment—some are baked and some are not, some are double-crust and some are single-crust, and so forth. I will begin by describing how to construct a basic double-crust pie using a pastry crust. Some of the procedures apply to all types of pies, so if pie-baking is a new experience, read the instructions carefully before embarking on the recipe that appeals to you.

PIE CRUSTS

 ## PASTRY CRUST

One 9-inch (23 cm) double crust

Anyone . . . who wants to make pastry, or any other perquisite of gourmandism, can comfort himself with the certainty that if he is not born with this inarticulate knowledge he can acquire it. —M. F. K. FISHER

The basic flaky pie crust. To help ensure success, always handle the dough as little as possible, have the cold ingredients *cold*, and the oven *hot*. Flakiness is caused by a cold crust containing unmixed bits of butter coming into contact with high heat. You can make pie dough in a food processor; just take care not to overprocess. To help avoid overprocessing, add all the ingredients at once rather than in three separate steps.

2 *cups (280 g) unbleached*
    white flour   ½ *teaspoon salt*

⅔ *cup (145 g) chilled unsalted*
    butter

5 *to* 5½ *tablespoons (65 to 85 ml)*
    cold water

1. Sift the flour and salt into a mixing bowl.
2. Cut the butter into small pieces and work into the flour with your fingers or a pastry cutter until the mixture resembles coarse meal—the goal is for the butter not to completely disappear into the flour. If using your fingers, work quickly so that your body temperature doesn't warm the butter.
3. Add the cold water. Stir with a fork; then, using your hands, gather the mixture into a ball that just holds together. Do not knead or otherwise work the dough.
4. Wrap the dough in plastic wrap or waxed paper and chill for at least 1 hour. You can also prepare the dough the night before and let it chill overnight.
5. Remove the dough from the refrigerator and allow to stand at room temperature for 15 to 30 minutes so it can be rolled out without unnecessary manipulation. Pie dough makes a more tender crust if it is allowed to rest before being rolled out. Lightly butter a 9-inch (23 cm) pie pan.
6. Divide the dough in half. Roll out one of the halves on a lightly floured board. For best results, roll away from your body rather than back and forth, which stretches the dough. Be careful that the dough does not stick to the board. Pick it up once or twice during the rolling and change position slightly. Check to see that there is still enough flour on the board. A good method that uses no extra flour is to roll out the dough between 2 sheets of waxed paper or kitchen parchment. Then you can just peel off the paper when you've finished rolling. Roll out ⅛ inch (3 mm) thick and 2 inches (5 cm) wider than the diameter of the *rim* of the pie pan.
7. To transfer the pie dough to the pan, roll the dough loosely around the rolling pin and then unroll it into the pan. If rolled out initially on waxed paper, peel off the top sheet of paper, reverse the crust over the pie pan, and peel off the remaining sheet.
8. Gently press the crust into place. Mend any tears by lightly moistening the dough surrounding the tear with water and applying a patch of dough. Gently press to seal. Trim the crust so that it hangs 1 inch (2.5 cm) over the edges of the pan. At this point I put the pie pan in the freezer to chill while I prepare the pie filling.
9. Place the desired filling in the crust and spread evenly. Roll out the remaining pie dough in the same manner as the bottom crust and place over the filling. Trim the crust evenly around the outside edge so that it slightly overlaps. There are pie-edge trimmers that do this in fancy patterns. Otherwise, seal by pressing the edges

together with the tongs of a fork to leave a fluted design, or pinch in even ridges for a ripple effect. Prick the top crust with a fork in a few places to serve as air vents.
10. Bake according to your selected pie recipe.

VARIATIONS

Whole Wheat Crust: Replace 1 cup (140 g) unbleached white flour with whole wheat pastry flour. A pie crust can be made from 100 percent whole wheat pastry flour, but it is difficult to work with. You may have to press it into a pan by hand rather than rolling it out. The waxed paper method is best for rolling it out.

Wheat Germ or *Cornmeal Crust:* Replace ½ cup (70 g) flour with wheat germ or cornmeal.

Spice Crust: Add ½ teaspoon ground cinnamon, cardamom, or ginger.

Sweet Crust: Add 1 tablespoon sugar.

Savory Crust: Replace the water with cold vegetable stock. Add 2 tablespoons sesame seeds and 2 teaspoons dried green herbs, such as basil.

 # PREBAKED SINGLE PASTRY CRUST

One 9-inch (23 cm) single crust

Single-crust pies and tarts containing unbaked fillings call for a prebaked crust.

½ recipe Pastry Crust (pp. 406–407)

1. Roll out the dough and press into a pan as directed in the recipe.
2. Trim and decorate the edges as indicated for sealing, although here it is simply for appearance. If the dough has softened considerably, chill in the freezer for 20 to 30 minutes.
3. Preheat the oven to 450°F (230°C). Lay over the crust a piece of baking parchment large enough to completely cover it. Fill with a layer of rice, dried beans, or, as the French do, with small pebbles to weight it down. This will keep the crust from losing its shape. (You can keep a jar of beans, rice, or pebbles on hand for this purpose and reuse them many times.)
4. Bake until the edges are delicately browned, about 9 minutes. Carefully remove the weights and parchment. Return the crust to the oven for 3 to 6 minutes to brown the bottom. If the edges are browning too much, cover with pieces of foil.

PARTIALLY BAKED CRUST

One 9-inch (23 cm) single crust

Single-crust pies and quiches in which the filling needs to bake for a shorter period of time than the crust call for a partially baked crust.

½ recipe Pastry Crust (pp. 406–407)

1. Prepare a single crust for baking as for Prebaked Single Pastry Crust (opposite), Steps 1 to 3.
2. Bake until it begins to become crisp but does not brown, 6 to 8 minutes.
3. Carefully remove the weights and waxed paper. Return the crust to the oven for about 3 minutes to cook the bottom a bit more. Do not allow to brown.

 # GHEE OR OIL CRUST

One 9-inch (23 cm) double crust

The only advantages of an oil crust are that it contains half the amount of fat of a pastry crust and uses ghee or oil rather than butter. Otherwise, it is not flaky and does not roll out well. I recommend it only for those who wish to reduce their fat intake.

STEP ONE

2 cups (280 g) unbleached white flour   *½ teaspoon salt*

STEP TWO

*6 tablespoons (85 ml) melted ghee   3 tablespoons cold water
  or oil*

1. Sift the flour and salt into a bowl.
2. Beat the ghee or oil and water until creamy. Pour over the flour and mix lightly with a fork until blended.
3. Divide in half. Roll out by the waxed paper method or simply crumble into the pan and press. Fill and bake according to your selected pie recipe.

 # CREAM CHEESE CRUST

One 9-inch (23 cm) double crust

An exceptionally flaky and rich crust.

STEP ONE

*1½ cups (210 g) unbleached   *½ teaspoon salt*
  white flour*

STEP TWO

½ cup (115 g) unsalted butter, at
   room temperature

½ cup (4 ounces/120 g) cream
   cheese, at room temperature

1. Sift the flour and salt into a bowl.
2. Cut in the butter and cream cheese. Mix just until all the ingredients hold together in a ball.
3. Wrap in plastic wrap and chill for at least 1 hour. To soften a bit, remove from the refrigerator 20 to 30 minutes before rolling out.
4. Roll out in the same manner as Pastry Crust (pp. 406–407) and bake according to your selected pie recipe.

 ## CRUMB CRUST

One 9-inch (23 cm) single crust

Vary the flavor by using different crackers or cookies. Gingersnaps and biscotti make lovely crusts. To obtain the necessary fine texture, crush the crackers or cookies in a blender or food processor in small batches. Or, when in a low-tech mood, crumble the cookies or crackers by placing in a plastic bag, closing tightly, and rolling a rolling pin over them until finely crushed.

1¼ cups (125 g) finely crushed
   graham cracker or cookie crumbs
3½ tablespoons melted ghee or butter

2 tablespoons raw or packed brown
   sugar

1. Mix all the ingredients together. Immediately press evenly into a buttered 9-inch (23 cm) pie pan. If you wait, the ghee or butter will harden and the mixture will be difficult to work with. Once hardened, you can never really soften it up again.
2. *To prebake if required by your recipe:* Bake in a 350°F (180°C) oven until lightly browned, 10 to 12 minutes.

VARIATION

   Replace ¼ to ½ cup (25 to 50 g) crumbs with ground nuts (30 to 60 g). Reduce the ghee or butter by 1 teaspoon.

 ## GRANOLA CRUST

One 9-inch (23 cm) single crust

Granola crust is usually used for single-crust pies. However, it can be sprinkled on as a topping to form a double crust pie. Double the recipe if a topping is desired. Since granola crusts tend to bake quickly, a shiny metal pie pan is a better choice than quick-baking glass or dull metal pans.

STEP ONE

½ cup (60 g) chopped nuts	¼ teaspoon salt
⅔ cup (80 g) rolled oats	¼ cup (40 g) whole wheat flour
⅔ cup (80 g) wheat germ	3 tablespoons raw or brown sugar
½ cup (40 g) grated dried unsweetened coconut	

STEP TWO

2 tablespoons melted ghee, butter, or oil	3 tablespoons water

1. Mix the nuts and dry ingredients together.
2. Add the ghee, butter, or oil, and the water, and gently toss to coat the dry ingredients.
3. Immediately press into a buttered 9-inch (23 cm) pie pan.
4. *To prebake if required by your recipe:* Bake in a 350°F (180°C) oven until lightly browned, about 20 minutes.

 ## RICE FLOUR-NUT CRUST

One 9-inch (23 cm) single crust

For people with wheat allergies.

¾ cup (105 g) rice flour	¼ cup (50 g) raw or packed brown sugar
¾ cup (85 g) ground walnuts or other nuts	¼ cup (60 ml) melted ghee, butter, or oil

1. Mix all ingredients together well. Press into a buttered 9-inch (23 cm) pie pan.
2. *To prebake if required by your recipe:* Bake in a 350°F (180°C) oven for 20 to 30 minutes.
3. *To prepare a fruit pie:* Fill an unbaked crust with the fruit filling. Cover the pie with an inverted pie pan. Bake in a 350°F (180°C) oven for 1 hour.

PIES AND TARTS

> *To be a perfect cook, one must first be a distinguished pastry-maker.*
> —CARÊME (1786–1833), "THE COOK OF KINGS AND KING OF COOKS,"
> CHEF TO PRINCE TALLEYRAND OF FRANCE, CZAR ALEXANDER I
> OF RUSSIA, AND BARON ROTHSCHILD OF ENGLAND

Pies were originally savory main dishes. Fruit pies were born during the reign of that notorious sweet tooth Elizabeth I of England. After tasting a gift of preserved cherries, she commanded the planting of a thirty-acre cherry orchard—the first in her country. Soon summer royal banquets were completed with cherry pies.

❖ Fill the crust just before baking so that it doesn't get soggy.
❖ Fruit fillings often dribble out during baking. It's a good idea to place a baking pan on the rack below the pie to catch any falling filling.

 # BERRY, CHERRY, OR YOU-NAME-IT PIE

One 9-inch (23 cm) pie

A general formula for fruit pies. Almost all fresh fruits can be used in fruit pies, and small amounts of dried fruit and crystallized ginger can be mixed in as well. A caution: When crystallized ginger is mixed with apples, the apples do not become soft. Finely slice whole fruits.

STEP ONE

Pastry Crust (pp. 406–407)

STEP TWO

4 cups (950 ml) ripe berries or pitted ripe cherries, or thinly sliced fruit
2 tablespoons arrowroot, cornstarch, or quick-cooking tapioca

⅔ cup (150 g) sugar
2 teaspoons lemon juice

STEP THREE

1 tablespoon ghee or butter

1. Preheat the oven to 450°F (230°C). Line a buttered 9-inch (23 cm) pie pan with half of the pie dough.
2. Mix all the ingredients for the filling. If using quick-cooking tapioca, let the mixture soak for 15 minutes.
3. Spoon into the crust and spread evenly. Dot with the ghee or butter. Roll out the second half of the dough and place on top. Seal and prick in a few places with a fork.
4. Bake for 10 minutes. Reduce the temperature to 350°F (180°C) and continue baking until the crust is golden, about 45 minutes.

VARIATION

Mix a little sour cream into the filling.

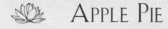 ## Apple Pie

One 9-inch (23 cm) pie

Good apple pies are a considerable part of our happiness.   —Jane Austen

Here are two ways to prepare this favorite, one with Pastry Crust and the other with Granola Crust. Granny Smith and other tart apples make full-flavored pies. Serve warm with whipped cream or ice cream.

STEP ONE

Pasty Crust (pp. 406–407) or 2 recipes
  Granola Crust (pp. 410–11)

STEP TWO

5½ to 6 cups (660 to 720 g) thinly   ¼ *teaspoon ground cinnamon*
  sliced peeled apples   *1 tablespoon arrowroot or*
⅓ *cup (70 g) sugar*   *cornstarch*
2 teaspoons lemon juice

STEP THREE

1 tablespoon ghee or butter

With Pastry Crust:
1. Preheat the oven to 450°F (230°C). Roll out half of the dough and line a buttered 9-inch (23 cm) pie pan with it.
2. Mix together the apples, sugar, lemon juice, cinnamon, and arrowroot or cornstarch.
3. Spoon into the crust and spread evenly. Dot with the ghee or butter. Roll out the second half of the dough and place on top. Seal and crimp the edges. Prick in a few places with a fork.
4. Bake for 10 minutes. Reduce the temperature to 350°F (180°C) and continue baking until the crust is golden, about 45 minutes.

With Granola Crust:
1. Preheat the oven to 350°F (180°C). Press half of it evenly into a buttered 9-inch (23 cm) pie pan.
2. Steam the apples until they start to become tender, about 5 minutes. Drain well. Mix with the remaining ingredients for the filling.
3. Melt the ghee or butter. Mix into the filling.
4. Spoon into the crust and spread evenly. Sprinkle the top with the remaining granola mixture.
5. Bake until the crust is lightly browned, 30 to 40 minutes.

COWHIG BLUEBERRY PIE

One 9-inch (23 cm) pie

With a pastry crust underneath and a streusel topping crowning the fruit filling, this style is known as a "Dutch pie." It is commonly filled with apples, and you can apply it to all manner of fruit fillings. This blueberry version is a family recipe from Mary Cowhig Zamarra, who recommends serving it with vanilla ice cream.

STEP ONE

Pastry Crust (pp. 406–407)

STEP TWO

4 cups (560 g) blueberries

STEP THREE

¾ to 1 cup (150 to 210 g) sugar *½ teaspoon ground cinnamon*
¼ cup (35 g) flour *½ teaspoon ground nutmeg*
⅛ teaspoon salt *1 teaspoon lemon juice*
½ to 1 teaspoon grated lemon zest

STEP FOUR

1 tablespoon ghee or butter

1. Preheat the oven to 400°F (200°C). Line a buttered 9-inch (23 cm) pie pan with half of the pie dough.
2. Spoon the berries evenly into the crust.
3. Mix the sugar, flour, salt, lemon zest, and spices in a bowl. Mix in the lemon juice.
4. Cut the ghee or butter into the dry mixture and work in until the mixture resembles coarse meal. Sprinkle over the berries.
5. Roll out the second half of the crust and place on top. Seal and prick in a few places with a fork.
6. Bake until the crust is golden, 40 to 50 minutes.

MANGO, PEACH, OR APRICOT PIE

One 9-inch (23 cm) pie

STEP ONE

Pastry Crust (pp. 406–407)

STEP TWO

5 cups (850 g) sliced peeled mangoes,
or sliced peaches or apricots,
blanched and peeled if desired
²/₃ cup (140 g) raw or packed
brown sugar

¼ teaspoon ground cinnamon
2 teaspoons lemon juice
1 tablespoon arrowroot or
cornstarch

STEP THREE

1 tablespoon ghee or butter

1. Preheat the oven to 450°F (230°C). Line a buttered 9-inch (23 cm) pie pan with half of the pie dough.
2. Drain the liquid from the fruit and mix the fruit with the sugar, cinnamon, lemon juice, and arrowroot or cornstarch.
3. Spoon into the crust and spread evenly. Dot with the ghee or butter. Roll out the second half of the dough and place on top. Seal and prick in a few places with a fork.
4. Bake for 10 minutes. Reduce the temperature to 350°F (180°C) and continue baking until the crust is golden, about 45 minutes.

VARIATION

Use a double recipe of Granola Crust (pp. 410–11). Bake for 30 to 40 minutes in a 350°F (180°C) oven.

Tapioca, derived from the *manioc* root, is a natural substance used in Ayurvedic cooking that can replace arrowroot or cornstarch in fruit sauces and pie fillings. Always use *tapioca flour* and *quick-cooking tapioca* to thicken sauces and pie fillings—not *pearl tapioca*. From 1 to 2 tablespoons of quick-cooking tapioca will thicken 4 cups of fruit mixture. Let the tapioca soak with the fruit mixture for 15 minutes before cooking.

 # RHUBARB PIE

One 9-inch (23 cm) pie

STEP ONE

Pastry Crust (pp. 406–407)

STEP TWO

4 cups (1 pound/500 g) rhubarb,
cut into ¾-inch pieces

1½ cups (310 g) sugar
¼ cup (35 g) unbleached white flour

STEP THREE

1 tablespoon ghee or butter

1. Line a buttered 9-inch (23 cm) pie pan with half of the pie dough.
2. Mix the rhubarb, sugar, and flour together. Allow to stand for 15 minutes.
3. Preheat the oven to 400°F (200°C). Spoon the rhubarb mixture into the crust and spread evenly. Dot with the ghee or butter. Roll out the second half of the dough and place on top. Seal and prick in a few places with a fork.
4. Bake for 10 minutes. Reduce the temperature to 350°F (180°C) and bake until the crust is golden, about 45 minutes.

VARIATION

Strawberry-Rhubarb Pie: Replace half the rhubarb with 2 cups (310 g) sliced strawberries.

 # MINCE PIE

ENGLAND   *One 9-inch (23 cm) pie*

King Henry VIII of England's Christmas *minc'd pye* was being escorted to the castle by Jack Horner. The temptation was too great, and he thrust a finger into it, hoping to pull out a plum. What he struck was paper—the title deeds to twelve manors. A nursery rhyme was born.

STEP ONE

Pastry Crust (pp. 406–407)

STEP TWO

3 cups (360 g) coarsely chopped apples
1 cup (125 g) raisins
⅔ cup (140 g) raw or packed brown sugar
¼ cup (70 g) chopped dates
¼ cup (40 g) chopped figs
¼ cup (40 g) chopped prunes
¼ cup (30 g) chopped crystallized orange rind

1 teaspoon finely grated lemon zest
⅓ cup (80 ml) orange juice
¼ cup (60 ml) lemon juice
2 tablespoons arrowroot or cornstarch
½ teaspoon ground cinnamon
¼ teaspoon ground cloves

1. Preheat the oven to 450°F (230°C). Line a buttered 9-inch (23 cm) pie pan with half of the pie dough.
2. Mix all the ingredients for the filling together. Spoon into the crust and spread

evenly. Roll out the second half of the dough and place on top. Seal and prick in a few places with a fork.

3. Bake for 10 minutes. Reduce the temperature to 350°F (180°C) and continue baking until the crust is golden, about 45 minutes.

VARIATION

Replace the arrowroot or cornstarch with tapioca. Allow the filling to sit for 15 minutes before placing in the crust.

 # AVOCADO-LIME PIE

One 9-inch (23 cm) pie

Lime pies usually obtain their green color from a bottle of chemicals; this one comes by its color honestly, along with its creaminess, from avocados. Use Key limes if you can find them.

STEP ONE

1 cup (250 g) chopped well-drained pineapple (optional)

Prebaked Crumb Crust (p. 410)

STEP TWO

½ cup (120 ml) lime juice
¼ cup (60 ml) water

1 tablespoon agar agar flakes*
¾ cup (150 g) sugar

STEP THREE

2 ripe medium avocados, pitted and peeled

½ teaspoon ground ginger

STEP FOUR

1 cup (240 ml) heavy (whipping) cream

STEP FIVE

¼ cup (35 g) grated unsweetened coconut, toasted

1. Spread the pineapple, if using, evenly over the pie shell.
2. Combine the lime juice and water in a saucepan. Bring to a boil. Add the agar agar flakes and simmer, stirring constantly, until dissolved, about 5 minutes. Stir in the sugar.
3. Place in a blender or food processor. Add the avocados and ginger and purée.
4. Whip the cream until it stands in soft peaks. Gently fold in the avocado mixture.
5. Spoon into the crust and spread evenly. Sprinkle the coconut over the top. Chill until firm.

---

*This measurement is for agar agar flakes of which 1 tablespoon flakes thickens 1 quart (1 l) liquid. If your brand requires more to thicken, increase the measurement to 4 teaspoons.

VARIATION

Replace the ground ginger with 2 or 3 pieces chopped crystallized ginger. Fold into the mixture in Step 4.

 # STRAWBERRY OR ANY FRUIT TART

FRANCE   *One 9-inch (23 cm) tart*

Doubtless God could have made a better berry, but doubtless God never did.
—WILLIAM BUTLER, DESCRIBING STRAWBERRIES

For those days when you are not having William Butler over for lunch, there are plenty of other berries that are also sumptuous in a tart. Also other fruits. Halved fresh figs are doubtless my favorite option during their fleeting season. Blanched peeled peach and apricot halves are classic and wonderful.

STEP ONE

Prebaked Single Pastry Crust (p. 408),
baked in a 9-inch (23 cm)
removable-bottom tart pan

STEP TWO

Cream Filling:

1 tablespoon arrowroot or
cornstarch
1 cup (240 ml) heavy (whipping)
cream or half-and-half
3 tablespoons sugar

STEP THREE

1 quart (620 g) strawberries, evenly
sized, with good color

STEP FOUR

Jam Glaze or Fresh Fruit Glaze
(see box opposite)

1. Allow the crust to cool completely. Carefully transfer from the pan to a serving plate.
2. Dissolve the arrowroot or cornstarch in half of the cream. Place in a saucepan with the remaining cream and the sugar. Heat slowly, stirring constantly with a whisk, until thickened. Let cool. Spread the cream filling evenly over the bottom of the crust.

3. Stud the filling with the strawberries, stem end down. Chill while preparing the glaze.
4. Spoon a little glaze over each strawberry to coat. Chill the tart to firm up the cream filling and the glaze.

Jam Glaze: Melt apricot jam and simmer for a few minutes over low heat, stirring constantly. Allow to cool for a few minutes before spooning over the tart.

Fresh Fruit Glaze:

⅓ cup (80 g) puréed steamed
   apricots (fresh or dried)
1 tablespoon lemon juice
¼ cup (50 g) sugar

Place all the ingredients in a saucepan. Bring to a boil and cook for 5 minutes over medium heat, stirring constantly. Allow to cool for a few minutes before spooning over the tart.

VARIATIONS
✪ Replace the dairy in the filling with thick coconut milk.
Instead of cream filling, use 1 cup (235 g) sweetened ricotta cheese, mascarpone, Hung Yogurt (p. 534), or Tofu Dessert Cream (p. 503).
Apricot, Nectarine, or Peach Tart: To prepare the fruit for the tart, drop into rapidly boiling water for 1 minute. Drain. Gently remove the skins. Cut into perfect halves and remove the pits. Carefully cover the cream mixture with the fruit halves, cut side down, in Step 3. Arrange them around the outside edge first and work inward.

 # TARTE AUX POMMES (APPLE TART)

FRANCE   *One 9-inch (23 cm) tart*

A friendly cow, all red and white,
I love with all my heart;
She gives me cream with all her might,
To eat with apple-tart.   —ROBERT LOUIS STEVENSON

STEP ONE

½ recipe Pastry Crust (pp. 406–407)
   baked in a 9-inch (23 cm)
   removable-bottom tart pan

STEP TWO

1 cup (215 g) sweetened
  Applesauce (pp. 463)

STEP THREE

2 cups (240 g) thinly sliced peeled   1 tablespoon lemon juice
  apples   1 teaspoon arrowroot or
3 tablespoons sugar   cornstarch
1 tablespoon melted ghee or butter

1. Preheat the oven to 375°F (190°C). Line a buttered 9-inch (23 cm) removable-bottom tart pan with the pie dough.
2. Spread the applesauce evenly over the bottom of the crust.
3. Mix the apples with the sugar, ghee or butter, lemon juice, and arrowroot or cornstarch. Arrange the apples in concentric circles around the outside edge. Fill the center with another concentric circle or with a nice design.
4. Bake until the crust is done, 45 to 50 minutes. Let cool thoroughly, then gently transfer from the pan to a plate.

 ## PECAN PIE

UNITED STATES   One 9-inch (23 cm) pie

Here it is—a pecan pie without eggs or corn syrup. The configuration looks a little strange when you put it together—but oh, how it works! Follow the recipe exactly—even slight variations can flounder. Believe me, I know. Serve with whipped cream or crème fraîche.

STEP ONE

½ recipe Pastry Crust (pp. 406–407)

STEP TWO

⅔ cup (90 g) unbleached white flour   2 teaspoons arrowroot or
⅔ cup (140 g) packed dark brown   cornstarch
  sugar   ¾ teaspoon baking powder

STEP THREE

6 tablespoons (85 g) butter   2 cups (180 g) pecan halves

STEP FOUR

1 cup (240 ml) water
⅔ cup (160 ml) rice or barley malt syrup

1. Preheat the oven to 375°F (190°C). Line a buttered 9-inch (23 cm) pie pan with the pie dough. Reserve in the freezer until ready to use.
2. Mix the flour, sugar, arrowroot or cornstarch, and baking powder together.
3. Cut the butter into small pieces and work into the flour mixture thoroughly until the mixture resembles cookie crumbs. A food processor does a good job. Stir in the pecans.
4. Mix the water and rice or barley malt syrup together thoroughly (a blender helps). Sprinkle ½ of the flour mixture into the pie crust. Pour ½ of the liquid over it. Repeat with the remaining flour mixture and liquid. Gently stir a few times so that the flour mixture is moistened, but do not mix thoroughly.
5. Place in the oven with a pan on the rack below it to catch any drips. Bake until the crust is golden and the top lightly browned, 50 to 60 minutes. Allow to cool for at least a few hours before serving.

 # TOTALLY NUTS FOR STEVE PIE

One 9-inch (23 cm) pie

Pecan pie laced with orange, crystallized ginger, and coconut. Replace ½ cup of the pecans with pistachios or macadamia nut halves to up the ante even more.

STEP ONE
½ recipe Pastry Crust (pp. 406–407)

STEP TWO

⅔ cup (90 g) unbleached white flour
⅔ cup (140 g) packed dark brown sugar
2 teaspoons arrowroot or cornstarch

¾ teaspoon baking powder
¼ cup (35 g) dried unsweetened grated coconut
1 tablespoon finely grated orange zest

STEP THREE

6 tablespoons (85 g) butter
1¾ cups (170 g) pecan halves

⅓ cup (55 g) coarsely chopped crystallized ginger

STEP FOUR

¾ cup (180 ml) orange juice
¼ cup (60 ml) water

⅔ cup (160 ml) rice or barley malt syrup

1. Preheat the oven to 375°F (190°C). Line a buttered 9-inch (23 cm) pie pan with the pie dough. Reserve in the freezer until ready to use.
2. Mix the flour, sugar, arrowroot or cornstarch, and baking powder together. Add the coconut and orange zest and mix well.
3. Cut the butter into small pieces and work into the flour mixture thoroughly until

the mixture resembles cookie crumbs. A food processor does a good job. Stir in the pecans and crystallized ginger.

4. Mix the orange juice, water, and rice or barley malt syrup together. Sprinkle ½ of the flour mixture into the pie crust. Pour ½ of the liquid over it. Repeat with the remaining flour mixture and liquid. Gently stir a few times so that the flour mixture is moistened, but do not mix thoroughly.

5. Place in the oven with a pan on the rack below it to catch any drips. Bake until the crust is golden and the top lightly browned, 50 to 60 minutes. Allow to cool for at least a few hours before serving. Refrigerate to hasten the process.

 # PUMPKIN PIE

One 9-inch (23 cm) pie

What moistens the lip and what brightens the eye?
What calls back the past, like the rich Pumpkin pie?

—JOHN GREENLEAF WHITTIER

You can substitute sweet potatoes for the pumpkin. All manner of winter squash also work well; kabocha squash has a particularly lovely color and texture. White sugar gives the pie best color.

STEP ONE

½ recipe Pastry Crust (pp. 406–407)

STEP TWO

3 tablespoons arrowroot or cornstarch	*⅛ teaspoon salt* (optional)
½ cup (120 ml) milk or cream	*2 tablespoons ghee or butter*
2¾ cups (400 g) puréed cooked pumpkin	*1 teaspoon ground cinnamon*
1 cup (210 g) sugar	*¼ teaspoon ground nutmeg*
	¼ teaspoon ground ginger
	⅛ teaspoon ground cloves

1. Preheat the oven to 350°F (180°C). Line a buttered 9-inch (23 cm) pie pan with the pie dough.

2. Dissolve the arrowroot or cornstarch in the milk or cream. Beat in with all the ingredients for the filling; a blender or food processor does a good job.

3. Pour the filling into the crust and spread evenly.

4. Bake for 1 hour. Let cool to room temperature to firm up the filling.

VARIATION

Unbaked Pumpkin Pie: Prepare Prebaked Single Pastry Crust (p. 408). Cook the above pie filling in a saucepan over low heat, stirring constantly, until it thickens. Pour into the crust and chill until firm.

Cookery, the most selfless of arts because the least enduring. A bite or two, a little gulp, and a beautiful work of thought and love is no more.

—SYBIL RYALL, *A Fiddle for Sixpence*

 ## SHOOFLY PIE

UNITED STATES   *One 9-inch (23 cm) pie*

A Pennsylvania Dutch creation, named for the action necessary to protect the molasses-sweetened confection from winged marauders while it cooled on a kitchen windowsill. The Vata-balancing filling is made by an unusual process and comes out like a gooey molasses brownie in a pie shell.

STEP ONE

½ recipe Pastry Crust (pp. 406–407)

STEP TWO

1¼ cups unbleached white flour (175 g) or whole wheat flour (190 g)
½ cup (100 g) sugar
½ teaspoon baking powder

½ teaspoon ground cinnamon
¼ teaspoon ground cloves
¼ teaspoon ground nutmeg
¼ teaspoon salt
⅓ cup (75 g) butter

STEP THREE

½ cup (120 ml) dark unsulphured molasses
1 cup (240 ml) strong herbal coffee (preferably made with Raja's Cup)

½ teaspoon baking soda

1. Preheat the oven to 375°F (190°C). Line a buttered 9-inch (23 cm) pie pan with the pie dough. Reserve in the freezer until ready to use.
2. Mix the flour, sugar, baking powder, spices, and salt together. Cut the butter into small pieces and work into the flour mixture thoroughly until the mixture resembles slightly moist crumbs. A food processor does a good job.
3. Mix the molasses, herbal coffee, and baking soda together. It's all right if the coffee is still hot—some cooks recommend it that way.

4. Sprinkle ⅓ of the flour mixture into the pie crust. Pour ½ of the molasses mixture over it. Repeat with ⅓ more of the flour mixture and the remaining molasses mixture. Sprinkle the remaining flour mixture on top. At this point, I usually can't help myself and attempt to stir them together a little, but it's really not necessary to do so.

5. Bake until the filling is set and the crust is lightly browned, about 45 minutes. Let cool thoroughly before serving.

 # COCONUT CREAM PIE

One 9-inch (23 cm) pie

Prebaked pie crusts can be filled with any of the arrowroot- or cornstarch-based puddings in the "Puddings" chapter. Chill and top with whipped cream.

STEP ONE

3 tablespoons arrowroot or *cornstarch*	*1 cup (210 g) sugar*
2¼ cups (540 ml) heavy (whipping) *cream or half and half*	*3 tablespoons ghee or butter* *2 cups (160 g) grated fresh or* *dried unsweetened coconut*

STEP THREE

Prebaked single pie crust, any type

STEP FOUR

¾ cup (180 ml) heavy (whipping) *cream*	*1 tablespoon or more confectioner's* *sugar or honey*

1. Dissolve the arrowroot or cornstarch in ¼ cup (60 ml) of the cream. Pour into a saucepan. Add the remaining cream, sugar, ghee or butter, and coconut.
2. Heat, stirring constantly, until thickened. Do not boil.
3. Pour into the crust. Chill until firm.
4. Just before serving, whip the second amount of cream until stiff. Sweeten with the confectioner's sugar or honey. Spread over the pie.

VARIATIONS

❂ Replace the cream with coconut milk. Replace the whipped cream topping with sliced fruit.

Tropical Pie: Cover the whipped cream topping with drained crushed pineapple, mango slices, and a sprinkling of toasted grated coconut.

Pastries

*The fine arts are five: Painting, sculpture, poetry, music, and architecture—
which has as its principal branch, pastry.* —Carême

 # Baklavá

GREECE *Thirty 2½-inch (6.5 cm) pieces*

Room can always be found for a delicacy. —Babylonian Talmud

There is evidence of baklavá in Constantinople during the reign of Emperor Justinian.
The Persian version was originally flavored with pussy willow and jasmine blossoms.
Today this food for the Olympian gods is associated with its adoptive country, Greece,
where it is prepared for New Year's and other celebratory occasions.

STEP TWO

*4 cups (420 g) ground walnuts or a
mixture of ground walnuts,
pistachios, and pine nuts*

*½ cup (100 g) sugar
2 teaspoons ground cinnamon*

STEP THREE

¾ cup (165 g) ghee or butter

¾ cup (180 ml) mild-flavored oil

STEP FOUR

*1 pound (500 g) frozen filo pastry
(24 sheets)*

STEP TEN

*2½ cups (520 g) sugar
1¼ cups (300 ml) water
2 tablespoons lemon juice*

*3 tablespoons honey
A few drops of rose water*

STEP ELEVEN

Chopped pistachios (optional)

1. Preheat the oven to 300°F (150°C).
2. Mix the ground nuts with the sugar and cinnamon. Set aside.
3. Melt the ghee or butter. Mix with the oil. Brush a 15 × 11-inch (38 × 28 cm) pan
   with the oil mixture. A broiling pan can be used if it has shallow sides. Cover it
   with foil to smooth out the grooves.
4. Lay 1 sheet of filo pastry flat in the pan. Brush with the oil mixture. It does not have
   to be coated completely; just make certain that most of the area has some oil on or

near it. Lay down another sheet and brush with oil again. Repeat until 6 sheets are in the pan.

5. Sprinkle 1 cup of the nut mixture over the pastry.

6. Lay down 6 more sheets of the pastry, brushing each with the oil mixture. Sprinkle 1 cup of the nut mixture over the pastry.

7. Repeat twice more, laying down 6 sheets of pastry and 1 cup of the nut mixture. Top with the remaining 6 sheets of pastry and pour any remaining oil over the top.

8. Score the top layer ¼-inch (8 mm) deep with a knife, making 2½-inch (6.5 cm) wide diamond shapes to guide later cutting. Sprinkle a little water over the pastry to make the dough lie flat.

9. Bake for 1 to 1¼ hours, until the pastry is a very pale gold—not browned.

10. While the baklavá is cooling, prepare the syrup. Boil the sugar, water, and lemon juice together for 5 minutes. Let cool to room temperature. Stir in the honey and rose water.

11. When the baklavá has cooled to room temperature, pour the syrup over it. If desired, sprinkle the top with pistachios. Let the baklavá soak in the syrup for at least 1 hour before serving. Cut into diamond shapes.

 ## PINEAPPLE SQUARES

24 squares

The wit who proclaimed "You can never be too thin nor too rich" could have been describing my mother-in-law's tour-de-force dessert. The pastry should be quite thin: a layer of pie dough spread with a thin layer of pineapple filling, topped with latticework pastry and a sprinkling of walnuts.

STEP ONE

4 cups (560 g) unbleached white flour	3 tablespoons arrowroot or cornstarch
2 tablespoons sugar	1 teaspoon salt

STEP TWO

1 pound (500 g) butter

STEP FIVE

2½ cups (615 g) well-drained finely chopped fresh pineapple	1 cup (210 g) sugar
3 tablespoons arrowroot or cornstarch	

STEP EIGHT

⅔ cup (65 g) finely chopped
walnuts

STEP TEN

Confectioner's sugar

1. Combine the flour, sugar, arrowroot or cornstarch, and salt in a bowl.
2. Cut the butter into little pieces, add to the dry ingredients, and work in with your fingers or a pastry cutter to form a pie dough.
3. Wrap and refrigerate for at least 2 hours. Remove the dough from the refrigerator to soften about 20 minutes before assembling the pastry.
4. Preheat the oven to 350°F (180°C). Lightly butter an 18- × 12-inch (46 × 32 cm) baking pan or cookie sheet.
5. Mix the pineapple, arrowroot or cornstarch, and sugar together until thoroughly blended. Set aside.
6. Roll out the pie dough ⅛ inch (3 mm) thick. Place in the pan and form a ¼ inch (6 mm) high rim around the edges. Trim and set aside the excess dough (there should be quite a bit) for the lattice top.
7. Spread the pineapple mixture evenly over the dough.
8. Roll out the reserved dough into a long piece ⅛ inch (3 mm) thick. Cut into strips ½ inch (1.5 cm) wide with a sharp knife or pie-edge trimmer. Place the strips diagonally in a lattice pattern over the pineapple. It is not necessary to interweave the strips; just lay them down flat. Sprinkle the walnuts over the entire pastry.
9. Bake until the pastry is golden, 35 to 40 minutes.
10. Let cool thoroughly. Place confectioner's sugar in a sieve and shake a light dusting onto the pastry. Cut into squares to serve.

 # JALEBIS (SWEET SPIRALS)

INDIA　　*About 40 spirals*

Deep-fried spirals of translucent pastry coated with a sweet syrup, *jalebis* are found in the Middle East as well as in India. A little practice is required to make perfect (or even imperfect) spirals; in the meantime, abstract squiggles à la Jackson Pollack are perfectly acceptable.

STEP ONE

3 cups (520 g) unbleached white flour	*1 Tablespoon baking powder*
¼ teaspoon saffron soaked in	*¼ cup (60 ml) yogurt*
¼ cup (60 ml) hot water	*1¾ cups (240 ml) water*

STEP TWO

1 cup (240 g)water   *1¾ cups (360 g)sugar*

STEP THREE

Oil for deep-frying

STEP SIX

A few drops of rose water

To prepare the batter:
1. Combine all the ingredients for the batter in a blender or food processor until smooth. Allow to stand at room temperature for 2 hours.

To prepare the syrup:
2. Combine the water and sugar. Bring to a boil, and boil for 5 minutes or until the syrup thickens slightly. Reduce the heat to a simmer.

To cook:
3. Heat oil for deep-frying. Have a platter covered with paper towels nearby.
4. Place a plain round nib on a pastry tube. Hold the nib shut and fill the bag halfway with batter. Pipe the batter in 3-inch (7.5 cm) spirals into hot oil. The batter will run out of the tube without having to be forced. If it is too difficult to pipe spirals, just pipe abstract patterns about 3 inches (7.5 cm) in width.
5. Deep-fry the jalebis on both sides until golden brown. Drain on paper towels.
6. Add the rose water to the syrup, and gently drop a few jalebis into the simmering syrup. Simmer for 2 to 3 minutes, making sure the jalebis are coated with the syrup. Remove to a plate. Repeat in small batches until all the jalebis are done. Serve when thoroughly dry and crisp.

Heaven . . . a treasury of everlasting joy.

—WILLIAM SHAKESPEARE, *Henry VI*

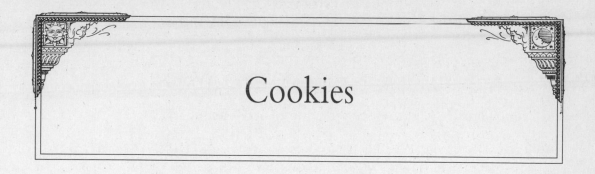

Cookies

The oven is the mother.   —OLD PROVERB

The word *cookie* comes from the Dutch, *koekje*. Along with fruit pies, cookies are a universal delight. Adding some dried cranberries, replacing nuts with pumpkin or sunflower seeds, and using spices will add a little balance for Kapha in an otherwise mostly Vata and Pitta cookie universe. Drier, crunchier cookies are also more balancing to Kapha than soft, moist ones. Preparing cookie dough is relatively simple, but baking eggless cookies requires alertness and attention.

Five Essential Elements of Eggless Cookies

I. Cookies made from 100 percent whole wheat flour are crumbly. I usually use unbleached white flour for smooth-textured cookies, reserving small additions of whole wheat for doughs containing wheat germ, ground nuts, and other textured ingredients.

II. Place cookies on thoroughly cooled baking sheets. If the sheets are hot, the dough will spread too much and the bottom of the cookies may burn. Wait between each batch for the baking sheets to cool—it is only a matter of a few minutes.

III. Eggless cookies tend to stick to the sheet if they are cooled on it. Therefore, even if soft and fragile, when they are done, transfer immediately to a plate using a spatula. The cookies will be too soft and floppy to use a standard cooling rack. A fine mesh rack is nice, but a plate works perfectly well.

IV. Do not stack cooling cookies or otherwise allow them to touch. Cookies that cool together stay together.

V. The fastest way to prepare cookie dough is in a food processor. Make the dough in the processor and stir in textured additions, such as nuts and raisins, by hand.

AT PLAY IN THE COOKIE UNIVERSE

You can use the same basic dough to make different styles of cookies.

❖ *Rolled cookies:* Roll out a fairly firm dough on a well-floured board ⅛ to ¼ inch (3 to 6 mm) thick and cut out with cookie cutters, the rim of a glass for round cookies, or a knife to make fancy individual shapes. Properly prepared rolled cookies hold their shape during baking and do not spread out very much.

❖ *Drop cookies:* Easy because you don't have to shape individual cookies. Add a little more liquid to make a thick, sticky batter. Place spoonfuls of batter 1½ inches (4 cm) apart on a buttered baking sheet. The cookies spread out during the baking.

❖ *Refrigerator cookies:* An easy solution for times when you need to make large amounts or when it's more convenient to prepare the dough and bake the cookies in two separate time periods. Roll firm cookie dough into a cylinder of the diameter desired for the cookies. Wrap in waxed paper or plastic wrap and chill in the refrigerator until very firm, 6 to 12 hours. When ready to bake, slice off cookies ⅛ to ¼ inch (3 to 6 mm) thick and bake.

Basic cookies, such as Butter Cookies and Oatmeal Cookies, are especially welcoming to additions:

Granola
Raisins, currants, and chopped dried fruit
Chopped crystallized ginger
Grated coconut
Sesame, sunflower, or pumpkin seeds and chopped or halved nuts
Finely grated citrus zest
Sweet spices: cinnamon, cardamom, nutmeg or mace, ground ginger, cloves, allspice
Herbal coffee substitute powder, preferably Raja's Cup

 # BUTTER COOKIES

4 dozen

Tender and buttery, these cookies can be served as is or used as a stage on which to entertain additions such as nuts and raisins. They can be prepared as rolled cookies or refrigerator cookies, or you can just form them into patties.

STEP TWO

2½ cups (570 g) unsalted butter   2¼ cups (260 g) sugar

STEP THREE

4⅓ cups (600 g) unbleached   1 teaspoon baking powder
   white flour   ½ to ¾ cup (120 to 180 ml)
1 teaspoon salt   nondairy milk

1. Preheat the oven to 350°F (180°C). Butter cookie sheets.
2. Cream the butter and sugar thoroughly.
3. Sift in the flour, salt, and baking powder. Add milk to make a soft dough. (Make a fairly firm dough for rolled cookies.)
4. Shape into ⅛-inch (3 mm) thick cookies by the desired method. Place on the cookie sheets ½ inch (1.5 cm) apart.
5. Bake until done, 12 to 15 minutes. Using a spatula, transfer immediately to a plate to cool and harden.

VARIATION

Raisin Cookies: Add 1 cup (125 g) or more raisins to the dough.

OATMEAL COOKIES

2½ to 3 dozen

Try preparing oatmeal cookies with pecan halves and chopped dates for something special.

STEP TWO

½ cup (115 g) unsalted butter
1¼ cups (260 g) raw or packed
   brown sugar

STEP THREE

1 cup (140 g) unbleached white   1 teaspoon ground cinnamon
   flour   ¾ teaspoon ground ginger
1 teaspoon baking powder   ¼ teaspoon ground cloves
½ teaspoon salt

STEP FOUR

3 cups (345 g) rolled oats   1 cup raisins (125 g) or chopped
¾ cup (180 ml) nondairy milk   dates (285 g)
½ cup (60 g) chopped nuts

1. Preheat the oven to 350°F (180°C). Butter cookie sheets.
2. Cream the butter and sugar thoroughly.

3. Sift all the dry ingredients except the oats together over the butter-sugar mixture.
4. Add the oats and the milk. Stir until blended. Beat in the nuts and raisins or dates.
5. Drop spoonfuls of batter onto a cookie sheet 1½ inches (3.5 cm) apart.
6. Bake until done, 12 to 15 minutes. Using a spatula, transfer immediately to a plate to cool and harden.

 # PUMPKIN COOKIES

3 dozen

You can prepare these cookies with any type of winter squash. Yams and kabocha squash give them a particular pretty orange color.

STEP TWO

½ *cup (115 g) unsalted butter*
1 *cup (210 g) raw or packed light brown sugar*

STEP THREE

2 *cups (280 g) unbleached white flour*
2 *tablespoons arrowroot or cornstarch*
½ *teaspoon baking powder*

⅛ *teaspoon salt*
¾ *teaspoon ground cinnamon*
¾ *teaspoon ground nutmeg*
½ *teaspoon ground cloves*

STEP FOUR

1¼ *cups (290 g) puréed cooked pumpkin*
1 *cup (95 g) coarsely chopped pecans*

⅓ *cup (55 g) chopped candied ginger*
⅔ *cup chopped dates (120 g) or raisins (90 g)*

STEP FIVE

Pecan halves

1. Preheat the oven to 350°F (180°C). Butter cookie sheets.
2. Cream the butter and sugar thoroughly.
3. Sift the dry ingredients together over the butter-sugar mixture.
4. Add the pumpkin and mix until the ingredients are blended. Beat in the chopped nuts, crystallized ginger, and dates or raisins.
5. Drop large spoonfuls of the batter onto the baking sheets about 1 inch (2.5 cm) apart. Flatten the top of each cookie slightly and press a pecan half into it.
6. Bake until done, 12 to 15 minutes. Using a spatula, transfer immediately to a plate to cool and harden.

ALMOND CRESCENTS

4 dozen

Little melt-in-your-mouth cookies that balance Vata and Pitta. The dough can also be pressed into a pan and baked in the same manner as shortbreads.

STEP ONE

1 cup (230 g) unsalted butter
1 cup (210 g) raw or packed
   light brown sugar

STEP TWO

2¼ cups (315 g) unbleached
   white flour
½ teaspoon salt

1⅓ cups (180 g) ground almonds
3 tablespoons water

STEP SIX

Confectioner's sugar

1. Cream the butter and sugar thoroughly.
2. Sift the flour and salt over the butter-sugar mixture. Add the almonds and water. Mix well.
3. Wrap in waxed paper or plastic wrap and chill for at least 1 hour.
4. Preheat the oven to 300°F (150°C). Butter baking sheets.
5. Roll into 1-inch (2.5 cm) balls. Gently shape into fat crescents. Bake until lightly browned, 20 to 25 minutes.
6. Immediately remove from the baking sheets and sift a light dusting of confectioner's sugar on them.

VARIATION
Replace the almonds with ground hazelnuts, walnuts, or other nuts.

 # RANGER COOKIES

2½ dozen

STEP TWO

½ cup (115 g) unsalted butter
1½ cups (310 g) raw or packed
   brown sugar

STEP THREE

1½ cups (165 g) rolled oats
¾ cup (60 g) dried grated
   unsweetened coconut
1 cup (150 g) whole wheat flour

1 teaspoon baking powder
½ teaspoon salt
¼ cup (60 ml) nondairy milk

1. Preheat the oven to 350°F (180°C). Butter cookie sheets.
2. Cream the butter and sugar thoroughly.
3. Add the oats and coconut. Sift the remaining dry ingredients over the mixture. Add the milk and mix well.
4. Roll into balls and place on the cookie sheets 1 inch (2.5 cm) apart. Press the tines of a fork against each cookie to form an indentation and flatten the cookie slightly.
5. Bake until done, 12 to 15 minutes. Using a spatula, transfer immediately to a plate to cool and harden.

CRAVINGS FOR SWEETS: AN AYURVEDIC UNDERSTANDING

Cravings are a warning signal that something is out of balance. One general understanding about sweets cravings is that the need to eat sweets can be caused by the body's response to aggravations of Vata and Pitta dosha, both of which are balanced by the sweet taste. People often reach for sweets when they are anxious or under a lot of pressure— a response to emotional conditions that aggravate Vata. Because movement is a quality of Vata dosha, travel and excessive exercise, both of which involve movement, can aggravate Vata and cause a sweets craving. Traumatic experiences such as an accident or surgery aggravate Vata and can trigger a desire for sweets. The onset of menses and menopause involve Pitta, which governs blood, and can trigger sweet cravings. Climatic changes, such as chilly winds or a heat wave, can increase Vata and Pitta respectively. And so forth. Ama, the toxic substance formed from improperly digested food, can also be a cause, as people tend to poop out more quickly when clogged up with ama and may reach for sweets to fortify their flagging energy. Such factors can result in occasional cravings for sweets, or they may tip the scales of a deeper imbalance and trigger the onset of a nonstop craving that can swoop down upon your life as if out of nowhere. Insatiable cravings indicate imbalances that are best identified and treated by a health-care practitioner trained in Maharishi Ayur-Veda.

One simple, general tactic that is helpful in dealing with sweets cravings is to make sure you get all six tastes in your meals. Pay particular attention to eating foods with pungent, bitter, and astringent tastes, which are often lacking in people's diets. Of the six tastes, the sweet, sour, and salty tastes are currently overemphasized, particularly in Western countries. According to the Ayurvedic theory of reducing a problem by using antidotes, eating foods with more pungent, bitter, and astringent tastes helps create balance by reducing cravings for the dissimilar flavors of sweet, sour, and salt.

NUT BUTTER COOKIES

4 dozen

These cookies are particularly sublime when prepared with Nut Butter made from toasted cashews. I've always tested the recipe with Nut Butter made with ghee by the blender method on pages 546–47. Commercial types also work well.

3 cups (720 g) *Nut Butter*
2 cups (280 g) *unbleached white flour*
½ cup (120 ml) *nondairy milk or buttermilk*

2½ cups (520 g) *raw or packed brown sugar*
1 teaspoon *baking powder*

1. Preheat the oven to 350°F (180°C). Butter cookie sheets.
2. Mix all the ingredients together well. Shape into flat, round cookies and place on the cookie sheets 1 inch (2.5 cm) apart.
3. Bake until done, 12 to 15 minutes. Using a spatula, transfer immediately to a plate to cool and harden.

 # GINGERBREAD PEOPLE

8 to 10 large cookies

We can thank Queen Elizabeth I of England for gingerbread people. Why? She ordered up ginger cakes formed into likenesses of her friends.

STEP ONE

¼ cup (55 g) *unsalted butter*
½ cup (100 g) *raw or packed brown sugar*

½ cup (120 ml) *dark unsulphured molasses*

STEP TWO

2¼ cups (340 g) *whole wheat flour*
½ teaspoon *baking powder*
1 teaspoon *ground cinnamon*

1 teaspoon *ground ginger*
¼ teaspoon *salt*
3 to 4 tablespoons *water*

STEP SEVEN

Confectioner's sugar
Water

Raisins

1. Cream the butter and sugar thoroughly. Beat in the molasses.
2. Sift the dry ingredients over the butter-sugar mixture. Add enough water to make a stiff dough that just holds together.

3. Wrap in waxed paper or plastic wrap and chill in the refrigerator for at least 1 hour.
4. Preheat the oven to 350°F (180°C). Butter cookie sheets.
5. Sculpt gingerbread people or roll out the dough ⅛ inch (3 mm) thick on a floured board and cut out the people with a knife or cookie cutter. You can cut out a paper pattern and lay it on the dough as a guide. Punch a small hole in the top of each cookie if you intend to hang them on a Christmas tree. Carefully transfer to the cookie sheets.
6. Bake until done, about 10 minutes. Using a spatula, transfer immediately to plates to cool and harden.
7. When the cookies are thoroughly cooled, make a glaze of confectioner's sugar and a few drops of water. Using a thin, clean paintbrush, apply like paint for decoration. Also use the glaze as glue to affix raisins for the eyes and buttons.

 # GINGERSNAPS

2½ dozen

We have all heard of bribing children with cookies. But political bribes? In pre–Revolutionary War Virginia, ginger cookies were used as friendly persuasion to steer the votes of sweet-toothed citizens toward wily candidates for seats in the House of Burgesses. This version gets its name from the Dutch *snappen,* "to seize quickly."

STEP TWO

¼ cup (55 g) unsalted butter
1 cup (210 g) raw or packed brown
  sugar

¼ cup (60 ml) dark unsulphured
  molasses

STEP THREE

2 tablespoons arrowroot or
  cornstarch
2 cups (300 g) whole wheat flour
2 teaspoons baking soda
1 teaspoon ground cinnamon

¾ teaspoon ground ginger
¼ teaspoon ground cloves
½ teaspoon salt
½ cup (120 ml) water

STEP FOUR

White sugar

1. Preheat the oven to 350°F (180°C). Butter cookie sheets.
2. Cream the butter and sugar thoroughly. Beat in the molasses.
3. Mix all the dry ingredients except the white sugar. Add to the molasses mixture. Add the water and mix.
4. Roll the dough into 1-inch (2.5 cm) balls. Roll the balls in the granulated sugar and place on cookie sheets 1½ inches (4 cm) apart.
5. Bake until done, 8 to 10 minutes. Using a spatula, transfer immediately to a plate to cool and harden.

Scottish Shortbread

20 pieces

Rich, buttery, and very, very easy to make to balance Vata and Pitta.

STEP TWO

1¼ cups (285 g) *unsalted butter,*
  at room temperature

1 cup (210 g) *raw or packed light*
  brown sugar

STEP THREE

2½ cups (350 g) *unbleached*
  white flour

¾ teaspoon *salt*

1. Preheat the oven to 300°F (150°C). Butter a 13 × 9-inch (33 × 23 cm) baking pan.
2. Cream the butter and sugar thoroughly.
3. Sift in the dry ingredients. Mix until blended.
4. Press evenly into the pan about ¼-inch (6 mm) thick.
5. For soft shortbreads, bake 25 to 30 minutes. For crunchy shortbreads, bake 35 to 40 minutes. Let cool thoroughly and cut into squares.

 # 'Swonderful Shortbread

16 pieces

Named after our favorite Gershwin song, this cookie is practically a staple in our home. The dough can be made in a few minutes by blending everything except the nuts in a food processor, and the recipe is open to many variations. The original recipe emigrated from Czechoslovakia in Grandmother Hospodar's recipe file—sans food processor and Gershwin—was passed along to my mother-in-law, and from her to me.

STEP TWO

1 cup (230 g) *unsalted butter, at*
  room temperature

¾ cup (150 g) *sugar*

STEP THREE

2 cups (280 g) *unbleached*
  white flour
1 teaspoon *salt*
1 teaspoon *lemon juice*

1 cup (115 g) *chopped nuts*
  (*walnuts, pecans, almonds,*
  or whole pine nuts)

1. Preheat the oven to 350°F (180°C). Butter a 9 × 9-inch (23 × 23 cm) square baking pan.
2. Cream the butter and sugar thoroughly.
3. Beat in the flour, salt, and lemon juice. Beat in the nuts.

4. Press evenly into the baking pan. Bake until golden brown, 25 to 30 minutes. Let cool thoroughly and cut into squares.

VARIATIONS

Reduce flour to 1½ cups (210 g). Add 1 cup (115 g) rolled oats.

Add chopped dried fruit in Step 3. Dried pineapple and crystallized ginger are particularly sumptuous.

 # FIG OR DATE BARS

About 16 bars

Ayurveda regards figs and dates as very nourishing, energy-giving, structure-building fruits. Homemade fig and date bars are entirely different from their packaged brethren. You can substitute dried apricots or peaches for the beat of a different drummer.

STEP TWO

1½ cups packed chopped
*   figs (240 g) or dates (430 g)*
⅔ cup (160 ml) apple juice

½ cup (100 g) sugar (optional)
2 tablespoons lemon juice

STEP THREE

1¾ cups unbleached white (245 g)
*   or whole wheat flour (265 g)*
½ cup (60 g) ground nuts
½ cup (60 g) wheat germ
2 tablespoons arrowroot or
*   cornstarch*

½ teaspoon salt
2 tablespoons raw or brown sugar
⅓ cup (80 ml) melted ghee or
*   butter*
2 tablespoons water

1. Preheat the oven to 400°F (200°C). Butter a 9-inch (23 cm) square baking pan.
2. *To prepare the filling:* Simmer the figs or dates, apple juice, sugar, and lemon juice in a small saucepan for 10 minutes. Purée in a food processor or mash with a fork.
3. *To prepare the dough:* While the filling is cooking, combine all the dry ingredients in a bowl. Add the melted ghee or butter and the water. Mix to a crumbly dough with your fingers.
4. *To assemble:* Press half the dough evenly in the pan. Spread the fruit filling evenly over the dough. Sprinkle the remaining dough over the filling to completely cover it.
5. Bake until lightly browned, 20 to 25 minutes. Let cool thoroughly and cut into squares.

VARIATION

Replace the wheat germ with rolled oats.

NEWPORT GOOD LUCK BENNE SQUARES

12 squares

Sesame seeds were brought to the United States from Africa. Called *benne* seeds after the Benue state of Nigeria, they were believed to be harbingers of good fortune. Traditional "Charleston Good Luck Cookies" featured benne seeds. Here is my offering for your bright and glorious future, named for its birthplace in the Yankee territory of Rhode Island.

1 cup (230 g) unsalted butter
1 cup (210 g) raw or packed
*   brown sugar*
½ teaspoon salt

½ cup (70 g) sesame seeds,
*   toasted*
2 cups (280 g) unbleached
*   white flour*

1. Preheat the oven to 350°F (180°C). Butter and lightly flour an 11 × 7-inch (28 × 18 cm) baking pan.
2. Cream the butter and sugar thoroughly. Beat in the remaining ingredients.
3. Press evenly in the pan. Bake for about 20 minutes, until lightly browned. Be careful not to let the mixture burn. Let cool thoroughly and cut into squares.

If you are ignorant of things of earth,
how can you know about things of heaven?

—THE TALMUD

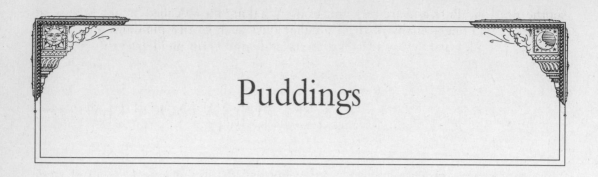

Puddings

Blessed be he that invented pudding, for it is a Manna that hits the Palates of all sorts of People; a Manna better than that of the Wilderness, because the People are never weary of it.

—FRANÇOISE MAXIMILIEN MISSION, 17TH CENTURY

Puddings are excellent Ayurvedic desserts—not as heavy as cakes and mostly balancing for Vata and Pitta. They play a wider variety of roles in Ayurvedic cooking than in the West, where they tend to be served mostly to the kindergarten set and the elderly, and are surreptitiously eaten by the adults in the middle as comfort food. In Ayurvedic households, all generations have equal access to puddings for dessert and sometimes as light suppers as well.

AYURVEDIC "MILKY GRAINS" FOR SUPPER

What's the matter with Mary Jane?
She's perfectly well and hasn't a pain,
And it's lovely rice pudding for dinner again!
—A. A. MILNE

Maharishi Ayur-Veda recommends light, nourishing foods for the evening meal that balance Vata and Pitta. Increased Vata can cause insomnia, and fiery Pitta can also keep you awake when overstimulated. Heavy foods are harder to digest with the reduced digestive fire, Agni, of evening. After sundown, during the Kapha time of day, Agni is reduced and less willing and able to fully process heavy foods. Besides, as we all probably know by experience, a meal that sits heavy on the tummy is hardly conducive to sleep. In addition to vegetable soups, mung dal, and khichari, grains cooked in milk soothe Vata and Pitta and are very nutritious. What are the so-called "milky grains" of Ayurveda? Puddings—many of them familiar ones such as rice puddings and noodle puddings. Besides making wonderful desserts, milk and grain puddings can make light Ayurvedic suppers.

FARINA OR SEMOLINA HALVA (SOOJI HALVA)

INDIA   *6 servings*

You can prepare this Vata- and Pitta-balancing halva from Cream of Wheat or from semolina. Very quick and easy, it is wonderful for breakfast as well as dessert.

STEP ONE

¼ cup (50 g) ghee or butter
¾ cup (140 g) farina (Cream of Wheat)
 or semolina

STEP TWO

2¼ cups (550 ml) water   *1 teaspoon ground cardamom*
¾ cup (150 g) sugar

STEP THREE

⅓ cup (50 g) raisins   *A few drops of rose water* (optional)

1. Melt the ghee or butter in a saucepan. Add the farina or semolina and cook over low heat, stirring constantly, until slightly darkened, 5 to 10 minutes.
2. Slowly stir in the water. Beat well. Add the sugar and cardamom. Cook until very thick, stirring constantly.
3. Remove from the heat. Mix in the raisins and, if desired, the rose water. Mound on a plate and serve warm. The halva can also be spread in a buttered rectangular pan, chilled to harden, and cut into squares.

VARIATIONS
 Add chopped almonds, cashews, or pistachios in Step 3.
 Replace the water with milk for a creamy pudding.

TOASTED VERMICELLI PUDDING (SEMILLA PAYASAM)

INDIA   *4 cups (1 l)*

Payasa is the name of a group of south Indian milk-based puddings. A wonderful, Vata-balancing payasa is made from very thin noodles called *seviya*, which can be found in

Indian markets. However, you can easily substitute vermicelli or capellini d'angelo or make the pudding from risoni or orzo pasta. In this recipe the milk is boiled down to two-thirds of its original volume to make it thicker; you can substitute 4 cups (1 l) of unreduced whole milk if you want to hasten your enjoyment of the finished product, though the finished pudding will be more liquid.

STEP ONE

6 cups (1.5 l) whole milk   ¼ teaspoon saffron threads

STEP TWO

1 tablespoon ghee
1 cup (100 g) untoasted seviya
  or vermicelli, broken into 1-inch
  (2.5 cm) pieces

STEP THREE

¼ cup (50 g) turbinado or white sugar   2 tablespoons slivered blanched
¼ cup (30 g) raisins   almonds (optional)
¾ teaspoon ground cardamom   Rose water

1. Bring the milk and saffron to a boil in a large saucepan. Reduce the heat and boil on as high a heat as possible without the milk boiling over, until the milk is reduced to 4 cups (1 l).
2. Heat the ghee in a skillet. Add the seviya or vermicelli and sauté over medium-low heat, stirring constantly, until the noodles are light brown.
3. Add the noodles to the milk. Add the sugar, raisins, and cardamom and simmer until the noodles are soft, about 5 minutes. Stir in the almonds if desired and a sprinkling of rose water. Serve warm.

 # BREAD PUDDING

4 to 6 servings

Bread, milk and butter are of venerable antiquity. The taste of the morning of the world.

—LEIGH HUNT, *The Seer*

Use whole grain bread for superior flavor and nutrition. Serve warm, with cream if desired.

STEP ONE

4 cups (200 g) cubed bread
3 cups (700 ml) milk or half-and-half

STEP THREE

1 medium apple, chopped	*¼ cup (30 g) raisins*
¼ cup (60 ml) melted ghee or	*1 teaspoon ground cinnamon*
butter	*1 cup (200 g) raw or packed*
¼ cup (70 g) chopped dates	*brown sugar*

1. Place the bread in a bowl. Pour the milk over it and let soak for 15 minutes.
2. Preheat the oven to 350°F (180°C). Butter a 2-quart (2 l) baking dish.
3. Mix the remaining ingredients into the bread mixture.
4. Spoon the mixture into the baking dish and spread evenly.
5. Bake until a light crust has formed, about 45 minutes. Serve warm or at room temperature.

VARIATION

❂ Replace the milk with nondairy milk.

 # SAFFRON TAPIOCA PUDDING WITH FIGS

6 servings

Though not technically a grain but a product of the manioc plant, tapioca serves the same function as a grain in a light, soothing milk pudding. Here is an eggless version. You can skip the saffron and replace the figs with raisins for a more traditional rendition.

STEP ONE

¼ teaspoon saffron threads	*3 tablespoons instant tapioca*
2 tablespoons hot water	*4 cups (1 l) milk*

STEP TWO

1 tablespoon arrowroot or cornstarch

STEP THREE

¼ cup (40 g) chopped dried	*Rose water*
white figs	
⅓ cup (70 g) raw or packed	
brown sugar	

1. Soak the saffron threads in the hot water. Soak the tapioca in the milk for 5 minutes.
2. Beat in the saffron and the arrowroot or cornstarch. Very slowly bring the mixture to a simmer, stirring gently but constantly.
3. As soon as the mixture boils, remove from the heat. Beat in the figs, sugar, and a sprinkling of rose water. Allow to cool without stirring. Serve at room temperature.

POLENTA INDIAN PUDDING WITH DRIED BLUEBERRIES

UNITED STATES   *6 servings*

I sing the sweets I know, the charms I feel,
My morning insence, and my evening meal—
The sweets of Hasty Pudding.
        —JOEL BARLOW (this was the inspiration for Harvard's Hasty Pudding Club)

Originally called "hasty pudding," Indian pudding was an attempt by creative American colonists to replicate English wheat-thickened puddings using New World corn. As such, it came to symbolize the rebellion against the British, and during the American Revolution, *tout Paris* demonstrated its support for the colonists by gamely downing the rustic New England dessert—but not without first smothering it with *crème Chantilly* to sweeten the patriotic gesture. You can substitute raisins for the blueberries and cornmeal for polenta for a more traditional version. However, I'd venture to guess that some New England Yankees used coarsely ground cornmeal and indigenous blueberries in their hasty puddings.

STEP TWO

½ *cup (75 g) polenta*	5 *cups (1.2 l) milk*

STEP THREE

⅓ *cup (80 ml) dark unsulphured molasses*	⅔ *cup (90 g) dried blueberries*
	1½ *teaspoons ground cinnamon*
⅓ *cup (70 g) raw or packed brown sugar*	½ *teaspoon ground ginger*
	2 *tablespoons melted ghee or butter*

1. Preheat the oven to 350°F (180°C). Butter a 2-quart (2 l) casserole dish.
2. Combine the polenta and milk in a saucepan and slowly bring to a boil, stirring frequently with a whisk. Reduce the heat and simmer for 15 minutes, until slightly thickened.
3. Remove from the heat and mix in the molasses, brown sugar, dried blueberries, spices, and ghee or butter. Pour into the baking dish. Bake until a dark brown skin has formed on top and the mixture is thick, about 1 hour.

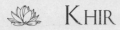

KHIR

INDIA   *About 3 cups (700 ml)*

"White rice with melted butter and white sugar is a dish not of this world," proclaimed al-Asma'i in the ninth century. Actually, it is a dish of virtually every continent of this world. In Central America and the South Seas, coconut milk replaces dairy milk. Benedictine monks in the Middle Ages prepared "rice soup" spiced with mace, cinnamon, and cloves. Khir is a rich, sweet, spiced east Indian rice pudding that is balancing for Vata and Pitta. Basmati rice makes the most sumptuous khir.

STEP ONE

¾ cup (150 g) white rice,   *6 cups (1.5 l) milk*
  preferably basmati   *1 tablespoon ghee*
⅛ teaspoon saffron threads

STEP TWO

⅔ cup (140 g) sugar   *½ teaspoon ground cardamom*

STEP THREE

A few drops of rose water   *Chopped pistachios* (optional)

1. Combine the rice, saffron, milk, and ghee in a saucepan. Simmer, stirring occasionally, until the mixture has a thick, soupy texture, about 1½ hours.
2. Add the sugar and cardamom. Simmer again until thick and soupy.
3. Remove from the heat and beat with a whisk to smooth out the mixture a little. Beat in a few drops of rose water. Pour into individual cups. If desired, sprinkle a few chopped pistachios on top of each serving. Serve warm or at room temperature.

VARIATIONS

    Replace 1 cup (240 ml) of the milk with cream in Step 1.

    Add chopped dates or raisins to the mixture in Step 2.

    Reduce the cardamom to ¼ teaspoon and add ¼ teaspoon ground cinnamon and ⅛ teaspoon ground ginger in Step 2.

BAKED RICE PUDDING

4 to 6 servings

Traditional Western rice puddings are prepared with short- or medium-grain rice, which is stickier and starchier than long-grain varieties and produces a more amalgamated result. Basmati rice produces a sumptuous, light pudding, and for those accustomed to cooking with it, short-grain rices will seem a little heavier and cruder. Here is a lighter version of the old classic, enhanced by the rich flavor and the energizing and nourishing value of dates.

3 cups (700 ml) milk or half-
and-half
⅓ cup (60 g) pitted dates
¾ cup (150 g) raw or packed
brown sugar

2 cups (500 ml) cooked
basmati rice

STEP TWO
½ teaspoon ground cinnamon
Pinch of ground nutmeg

STEP THREE
⅓ cup (50 g) raisins

1. Preheat the oven to 350°F (180°C). Butter a 1½-quart (1.5 l) baking dish.
2. Mix the milk or half-and-half, dates, sugar, and spices in a blender until smooth.
3. Place the rice and raisins in the baking dish. Add the milk mixture and stir gently.
4. Bake until a light brown skin has formed on the top, about 1 hour. Serve warm or at room temperature.

VARIATION
✿ Use nondairy milk and blend one ripe banana into it.

MILK PUDDINGS

 # BANANA PUDDING

5 cups (1.2 l)

Puddings made with arrowroot or cornstarch thicken somewhat during cooking and then become even thicker in the refrigerator. They can be prepared with anything from heavy cream to nonfat milk to nondairy milk, can be used as fillings for cream pies, and can be churned and frozen to make ice cream. Arrowroot is preferable to cornstarch for both its delicate texture and nutritive value. Pudding made with real bananas never comes out true banana yellow. Use white or turbinado sugar and add a pinch of saffron to the mixture if you wish to create that illusion.

STEP ONE
2½ cups (600 ml) nondairy milk
2 tablespoons ghee or butter
2 cups (480 g) mashed ripe
bananas

3½ tablespoons arrowroot or
cornstarch
½ teaspoon ground cardamom
⅛ teaspoon salt

STEP TWO
¾ cup (150 g) raw or packed
brown sugar

1. Combine the nondairy milk, ghee or butter, bananas, arrowroot or cornstarch, cardamom, and salt in a blender.
2. Pour into a saucepan and bring to a simmer, stirring constantly with a whisk. Simmer until thickened. Remove from the heat and stir in the sugar. Pour into individual bowls and chill to thicken.

VARIATION

Add chopped dates or dried apricots in Step 1.

 # BUTTERSCOTCH-COCONUT PUDDING

5 cups (1.2 l)

STEP ONE

5 tablespoons arrowroot or cornstarch

3½ cups (850 ml) milk

1⅓ cups (280 g) raw or packed brown sugar

1 tablespoon dark unsulphured molasses

¾ cup (60 g) grated unsweetened coconut, fresh or dried, toasted

2 tablespoons ghee or butter

STEP THREE

Whipped cream (optional)

Chopped toasted cashews (optional)

1. Dissolve the arrowroot or cornstarch in ½ cup (120 ml) of the milk. Pour into a saucepan and add the sugar, molasses, coconut, and ghee or butter.
2. Heat to a simmer, stirring constantly with a whisk. Simmer until thickened.
3. Pour into cups and chill to thicken. If desired, top with whipped cream and cashews before serving.

 # CARROT HALVA (GAJAR HALVA)

6 to 8 servings

Halvas are a cross between a pudding and a candy found throughout the Middle East and India. On special occasions they are coated with gold or silver leaf. After you try *gajar halva*, you'll want to make it (or rather, eat it) again and again. The bright orange color makes it particularly attractive, and the contrast with a garnish of green chopped pistachios is very special. Carrot Halva is Vata balancing, especially when served warm.

STEP ONE

½ cup (120 g) ghee or butter

3 cups (270 g) finely grated carrots

STEP TWO

4 cups (950 ml) milk

STEP THREE

1 cup (210 g) sugar

STEP FOUR

¼ to ½ teaspoon ground
cardamom

A few drops of rose water
Chopped pistachios (optional)

1. Melt the ghee or butter in a saucepan. Add the carrots and cook, stirring constantly, until the carrots are slightly mushy, about 10 minutes.
2. Add the milk. Bring to a boil, stirring constantly. Reduce the heat to a low boil and cook, stirring frequently, until the mixture is very thick, 1½ to 2 hours.
3. Add the sugar and cook again until thick. Stir constantly to avoid scorching.
4. Add the cardamom and rose water. Mound on a plate. Decorate with chopped pistachios if desired. Serve warm or at room temperature.

VARIATION

Replace 1 cup (250 ml) of the milk with cream.

RIS À LA MANDE (RICE PUDDING WITH WHIPPED CREAM AND ALMONDS)

DENMARK   *4 to 6 servings*

STEP ONE

1½ cups (350 ml) cooked rice,
cooled
3 tablespoons honey or ¼ cup
(50 g) sugar
⅓ cup (45 g) slivered blanched
almonds

¼ cup (30 g) raisins
¼ teaspoon ground ginger
¼ teaspoon ground cardamom
1 piece of fruit, cut into small pieces
(apple, banana, pear, peach,
orange, etc.)

STEP TWO

1 cup (250 ml) heavy (whipping) cream

1. Mix the rice with the honey or sugar, almonds, raisins, spices, and fruit.
2. Whip the cream until stiff. Fold into the rice mixture.

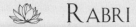 # RABRI

INDIA   *6 to 8 servings*

A rich, Vata- and Pitta-balancing pudding made from *khou*, milk boiled and reduced until thick.

STEP ONE

½ gallon (2 l) whole milk

STEP TWO

⅔ cup (140 g) sugar   *A few drops of rose water*
¼ teaspoon ground cardamom   *Chopped almonds or pistachios*

1. Bring the milk to a boil, stirring frequently. Boil on the highest heat possible without causing the milk to boil over for 1½ to 2 hours, stirring frequently, and toward the end stirring constantly, until the mixture thickens to a pudding texture.
2. Add the sugar and cardamom. Cook, stirring constantly, until the mixture is thick again. Add the rose water. Pour into bowls and sprinkle with nuts. Let cool to room temperature.

STEAMED PUDDINGS

Puddings can be steamed in a pudding mold or in a lidded baking dish. I have also used a stainless-steel bowl, covering the top with foil or inverting an identical bowl over it as a lid. Butter the mold or dish very well so that the pudding can be unmolded easily.

 # STEAMED DATE OR FIG PUDDING

10 to 12 servings

Soak hard figs in hot water to soften before using. I have also used fresh figs with great success.

STEP TWO

⅓ cup (75 g) butter
1 cup (210 g) raw or packed brown sugar

STEP THREE

1¾ cups (250 g) unbleached   *½ teaspoon baking soda*
*   white flour*   *1 tablespoon arrowroot or*
½ cup (75 g) whole wheat flour   *   cornstarch*
1 teaspoon baking powder

STEP FOUR

½ cup (120 ml) buttermilk
½ cup (120 ml) water
1 cup packed chopped dates (285 g)
  or chopped soft figs (160 g)

1 cup (100 g) chopped walnuts
(optional)

STEP SIX

Heavy (whipping) cream (optional)

1. Preheat the oven to 350°F (180°C). Generously butter a 1-quart (1 l) mold or lidded casserole dish.
2. Cream the butter and sugar thoroughly.
3. Mix the dry ingredients together and beat into the butter-sugar mixture.
4. Add the buttermilk and water, and mix. Stir in the dates and nuts.
5. Spoon the mixture into the mold or baking dish and spread evenly. Cover, place in a larger pan, and add boiling water to come ⅓ of the way up the sides of the mold or baking dish.
6. Bake for 2 hours, replenishing the water occasionally as it evaporates. Carefully unmold onto a plate. Serve warm with cream if desired.

 HOLIDAY PUDDING

10 to 12 servings

Delicious served with whipped cream or Caramel Sauce.

STEP TWO

1½ cups (135 g) grated carrots
1 cup (130 g) raisins

1½ cups (180 g) grated apples

STEP THREE

1 cup (140 g) unbleached
  white flour
¼ cup (40 g) whole wheat flour
¾ cup (150 g) raw or packed
  brown sugar
½ teaspoon ground cinnamon

Pinch of cloves
⅛ teaspoon ground nutmeg
1½ teaspoons baking powder
2 tablespoons arrowroot or
  cornstarch
½ teaspoon salt

1. Preheat the oven to 350°F (180°C). Generously butter a 1-quart (1 l) mold or lidded casserole dish.
2. Mix the carrots, raisins, and apples in a bowl.
3. Mix the dry ingredients together and add to the carrot mixture. Mix well.
4. Spoon the mixture into the mold or casserole dish and spread evenly. Cover, place

in a larger pan, and add boiling water to come ⅓ of the way up the sides of the mold or casserole.

5. Bake for 1½ hours, replenishing the water occasionally as it evaporates. Carefully unmold onto a plate. Serve warm.

 # PERSIMMON PUDDING
10 to 12 servings

A stellar dessert for persimmon season, worthy of gracing any autumn holiday table. Because it contains spices and Kapha-balancing persimmons and does not contain oil, this is somewhat in the direction of being a more Kapha-balancing dessert.

STEP TWO

1¼ cups (175 g) unbleached white flour
½ cup (75 g) whole wheat flour
½ cup (100 g) raw or packed brown sugar
1 teaspoon baking powder

¼ teaspoon baking soda
2 tablespoons arrowroot or cornstarch
½ teaspoon salt
¾ teaspoon ground cinnamon
¼ teaspoon ground cloves

STEP THREE

1½ cups (360 g) puréed persimmon pulp (3 to 4 medium persimmons)
½ cup (65 g) raisins

¼ cup (40 g) chopped crystallized ginger
Lightly whipped cream (optional)

1. Preheat the oven to 350°F (180°C). Butter a 1-quart (1 l) mold or covered baking dish.
2. Sift all the dry ingredients together.
3. Stir in the persimmon purée and mix until all the ingredients are well combined. Stir in the raisins and crystallized ginger.
4. Spoon the mixture into the mold or baking dish and spread evenly. Cover, place in a larger pan, and add boiling water to come ⅓ of the way up the sides of the mold or baking dish.
5. Bake for 2 hours, replenishing the water occasionally as it evaporates. Carefully unmold onto a plate. Serve hot or at room temperature with lightly whipped cream if desired.

Heaven does not speak. —MENCIUS

Candies and Dessert Sauces

The love of sweetmeats comes from the faith. —Muhammad

CANDIES

The word *candy* is derived from the Sanskrit *khanda*, "rock sugar."

 ## LOUISIANA PRALINES

UNITED STATES   *About 20*

A Frenchwoman residing in New Orleans longed for a type of almond candy of her homeland invented by the chef of Marechal, Duc de Duplessis-Praslin (and obviously named to honor the master, not the chef). And so it came to pass that madame's cook recreated the candies for her using native pecans. Voilà! A Vata-balancing star was born, and pralines are now completely associated with—and claimed by—New Orleans.

STEP ONE

1 cup (200 g) white sugar
1 cup (200 g) packed dark brown
  sugar

1 cup (250 ml) heavy (whipping)
  cream

STEP THREE

2 cups (200 g) coarsely chopped pecans

1. Combine the sugars and cream in a saucepan. Bring to a boil, stirring constantly.
2. Boil, without stirring, to the soft ball stage, 5 to 7 minutes.

452

3. Remove from the heat and let cool to lukewarm. Beat until creamy. Beat in the nuts. When cool enough to shape, form 1½-inch (4 cm) patties and place on a buttered tray. Do not wait too long, or the mixture will harden completely. Allow to cool and harden.

VARIATION

Replace the pecans with walnuts or toasted blanched almonds—not authentically Creole, but the Duc de Duplessis-Praslin's chef would have approved.

A cooking term used often in candy making is the *soft ball stage*: the point at which a mixture of water and sugar reaches a temperature between 234° and 240°F (112° and 115°C) and forms a syrup that will harden when cooled. The syrup reaches the soft ball stage after 5 to 7 minutes of boiling. The surface will usually have a mixture of large and small bubbles, and will pass the following test:

Drop a little of the syrup into a cup of cold water. The drops will hold their shape instead of dispersing in the water. They will feel rubbery to the touch. The drops may not hold the round shape of balls, but there will be an obvious difference between them and a syrup that simply dissolves in the water.

 # MARZIPAN

1¾ cups (450 g)

Marzipan is so associated with Europe that we forget that originally it was a prized delicacy of the Middle East, unknown in Europe until Crusaders brought it back from their travels to the Holy Land. Records tell of marzipan centerpieces depicting a castle with a moat filled with orange drink, and even a sculpture enclosing a twenty-eight-man orchestra! On a lesser scale, marzipan is great for sculpting into figures and flowers for cake decorations. It also can be used as a rich filling between cake layers. Use a meat grinder to pulverize the almonds. If you don't have one, a blender is second best, and a food processor produces an undesirable, coarsely textured result.

STEP ONE

2 cups (280 g) blanched almonds

STEP TWO

¾ cup (90 g) confectioner's sugar
¼ cup (20 g) noninstant milk powder

2 to 3 tablespoons water
1 tablespoon lemon juice
A few drops of rose water

1. Grind the almonds to a completely smooth paste, or pulverize to a fine powder.
2. Mix the paste with the other ingredients. Shape as desired.

VARIATIONS

For golden-colored marzipan, soak saffron in the water (use hot water) before preparing the candy.

Replace the sugar with ⅓ cup (80 ml) honey. Omit the water.

 ## Laddu

INDIA   *3 dozen*

These crumbly Vata- and Pitta-balancing sweets melt in your mouth. They are very popular in India and are served at celebrations and in temples.

STEP ONE

¾ cup plus 2 tablespoons (210 ml) melted ghee or butter	*2 cups (240 g) besan (chickpea flour)*

STEP TWO

½ cup (60 g) ground almonds	*½ teaspoon ground cardamom*
2 cups (230 g) confectioner's sugar	

1. Melt the ghee or butter in a saucepan or a large cast-iron skillet. Add the besan and cook over low heat, stirring constantly, for 20 to 40 minutes, until slightly darkened.
2. Remove from the heat. Stir in the nuts, confectioner's sugar, and cardamom. When just cool enough to handle, squeeze into 1-inch (2.5 cm) balls. The balls should just barely hold together. Do not wait for the mixture to cool completely; the ghee will harden and you won't be able to form the laddus.

VARIATION

Add grated coconut in Step 2.

 ## Crystallized Ginger

4 cups (660 g)

These sugared slices of fresh ginger have the side benefit of being a digestive aid. Besides being eaten like a candy, they are delicious chopped and added to baked goods in the manner of dried fruit. When you make them at home, you'll also end up with a ginger infusion to use in soup stock or beverages, plus a scrumptious ginger-flavored syrup.

STEP ONE

4 cups (500 g) fresh ginger,
   peeled and cut diagonally into
   ¼-inch (5 mm) slices

6 cups (1.5 l) water

STEP THREE

8 cups (2 l) water

2 cups (400 g) white sugar

STEP FIVE

White sugar

1. Place the ginger and water in a saucepan and bring to a boil. Reduce the heat and simmer for 40 minutes.
2. Drain, catching the water in a pot for other uses. Rinse the ginger slices.
3. Mix the 8 cups (2 l) water and the sugar together in a large pot. Add the ginger and bring to a boil. Reduce the heat to medium-low, so that the water is at a low boil. Cook until the liquid is reduced to a syrup, about 3½ hours.
4. Drain off the syrup into a bowl and save for other uses.
5. Spread a 13 × 9-inch (33 × 23 cm) baking pan with a ¼-inch (6 mm) thick layer of sugar. Add the ginger slices and toss to coat thoroughly. Spread them out in the pan and allow to dry overnight. Store in an airtight container.

SESAME HALVAH

About 20 pieces

In cooking, as in all the arts, simplicity is the sign of perfection. —CURNONSKY

Unlike India halvas, which are thick puddings, and Middle Eastern halvah, which is dense and crunchy, this version is somewhat soft and has the more complex flavor of toasted sesame seeds.

STEP ONE

1½ cups (200 g) sesame seeds

STEP THREE

½ cup (120 ml) honey

3 tablespoons butter

1. Toast the sesame seeds in a dry skillet over medium heat, stirring constantly, until they turn golden brown and begin to pop.
2. Grind to a coarse powder in a blender. Allow to cool.
3. Mix in the honey and butter. Press into a buttered pan. Chill to harden. Cut into squares or, with oiled hands, roll the mixture into balls. Chill again.

VARIATIONS
Add a little cardamom, cinnamon, or anise in Step 3.
Replace some of the sesame seeds with pine nuts or pistachios.

WHERE'S THE CHOCOLATE?

If you have been trawling the dessert sections in *Heaven's Banquet* in search of the elusive chocolate recipe, by now you must have noticed a conspicuous absence. The sad story is that chocolate is not a favored food in Ayurveda. Dr. Rama Kant Mishra, an expert vaidya of Maharishi Ayur-Veda, explains that chocolate contains theobromide, a stimulant similar to caffeine. Stimulants can be hard on the body, particularly for Vata and Pitta types, and the sugar in chocolate dishes affects the metabolization of theobromide in a manner that can leave deposits of toxic impurities, ama, in the body.

DESSERT SAUCES

 ## FRESH SUMMER FRUIT SAUCE

1½ cups (360 ml)

Know that by knowing which nothing else remains to be known.
—THE VEDAS

By knowing this, one knows the only sauce that remains to be known for ice creams and fruit salads: a purée of fresh fruit. The best combinations are mixtures of berries with sliced fruit. Try raspberries and peaches for the classic Melba combination. You can also choose a single type of fruit to stand alone.

2 cups (500 ml) pitted cherries, berries, sliced strawberries, finely cut peaches, apricots, mangoes, or peeled persimmons

2 tablespoons honey or *3 tablespoons sugar*
2 to 3 tablespoons lemon juice

Purée all the ingredients in a blender or food processor. Add more sweetening if desired.

APRICOT, PEACH, OR MANGO SAUCE

About 1½ cups (360 ml)

3 cups (650 g) chopped ripe
   apricots, peaches, or peeled
   mangoes
¼ cup (60 ml) water

2 tablespoons lemon juice
¼ to ½ cup (50 to 100 g) sugar
½ teaspoon ground ginger
½ teaspoon ground cardamom

1. Simmer all the ingredients in a covered saucepan until very soft, 10 to 15 minutes.
2. Purée in a food mill, blender, or food processor. Add more sugar if necessary.

 # BERRY OR CHERRY SAUCE

About 1½ cups (360 ml)

A thickened sauce that becomes somewhat glossy and firm if chilled, making it a nice topping for cheesecake. Serve warm over ice cream, blintzes, and pancakes.

STEP ONE

1½ cups (350 ml) whole
   blueberries, blackberries,
   raspberries, or sliced
   strawberries, or halved and
   pitted cherries

3 to 4 tablespoons sugar
1 tablespoon lemon juice
½ cup (120 ml) water

STEP TWO

1 tablespoon arrowroot or
   cornstarch

2 tablespoons water

1. Cover and simmer the berries or cherries, sugar, and lemon juice in the water until tender, about 10 minutes.
2. Dissolve the arrowroot or cornstarch in the water. Stir into the sauce and simmer until thickened, stirring constantly, about 1 minute.

 # LEMON OR LIME SAUCE

1½ cups (360 ml)

Serve warm over ice cream, pancakes, or crêpes. When chilled, the sauce has the texture of a light pudding.

1½ tablespoons arrowroot or
  cornstarch
1¼ cups (300 ml) water
¼ cup (60 ml) lemon or lime juice
1 teaspoon finely grated lemon or
  lime zest

3 tablespoons ghee or butter
⅔ cup (140 g) sugar
Pinch of salt

Mix the arrowroot or cornstarch into ¼ cup of the water until smooth. Combine all the ingredients in a saucepan. Bring to a simmer over low heat, stirring constantly with a whisk. Simmer for a few minutes, until thickened.

 # CARAMEL SAUCE

2 cups (480 ml)

Preparing caramel sauce is an adventure. It looks as if it is not going to come out right—the ghee or butter separates from the sugar, and the sugar masses together in the cream—and then, at the very last moment, it transforms into a smooth, creamy sauce. Try it over Nut Ice Cream.

STEP ONE

⅓ cup (75 g) ghee or butter   2 cups (420 g) white sugar

STEP THREE

1 cup (250 ml) heavy (whipping)
  cream

1. Melt the ghee or butter in a saucepan with high sides. Add the sugar. Cook over medium heat, stirring constantly, until the sugar turns brown. (The ghee or butter will separate from the sugar at this point.)
2. Remove from the heat for a few minutes, continuing to stir.
3. Pour in the cream and stand back! The cream will bubble up and the sugar will turn into a solid mass.
4. When the bubbling subsides, return the mixture to low heat. Simmer and stir until the sugar melts to form a smooth sauce, about 5 minutes.
5. Strain the sauce to remove the few chunks of hardened sugar that inevitably remain in the bottom of the pot. Sprinkle the chunks on ice cream, like candy.

A gourmet is a being pleasing to heaven.

—CHARLES MONSELET

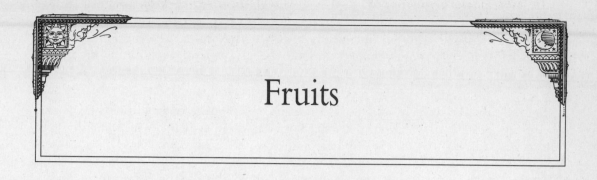

Fruits

What wond'rous is this life I lead!
Ripe Apples drop about my head;
The Luscious clusters of the Vine
Upon my Mouth do crush their Wine;
The Nectaren and curious Peach
Into my hands themselves to reach;
Stumbling on Melons as I pass,
Insnar'd with Flow'rs, I fall on Grass.

—ANDREW MARVELL

The word *fruit* comes from the Latin *fructus*, meaning "enjoy." It has long inspired writers, artists, and philosophers with its beauty and its symbolism of sweetness and abundance. It signifies accomplishment, as in "the fruits of one's labors," or whether or not a project will "bear fruit." Indeed, the fruit of a plant is the culmination of a lengthy growth process—and also the potential beginning of a new one, as it contains the seeds for a new plant.

According to Ayurveda, fruit is a food that is both nourishing and purifying. It is treated differently from vegetables in that sun-ripened fruit is considered a cooked food, with Mother Nature the *chef de cuisine*. Therefore, uncooked fruit is not a raw food and is wonderfully digestible. Also, unlike vegetables, fruit can be healthfully preserved with sweetenings, making fruit jams and chutneys part of an Ayurvedic diet. Fruits are best for eating when fully ripe, and best for cooking when just ripe but not overly so. Otherwise, you are cooking an already "cooked" food—which amounts to overcooking!

Fruit out of season, sorrow out of reason.   —HENRY FRIEND

❖ Fruits shipped across country or imported have probably been picked unripe and allowed to ripen while in storage or shipping—often with the encouragement of chemical gases. Such fruit is often stored for days, weeks, or even months before it sees the light of day again. Farmers' markets are excellent sources of tree-ripened, seasonal, locally grown, organically grown (gasp) fruits. The farmers generally grow smaller amounts than those who supply supermarkets, and often have unusual produce that mass distributors would balk at.

Stewed fruit: For best results, use dried fruits or a mixture of fresh sliced fruits and dried fruits. Simmer in water or apple juice until tender. Juicy fruits, which literally stew in their own juices, need only a small amount of water to get them started. Add sweetening if desired. Serve with the cooking water.

Grilled fruit: Choose fruits that are firm and hold their shape rather than mushy, extremely juicy types. Melon, pineapple, peach, papaya, and mango slices all work well. Wipe the fruit slices dry. Brush with melted ghee or oil. Place on a lightly oiled grill 4 to 6 inches (10 to 15 cm) above the coals. Grill on each side until sear marks form. Brush the fruit with melted apricot preserves or sprinkle with a little lemon juice. Serve hot or at room temperature.

Broiled fruit: Use the same fruits as for Grilled Fruit, plus halved grapefruits. Sprinkle the cut surfaces with raw sugar. Place under the broiler for a minute, until the sugar is melted and bubbly.

 # FRUIT CRISP

UNITED STATES   *6 servings*

Fruit crisps are simple to prepare and universally loved. I make the topping by throwing everything in a food processor. Here are three ideas for toppings and fillings, plus ways to vary them to make even more creations.

Apple Filling:

5½ cups (660 g) *thinly sliced*
    apples (peeled or unpeeled)
½ teaspoon *ground cinnamon*

½ cup (65 g) *raisins*
1 tablespoon *lemon juice*

Berry, Cherry, Peach, or Apricot Filling:

5 cups (1.2 l) *berries, pitted*
    cherries, or sliced peaches or
    apricots
2½ tablespoons *arrowroot or*
    cornstarch

1 tablespoon *lemon juice*
2 tablespoons *sugar*

Rhubarb Filling:

Filling for Rhubarb Pie (pp. 415–16)—
    reduce sugar to ¾ cup (150 g)

Streusel Topping:

1 cup (140 g) unbleached white or
  whole wheat flour
½ cup (100 g) raw or packed
  brown sugar

½ teaspoon salt
¾ cup (165 g) unsalted butter

Nut Topping:

½ cup (100 g) raw or packed
  brown sugar
¾ cup (110 g) unbleached white or
  whole wheat flour

½ cup (60 g) ground nuts
¼ cup (30 g) wheat germ
½ teaspoon salt
½ cup (115 g) unsalted butter

Oatmeal topping:

½ cup (100 g) raw or packed
  brown sugar
⅔ cup (90 g) unbleached white or
  whole wheat flour

1¼ cups (145 g) rolled oats
½ teaspoon salt
¾ cup (165 g) unsalted butter

1. Preheat the oven to 375°F (190°C). Butter an 8-inch (22 cm) square baking dish or 9½ × 6½-inch (24 × 18 cm) pan.

To prepare the filling:

2. Mix all the ingredients for the desired filling together and spread evenly in the baking dish.
3. *To prepare the topping by hand:* Combine the dry ingredients for the desired topping in a bowl. Cut the butter into small pieces, add to the dry ingredients, and work in with your fingers or a pastry cutter until the mixture resembles coarse meal.
4. *To prepare the topping in a food processor:* Process everything together except the oats, then stir them in by hand.
5. Crumble the topping evenly over the fruit.
6. Bake until the topping is lightly browned and the fruit is tender, about 45 minutes.

VARIATIONS
   Add a handful of finely chopped nuts to the streusel or oatmeal topping.
   Add a handful of shredded coconut to any of the toppings.

DRIED FRUIT

In 300 B.C., the government of Greece received a communiqué from an Indian raja, requesting a shipment of dried figs, grape syrup, and one philosopher. The dried fruits were duly sent, but the raja was informed that "it is against the law to trade in philosophers."

Drying methods today can be peppered with all sorts of shenanigans to increase shelf life and make the goods look enticing. The most questionable is treating dried fruits with sulphur dioxide to keep their colors bright. Fruits naturally turn brown when exposed to air; fiery-colored dried apricots and peaches and golden raisins are sulphur treated. Soft, plump, juicy dried fruits have often been treated with preservatives. Occasionally, dried fruits are coated with mineral oil. And lo—anything labeled "honey-dipped" is, in actuality, dipped in sugar! (Ever wondered why those fruits weren't sticky?)

What to do? Select carefully. Naturally dried fruits have faded color and, with the exception of dates, can be somewhat on the leathery side. Soak hard dried fruits in water overnight or simmer for a few minutes in water or fruit juice to soften. This also helps render them more balancing for Vata (the dry quality is a tipoff that they could aggravate Vata dosha). If you can obtain only sulphured fruits, exposure to air dissipates most of the sulphur. Leave them out overnight, then rinse them off.

❖ *Dried fruit purées* have highly concentrated flavor and sweetness. They can be used as a substitute for sugar or honey in some desserts and as a natural frosting for cakes and cookies. Also use like jam and in Fruit Fool. Either grind softened, pitted, dried fruits to a paste in a meat grinder, or simmer in a little water until tender and purée in a food processor or through a food mill.

COMMON FRUITS IN AYURVEDIC COOKING

Amalaks, or Myrobalans

Amalaks are native to India, where lived the great enlightened saint Hastamalaka—"hand-amalak"—to whom the truth of life was as apparent as an amalak fruit in the palm of his hand. Amalaks were briefly in fashion in eighteenth-century France but otherwise have kept a low profile in the West. They are highly praised by Ayurveda and used in many *rasayanas* (rejuvenation formulations). You can find them preserved in sugar syrup in Indian markets. Chop them up and use as you would dried fruits in desserts, or purée and use as jam.

Apples

> *Beauty diffuses itself in the world as an apple.* —ZOHAR, *The Book of Light*

Of all the apple's inestimable qualities, the one most prized by Cézanne was inertness: "Sit still, like an apple!" he harangued his models. Apples are Kapha-balancing. There are over seven thousand varieties of apples, of which only about fifteen are widely available. If you even encounter a *lady apple*, know it to be the most ancient known species still in existence, the *api* of the Etruscans. Apples ripen ten times faster at room temperature than in the refrigerator. They can be stored in the refrigerator for months, for which reason you should check your source; you don't want to buy something that has already been the resident of a cooler long enough to apply for citizenship.

APPLESAUCE OR PEAR SAUCE

About 2 cups (500 ml)

Apples and pears are both Kapha-balancing fruits, and their sauce is a welcome sweet treat for those who want to reduce Kapha but are Desperately Seeking Desserts. Often no additional sweetening is necessary. I like to cook a handful of dried fruit, such as cherries or apricots, with the apples, then purée the sauce. This adds a small, still voice of balance for Vata and Pitta.

STEP ONE

4 cups sliced apples (480 g) or pears (640 g), peeled or unpeeled

STEP TWO

½ to 1 teaspoon ground cinnamon   *Sugar*
⅓ cup (50 g) raisins or other dried fruit (optional)

1. Place the apples in a saucepan in ½ inch (1.3 cm) of water. Cover and simmer until soft, 15 to 20 minutes.
2. Mash or purée in a blender or food processor with the cinnamon. Add the raisins if desired, and sugar to taste.

VARIATIONS

Let the applesauce cool to room temperature and stir in honey.
Add cranberries or other fruits. Quinces were popular additions in colonial America.
Add ¼ teaspoon ground ginger.

Bananas

Bananas and plantains do not grow on trees; therefore botanists classify them as herbs. The botanical name for bananas, *Musa sapientum,* "wise men's fruits," comes from descriptions, originating with Alexander the Great's army, of Indian holy men who meditated in the shade of banana plants and reached up to pick a fruit whenever sustenance was desired. Although bananas taste sweet, they are identified as having a sour Ayurvedic taste and therefore do not combine well with milk. Such dishes as banana milk shakes, banana ice cream, or bananas atop cold cereal with milk contain incompatible ingredients and could cause ama, toxins from incomplete digestion.

 ## BAKED BANANAS

4 servings

	STEP TWO
4 ripe bananas	*¼ cup (20 g) grated fresh or dried*
½ cup (120 ml) orange juice	*unsweetened coconut* (optional)
3 tablespoons raw or brown sugar	*Ghee or butter*

1. Preheat the oven to 375°F (190°C). Butter a baking dish.
2. Cut the bananas in half lengthwise. Arrange cut side up in the baking dish. Pour the orange juice over them. Sprinkle with the sugar. Sprinkle with the coconut if desired. Dot liberally with ghee or butter. Bake for 15 to 20 minutes. Serve warm.

 ## BANANAS ALEXANDER

4 servings

This sauce contains simple ingredients, is prepared in 5 minutes, yet has a special flavor that seems to speak of some secret ingredient.

	STEP ONE
¼ cup (55 g) ghee or butter	*2 tablespoons lemon juice*
2 cups (480 g) mashed bananas	

	STEP TWO
1 teaspoon ground cinnamon	*Approximately ¼ cup (60 ml) honey*

1. Melt the ghee or butter in a skillet. Add the bananas and sauté for 5 minutes, mashing them as they cook. Sprinkle the lemon juice over the bananas while cooking.
2. When the bananas are tender, remove from the heat and let cool to lukewarm. Mix in the cinnamon and honey to taste.

Dates

Ayurveda prizes dates as excellent sources of energy, and some vaidyas recommend eating one or two every day. In Mesopotamia cultivated date palms have been carbondated to 50,000 B.C. They have also been found in Mohenjo Daro.

❖ There are more than one hundred varieties of dates. Most popular by far is the *deglet noor*, a good all-purpose date. *Zahidi* is a medium-sized, slightly less sweet variety that is also versatile. *Medjools* are very large and very sweet and are excellent for eating plain or removing the pit and stuffing with nuts or marzipan. *Barhi* are squishy soft and sweet—great for puréeing into candies and frostings and a real treat to eat plain.

Figs

The fig is the most useful of all the fruits which grow on trees.   —ATHENAEUS

❖ Dried figs and fig syrup were common sweeteners of the ancient world.
❖ Ayurveda particularly recommends the dried *white, Smyrna,* and *Calimyrna* varieties for vitality.
❖ Fresh figs, in theory, are plump, juicy, and smooth skinned at the peak of ripeness. However, in practice they are often a little withered or a little bruised and cracked, and you have to allow some leeway in selection unless you are prepared to search to the ends of the earth for the perfect ripe fig. Allow firm figs to ripen at room temperature, then eat them. They do not store well.

Grapes and Raisins

Says the ancient Ayurvedic text *Ashtanga Hridaya,* "Grapes are the best among fruits."
Raisins are highly recommended in Ayurvedic cooking. They are most commonly made from *Thompson seedless* grapes. Beware of *golden raisins*: they are ordinary brown raisins that have been treated with sulfur dioxide to maintain their color. *Monukka* raisins are large and often crunchy from tiny seeds. *Zante currants* are actually small grapes, also called *black Corinths*. Store raisins in the refrigerator so they don't ferment.

Mangoes

I consider the mango . . . one of the most delectable fruits with which God graced an already bountiful world.   —EUELL GIBBONS

As apple is the king of fruits in colder climates, mango rules supreme in tropical areas and is highly appreciated in Ayurvedic cooking. It comes from a noble Indian family that includes pistachios and cashews.

❖ Small, unripe mangoes are used for making *achar*, a spicy cooked relish. Otherwise, they must be completely ripe or they taste like turpentine and aggravate the doshas. Look for mangoes that are fairly soft but not mushy to the touch. The skins can be yellow-orange or light green. Allow mangoes to ripen at room temperature. Store them ripe in the refrigerator for up to about three days.

MANGO FOOL

ENGLAND   *4 servings*

*Soft, pale, creamy, untroubled, the English fruit fool is the most frail and
insubstantial of English summer dishes. That at any rate is how it should be,
and how we like to think it always was. . . . Gradually the delicacy now
regarded as the traditional English fruit fool came to be accepted as a purée of
fruit plus sugar, plus thick cream, and nothing more.*

—ELIZABETH DAVID, *Syllabubs and Fruit Fools*

The name *fool* comes from the French *fouler*, "to press," from the action of pressing the
cooked fruit through a sieve to purée it. As my mother would say, this is "a simple but
eloquent" dish. When using fresh fruit, be sure it is very ripe and sweet; according to
Ayurveda, sour fruit is incompatible with sweet cream.

STEP ONE

2 large mangoes, coarsely chopped   ¼ teaspoon ground ginger
   (about 2½ cups/530 g)   ½ teaspoon ground cardamom
⅓ cup (70 g) sugar

STEP TWO

1 cup (240 ml) heavy (whipping)   A few drops of rose water
   cream   (optional)

1. Place the mangoes, sugar, ginger, and cardamom in a saucepan. Cover and simmer
   for about 10 minutes, until the mangoes are tender. Purée in a food processor. Let
   cool to room temperature.
2. Just before serving, whip the cream until it stands in soft peaks. Sprinkle with rose
   water and gently fold in the mango purée. Adjust the sweetening. Mound up in
   individual custard cups or bowls.

VARIATIONS

Substitute ripe berries, apricots, or peaches for the mangoes.
Substitute 2½ cups (600 ml) sweet fruit sauce made of fresh or dried fruits for the mangoes.

Melons

*When one has tasted watermelons, one knows what angels eat. It was not a
southern melon that Eve took; we know it because she repented.* —MARK TWAIN

Melons are defined as sweet, cooling foods in Ayurveda. *Watermelons*, excellent for
cooling Pitta, are members of the gourd family, while virtually all other melons are classified together as *muskmelons*.

The only melons worth eating are vine ripened. Picking them this way is labor-intensive; melons growing on the same vine ripen at different times. Mass-marketed melons are strip harvested—all picked unripe at the same time—and sit in storage for a week or two to ripen a little more before they reach you. Beware! Buy from farmers' markets or grow them yourself if you want a melon that really tastes good. How to choose a ripe melon? Taste is the only reliable test. Generally, a ripe melon will be fragrant and the stem end will be slightly soft and indented (though this is so well known that sometimes the stem end will be soft from all the people pushing on it to find out).

Oranges and Mandarins

> *Probably the best way to eat an orange is to pick it dead-ripe from the tree, bite into it at once to start the peeling, and after peeling eat a section at a time.*
> —M. F. K. FISHER

The name comes from the Sanskrit *naranga*, and oranges, with their sweet-and-sour flavor, are generally a Vata-balancing fruit. Pitta can be balanced by very sweet oranges. Ayurveda considers oranges to be a very life-supporting food.

Mandarins, named for the yellow-orange button that crowned the hats of imperial Chinese officials, include *tangerines*; *tangelos*, a cross between a tangerine and a pomelo; *clementines*, either a type of tangerine or a tangerine-orange hybrid; and *mandarin oranges*. These fruits resemble oranges but relinquish their peels and divide into sections much more easily.

❖ The majority of oranges in the Americas are grown in Florida and California. Florida's climate produces the best oranges for juicing; *Valencias* are the top-of-the-line juicy oranges. *Navel oranges,* grown in California, are the best for eating. *Blood oranges,* grown in the Mediterranean regions, enjoy great popularity because of their ever-appealing red color and their sweet juice. There are many other varieties.

❖ The brightness of the orange color can be deceiving; some skins are dyed. Ripe oranges can have some green on their skins. Store oranges at room temperature for about a week and in the refrigerator for about two weeks.

Papayas

In Ayurvedic cooking, papayas are served both as a nourishing fruit and as a cooked vegetable. Columbus dubbed papayas "fruit of the angels." Cortez saw native Mexicans eating papayas after their meals as a digestive aid. Indeed, they contain *papain*, an enzyme that helps break down proteins. *Solo* papayas, smallish fruits with yellow-green skins and golden flesh, are the usual type grown for export. Those grown in Hawaii are often heavily treated with pesticides or irradiated to get rid of a tropical fly that infests the crop. A large type of papaya called *Mexican* but grown in tropical countries around the world has green skin, red-orange flesh, and can weigh in at 10 pounds (5 kg). Most papayas are sold unripe and firm. Allow papayas to ripen at room temperature until slightly soft. Store in the refrigerator for not more than a few days.

Peaches and Nectarines

An apple is an excellent thing—until you have tried a peach!
—GEORGE DU MAURIER

To the Chinese, peaches symbolize immortality. *Shou fao,* "long life peach," is frequently depicted in painting and poetry. Peach-shaped steamed buns are featured at birthdays of elderly people. Very sweet, ripe peaches are balancing to Vata and Pitta. If unripe peaches are left to languish in cold storage, their texture is virtually ruined. Sometimes you can ripen them in a paper bag at room temperature over a few days, but often they will remain hard and simply go bad. Store ripe peaches in the refrigerator for no more than a few days. If you wish to remove the skins without cutting into the flesh, drop peaches into boiling water for about 30 seconds, drain, and immediately peel off the skin.

Talking of Pleasure, this moment I was writing with one hand, and with the other holding to my Mouth a Nectarine—good God how fine. It went down pulpy, slushy, oozy—all its delicious embonpoint melted down my throat like a large beatified Strawberry.   —KEATS, IN A LETTER TO A FRIEND

Commonly believed to be a cross between a peach and a plum, nectarines claim neither as parents. They have stood on their own two feet, as it were, in the plant kingdom for at least five thousand years. The name is derived from the Greek *nektar,* beverage of the gods. Nectarines, along with peaches, have been bred to exhibit two qualities supposedly most precious to consumers: largeness and red color. They now resemble peaches quite closely and can be selected and prepared in the same manner as peaches.

Pears

The pear is the grandfather of the apple, its poor relation, a fallen aristocrat, the man-at-arms of our domains, which once, in our humid land, lived lonely and lordly, preserving the memory of its prestige by its haughty comportment.
—FRANÇOIS DE LA VARENNE, 1650

Kapha-balancing pears, like apples, are members of the rose family. There are two categories of pears now available: European and Asian. Of the European pears, there are types for both summer and winter seasons: the *Bartlett* and *Comice* of summer and the *Bosc* and *d'Anjou* of winter. Winter pears are hard, and summer pears soft and juicy. Asian pears are round, with a crunchy texture like apples. According to type, a ripe pear could be either hard or soft. Pears can be ripened in a paper bag at room temperature. It can take up to a week. Store ripe pears in the refrigerator for about three days, tops. European pears can be poached, stewed, grilled, sautéed, or baked. Asian pears are best eaten uncooked.

 # BAKED STUFFED PEARS

4 servings

A gift of the gods.   —HOMER, DESCRIBING PEARS IN THE *ODYSSEY*

Other nuts and dried fruits can be mixed for the stuffing, but the suggested ones marry particularly well with pears. If you are using tough, unsulphured dried apricots, simmer them for 5 minutes in the ¼ cup (60 ml) orange juice before blending in Step 3.

STEP TWO

4 ripe pears (not Asian pears)

STEP THREE

⅓ cup (40 g) finely chopped   *¼ cup (60 ml) orange juice*
dried apricots   *⅓ cup (50 g) pine nuts*

STEP FOUR

¼ cup (60 ml) orange juice   *Honey*
Ghee or butter

1. Preheat the oven to 350°F (180°C). Butter a baking dish.
2. Halve the pears lengthwise. Remove the stem and the seeds, leaving a small hollow in each half.
3. Purée the apricot pieces and orange juice in a blender until smooth. Mix in the pine nuts. Place a spoonful in the hollow in each pear.
4. Place the pear halves in a baking dish and pour the orange juice over them. Dot liberally with ghee or butter. Cover and bake until tender, about 1 hour. Let cool to lukewarm. Drizzle with a little honey before serving.

Persimmons

If it is not ripe it will drive a man's mouth awrie with much torment; but when it is ripe, it is as delicious as an apricock.
        —CAPTAIN JOHN SMITH, JAMESTOWN SETTLEMENT

An astringent and therefore Kapha-balancing fruit. Persimmons are indigenous to both North America and Asia. Wild North American persimmons are tiny—the size of walnuts—and are delicious. The cultivated persimmons now available in the United States have been bred from Japanese persimmons and a Himalayan variety called *date plum*. Persimmons ripen the most slowly of all sweet fruits, not reaching the peak of succulence until October. They must be fully ripe to offer their sweet, mild flavor; otherwise, they are excruciatingly puckery, as Captain John Smith discovered. Allow persimmons to ripen in a closed paper bag at room temperature.

Pineapples

I can with justice call it the king of fruits because it is the most beautiful and the best of all those of the earth. It is doubtless for this reason that the King of Kings has put a crown upon its head, which is like the essential mark of its royalty.

—PÈRE DU TERTRE

Pineapples are native to the Americas, where they were called *ananas*. The inhabitants of the Caribbean traditionally hung them over their doors, symbolizing hospitality—a custom adopted by American sailors. A pineapple over the door meant the seaman was home from a journey, and all were welcome to stop by.

Pineapples, with their sweet-and-sour flavor, are balancing to Vata and must be very very sweet to make Pitta happy as well. Most pineapples sold in the United States come from Hawaii, where they are grown by virtually one company, which uses heavy amounts of pesticides and inorganic fertilizers. Pineapples achieve their final amount of sweetness before they are picked. To select a ripe pineapple, sniff to see if it has a fragrance. Next, pull on a leaf. If it comes out fairly easily, the pineapple is probably ripe. Store at room temperature but not for too long; pineapples go bad quickly.

Pomegranates

Eat the pomegranate, for it purges the system of envy and hatred.

—MUHAMMAD

"Pomegranate mitigates greatly increased Pitta," says the ancient Ayurvedic text, *Ashtanga Hridaya*. Excessive anger indicates a Pitta imbalance. Eat pomegranates plain, juice them—which can be accomplished with a citrus juicer—and use the seeds as garnishes.

*Though in Heav'n the trees
Of life ambrosial fruitage bear, and vines
    Yield nectar.*

—JOHN MILTON, *Paradise Lost*

Frozen Desserts

*My advice to you is not to inquire why or whither, but just enjoy
your ice cream while it's on your plate.* —THORNTON WILDER

ICE CREAM

Ice cream is technically most balancing when taken as a warm weather delight for
people with predominantly Pitta constitutions. However, I listened to a group of
vaidyas in India who were discussing how ice cream is balancing only for Pittas, and
the most respected Ayurvedic expert among them chuckled, "So how can we make
everyone a Pitta?"

The earliest known frozen desserts were made in India from frozen condensed milk,
and in the Chinese imperial court from frozen ground rice, cream, and fruits. During
World War I ice cream was categorized by the U.S. government as an "essential food-
stuff." To spread the gospel and welcome immigrants, it was served to new arrivals on
Ellis Island, and those who had never before been confronted with this necessity of life
promptly slathered it on their bread.

❖ There are two basic methods of freezing ice cream. *Still-frozen* ice creams are
made by placing a prepared mixture in the freezer. *Churn-frozen* ice creams are
frozen in an ice cream maker that stirs the mixture while it freezes. It has a
smoother texture than its still-frozen relatives. The stirring motion also incorporates air into the mixture, making it a bit lighter and greater in volume.

❖ Most commercial products contain emulsifiers, such as eggs, gelatin, and car-
rageen, to prevent ice crystals from forming, as the ice cream may sit for weeks or
months before it is served. All still-frozen ice creams need an emulsifier. Agar agar
flakes are excellent. Arrowroot or cornstarch can also be used as emulsifiers when
cooked into ice cream mixtures. However, with the ease provided by modern ice

471

cream makers, I suggest preparing ice cream the day it is to be served, eliminating the need for any emulsifier in churn-frozen mixtures.

❖ Make ice cream mixtures slightly sweeter than your taste dictates; extreme cold dulls the sensation of sweet after freezing.

❖ Replace sugar with ⅔ the amount of honey. Blend in the honey only when the mixture is cool.

❖ It is best to cook fruit, as it can discolor, taste off, or not impart sufficient flavor when added uncooked. Cooking with sugar lessens any sourness, making fruit more compatible with milk and cream.

❖ The ratio of milk to cream is entirely up to you. The recipes here suggest equal parts milk and cream for a rich-but-not-too-rich texture. Increase the cream and reduce the milk if desired, but keep in mind that ice creams made entirely from cream can have a greasy texture, like butter. For less richness, increase the milk and reduce the cream. You can make ice cream entirely from milk and even use low-fat or nonfat milk. The texture will be less rich and slightly granular.

❖ *Frozen pudding:* Prepare any arrowroot- or cornstarch-based pudding and either still-freeze or churn-freeze.

❖ *Mousse:* A rich dessert with the texture of mousse can be created by chilling, rather than freezing, still-frozen ice cream mixtures. See the pages that follow for ideas. Variations for the appropriate ice cream mixtures contain instructions.

❖ *Frozen yogurt* can be prepared from any ice cream recipe by replacing the milk and cream with yogurt. The flavor will be more tart than that of commercial varieties, in which milk solids and other fillers, plus copious amounts of sweeteners, counteract yogurt's sourness. Homemade yogurt is the sweetest and therefore the most desirable for frozen desserts.

❖ *Buttermilk ice cream* is delicious in fruit-flavored mixtures. Replace the milk and cream in any recipe with buttermilk.

How to Still-Freeze Ice Cream

❖ Freeze the mixture until semisolid. Stir to distribute the ingredients—nuts and textured additions tend to sink to the bottom. Freeze again until the desired texture is achieved.

❖ Ice cream freezes in approximately 6 hours. This time can vary by 1 to 2 hours, depending on the temperatures of the freezer and the ice cream mixture.

❖ Don't freeze the mixture much longer than necessary—and don't prepare ice cream more than a day in advance. It can become solid, and trying to melt it back to the desired texture usually results in a mixture of partially melted and partially rock-solid ice cream.

DAIRY-FREE ICE CREAM

❖ Replace the milk and cream in ice cream recipes with nut milk or coconut milk. To use soy milk, replace each cup of milk and cream with 1 cup (250 ml) soy milk, 1 tablespoon mild-flavored oil, and ⅛ teaspoon salt.

❖ *Tofu Ice Cream:* Replace each cup of milk and cream with ½ cup (110 g) soft tofu, ½ cup (120 ml) soy milk, 2½ tablespoons mild-flavored oil, and ⅛ teaspoon salt combined in a blender until smooth. It will have less volume and a denser texture than ice cream made with dairy cream.

> *It's a very odd thing—*
> *As odd as can be—*
> *That whatever Miss T. eats*
> *Turns into Miss T.* —WALTER DE LA MARE

RICE CREAM FOR ICE CREAM

2 cups (500 ml)

Chinese emperors of yore feasted on frozen ground rice. You can use this mixture to replace the milk and cream in any ice cream recipe. When preparing it for a Chinese emperor, see the Variation for a rich dairy version.

1⅓ *cups (300 ml) water*	2 *tablespoons mild-flavored oil*
⅓ *cup (70 g) white rice, preferably basmati*	¼ *teaspoon salt*

1. Bring all the ingredients to a boil. Cover, reduce the heat, and simmer until the water is just barely absorbed and the rice is very tender.
2. Place in a measuring cup. Add water to bring the mixture up to 2 cups (500 ml), and purée thoroughly in a blender. Chill.

VARIATION

Omit the oil and salt. Replace the water with milk, and use cream or more milk when adding more liquid in the measuring cup in Step 2.

Coffee Ice Cream

Churn-Frozen

(6½ cups/1.5 l)

STEP ONE

½ cup (120 ml) water
4 teaspoons herbal coffee
substitute powder (preferably
Raja's Cup)

⅔ cup (140 g) raw or packed
brown sugar

STEP TWO

1½ cups (350 ml) milk
2 cups (500 ml) heavy (whipping)
cream

1. Bring the water, herbal coffee substitute powder, and sugar to a boil, stirring until the sugar is dissolved.
2. Remove from the heat and stir in the milk and cream. Chill. Churn according to the directions for your ice cream maker.

Still-Frozen

(4¼ cups/1 l)

STEP ONE

2 cups (500 ml) water
4 teaspoons herbal coffee
substitute powder (preferably
Raja's Cup)

⅔ cup (140 g) raw or packed
brown sugar
*1 tablespoon agar agar flakes**

STEP TWO

1 cup (70 g) milk powder

STEP THREE

2 cups (500 ml) heavy (whipping)
cream

1. Bring the water, herbal coffee substitute powder, and sugar to a boil. Add the agar agar. Reduce the heat and simmer until the agar agar is dissolved, about 5 minutes. Let cool to lukewarm.
2. Place in a blender or food processor and add the milk powder. Blend until smooth.

*This measurement is for agar agar flakes of which 1 tablespoon flakes thickens 1 quart (1 l) liquid. If your brand requires more to thicken, increase the measurement to 4 teaspoons.

3. Whip the cream until it stands in soft peaks. Gently fold in the coffee mixture.
4. Place in a 1-quart (1 l) bowl or mold and freeze according to the directions on page 472.

VARIATIONS

Coffee Crunch Ice Cream: Add 1 recipe for praline from Steps 1 and 2 of Pecan Praliné Hung Yogurt Frosting (pp. 392–93) when halfway churned.

Coffee Mousse: After Step 3 in the still frozen recipe, spoon the mixture into individual bowls. Chill for at least 1 hour. Top with Caramel Sauce (p. 458), whipped cream, and a dusting of chopped nuts if desired.

Nut Ice Cream: Reduce herbal coffee substitute powder to 1 teaspoon. Add 1 cup (110 g) coarsely chopped toasted nuts before freezing. Prepare with toasted almonds, pecans, cashews, pistachios, or other nuts for completely different, completely sumptuous flavors. To gild the lily, serve with Caramel Sauce.

Pralines and Cream Ice Cream: Reduce herbal coffee substitute powder to 1 teaspoon. Add Louisiana Pralines (pp. 452–53), broken into pieces.

MANGO ICE CREAM

You can substitute very ripe peaches or apricots for the mangoes.

CHURN-FROZEN

(6½ cups/1.5 l)

STEP ONE

3 cups (350 g) chopped peeled mangoes, peaches, or apricots
¾ cup (150 g) sugar

½ teaspoon ground ginger
½ teaspoon ground cardamom
1 tablespoon water

STEP TWO

1 cup (250 ml) milk
1 cup (250 ml) heavy (whipping) cream

1. Bring the fruit, sugar, ginger, cardamom, and water to a boil. Reduce the heat and simmer for 5 minutes. Chill.
2. Stir in the milk and cream. Churn according to the instructions for your ice cream maker.

STILL-FROZEN

(5 cups/1.2 l)

STEP ONE

1 cup (250 ml) water
4 cups (450 g) chopped peeled
   mangoes, peaches, or apricots
¾ cup (150 g) sugar

½ teaspoon ground ginger
½ teaspoon ground cardamom
2 tablespoons lemon juice
1 tablespoon agar agar flakes*

STEP TWO

½ cup (35 g) milk powder

STEP THREE

2 cups (250 ml) heavy (whipping)
   cream

1. Bring the water, fruit, sugar, ginger, cardamom, and lemon juice to a boil. Add the agar agar. Reduce the heat and simmer until the agar agar is dissolved, about 5 minutes. Let cool to lukewarm.
2. Place in a blender or food processor with the milk powder and blend until smooth.
3. Whip the cream until it stands in soft peaks. Gently fold in the fruit mixture.
4. Place in a 1½-quart (1.5 l) mold or bowl and freeze according to the directions on page 472.

VARIATIONS

Top the ice cream with Fresh Summer Fruit Sauce (p. 456) made with peaches, mangoes, or fresh berries. How about peach ice cream with raspberry sauce?

Fruit Mousse: After Step 3 of the still-frozen version, spoon the mixture into individual bowls. Chill for at least 1 hour. If desired, top with whipped cream or Fresh Summer Fruit Sauce.

 # DATE ICE CREAM

CHURN-FROZEN

(5 cups/1.2 l)

STEP ONE

1½ cups (350 ml) water
1 cup (285 g) packed pitted dates

⅓ cup (70 g) raw or packed
   brown sugar

---

*This measurement is for agar agar flakes of which 1 tablespoon flakes thickens 1 quart (1 l) liquid. If your brand requires more to thicken, increase the measurement to 4 teaspoons.

STEP TWO

1½ cups (350 ml) milk
1½ cups (350 ml) heavy
  (whipping) cream

½ cup (60 g) chopped nuts, toasted
  (optional)

1. Bring the water, dates, and sugar to a boil. Reduce the heat and simmer until the dates are very soft and the water is absorbed, about 10 minutes.
2. Place in a blender or food processor with the milk and cream and blend until smooth. Strain the mixture. Chill. Churn according to the instructions for your ice cream maker, adding the nuts when halfway churned.

STILL-FROZEN

(4¼ cups/1 l)

STEP ONE

2 cups (500 ml) water
1 cup (285 g) packed pitted dates
⅓ cup (70 g) raw or packed
  brown sugar

1 tablespoon agar agar flakes*

STEP TWO

1 cup (70 g) milk powder

STEP THREE

2 cups (500 ml) heavy (whipping)
  cream

½ cup (60 g) chopped nuts, toasted
  (optional)

1. Bring the water, dates, and sugar to a boil. Add the agar agar. Reduce the heat and simmer until the agar agar is dissolved and the dates are very soft, about 10 minutes. Let cool to lukewarm.
2. Place in a blender or food processor with the milk powder and blend until smooth. Strain the mixture.
3. Whip the cream until it stands in soft peaks. Gently fold in the date mixture and the nuts.
4. Place in a 1½-quart (1.5 l) mold or bowl and freeze according to the directions on page 472.

VARIATION

  Date Mousse: After Step 3 of the still-frozen version, spoon the mixture into individual bowls. Chill for at least 1 hour.

*This measurement is for agar agar flakes of which 1 tablespoon flakes thickens 1 quart (1 l) liquid. If your brand requires more to thicken, increase the measurement to 4 teaspoons.

AMRITA AMBROSIA ICE CREAM

6 cups (1.4 l)

A churn-frozen ice cream with a flavor resembling that of Kulfi (next recipe).

STEP ONE

½ cup (120 ml) milk   *½ cup (100 g) sugar*

STEP TWO

1½ cups (350 ml) milk   *¼ cup (30 g) coarsely chopped*
2 cups (500 ml) heavy (whipping)   *pistachios*
  cream   *¼ cup (35 g) coarsely chopped*
½ teaspoon ground cardamom   *blanched almonds*
A few drops of rose water

1. Bring the milk and sugar to a boil, stirring constantly until the sugar dissolves. Chill.
2. Add the remaining milk, cream, cardamom, and rose water. Churn according to the directions for your ice cream maker, adding the pistachios and almonds when halfway churned.

VARIATIONS

Add about ¼ teaspoon saffron threads in Step 1. Cook until the saffron colors the milk.

Replace the milk and cream with 4 cups (1 l) Khoa (p. 531).

 ## KULFI

INDIA   *2½ cups (600 ml)*

A sumptuous frozen dessert prepared with *khoa*, freshly condensed milk. Rather than airy, like Western ice creams, it is dense and intensely flavored. Traditionally, kulfi is made in cone-shaped molds. More widely available muffin tins also suffice.

STEP ONE

8 cups (1.9 l) whole milk

STEP TWO

½ cup (100 g) sugar   *A sprinkling of rose water*
½ teaspoon ground cardamom
¼ cup (30 g) coarsely chopped
  pistachios

1. Bring the milk to a boil. Continue to boil the milk at the highest heat possible without boiling over for 1 hour. Stir occasionally.
2. Stir in the sugar. Continue to cook until the mixture resembles thin cream, about 45 minutes. Stir in the cardamom, pistachios, and rose water.
3. Pour into kulfi molds or a muffin tin. You should have about 8 full muffin cups. Freeze. To unmold, gently run a sharp knife around the edges and pry out. Allow to stand at room temperature for 5 to 10 minutes before serving.

VARIATION
Add about ¼ teaspoon saffron threads in Step 1.

 # GINGER ICE CREAM

6½ cups (1.5 l)

A churn-frozen rendition.

STEP ONE

½ cup (120 ml) water
⅔ cup (140 g) sugar
1 tablespoon ground ginger

STEP TWO

1½ cups (350 ml) milk   *½ cup (80 g) chopped crystallized*
2 cups (500 ml) heavy (whipping)   *ginger*
  cream

1. Heat the water, sugar, and ginger, and stir until the sugar is dissolved. Chill.
2. Combine with the milk and cream. Churn according to the instructions for your ice cream maker, adding the crystallized ginger when halfway churned.

 # RICOTTA SPUMONI (SPUMONI DI RICOTTA)

ITALY   *4 cups (1 l)*

This has a particularly beautiful appearance when frozen in a mold and served in slices.

STEP ONE

3 cups (700 g) ricotta cheese   *1 tablespoon finely grated*
½ cup (120 ml) coconut milk   *orange zest*
¾ cup (150 g) sugar or ½ cup
  (120 ml) honey

1 cup (150 g) sliced cherries or strawberries

¾ cup (90 g) coarsely chopped pistachios

¼ cup (30 g) dried cherries or raisins

½ cup (40 g) grated dried unsweetened coconut

Walnut halves

1. Beat the ricotta, coconut milk, sugar or honey, and orange zest together.
2. Mix in the cherries or strawberries, pistachios, raisins, and coconut.
3. Pour into individual cups and decorate the tops with walnut halves. Or pour into a 1-quart (1 l) mold and decorate after unmolding.
4. Freeze until firm, about 6 hours. If prepared in a mold, unmold and serve by slicing with a sharp knife.

VARIATION

For a rich pudding, chill the mixture instead of freezing it.

ICES, GRANITE, AND SORBETS

Sharbat—a sweet slushy water ice—was a feature of luxurious living in old Arabia and Turkey. By the 1500s it was hawked in the streets of Europe by merchants dressed in Armenian or Turkish costumes. In the hands of European chefs, sharbat took a less liquid, firmer textured turn, to becoming reincarnated as Italian *granite*, French *sorbet*, and American *ice* or *sherbet*.

❖ In the still-frozen recipes, agar agar flakes are used to prevent large crystals of ice from forming.

❖ Serve sorbet plain, over fruit salads, or in the hollowed-out portions of halved, seeded melons.

How to Still-Freeze Sorbet:
1. Pour the mixture into a bowl. Freeze until semisolid.
2. Beat with a whisk or an electric mixer to break up the ice crystals.
3. Beat again every half hour until the mixture has reached the desired frozen consistency. The beating helps to refine the texture of the final product. Total freezing time will be approximately 6 hours.

How to Still-Freeze Sorbet with a Food Processor:
Freeze the mixture in ice cube trays. Just before serving, process the frozen cubes until puréed.

CELESTIAL SORBETS

Fruit or Flavoring	Sugar (cups/grams)	Water (cups/ml)	Lemon Juice (Tbsp or cups)	Yield (cups/ml)	Agar Agar (for still-frozen)
Berry or Cherry	½ (100 g)	1 (250 ml)	2 Tbsp	6 (1.4 l)	1 Tbsp
3 cups (700 ml) sliced strawberries, whole blueberries or raspberries, or halved cherries					
Herb Tea	to taste	none	¼ cup (60 ml)	6 (1.4 l)	2 tsp
3¾ cups (900 ml) strong herb tea					
Kiwi or Cherimoya	⅓ (70 g)	¾ (200 ml)	2 Tbsp	2½ (600 ml)	2 tsp
2 cups (380 g) sliced kiwis or seeded peeled cherimoyas					
Lemon or Lime	½ (100 g)	2¾ (650 ml)	no extra	5 (1.2 l)	1 tsp
½ cup (120 ml) lemon or lime juice (*Lemon- or Lime-Mint:* replace water with mint tea)					
Orange	2 Tbsp	none	2 Tbsp	5 (1.2 l)	1 tsp
3 cups (700 ml) orange juice					
Peach, Apricot, or Mango	½ (100 g)	¾ cup (200 ml)	2 Tbsp	6 (1.5 l)	1 Tbsp
3 cups (650 g) peeled, sliced fruit					
Persimmon	½ (100 g)	none	none	4 (1 l)	2 tsp
2 cups (480 g) pulp, 3 Tbsp chopped crystallized ginger, and 1¼ cups (300 ml) orange juice					
Pineapple	¾ (150 g)	1¾ (400 ml)	¼ cup (60 ml)	5 (1.2 l)	1 Tbsp
3 cups (750 g) crushed					
Rhubarb	¾ (150 g)	1¼ (300 ml)	none	5 (1.2 l)	2 tsp
4 cups (460 g) 1-inch (2.5 cm) pieces					

Directions
1. Bring the water and sugar to a boil. If using agar agar, stir in now.
2. Reduce the heat and simmer for 5 minutes.
3. Place in a blender or food processor with the fruit, if applicable, and blend until smooth.
4. Freeze in your ice cream freezer or, for still-frozen sorbet, freeze according to the instructions for still-frozen ice cream on page 472.

INSTANT SORBET

Make haste slowly.   —BENJAMIN FRANKLIN

Instant sorbet is very flexible and easy to make. The principle is to freeze fresh, juicy fruit and then blend it in a food processor or blender with a little liquid to a slushy sherbet texture. Serve immediately—instant sorbet waits for no man and, unfortunately, for no woman either.

1. Freeze:

   Pieces of fresh fruit, *or*
   Fruit juice or fruit sauce poured into ice cube trays.

2. Just before serving, place the fruit or frozen cubes in a food processor or blender and process just until the mixture is puréed. To assist in blending, add a small amount of:

   Cream, crème fraîche, coconut milk, yogurt, *or*
   Juicy, unfrozen fruit or fruit juice, *and*
   Sweetening if desired.

> *Heaven and earth last forever.*
> *Why do heaven and earth last forever?*
> *They are unborn,*
> *So ever living.*
> *The sage stays behind, thus he is ahead.*
> *He is detached, thus at one with all.*
> *Through selfless action, he attains fulfillment.*
>
> —LAO-TZU, *Tao Te Ching*

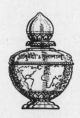

Beverages

They eat, they drink, and in communion sweet
Quaff immortality and joy.

—JOHN MILTON, *Paradise Lost*

WATER

Water is referred to throughout the Vedas as a primary life-giving substance. Ayurveda recommends drinking plenty of water throughout the day and sipping it with meals. Very warm water is light and especially beneficial. It aids digestion, helps remove toxic impurities, such as ama, and keeps ama from forming. Boil water first, then allow it cool to drinking temperature. It may sound strange at first to drink plain warm water, but it feels great—it's soothing, and you'll notice that you feel better throughout the day. Ice cold water extinguishes the digestive fire, Agni, hindering digestion. At least take water at room temperature and not loaded with ice.

If your water is free of pollution, you are well ahead in managing the entrée of environmental toxins into your body. For most of us this means using purified water. Tap water often harbors manmade additions, some intentionally added to kill bacteria and others the discarded wastes of civilization.

Unfiltered tap water containing large quantities of natural minerals and salts (hard water—you know if you've got it) can affect cooking in ways that require adjusting your *modus operandi*. White and light-colored foods cooked in hard water may yellow. (Adding a teaspoon of lemon juice to the cooking water solves this problem in most cases.) Most hard waters strengthen the gluten in flour, making baked goods tough. However, highly alkaline waters dissolve gluten and cause baked goods to shrink. Also, legumes and fruits cooked in hard water may become tough.

❖ *Filtered water:* At present the most effective purifiers work by reverse osmosis (RO) and cost considerably more than other systems. They remove everything from the water, leaving pure H_2O. Doctors trained in Maharishi Ayur-Veda recommend RO filters.

❖ *Spring water:* Some spring waters are indeed better than some tap waters, although they are not as pure as RO water. Ask for a water analysis from the company before investing in a monthly supply of spring water for the sake of its purity. Springs can be just as polluted as any other water sources; also, some bottled waters actually come from the same spring that supplies tap water at considerably less cost!

❖ *Bottled mineral waters* may contain health-enhancing minerals, and some contain fewer pollutants than tap water. Ayurveda does not agree with the claim that carbonation aids digestion—in fact, it states that the opposite effect takes place and recommends avoiding carbonated beverages in general.

Since, Waters, you are the sources of happiness, grant to us to enjoy abundance, and great and delightful perception.

May the divine waters be propitious to our worship; [may they be good] for our drinking; may they flow round us, and be our health and safety.

Waters, bring to perfection all disease-dispelling medicaments for the good of my body, that I may long behold the sun.

—*RIK VEDA* X.1.9

JUICES AND JUICE-BASED BEVERAGES

In Ayurveda freshly pressed juices are described as being both nutritive and purifying. While raw vegetables are difficult to digest, uncooked juices, which have the cellulose and other rough portions removed, are easily accepted by the body. Have the fruits and vegetables to be juiced at room temperature and serve juice immediately after preparing for the best flavor and effects. There are three basic tools for extracting juice at home: (1) Juicers or juice extractors are for vegetables and some fruits. Look for juicers that separate the pulp from the juice rather than mixing the two together. (2) Citrus juicers are used for citrus fruits and also work for pomegranates. (3) Blenders and food processors can be used to purée very juicy fruits so that the juice can be strained out.

Grape, pineapple, or watermelon juice: Blend seedless grapes or small chunks of ripe pineapple or watermelon to a mush in a blender or food processor. Strain through a sieve. Serve immediately.

PEACH, APRICOT, OR MANGO NECTAR

2 to 2½ cups (500 to 600 ml)

STEP ONE

3 cups (650 g) crushed peaches,   1 tablespoon lemon juice
  apricots, or mangoes   1 cup (250 ml) water

STEP THREE

Sugar or honey to taste

1. Combine the fruit, lemon juice, and water in a blender or food processor.
2. Place in a saucepan. Bring to a boil, cover, reduce the heat, and simmer for about 10 minutes.
3. Add sugar to taste; if using honey, wait until the mixture is cool before adding. Add more water to thin if necessary. Let cool.

 # CRANBERRY JUICE

1 quart (1 l)

STEP ONE

3½ cups (400 g) cranberries   3½ cups (850 ml) water

STEP THREE

1 tablespoon lemon juice   ⅓ to ½ cup (70 to 100 g) sugar
½ cup (120 ml) orange or
  apple juice

1. Bring the cranberries and water to a boil. Reduce the heat and simmer until the skins pop, 5 to 7 minutes.
2. Mash lightly and strain.
3. Mix in the remaining ingredients with sugar to taste. Let cool to drinking temperature.

 # LEMONADE OR LIMEADE

1 cup (250 ml)

Life is a difficult thing in the country, and it requires a good deal of forethought to steer the ship, when you live 12 miles from a lemon.   —SYDNEY SMITH

When life hands you a lemon—or lime—here's what to do with it. Lemonade prepared with honey is purifying, Kapha reducing, and energizing. Ayurveda recommends drinking it several times a day for reducing ama and Kapha conditions. Unsweetened lemon juice and water taken as many times during the day as desired also reduces ama, toxic deposits formed from incompletely digested food. Prepared with raw sugar, lemonade is energizing for Vata types and is particularly restorative during hot weather.

2 tablespoons lemon or lime juice	*Honey or raw sugar*
1 cup (250 ml) water	

Mix all the ingredients together with sweetening to taste.

VARIATION

Mint Lemonade: Replace the water with mint tea or add chopped fresh mint leaves.

 # SPICE NECTAR

1 quart (1 l)

Adapted from a recipe idea by Ellen Finkelstein, this lovely beverage has a flavor reminiscent of good-quality ginger ale. It is wonderful both hot and cool.

STEP ONE

5 cups (1.2 l) water	*½ cup (120 ml) chopped fresh mint*
6 whole cloves	*or 1 mint tea bag*
1 cinnamon stick	
1 tablespoon minced fresh ginger	

STEP TWO

½ cup (100 g) sugar

STEP THREE

1 lemon

1. Combine the water, cloves, cinnamon stick, ginger, and mint in a saucepan. Bring to a boil. Continue to boil until the water is reduced to 4 cups (1 l).
2. Add the sugar and stir until blended. Remove from the heat.
3. Cut the lemon in half and squeeze the juice of one half into the drink. Strain. Salvage the cinnamon stick and return to the drink for decoration. Thinly slice the other lemon half and add.

MILK

When overcome by bodily fatigue or exhausted by brain labor no stimulant, so-called, serves so well the purpose of refreshment and rest both bodily and mentally as milk. When heated as hot as one can readily take it, it may be sipped slowly from a tumbler and as it is easily digested one feels very soon its beneficial effect. Few persons realize the stimulating qualities of this simple pure beverage.
—THE SHAKERS, *Manifesto*, 1899

"Milk is the best among vitalizers," declares the *Charaka Samhita*. Ayurveda considers cow's milk to be one of the most nourishing and beneficial foods—something that is life-supporting for virtually everyone. The untoward symptoms some people experience from drinking it are often caused by the standard-issue manner in which it is imbibed: ice cold from the fridge and accompanied by other foods.

❖ Ayurveda recommends boiling milk before drinking. Unboiled milk increases Kapha. Increased Kapha causes the excess mucus and congestion many people experience after taking milk. It also accounts for many cases of lactose intolerance. Even if you wish to drink cool milk, boil it first and then cool it to room temperature. You can further reduce milk's Kapha-increasing tendencies by adding a slice of fresh ginger or a pinch of powdered ginger or turmeric while boiling.

❖ If your mind-body type is predominantly Kapha, Ayurveda recommends drinking low-fat or nonfat milk. People with predominantly Pitta constitutions may find they also feel more balanced drinking low-fat milk. Vata types are usually more balanced by whole milk.

❖ Milk is unique with regard to the six tastes: it is the only food that contains all six. However, it is a predominantly sweet food and doesn't mix well with the other five tastes. According to Ayurveda, mixing milk with any of the other five tastes can cause impurities, or ama, and illness. Milk and cookies—or hot cereal, grains, bread, etc.—are fine, but for a meal containing any taste other than sweet, allow *twenty minutes* before or after to drink milk.

❖ *Unhomogenized milk* is much easier on the tummy. Homogenized milk has been subjected to a process that breaks down the fats and distributes them throughout the milk so that the cream is permanently mixed in. This process renders milk indigestible for some people and leads them to conclude that they have lactose intolerance.

❖ *Skim* or *nonfat milk* has the fat removed—along with the vitamins. The protein and mineral content remain intact, and many of the nourishing qualities of milk extolled by Ayurveda are still present.

❖ Ayurveda recommends drinking fresh milk over powdered. I certainly noticed a difference in my vitality when I lived for seven months in a village in the Philippines where only powdered milk was available. When my husband and I returned to Manila we each drank about ten glasses of fresh milk a day for a week—our bodies were so starved for its nourishment that the cravings didn't calm down until we'd each gained five pounds from milk alone!

❖ *Goat's milk* is described by the Ayurvedic texts as being sweet and astringent. Its fat globules are smaller than those of cow's milk, so it "homogenizes" naturally and is easy to digest. Some people who are allergic to cow's milk can drink goat's milk without problems. Goat's milk should be very fresh for best flavor.

AMRITAM

INDIA   *2 cups (500 ml)*

A soothing beverage to drink at bedtime. Many people take it nightly as a Vata-balancing aid to sound sleep. People with Kapha constitutions could prepare it with low-fat milk and omit the sugar.

2 cups (500 ml) milk   *Pinch of ground cinnamon*
Pinch of saffron   *Pinch of ground cardamom*
2 tablespoons sugar   *1 teaspoon or more ghee*

Bring the milk and saffron to a boil. Reduce heat and simmer for a few minutes. Stir in the remaining ingredients.

TAHINI MILK

1 cup (250 ml)

Prepare with hot or cool milk. When serving hot, sweeten with sugar.

1 cup (250 ml) milk   *1 tablespoon honey or sugar*
1 tablespoon Tahini (p. 512)

Combine all the ingredients together in a blender.

ALMOND MILK

2 cups (480 ml)

A delightful, nutritive, and energizing beverage found in both classical Indian and French cooking. Most balancing to Vata and Pitta when prepared with sugar. Nuts are more digestible when soaked overnight in water.

½ cup (70 g) soaked blanched almonds   1½ tablespoons honey or sugar
2 cups (480 ml) milk

Combine the ingredients in a blender. Soak for a few hours or overnight in the refrigerator. Strain out the almond meal through a fine muslin cloth. Serve hot or at room temperature. When serving hot, sweeten with sugar.

LASSI

Lassi is an excellent Ayurvedic digestive aid to serve during or after a meal. Many people drink lassi on a daily basis. It is the one curd-based dish that is good for all doshas, as lassi is treated as a different food from yogurt. Mixing yogurt with water makes it digestible even in the evening. Fresh, homemade yogurt has the best effect, and lowfat yogurt is better for Pitta and Kapha.

 # SWEET LASSI (MITHA LASSI)

INDIA

Use sugar to balance Vata and Pitta, and honey to balance Kapha.

1 cup (250 ml) yogurt   *3 tablespoons sugar or*
2 to 5 cups (500 ml to 1.2 l)   *2 tablespoons honey*
  water   *A few drops of rose water*
Pinch of ground cardamom   *(optional)*

Mix the ingredients well. Add more sugar or honey if desired.

VARIATIONS

Saffron Lassi: Add a pinch of saffron soaked in 1 tablespoon hot water for 10 minutes.

Rose Petal Lassi (Gulab Lassi): Replace the sweetening with 2 tablespoons rose petal conserve. Blend for 1 to 2 minutes and strain. Great for cooling down Pitta. An excellent rose petal conserve is available from the sources listed for Ayurvedic products in Appendix B.

SALT LASSI (NAMAK LASSI)

INDIA/MIDDLE EAST

In Armenia this popular drink is known as *tan*, and in Lebanon it goes by the name *ayran*. This version is cooling on a hot day and is an excellent digestive aid.

STEP ONE

1 teaspoon ground cumin

STEP TWO

1 cup (250 ml) yogurt

½ teaspoon salt

2 to 5 cups (500 ml to 1.2 l)
water

Black pepper (optional)

1. Toast the cumin in a small dry skillet over low heat, stirring frequently, until fragrant and lightly browned.
2. Mix the cumin and the remaining ingredients together well. Add a grinding of black pepper if desired.

VARIATIONS

Add a pinch of ground ginger to further aid digestion.
Replace the salt with black salt (see introduction to Mint Lassi).

MINT LASSI (PODINA LASSI)

INDIA

A refreshing, nonsweet lassi that serves especially well as an aid to digestion. Black salt, a slightly sulfurous mineral salt compound available in Indian markets, is traditionally used in this drink. Black salt is particularly beneficial to digestion. Appreciation of its flavor is an individual matter, but there are definitely those who have a taste for it, myself included.

STEP ONE

1 teaspoon ground cumin

STEP TWO

1 cup (250 ml) yogurt

½ cup (120 ml) loosely packed
fresh mint leaves

2 to 5 cups (500 ml to 1.2 l)
water

Dash of black pepper

½ teaspoon salt (black salt if
possible)

1. Toast the cumin in a small dry skillet over low heat, stirring frequently, until fragrant and lightly browned.
2. Combine all the ingredients in a blender at high speed until the mint is well blended in.

MANGO-DATE LASSI (AM KHAJUR LASSI)

1 cup (250 ml) yogurt
2 to 5 cups (500 ml to 1.2 l)
*   water*
1 mango, peeled and pitted

4 soft dates
1 to 2 pinches of ground cardamom
Raw sugar or honey

Combine all the ingredients in a blender or food processor, using sweetening to taste.

SEED AND GRAIN BEVERAGES

CEBADA

CENTRAL AMERICA   *5½ cups (1.3 l)*

A lightly thickened and sweetened barley drink. El Salvadorans whip it to a froth in a blender. To balance Kapha, omit the sugar and replace with honey to taste when the mixture is lukewarm.

STEP ONE

5 cups (1.2 l) water
1½ sticks cinnamon

1 tablespoon minced fresh ginger

STEP TWO

⅓ cup (45 g) barley flour
3 tablespoons water

½ cup (100 g) sugar

1. Bring the water, cinnamon sticks, and ginger to a boil.
2. Meanwhile, mix the barley flour, water, and sugar to a smooth paste.
3. Slowly add the barley paste to the boiling water, vigorously mixing it in with a whisk. Return the water to a boil, whisking constantly.
4. Remove from the heat. Pour the mixture through a fine-meshed strainer. Serve hot or at room temperature.

Chan con Limón
(Chia Seeds with Lemon)
CENTRAL AMERICA   *1 quart (1 l)*

Ana Cecilia Rosales of El Salvador described this nourishing beverage made with chia seeds, tiny seeds that gel slightly when soaked in water. You can find them in natural foods stores.

½ cup (70 g) chia seeds   *3 tablespoons lemon juice*
3½ cups (850 ml) water
¼ cup (50 g) sugar or
    3 tablespoons honey

Mix all the ingredients together well. Adjust the sweetening and lemon juice to taste. Allow to stand at room temperature for at least 10 minutes for the chia seeds to swell up. Stir well before serving.

VARIATION
    Replace part or all of the water with fruit juice. Add the sweetening and lemon juice to taste.

 # Seed Horchata (Horchata de Semilla)
MEXICO   *3 cups (700 ml)*

Horchata is a pre-Columbian beverage—essentially spiced, sweetened nondairy milk. Seed-based horchata is traditionally made from melon, sunflower, or pumpkin seeds. I like the tri-doshic pumpkin seed version best. Before using melon seeds, rinse off the fruit residue and dry them in the sun or in a 300°F (150°C) oven. Use soft Mexican cinnamon sticks, if you can obtain them, which are real cinnamon, instead of the more commonly available cassia.

STEP ONE

⅔ cup (90 g) sunflower,
    pumpkin, or melon seeds

STEP TWO

1 stick cinnamon   *Raw or dark brown sugar*
3 cups (700 ml) water

1. Soak the seeds in water overnight. Drain.

2. Purée the seeds, cinnamon stick, and water in a blender for 2 to 3 minutes, until as smooth as possible. Strain through cheesecloth or a fine-meshed tea strainer. Sweeten to taste. The mixture will separate if not served immediately. No matter; just shake well before serving.

 ## RICE HORCHATA (HORCHATA DE ARROZ)

MEXICO   *1½ cups (350 ml)*

A New World beverage adapted to the rice introduced by Old World folk. Prepare with Mexican cinnamon and *piloncillo*, Mexican raw sugar, if you can obtain them.

STEP ONE

*⅓ cup (70 g) long-grain white
   rice, preferably basmati*

STEP TWO

3 cups (700 ml) boiling water   Raw or dark brown sugar
1 stick cinnamon   Grated nutmeg

1. Soak the rice in the water overnight. Drain.
2. Purée. Combine the rice, boiling water, and cinnamon stick in a blender for 2 to 3 minutes, until as smooth as possible. Strain through cheesecloth or a fine-meshed tea strainer. Add sugar to taste and a grating of nutmeg. The rice will settle if not served immediately. No matter; just shake well before serving.

NONDAIRY MILKS

 Milk is a complete food, and there is no substitute for all its good effects. Nondairy milks are useful in dishes containing any of the six tastes other than sweet, which Ayurveda recommends not combining with dairy milk. Dishes such as cream sauces and soups can be made successfully with nondairy milks.

SOY MILK

CHINA   *1 quart (1 l)*

Soy milk balances Vata and Pitta. The Chinese serve freshly made soy milk hot for breakfast like a soup, garnished with a little toasted sesame oil. If you are preparing soy milk for drinking, it improves the flavor to blend a little mild-flavored oil into the finished milk.

STEP ONE

1 cup (170 g) dried soybeans

STEP TWO

1 quart (1 l) water

1. Clean the beans. Place them in a bowl with at least 3 cups of water and soak overnight. Drain.
2. Purée the beans in the water in a blender.
3. Line a sieve with a piece of muslin. Place over a bowl and strain the liquid through it. Gather up the corners of the muslin and squeeze out any remaining liquid. Store in the refrigerator for up to a week.

 # COCONUT MILK

SOUTHEAST ASIA   *2 cups (500 ml)*

Coconut milk balances Vata and Pitta. Asians never use the liquid from the coconut for cooking; instead, they prepare this milk and use the rich liquid throughout their cuisine—from soup to (coco)nuts. It can be made with either fresh or dried unsweetened coconut. Make coconut milk fresh for each use or day—it doesn't keep well.

2 cups (500 ml) hot water
2 cups (180 g) grated fresh or
  dried unsweetened coconut

1. Purée the water and coconut in a blender until fairly smooth. Allow to stand for 30 minutes.
2. Line a sieve with a piece of muslin. Place over a bowl and strain the liquid through it. Gather up the corners of the muslin and squeeze out any remaining liquid.

 # COCONUT CREAM

INDONESIA   *About ⅔ cup (160 ml)*

4 cups (360 g) grated fresh   *1 quart (1 l) water*
  coconut

1. Bring the coconut and water to a boil in a 3-quart pot. Reduce the heat, cover, and simmer for 20 minutes.

2. Purée in a blender 2 cups at a time, holding the lid firmly shut with a folded towel. Strain.
3. Allow the liquid to stand undisturbed at room temperature until cool. The cream will rise to the top; carefully skim it off with a spoon. Serve the same day at room temperature.

 # Nut or Seed Milk

2 to 3 cups (500 to 700 ml)

Nut milk has enjoyed wide popularity in times and places where dairy milk was scarce. Native Americans made nut milk from wild hickory nuts and pecans, and almond milk was a delicacy in medieval Europe. Nut milks do not hold up well to long cooking. Use them for drinking and for quick-cooking soups, sauces, and puddings. Soaking the nuts makes them more digestible.

½ cup (60 g) blanched almonds, raw cashews, pecans, walnuts, or hazelnuts, or pumpkin or sunflower seeds, or ⅓ cup (45 g) sesame seeds

2 to 3 cups (500 to 700 ml) water

1. Soak the nuts overnight in water to cover. Drain.
2. Combine the nuts and water in a blender until smooth. Allow to stand in the refrigerator for 1 to 2 hours. Strain through a muslin cloth. Store in the refrigerator for up to 5 days.

VATA, PITTA, AND KAPHA HAVE A JAVA

The stimulating qualities of coffee and black tea are sometimes used in Ayurvedic medicine to enhance the effectiveness of an herbal formula. However, drinking caffeinated beverages is overstimulating to many, and caffeine combined with sugar really packs a wallop that can create toxins and other havoc within. It's pretty easy to go by your feelings: If you're climbing the walls after drinking a caffeinated beverage, maybe it's time to cut back. Also, if you need several cups of coffee or tea in the morning to feel human, it's a pretty safe bet that there is an imbalance in your system that needs attention. Some people, typically with a high proportion of Kapha dosha, can drink a cup of tea or coffee without feeling untoward effects. Adding boiled milk slightly reduces the effects of caffeine.

TEAS

 ## SALABAT (GINGER TEA)

PHILIPPINES   *1 quart (1 l)*

Dark raw sugar gives this spicy, refreshing beverage the most authentic flavor.

STEP ONE

¼ cup (30 g) coarsely chopped   6 cups (1.4 l) water
fresh ginger

STEP TWO

⅓ cup (70 g) raw or packed dark brown sugar

1. Bring the ginger and water to a boil. Continue to boil until the water is reduced to 4 cups.
2. Add the sugar. Stir until dissolved. Strain. Serve hot or cold.

 ## MASALA CHAI (SPICE TEA)

INDIA   *1 quart (1 l)*

Decaffeinated orange pekoe or Darjeeling teas are ideal for this recipe.

STEP ONE

2 cups (500 ml) water   4 whole cloves
4 teaspoons black tea leaves   2 tablespoons minced fresh ginger
⅛ teaspoon ground cardamom   ⅛ teaspoon saffron (optional)

STEP TWO

2 cups (500 ml) milk   Sugar

1. Bring the water, tea, and spices to a boil. Boil for 1 minute.
2. Add the milk. Return to a boil for another minute. Remove from the heat and add sugar to taste. Strain out the spices and tea leaves before serving.

VARIATION
Replace some of the milk with cream.

> *For he on honey-dew hath fed,*
> *And drunk the milk of Paradise.*
>
> —SAMUEL TAYLOR COLERIDGE, "Kubla Khan"

Sauces, Condiments, and Chutneys

It is the sauce that distinguishes a good chef. The saucier is a soloist in the orchestra of a great kitchen.

—FERNAND POINT

SAUCES

The name *sauce* is derived from the Latin *saltus*, or "salted." In the European tradition *sauciers*, chefs who prepare sauces alone, undergo long study and apprenticeship before they ever produce their own creation for public consumption. In India it is much the same; the preparation of *masalas*, spice mixtures for sauces, and chutneys are culinary arts in themselves. Sauces and chutneys are useful in Ayurveda for adding more tastes to a meal that does not contain all of the six. They can also add a moist, unctuous element to inherently dry dishes, such as nut and bean loaves, making them more balanced. Sauces and chutneys also offer a solution for families in which some members prefer their foods plain and others like them more dressed up or in which different Ayurvedic constitutions must be satisfied.

Roux-Based Sauces

An effective method of thickening liquids with flour is to make a *roux*, which is considered one of the foundations of Western cooking. The name comes from the French word meaning "red," which refers to cooking the flour until it changes color—which is not usually done, as a roux is usually used to thicken "white sauce." Go figure. There are many alternatives to the classic combination of white flour, butter, and milk. I use nondairy milk in all roux-based sauces to avoid mixing milk with salt, and I substitute ghee for butter.

❖ A roux can be prepared with unbleached white or whole wheat flour. You can also use besan (chickpea flour), when herbs or strong-tasting ingredients are included. Sauté besan in ghee, stirring frequently, for 10 minutes over low heat to soften its flavor.

497

❖ A whisk is an essential tool-of-the-trade for preventing or removing lumps. A wooden spoon is also good for stirring sauces gently. However, if in spite of your best efforts lumps do appear, a whirl on the spin cycle in a blender or food processor will take care of them.

OIL-FREE AND FLOUR-FREE ALTERNATIVES TO ROUX-BASED SAUCES

❖ Omit the flour and oil in Béchamel Sauce (recipe follows). Mix 2 tablespoons arrowroot or cornstarch or 4 teaspoons kudzu powder into ¼ cup (60 ml) of the nondairy milk. Add the rest of the liquid. Heat the mixture to a simmer over low heat, stirring constantly. Simmer until thickened. Add the salt and nutmeg.

❖ Replace Béchamel Sauce with Creamy Cauliflower Soup with Cashews (p. 238), both of which contain oil but not flour.

He is always different, like a sauce.   —SICILIAN EXPRESSION

BÉCHAMEL SAUCE
(WHITE SAUCE OR CREAM SAUCE)

FRANCE   *2 cups (480 ml)*

Historical records have it that this classic sauce was invented by Orion, a chef in ancient Greece. It is named, however, for the Marquis de Béchameil, steward of Louis XIV of France and superintendent of the royal kitchens. Classic béchamel sauce is simmered in a double boiler for one hour, which makes it exquisitely smooth and slightly thinner. However, the long cooking is rarely undertaken by those who don't have access to the royal kitchen staff and is not necessary to achieve a decent sauce by most standards.

STEP ONE

¼ to ⅓ cup (60–75 g) ghee or butter   *3 tablespoons flour*

STEP TWO

2 cups (480 ml) nondairy milk

STEP THREE

½ teaspoon salt   *Pinch of ground nutmeg* (optional)

1. Melt the ghee or butter in a saucepan. Add the flour and cook for 1 minute, stirring constantly with a whisk to eliminate all lumps.
2. Gradually add the milk, stirring constantly. Return to the heat. Bring to a simmer, stirring constantly with the whisk. Do not boil.
3. Add the salt. Simmer for a few minutes until fully thickened. Add the nutmeg.

VARIATIONS

Sauté a pinch of hing in the ghee or butter for 30 seconds before adding the flour. Stir in chopped fresh herbs before serving.

Béchamel with Stock: Replace the milk with 1½ cups (360 ml) vegetable stock and ½ cup (120 ml) crème fraîche.

Curried Béchamel Sauce: Omit the nutmeg. Add 1 to 1½ teaspoons curry powder or Maharishi Ayur-Veda churnas to the ghee or butter in Step 1.

Dark Béchamel: Cook the flour and ghee or butter, stirring constantly, until the mixture turns golden brown. Remove from the heat for 5 minutes, then add the milk as above. The holding power of the flour is slightly reduced, but the flavor is distinctive.

Sauce Béchamel aux Herbes (Béchamel-Herb Sauce): Omit the nutmeg. Sauté 1 teaspoon dried green herbs in the ghee or butter before adding the flour. Replace the salt with celery salt or seasoned salt.

Sauce Mornay: A sauce ascribed to Prime Minister Philippe de Mornay, which he invented for his king, Henri IV of France. Add ½ cup (50 g) grated Swiss or Gruyère cheese to the simmering sauce. Stir constantly until the cheese is completely melted and blended. Remove from the heat immediately.

Sauce Aurore: The name means "dawn," for the dawn-pink color of the sauce. Simmer 1 cup (230 ml) puréed tomatoes, covered, for 20 minutes. Place in a measuring cup and add nondairy milk until there are 2 cups (480 ml) of liquid. Replace the 2 cups (480 ml) milk with this mixture.

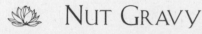 # NUT GRAVY

3 cups (720 ml)

The word *gravy* comes from the Latin *granatus*, meaning "made from grains." Today's gravies are more likely to be spooned over grains than contain them. Here is a basic vegetarian version—delicious over stuffings, burgers, nut and bean loaves, or mashed potatoes. Vary the flavor by using different types of nuts. Pistachios contribute a beautiful green color, and toasted cashews and almonds give particularly excellent flavor.

STEP ONE

2 tablespoons ghee, butter, or oil *3 tablespoons unbleached white or*
Pinch of hing (optional) *whole wheat flour*

STEP TWO

2 cups (480 ml) nondairy milk *Salt*
1 cup (120 g) ground toasted nuts* *Black pepper*

---

*Oily nuts such as pecans, which grind to a moist mixture, weigh more than drier nuts, such as pistachios, which grind to a dry powder. If using metric measurements, you may have to adjust 15 to 20 grams up or down from the suggested amount.

1. Heat the ghee, butter, or oil in a saucepan. Add the hing if desired and sauté over low heat until fragrant, about 30 seconds. Add the flour and cook for 1 minute, stirring constantly with a whisk to remove all lumps. For best results, remove from the heat for a few minutes before proceeding to the next step.
2. Add the milk and nuts. Bring the gravy to a simmer, stirring constantly. Simmer for a few minutes, until thickened. Add salt and pepper to taste.

VARIATIONS
  Add Miriam's Sofrito (p. 218) to the gravy.
  Replace the milk with vegetable stock.

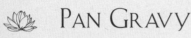 # PAN GRAVY

2 cups (480 ml)

STEP ONE

1 tablespoon ghee or oil	*2 tablespoons minced fresh parsley*
Pinch of hing (optional)	*1 teaspoon dried thyme*
½ bell pepper, finely chopped	*¼ teaspoon dried sage*
1 stalk celery, thinly sliced	

STEP TWO

¼ cup (60 ml) ghee or oil
¼ cup (35 g) unbleached white
  or whole wheat flour

STEP THREE

2 cups (480 ml) stock or water	*Black pepper*
Liquid seasoning or salt	

1. Heat the ghee or oil in a saucepan. Add the hing if desired and sauté over low heat until fragrant, about 30 seconds. Add the bell pepper, celery, and herbs and sauté, stirring frequently, until the bell pepper and celery are tender.
2. Add the remaining ghee or oil. When hot, add the flour and cook, stirring constantly with a whisk, until golden brown. If using whole wheat flour, be especially alert not to burn.
3. Remove from the heat for a few minutes. Add the stock or water and beat with a whisk. Return the gravy to the heat. Bring to a simmer, stirring constantly. Add liquid seasoning or salt and pepper to taste, and simmer for a minute or two until thickened.

GHEE AND LEMON SAUCE

Mix two parts melted ghee with one part lemon or lime juice as a perfect simple sauce for vegetables and for dipping artichoke leaves.

> *All's well that ends with a good meal.* —ARNOLD LOBEL

 # SAUCE NOISETTE
(BROWNED BUTTER WITH NUTS)
FRANCE   *½ cup (120 ml)*

Try tossed with steamed green beans. Hazelnuts and almonds are particularly good.

½ cup (115 g) ghee or butter   *3 tablespoons ground nuts*

Combine the ingredients in a saucepan. Bring to a boil over low heat and cook until light brown, stirring constantly.

 # CREAM CHEESE HOLLANDAISE
A little over 1 cup (250 ml)

Classic Hollandaise was created by French Huguenot chefs exiled in Holland. Warm, it is a tart, creamy sauce for vegetables. At room temperature this version takes on a sour cream–like texture and is a delicious dip for artichokes.

½ cup (120 ml) melted ghee or butter   *1 tablespoon chopped fresh*
¼ cup (60 ml) lemon juice   *tarragon or ½ teaspoon dried*
½ cup (4 ounces/115 g) cream
* cheese, softened*

Mix the ingredients together in a blender or food processor. Transfer to a saucepan and heat to serving temperature. The mixture will separate, but it doesn't matter. Just before serving, remix in a blender or food processor.

VARIATION
   ✪ Substitute crumbled tofu for the cream cheese.

CREAMY HORSERADISH SAUCE (SAHNIGE MEERRETICH SOßE)

GERMANY   *1 cup (240 ml)*

You have some textural choices with this tangy mixture. For a sauce with the consistency of cream that can also be used as a salad dressing, prepare with buttermilk. For a thick, spoonable consistency that is great for baked potatoes and can be used as a dip, prepare with sour cream. Either way, it can be tossed with steamed vegetables.

*2 tablespoons finely grated
  horseradish
1 tablespoon lemon juice
1 tablespoon sugar or honey*

*¼ teaspoon salt
⅔ cup (160 ml) buttermilk or sour
  cream*

Mix the horseradish, lemon juice, sugar or honey, and salt together thoroughly. Gently fold in the buttermilk or sour cream. For best results, chill for at least 1 hour.

VARIATIONS
  Escoffier's Horseradish Sauce: Add 2 tablespoons finely ground walnuts.
  Substitute crème fraîche for the buttermilk or sour cream.
  Add 1 tablespoon finely grated beets.
  ❂ Substitute Tofu, Cashew, or Avocado Mayonnaise (recipes follow, pp. 503–504) for the dairy.

MOCK MAYONNAISES

Condiments are like old friends—highly thought of, but often taken for granted.
—MARILYN KAYTOR

In 1628 on the Spanish island of Minorca, the Duc de Richelieu sampled a sauce called *ali-oli,* known today as *aïoli.* Upon his return home, he had it prepared in Versailles, minus the olive oil and garlic. He christened it *Sauce Mayonnaise,* after Minorca's principal city, Mahon. Here the noble sauce receives a complete overhaul, making it accessible to those who don't want the eggs, the potentially rancid oils, and other dubious ingredients included in today's bottled "mayo."

FLAVORINGS FOR MOCK MAYONNAISES

A pinch of hing sautéed in 1 tablespoon of oil
Dried Tomato Paste (p. 506)
Sweet Red Pepper Purée (p. 513)
Pesto
Chutney or salsa
Fresh or dried herbs
Curry powder or Maharishi Ayur-Veda churnas
Flavorful oils such as olive or hazelnut
A few drops of toasted sesame oil

 # TOFU OR PANIR MAYONNAISE

A little over 1 cup (250 ml)

A very flexible mixture that can be used as a mayonnaise, a cream sauce, or in place of sour cream.

*1 cup (240 ml) drained, crumbled
   tofu (soft tofu is best) or soft
   panir
¼ cup (60 ml) mild-flavored oil*

*2 tablespoons lemon juice
Liquid seasoning or salt
White pepper*

Purée the tofu or panir, oil, and lemon juice in a food processor or blender until smooth and creamy. Add liquid seasoning or salt and pepper to taste. If a thinner consistency is desired, add water.

VARIATION

❂ *Tofu Dessert Cream:* A nondairy creamy topping for desserts and fruit salads. It is firmer when made with sugar than with honey. Reduce the lemon juice to 1 tablespoon. Blend in 2 to 3 tablespoons honey or 3 to 4 tablespoons raw sugar and a pinch of salt. If desired, flavor with dried fruit purée, lemon and orange zests, herbal coffee substitute powder, or sweet spices.

 # CASHEW MAYONNAISE

1 cup (240 ml)

You can thin this mixture to serve as a creamy sauce—my mother pours it over asparagus—or chill to make it slightly thicker. To add balance for Kapha, and remain balancing for Pitta and Vata, replace the cashews with raw sunflower seeds, which are tri-doshic.

STEP ONE

⅓ *cup (45 g) raw cashews*
½ *cup (120 ml) water*

¼ *teaspoon salt*
¼ *teaspoon paprika*

STEP TWO

⅔ *cup (160 ml) mild-flavored oil*

STEP THREE

3 *tablespoons lemon juice*

1. Purée the cashews, water, salt, and paprika in a blender on high speed until completely smooth.
2. Reduce to the lowest speed. Carefully remove the lid. While the mixture is spinning, pour the oil into it in a steady drizzle.
3. When all the oil has been added, turn off the blender. Add the lemon juice, replace the cover, and return to high speed until the mixture is thick.

It is the duty of a good sauce to insinuate itself all around the maxillary glands, and imperceptibly awaken into activity each ramification of the organs of taste; if not too sufficiently savory it cannot produce this effect, and if too piquant, it will paralyze, instead of exciting, those delicious titillations of tongue and vibrations of the palate that only the most accomplished philosophies of the mouth can produce on the highly-educated palates of thrice happy grands gourmets!

—GRIMOD DE LA REYNIÈRE

 # AVOCADO MAYONNAISE

A little over 1 cup (250 ml)

A very creamy sauce with no added oil. Avocado is quite perishable; for best results, prepare the mayonnaise just before using. Try the variation to add a little zip to the otherwise neutral flavor.

1 *cup (220 g) mashed ripe*
  avocado
1 *tablespoon plus 1 teaspoon*
  lemon juice

Water
Liquid seasoning or salt

Purée the avocado and lemon juice in a blender or food processor. Add water in 1-tablespoon increments until the desired texture is achieved. Add liquid seasoning or salt to taste.

VARIATION

Blend in ½ teaspoon honey and 1 tablespoon minced fresh ginger.

TOMATO SAUCES

Tomatoes are a bit questionable in Ayurveda, as they aggravate all the doshas, but like all plants, they have some health-giving qualities as well. Using fresh, ripe tomatoes in season will always offer better effects than using the canned article, and serving at meals that do not include other acidic foods will be more balancing.

> While some enjoy their tomatoes straight up in sauces, others prefer to eliminate seeds and annoying little curls of skin in the sauce. Skins and seeds can easily be banished by blanching the tomatoes, chopping them, and passing them through an old-fashioned food mill.

TOMATO SAUCE

ITALIAN AMERICAN   *4 to 5 cups (900 ml to 1.2 l)*

Long-cooking tomato sauces were prepared by Italian immigrants in America who adapted to the shorter growing season in their new home by finding ways to preserve tomatoes. The rich flavor of this sauce will be a pleasant surprise to those accustomed to cooking with a canned sauce base. The final amount of sauce depends on whether the cooking stops when the sauce is thick but still liquid or when it is cooked to a very thick paste with no separated liquid.

STEP ONE

¼ cup (60 ml) olive oil
Pinch of hing (optional)
1 bell pepper, cut into small
* pieces*
1 carrot, sliced

1 stalk celery with leaves, sliced
¼ cup (60 ml) minced fresh parsley
2 teaspoons dried basil
1 teaspoon dried thyme
½ teaspoon rosemary

STEP TWO

9 cups (2.1 kg) chopped ripe
* tomatoes*

¾ cup (180 ml) water
2 bay leaves

STEP THREE

Liquid seasoning or salt
Black pepper

1 to 2 teaspoons sugar (optional)

1. Heat the olive oil and hing in a large pot over low heat. Add the bell pepper, carrot, celery, and herbs and sauté for 5 minutes, stirring frequently.
2. Add the tomatoes, water, and bay leaves. Cover and simmer over medium-low heat

for 2 hours or more, or over the lowest heat for 4 to 5 hours or more until very thick. Stir occasionally.

3. Add liquid seasoning or salt and pepper to taste and simmer for a few minutes more. If the sauce is too tart, add 1 to 2 teaspoons sugar.

VARIATIONS

For a sweeter sauce, substitute 2 grated carrots for the celery and bell pepper.
Oil-Free Tomato Sauce: Eliminate the olive oil and cook all the ingredients together.

 # DRIED TOMATO PASTE

1½ cups (360 ml)

Dried tomatoes make a thick sauce similar to canned tomato paste, and you can use it just like the canned article to add flavor and thickness. Its intense flavor also works well as a sandwich spread and a topping for canapés and pizzas. Add the paste to dips and to sauces such as the mayonnaises and Béchamel Sauce.

STEP ONE

One 8-ounce (230 g) jar oil-
packed dried tomatoes, drained, or
1½ cups (120 g) packed
dry-packed dried tomatoes

¾ cup (180 ml) water

1. Bring the tomatoes and water to a boil in a saucepan. Cover, reduce the heat, and simmer for 10 minutes.
2. Purée in a blender or food processor until smooth. Add more water to achieve the desired texture if necessary.

SALSAS

Salsa means "sauce." Since ancient times in Mexico, mixtures of spiced chopped fruits and vegetables have been spooned over dishes to flavor them in the same manner as the chutneys of India.

Make hunger thy sauce, as a medicine for health. —THOMAS TUSSER

SALSA CRUDA

MEXICO   *1¾ cups (420 ml)*

The name *cruda,* or "crude," refers to both the uncooked ingredients and the rustic texture. The ingredients should be chopped—not puréed. I've used ginger and black pepper instead of the usual chilies to give it a gentle kick.

Pinch of hing (optional)
1 teaspoon oil (optional)
1½ cups (2 medium/350 g) finely chopped tomatoes
¼ cup (40 g) finely chopped green bell pepper

¼ cup (60 ml) finely chopped fresh cilantro
1 tablespoon minced fresh ginger
1 tablespoon lemon juice
¼ teaspoon salt
Black pepper

If desired, sauté the hing in the oil over low heat until fragrant, about 30 seconds. Toss with the remaining ingredients, including a generous amount of black pepper. Serve at room temperature.

VARIATION
Add chopped jalapeños to taste.

 ## MANGO SALSA

About 2 cups (480 ml)

When the mangoes are ripe on the tree, then the branches bow down.
      —ANCIENT INDIAN SAYING DESCRIBING THE HUMILITY OF ENLIGHTENED PEOPLE

Salsa or chutney? You could serve this with either Mexican- or Indian-style dishes.

STEP ONE
1 tablespoon mild-flavored oil
½ teaspoon brown mustard seeds

1 tablespoon minced fresh ginger

STEP TWO
2 cups (230 g) coarsely chopped mangoes
2 tablespoons lime juice

2 tablespoons finely chopped cilantro
⅛ teaspoon salt

1. Heat the oil in a small skillet over low heat. Add the mustard seeds and sauté until they "dance." Turn off the heat, add the ginger, and stir a few times to coat with the oil.
2. Toss with the mangoes, lime juice, cilantro, and salt.

VARIATION
Add finely chopped green chilies.

 ## ROASTED TOMATO SALSA

MEXICO   *2 cups (480 ml)*

A chunky cooked salsa with distinctive spices that you could serve with Indian-style food as well as with Mexican dishes. It is difficult to determine the exact measurement from the raw tomatoes, so be prepared to have a little leftover roasted tomato or to throw one more in the oven.

STEP ONE

Olive oil   *Pinch of hing* (optional)

STEP TWO

*Approximately 4 large or
  6 medium tomatoes*

STEP THREE

1 tablespoon lemon juice   *½ teaspoon salt*
1½ teaspoons sugar   *½ teaspoon ground ginger*
1½ teaspoons ground cumin,   *¼ teaspoon ground cinnamon*
  toasted   *¼ teaspoon ground coriander*
¾ teaspoon paprika   *Pinch of ground cloves*

1. Preheat the oven to 450°F (230°C). Generously coat a baking pan with olive oil and sprinkle a pinch of hing on the bottom if desired.
2. Cut the stem out of each tomato with a paring knife, place the tomatoes in the baking pan, and bake until the skins begin to brown and split and the tomatoes are fairly soft, about 15 minutes.
3. As soon as the tomatoes are cool enough to handle, remove the skins. Place the tomatoes and all the juices remaining in the baking pan in a food processor and pulse once or twice to make a chunky sauce. Alternatively, coarsely chop the tomatoes. Place in a measuring cup and measure 2 cups (480 ml) of sauce. Stir in the remaining ingredients.

VARIATIONS
For a *salsa picante*, replace the paprika with cayenne, crumbled red chilies, or chopped fresh chilies.
Add chopped fresh cilantro.

Papaya-Jicama Salsa

2 cups (480 ml)

Sweet-and-sour fresh salsa that gets its kicks from ginger and pepper.

*1 cup (150 g) very finely diced
  papaya*
*1 cup (140 g) very finely diced
  jicama*
*3 tablespoons finely chopped
  fresh cilantro*

2 tablespoons lemon juice
1 tablespoon minced fresh ginger
1 teaspoon sugar
½ teaspoon salt
Black pepper to taste

Mix all the ingredients together. Allow to stand at room temperature for at least 10 to 15 minutes before serving to allow the flavors to blend.

VARIATIONS
  Replace the ginger and black pepper with finely chopped fresh chilies added to taste.
  Papaya Salsa: Replace the jicama with papaya.

Pesto

The name *pesto* is derived from *pestare*, to "pound" or "grind." The simplest ones contain fresh herbs ground with olive oil. Traditionally, pesto is prepared in a *mortare*, a large stone mortar with a heavy wooden pestle. Hand-grinding coaxes the most exquisite flavors from the ingredients. However, it is possible to produce an acceptable version in a food processor in a matter of minutes. In fact, pasta with pesto is sublime fast food. The following recipes will give you a good idea of the basic theory and technique. They are highly flexible propositions with lots of room to exercise your creativity. My pesto recipes are quite thick and contain less oil than some other versions. If you like a more liquid sauce, thin with water or stock, crème fraîche or sour cream, or more oil.

To make a classic pesto with a mortar and pestle, finely chop the ingredients, such as herbs and nuts, and grate the cheese if using. Pound the ingredients in a mortar, adding the oil drizzle by drizzle to lubricate the mixture, until the consistency of a paste is achieved. You may end up needing less oil than the recipe recommends, as the pounding will more thoroughly release the nuts' oils.

PESTO ALLA GENOVESE

ITALY   *1¼ cups (300 ml)*

An emerald green, flavorful sauce from Genoa, where it is traditionally served in a dish combining pasta with new potatoes and green beans.

1 cup (240 ml) minced fresh parsley
1 cup (240 ml) minced fresh basil
¼ cup (30 g) pine nuts or
   chopped walnuts

⅔ cup (160 ml) olive oil
½ cup (50 g) grated Parmesan
   cheese (optional)
Salt

Purée all the ingredients in a blender or food processor, adding salt to taste.

VARIATIONS
   Replace some or all of the basil with spinach, watercress, or other fresh green herbs.
   Omit the nuts.
   Sauté a pinch of hing in the olive oil for a minute.

DRIED TOMATO AND WALNUT PESTO

1 cup (240 ml)

Intensely flavored, this pesto is an excellent pasta and pizza sauce. Double the amount for spreading on a large pizza. It is also a tasty spread for sandwiches and for topping baked or grilled eggplant slices.

STEP ONE
½ cup (120 ml) drained
   oil-packed dried tomatoes

½ cup (120 ml) water

STEP TWO
⅓ cup (80 ml) olive oil
Pinch of hing (optional)

⅓ cup (35 g) coarsely chopped
   walnuts

STEP THREE
⅔ cup (160 ml) coarsely chopped
   fresh flat-leaf parsley
⅓ cup (35 g) grated Parmesan
   cheese (optional)

Salt

1. Bring the tomatoes and water to a boil in a small saucepan. Cover, reduce the heat, and simmer until the tomatoes are soft, about 10 minutes. Set aside.

2. Heat the oil in a small skillet. Add the hing if desired and the walnuts and cook over low heat, stirring frequently, until lightly browned.
3. Purée with the remaining ingredients in a blender or food processor, adding salt to taste.

 # SPINACH AND TOASTED ALMOND PESTO

About 1 cup (240 ml)

STEP ONE

½ cup (120 ml) olive oil
Pinch of hing (optional)

⅓ cup (45 g) whole blanched almonds

STEP TWO

2 cups (190 g) packed chopped spinach leaves
½ cup (50 g) grated Parmesan cheese (optional)

Salt

1. Heat the oil in a small saucepan. Add the hing if desired and the almonds and cook over low heat until the almonds are lightly toasted. Remember that they will continue to toast for a minute after you remove them from the heat. Allow to cool for a few minutes.
2. Purée with the remaining ingredients in a blender or food processor, adding salt to taste.

VARIATIONS

Replace the spinach partially or totally with basil leaves, watercress, or other fresh green herbs.

Replace the almonds with pine nuts, walnuts, or other nuts.

 # PISTACHIO PESTO FOR EDITH

1½ cups (360 ml)

In honor of Edith Kasin, my mother. Sublime on pasta or spread on crusty bread slices, this creamy mixture can also be served as a dip. It can be prepared with any creamy cheese—or even with tofu—but it tastes especially special made with a creamy chèvre such as Montrachet.

STEP ONE

½ cup (120 ml) olive oil
Pinch of hing (optional)

⅔ cup (80 g) pistachios

STEP TWO

⅔ cup (60 g) *creamy cheese, such*
   as chèvre, panir, or cream
   cheese
1 cup (240 ml) *coarsely chopped,*
   loosely packed fresh basil

½ cup (120 ml) *coarsely chopped,*
   loosely packed fresh flat-leaf parsley
Salt

1. Heat the oil in a small skillet. Add the hing if desired and the pistachios and cook over low heat, stirring constantly, until fragrant, about 30 seconds. Remove from the heat and allow to cool to room temperature.
2. Purée with the remaining ingredients in a blender or food processor, adding salt to taste. When adding to pasta, gently toss with the pasta over low heat until the cheese melts slightly. If too thick, thin with vegetable stock or water to the desired consistency.

VARIATION

Replace the parsley with spinach, arugula, tarragon, chervil, or other fresh green herbs.

MISCELLANEOUS SAUCES

 ## TAHINI (SESAME BUTTER)

Grinder method (pure, thick tahini): Put raw or toasted sesame seeds through the finest blade of a meat grinder. Grind several times if necessary to produce a smooth paste.

Blender method, about ¾ cup (180 ml): Blenders produce rough-textured, thinner tahini, as oil must be added. Toast ½ cup (70 g) sesame seeds in ⅓ to ½ cup (80 to 120 ml) mild-flavored oil over medium heat. Shake the pan and stir until the seeds are golden and begin to pop. Remove from the heat immediately—they will continue to brown for a few seconds more. Blend until smooth in a blender. The oil and sesame seeds may separate a little during storage—just stir a bit before using.

 ## TARATOOR SAUCE

MIDDLE EAST   *⅔ cup (160 ml)*

Traditionally served on falafel sandwiches, taratoor sauce also goes well with vegetables and salads and can be mixed into casseroles and dips.

½ cup (120 ml) Tahini
  (recipe follows)
¼ cup (60 ml) lemon juice

2 tablespoons minced fresh ginger
Liquid seasoning or salt

Combine the tahini, lemon juice, and ginger in a blender or food processor. Add liquid seasoning or salt to taste.

VARIATIONS
  Add a little cayenne or ground red chilies.
  Blend in a handful of chopped fresh cilantro.

 # SWEET RED PEPPER PURÉE

An intensely flavored and colored thick purée that is sublime over pasta. Place a spoonful in a bowl of thick soup, such as Cream of Corn Soup, for a beautiful contrast of colors and flavors. You can also use yellow or green bell peppers.

Sweet red bell peppers (5 peppers
  will yield about ⅔ cup/160 ml
  of sauce)

STEP TWO
Olive oil
Salt

Lemon juice
Olive oil

STEP THREE
Sugar (optional)
Salt

1. Preheat the oven to 350°F (180°C).
2. Seed and slice the peppers into large chunks. Place on a baking sheet. Drizzle with olive oil and sprinkle with salt. Bake until tender, 20 to 30 minutes.
3. Purée the peppers in a blender or food processor with a sprinkling of lemon juice and enough olive oil to form a fairly smooth, thick sauce. If too tart, add a pinch of sugar. Add salt to taste.

VARIATION
  Instead of baking the peppers, grill them, or cook in olive oil in a covered skillet over low heat until tender.

SALSA DI NOCI (LIGURIAN WALNUT SAUCE)

ITALY   *1 cup (240 ml)*

This recipe can also be beautifully rendered with pistachios or hazelnuts.

STEP ONE

⅓ cup (80 ml) olive oil
Pinch of hing (optional)

¾ cup (75 g) walnut pieces

STEP TWO

⅓ cup (80 ml) sour cream or
*   thick coconut milk*
⅔ cup (160 ml) loosely packed
*   chopped fresh flat-leaf parsley*

¼ teaspoon salt
Black pepper

1. Heat the oil in a small skillet. Add the hing if desired and the walnuts and cook over low heat, stirring frequently, until the walnuts are very lightly browned. Remove from the heat and let cool to room temperature.
2. Purée with the remaining ingredients except the pepper in a blender or food processor. Adjust the salt and add pepper to taste.

VARIATION
Replace the parsley partially or totally with other fresh green herbs, such as basil.

SWEET-AND-SOUR SAUCE

ASIA   *About ¾ cup (180 ml)*

A very simple rendition. Other herbs and spices, such as fresh ginger, hing, and cilantro, should be cooked with the vegetables in the main dish before this sauce is added as a finishing touch.

1 tablespoon arrowroot or
*   cornstarch*
⅔ cup (160 ml) orange or
*   pineapple juice*

1 tablespoon sugar
1 to 3 tablespoons lemon juice
Liquid seasoning

Mix the arrowroot or cornstarch in a little of the juice. Add the sugar, lemon juice, and liquid seasoning to taste. Add to stir-frying vegetables and stir for a minute until thickened.

PINEAPPLE SWEET-AND-SOUR SAUCE

SOUTHEAST AND EAST ASIA   *1¾ cups (420 ml)*

This sauce finishes a dish that presumably already contains whatever spices you are using, such as fresh ginger, hing, and cilantro. For a beautiful presentation, serve stir-fried vegetables in this sauce in a scooped-out pineapple shell.

STEP ONE

*2 cups (460 g) chopped ripe
  tomatoes*
1 cup (245 g) finely diced pineapple
¼ cup (60 ml) water

1 tablespoon raw or brown sugar
2 tablespoons lemon juice
½ teaspoon salt

STEP TWO

*1 tablespoon arrowroot or
  cornstarch*

¼ cup (60 ml) water
White pepper

1. Combine the tomatoes, pineapple, water, sugar, lemon juice, and salt in a saucepan. Simmer, covered, until the pineapple and tomatoes are tender, about 30 minutes.
2. Mix the arrowroot or cornstarch into the remaining water. Add to the sauce and stir for 2 to 3 minutes to thicken. Adjust the salt and sprinkle with a little white pepper.

 ## SAMBAL (INDONESIAN-STYLE SAUCE WITH CASHEWS)

1⅔ cups (400 ml)

There are numerous versions of coconut milk and peanut butter–based sauces throughout Southeast Asia. I have adapted a sauce to include Ayurvedic ingredients, and it has a marvelous, subtle flavor of its own. You can use commercial cashew butter to hurry up the preparation (see the second variation). Serve over stir-fried or steamed vegetables, tossed with noodles, or for an ethnically mixed-up presentation, as a dipping sauce for Tempura or Spring Rolls.

STEP ONE

¼ cup (60 ml) mild-flavored oil

⅔ cup (90 g) coarsely chopped cashews

STEP TWO

Pinch of hing (optional)
*½ cup (70 g) coarsely chopped
  bell pepper*

*1 tablespoon finely chopped
  fresh ginger*
½ teaspoon curry powder

STEP FOUR

1 cup (240 ml) coconut milk   ¾ teaspoon salt
2 tablespoons lime or lemon juice   ¼ teaspoon ground cinnamon
4 teaspoons raw or brown sugar

1. Heat the oil in a small saucepan. Add the cashews and cook over low heat, stirring frequently, for about 2 minutes.
2. Add the hing if desired and the bell pepper, ginger, and curry powder. Continue stirring for a few minutes until the cashews are golden brown.
3. Grind the cashew mixture in a food processor as smooth as possible to make cashew butter.
4. Combine the cashew butter with the remaining ingredients in the saucepan over low heat. Simmer, stirring, for 10 minutes. Adjust the salt if necessary.

VARIATIONS

To be true to the original, fire up the sauce by adding crumbled dried red chilies to the oil in Step 2.

Sambal à la Less Work: Omit Step 1. Begin at Step 2, using ⅔ cup (170 g) roasted cashew butter and 2 teaspoons oil in Step 3. If the cashew butter is salted, add salt to taste instead of the ¾ teaspoon measurement given in Step 4.

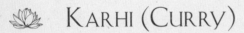 # KARHI (CURRY)

INDIA   *A little over 2 cups (500 ml)*

Here is one of the original forms of curry, a light, thin sauce to be served over rice. Cook some finely cut vegetables in the sauce, or float plain Pakoras in it after cooking.

STEP ONE

¼ cup (55 g) ghee   1 tablespoon minced fresh ginger
Pinch of hing (optional)   ½ teaspoon cumin seeds

STEP TWO

2 ripe tomatoes, chopped

STEP THREE

2 tablespoons besan (chickpea flour) or wheat flour

STEP FOUR

2 cups (480 ml) buttermilk   ½ teaspoon ground coriander
1 teaspoon salt   ¼ teaspoon ground fenugreek
½ teaspoon turmeric   ⅛ teaspoon ground cloves

1. Heat the ghee in a small saucepan on a low heat. Add the hing if desired, the ginger, and cumin and sauté for 1 minute, stirring constantly.
2. Add the tomatoes and cook, stirring frequently, until they are mushy, 3 to 4 minutes.
3. Stir in the besan or wheat flour. Beat with a whisk and cook for 2 minutes, stirring constantly.
4. Pour in the buttermilk. Add the salt and remaining spices. Bring to a simmer, stirring constantly with the whisk. Do not boil. Cover and simmer over very low heat for 20 minutes, stirring occasionally. Adjust the seasoning.

VARIATIONS

Add cayenne or ground red chilies to the ghee or butter in Step 1.
For a thicker sauce, add 1 more tablespoon flour.

Chutneys

Spice a dish with love and it pleases every palate.   —Plautus, *Casina*, 200 B.C.

A chutney can contain three or four tastes, such as a cooked fruit chutney that is sweet, sour, salty, and pungent. Chutneys originated in India. They became popular in England and were translated into spicy preserved fruits in vinegar. Indian chutneys do not contain vinegar, and not all are sweet. There are also many fresh chutneys prepared the day they are to be served. Some are cooked and others are not.

 ## Date Chutney (Khajur Chatni)

INDIA   *1¾ cups (420 ml)*

STEP ONE

1 tablespoon oil   *¼ teaspoon black mustard seeds*

STEP TWO

1 cup (285 g) packed pitted dates   *¼ teaspoon ground cardamom*
½ cup (120 ml) orange juice   *⅛ teaspoon ground cloves*
¼ cup (60 ml) lemon juice   *¼ teaspoon salt*
¼ teaspoon ground coriander

1. Heat the oil in a saucepan. Add the mustard seeds and sauté over low heat until they "dance."
2. Add the remaining ingredients. Cover and simmer for 10 minutes.
3. Purée in a blender or food processor until smooth.

VARIATIONS
  Add ½ cup (40 g) grated unsweetened coconut.
  Replace the orange and lemon juices with strong mint or hibiscus tea.

 # COCONUT CHUTNEY (NARIYAL CHATNI)

INDIA   *1 cup (240 ml)*

My favorite, and a pleasant surprise for those who associate coconut only with sweet dishes. It is traditionally served in south India with dosas for breakfast and *tiffin*— afternoon snack time.

STEP ONE

1 cup (90 g) grated fresh coconut
2 tablespoons fresh ginger, peeled
  and chopped

½ teaspoon salt
3 tablespoons yogurt
2 to 3 tablespoons water

STEP TWO

1 teaspoon oil
Pinch of hing (optional)

½ teaspoon brown mustard seeds
1 teaspoon urad dal (optional)

1. Combine the coconut, ginger, salt, and yogurt in a blender or food processor with just enough water to grind to a paste.
2. Heat the oil in a small skillet. Add the hing if desired, the mustard seeds, and urad dal and sauté over low heat until the mustard seeds "dance" and the urad dal turns reddish brown. Stir into the coconut mixture.

VARIATIONS
  Add a handful of chopped fresh cilantro in Step 1.
  Add crumbled dried red chilies or chopped green chilies to the oil in Step 2.

 # PINEAPPLE CHUTNEY (ANANAS CHATNI)

INDIA   *1½ cups (360 ml)*

The gods might luxuriate on it and it should only be gathered by the hand of Venus.   —JEAN DE LÈRY, DESCRIBING PINEAPPLE

STEP ONE

¼ cup (60 ml) ghee or oil
1 tablespoon minced fresh ginger

⅛ teaspoon ground cumin

STEP TWO

3 cups (735 g) chopped pineapple
with its juice
1 cup (210 g) raw or packed
brown sugar
2 tablespoons lemon juice

⅓ cup (45 g) raisins
⅛ teaspoon ground cardamom
⅛ teaspoon ground cinnamon
½ teaspoon salt

1. Heat the ghee or oil in a large saucepan. Add the ginger and cumin and sauté for 1 minute over low heat, stirring frequently.
2. Add the remaining ingredients. Cover and simmer until the mixture has a jamlike consistency, 1½ to 2 hours. The pineapple never breaks down entirely, but the sugar should bind the mixture together. Let cool to room temperature.

VARIATION

Add cayenne or dried red chilies in Step 1.

 ## PLUM CHUTNEY

2 cups (480 ml)

A westernized chutney that my brother Peter likes to spread on burritos. Fresh prunes are available in late summer and early autumn.

3½ cups (700 g) halved pitted
fresh prunes (prune plums)
1 cup (125 g) raisins
1 cup (210 g) raw or packed
brown sugar
½ cup (80 g) slivered crystallized
ginger or 1 tablespoon ground
ginger

⅓ cup (80 ml) water
⅓ cup (80 ml) lemon juice
2 teaspoons salt
2 teaspoons brown mustard seeds

Combine all the ingredients in a large saucepan. Bring to a boil. Cover and simmer, stirring occasionally, until the mixture becomes jamlike, about 1 hour. Let cool to room temperature.

VARIATION

Add cayenne or dried red chilies.

MIXED FRUIT CHUTNEY

1½ cups (360 ml)

Another anglicized chutney that can be prepared with anything from apples to mangoes.

3½ cups (840 ml) finely chopped
    mixed fruit
½ cup (65 g) raisins
¾ cup (150 g) sugar
¼ cup (60 ml) water
¼ cup (60 ml) lemon juice

2 teaspoons salt
2 teaspoons ground ginger
1½ teaspoons brown mustard seeds
1 teaspoon ground coriander
2 whole cloves

Combine all the ingredients in a large saucepan. Bring to a boil. Cover and simmer, stirring occasionally, until the mixture becomes jamlike, about 1 hour. Let cool to room temperature.

VARIATIONS

Add cayenne or dried red chilies.
Replace the ground ginger with ¼ cup (40 g) slivered crystallized ginger.

 ## RAISINS AND ROSE WATER (KISHMISH GULAB JAL CHATNI)

INDIA   *1 cup (240 ml)*

Subtle rose water–flavored raisins to serve as a condiment.

¾ cup (95 g) washed seedless raisins
1 teaspoon sugar

1 cup (240 ml) water
1 teaspoon rose water

Simmer the raisins and sugar in the water, covered, for 20 minutes. Let cool to room temperature. Stir in the rose water.

 ## MINT CHUTNEY (PODINA CHATNI)

INDIA   *½ cup (120 ml)*

A cooling, emerald green chutney that aids digestion.

1 cup (240 ml) packed fresh mint
   leaves
2 tablespoons lemon juice
2 tablespoons water

1 tablespoon honey or 4 teaspoons
   sugar
½ teaspoon salt

Purée all the ingredients in a blender until smooth. Add more water if necessary for blending.

VARIATIONS

Parsley Chutney (Khatte Chatni): Substitute parsley for the mint. Add fresh green chilies.

 # PARSLEY-CASHEW CHUTNEY (KHATTE KAJUR CHATNI)

About ½ cup (120 ml)

The nuts give this chutney a rich texture. It contains a little bit of all six tastes.

1½ cups (360 ml) coarsely
   chopped fresh parsley
½ cup (65 g) raw cashews
1 tablespoon minced fresh ginger

1 or more tablespoons yogurt
2 tablespoons lemon juice
2 teaspoons sugar or honey
½ teaspoon salt

Purée all the ingredients in a blender until smooth. Add more yogurt if necessary for blending.

VARIATIONS

Add fresh green chilies.
✪ Replace the yogurt with water.
Cilantro Chutney (Hari Dhania Chatni): Replace the parsley with cilantro. Alternatively, prepare Mint Chutney (preceding recipe), replacing the mint with cilantro.

 # MINT, CILANTRO, AND TOMATO CHUTNEY (PODINA, HARI DHANIA, TAMATAR CHATNI)

INDIA   *1 cup (240 ml)*

A fresh, bright, uncooked chutney you can prepare in minutes.

2 cups (480 ml) loosely packed,
  coarsely chopped fresh mint
2 cups (480 ml) loosely packed,
  coarsely chopped fresh cilantro
2 Roma tomatoes

1 tablespoon minced fresh ginger
2 tablespoons lemon juice
½ teaspoon salt
¼ teaspoon black pepper

Purée all the ingredients in a blender or food processor until smooth.

SALT AND AYURVEDA

Salt is born of the purest of parents: the sun and the sea.   —PYTHAGORAS

The word *salt* is derived from the name of the Roman god of health, Salus, the root of such words as *salutary*, *salubrious*, and *salvation*. Sharing salt signifies human relationships—the sharing of basic nourishment. The Russian word for hospitality, *khebosolstvo*, translates as "bread-salt." When one contemplates the history of salt, a substance inextricably linked with practically the entire history of humankind, it is puzzling to even conceive of the modern trend toward condemning and abolishing it. The Ayurvedic text *Charaka Samhita* states, "Salt is the best among those [substances] producing relish in food." Maharishi Ayur-Veda provides a wise approach: it is not salt in itself but the improper use of salt that causes problems.

❖ Salt is one of the six major tastes described in Ayurveda as important for maintaining balance. It is recommended that all six tastes be included in every meal. In that context, a little salt is part of a balanced diet.

❖ The amount of salt you can healthfully consume—or avoid—depends on your mind-body type. In general, predominantly Vata types thrive on salty foods, while predominantly Pitta and Kapha types are better off reducing them. In Vata season it is beneficial to eat more salt; in Pitta and Kapha seasons, to eat less. These are general principals; each individual is different. Individuals with specific health concerns should particularly avoid self-doctoring in this area and seek advice from a health care practitioner trained in Maharishi Ayur-Veda.

❖ A universal recommendation of Ayurveda is to add salt to food while it is cooking. The cooking process allows salt to dissolve and be absorbed by the food. According to Ayurveda, it is much easier to digest salt in this form than when it is poured straight from the shaker onto already-cooked food.

❖ There are different types of salt, and some are superior to others. This may sound a little picky, but remember that pure sodium chloride is hardly ever what we eat. Salt comes from different sources and has different ingredients added to it, some by Nature herself, and others by Nature's sometimes erring children. The type of salt recommended most highly in Ayurvedic texts is *mineral salt* or *rock salt* from salt deposits in the earth. It contains trace minerals that exhibit themselves in the pinkish color of the salt. You can find it in Indian markets, often in blocks that must be pulverized, and sometimes in a ready-to-use form in natural foods stores.

❖ *Black salt* is a compound with a sulfurous flavor. While its odor may at first be a turnoff, its unique taste can grow on you. Ayurveda recommends black salt as a digestive aid. It is available in Indian markets.

Salt is pure and white—there is something holy in salt.

—NATHANIAL HAWTHORNE

As much of heaven is visible as we have eyes to see.

—WILLIAM WINTER

Dairy Products

I nourish you gods, who are everywhere present, with curds, with butter, with milk.

—*RIK VEDA* X.2.4

Dairy products have been enjoyed throughout history by virtually all civilizations that domesticated animals. Even nomadic tribes deprived of all other perishable and cultivated foods kept herds of milk-giving animals and developed ways to preserve milk during travel and hot weather. Dairy products have received some bad press in recent years because of their fat and cholesterol contents. I believe that the bad rap on dairy is a temporary situation that, in retrospect, will be far outweighed by the thousands of years in which milk and milk products have nourished millions.

Ayurvedic texts describe milk as a perfect food. According to Maharishi Ayur-Veda, it is improper preparation and misuse of dairy products that causes most problems. Ayurveda describes specific ways to treat dairy products for optimum benefit, explains which dairy foods are the most nourishing for each mind-body type, and notes in which seasons and times of day it is most beneficial to eat them.

Some people eschew dairy products because of the mistreatment perpetrated on cows to obtain their milk. Fortunately, there are an increasing number of dairies that recognize that mistreating their bovines is biting the hand that feeds them, so to speak. They take pride in the life-supporting environment and organic food they provide for their cows, and advertise their refusal to administer hormones and antibiotics. Products from compassionate, "organic" dairies are the most highly recommended for Ayurvedic cooking.

GHEE

"I have the simplest tastes. I am always satisfied with the best," proclaimed Oscar Wilde. I hope that somehow he tasted ghee, for it is the finest cooking oil in the world.

Charaka Samhita says that "regular use of ghee is among the best rasayanas" (rejuvenating and longevity-promoting foods), and extols its numerous health-giving properties. Ghee's rate of absorption by the body is higher than that of any other cooking oil, making it an excellent medium for transporting nutrients to the tissues. It is therefore utilized in medicinal formulas for assisting the absorption of herbs and minerals. Ghee stimulates digestion without aggravating the digestive fire. Vata is balanced by any reasonable amount of ghee, while Pitta enjoys a little less and Kapha is balanced by small amounts.

Ghee can be heated to high temperatures without burning. You can even deep-fry foods in ghee. Substitute ghee for butter or oil in any recipe using them for *cooking*. You can't replace oil with ghee in cooler dishes, as, like butter, it is solid when chilled, semisolid at moderate room temperature, and liquid when heated. Theoretically, ghee keeps for two months without refrigeration; in my experience it can go rancid in warmer weather. Ghee can be purchased from the sources listed in Appendix B.

> To early Chinese Buddhists, the progression of obtaining cream from milk, churning the cream into butter, and refining the butter into ghee was representative of spiritual evolution; ghee symbolized the finest essence of life, the attainment of enlightenment.

Creating Delicious Ghee

Ghee is made by simmering butter until the water evaporates and the solids separate from the oil. The solids are then strained out, and the pure, golden oil that remains is ghee. The yield of each batch depends on the amounts of water and solids in the butter. Two pounds (900 g) butter yield approximately 1½ pounds (675 g) ghee. However, this is an average figure—your yield could be quite a bit more or less.

❖ Always use unsalted butter. It is possible to make ghee from salted butter, but do so only when your back is to the wall. The only such wall I've been backed against was in a small village in Taiwan, where the only butter was a heavily salted product "of a certain age" imported from New Zealand.

❖ Slow cooking over very low heat allows the milk sugars to caramelize and is the secret to spectacular ghee. Because it takes a long time, you may want to make large amounts. In any case, don't go for any less than 1 pound (500 g) of butter; smaller amounts burn easily. Do not stir cooking ghee. (Dark—not burned—ghee is delicious; it's just not the ideal.)

❖ One Ayurvedic recommendation that differs from other methods of ghee preparation is to refrain from skimming off the foam that forms at the top during cooking. This foam has medicinal properties that enhance the finished product. Leaving it on requires an extra measure of alertness when the end of cooking is in sight, to ensure that the solids don't burn.

Crock-Pot method: Crock-Pots are ideal for making large amounts of ghee. They heat slowly, freeing you from having to watch them constantly. I use 6 pounds (2.7 kg) of butter, which just fit into a standard 3½-quart (4 l) Crock-Pot. I start the ghee in the evening, and it is ready the afternoon of the following day.

1. Melt the butter using the high setting. You may have to melt 5 pounds (2.3 kg) first and then add the remaining butter.
2. When cooking ghee overnight or otherwise leaving it unattended, turn the setting to low. If you are around to keep an eye on it and see that it doesn't burn, continue with the high setting. Leave uncovered. Most of the solids will sink to the bottom, but some will remain on top. They will brown, which adds to the flavor of the ghee, but be careful that they don't burn. If you use 4 to 6 pounds (1.8 to 2.7 kg) butter, the process will take at least 12 and up to 24 hours. The finishing point to look for is when the liquid is clear and golden colored. If it starts to darken, remove it from the heat.
3. Line a large sieve with 3 layers of clean cotton cloth. Pocket handkerchiefs work well, as do pieces of unbleached muslin. Set it over a pot and pour the ghee through it while still hot. Carefully transfer the ghee to clean glass jars with lids.

Oven method: By this method ghee cooks in a slow, even heat that surrounds the cooking vessel. It does not require constant attention. It is faster than the Crock-Pot technique, but preparing a large amount is still an all-day affair.

1. Place butter in a casserole. Allow some room at the top for the butter to bubble up and foam. Place the uncovered casserole in a 275°F (140°C) oven.
2. Cook until most of the solids sink to the bottom. The finishing point to look for is when the ghee is clear and golden. Be careful not to let the solids burn or the ghee darken.
3. Line a large sieve with 3 layers of clean cotton cloth. Pocket handkerchiefs work well, as do pieces of unbleached muslin. Set it over a pot and pour the ghee through it while still hot. Carefully transfer the ghee to clean glass jars with lids.

Stovetop method: For small batches this is the fastest method, mostly because it is difficult to lower the heat sufficiently to match the leisurely simmering of the other two techniques. One pound of butter takes under an hour to prepare. Use the heaviest pot you can find. Placing a heat diffuser on the burner to raise the pot is also helpful.

1. Melt the butter over low heat in an uncovered pot with high sides. Make sure the pot is completely dry before adding the butter, and allow some room at the top for the butter to bubble up and foam.
2. Turn the heat as low as possible and cook the butter until it is clear and golden. Do not skim off the foam. The solids may brown, but take care that they don't burn. Check the butter frequently. The finishing point to look for is when the liquid is clear and golden colored. If it starts to darken, remove from the heat.

3. Line a large sieve with 3 layers of clean cotton cloth. Pocket handkerchiefs work well, as do pieces of unbleached muslin. Set it over a pot and pour the ghee through it while still hot. Carefully transfer the ghee to clean glass jars with lids.

Butter

Eat butter first and last,
and live till a hundred years be past.   —Old Dutch proverb

In North Carolina our neighbors would bring us what they called "country butter." It was churned from the raw cream of their own cows and pressed into molds with lovely designs. The flavor was indescribable, containing the essence of sweet Appalachian air and pastures. If your neighbors live in Apartment 14-E and their only pet is a Pekingese, your best bet is to purchase *organic, unsalted butter* in a natural foods store. *Cultured butter,* churned from cream to which a bacterial culture has been added, has a stronger flavor, closer to that of the product churned from "ripened" cream that was much preferred in days gone by. It is available in natural foods stores.

❖ Store unsalted butter in the freezer and bring it out a stick at a time.
❖ Always keep butter covered when not using. Prolonged exposure to air causes oxidation, which can create health problems.
❖ *To substitute melted butter in recipes containing oil:* If a standard-sized recipe calls for more than ¼ cup (60 ml) oil, when substituting melted butter, increase the amount by 20 percent. This compensates for the milk solids in the butter.

Ayurveda, Butter, Fats, and the C Word

Cholesterol—a word used to strike fear literally into our hearts. There's good cholesterol and bad cholesterol and exceptionally authoritative, well-explained theories of the life-and-death consequences of eating correctly—whatever eating correctly happens to mean in a particular school of thought. As theories do, they change regularly and send us scrambling in ever-changing directions in search of clear arteries and healthy hearts.

According to Ayurveda, arterial plaque is one of the many forms that ama can take. Ama is created from improperly digested substances of many types—not just fat. When the health-promoting or health-damaging effects of fats are analyzed, the same Ayurvedic factors that determine the wholesomeness of any food must be addressed, including an individual's ability to process fats and the qualities of the fat itself.

In general, Ayurveda maintains that those high-quality fats and oils that are most balancing for an individual's doshas, taken in the recommended amounts (more for Vata, less for Pitta, and least for Kapha) and eaten in the context of a wholesome and balanced diet and lifestyle, are very nourishing and life-supporting. As always, if you have a specific concern about cholesterol and heart disease, you would be wise to consult with a health-care practitioner trained in Maharishi Ayur-Veda to determine the best use of fats and oils in your diet.

BUTTER

Approximately 1⅔ cups (380 g)

Although ghee is the generally preferred oil of Ayurvedic cooking, butter is also extolled in Ayurvedic texts as a very good food. If you have access to good-quality cream and not-so-good quality butter, you may wish to make your own butter at home. With the modern-day answer to the butter churn, the food processor, it's an easy proposition. Make butter in small batches so that the metal blade of the processor will move through most of the cream. The process is lightning fast, and you can make a large amount in several batches in no time.

1 quart (1 l) heavy (whipping) cream

1. Process the cream with the metal blade. It will become very thick, stay that way for a while, then the whey will separate from the pale yellow butter.
2. Scrape out the butter into a colander with small holes. (You may want to catch the whey in a bowl—it's the original form of buttermilk.) Squeeze the butter with your hands to release all the whey. Rinse off any remaining whey with cold water.
3. Squeeze the butter into a ball or press into a butter mold. Store in a closed container in the freezer, where it can be kept for several months. Keep the amount you want to use for just a few days at a time in the refrigerator.

Flavored Butter and Ghee for the Table

Flavored butter and ghee make wonderful, subtle sauces for vegetables and pasta. At the table they can provide unexpected delight for someone you love who is reaching to butter the morning toast for the 27,000th time. Most flavorings can be beaten into room-temperature ghee or butter (a food processor works well) in amounts to suit your taste. (Recipes for flavoring butter and ghee *for cooking* are on pp. 566–67.)

Flavorings for Butter and Ghee

Finely grated lemon, lime, or orange zest
A sprinkling of toasted sesame oil
Honey (do not add in an equal amount to ghee) or other sweeteners
Pesto alla Genovese (p. 510)
Dried Tomato and Walnut Pesto (pp. 510–11)
Spinach and Toasted Almond Pesto (p. 511)
Dried Tomato Paste (p. 506)
Dried Fruit Purée (p. 462)
Jams and preserves
Lemon or lime juice
Minced fresh herbs
Dried green herbs sautéed briefly in a small portion of the ghee or butter
  to enhance their flavors
Freshly ground pepper
Sweet spices, such as cinnamon and cardamom
Maharishi Ayur-Veda churnas

HERBED GHEE OR BUTTER

½ cup (115 g)

½ cup (115 g) ghee or butter,   *Salt*
  softened
Pinch of hing (optional)
¼ cup (60 ml) minced fresh
  parsley, cilantro, basil, tarragon,
  or other fresh green herbs, or
2 tablespoons dried herbs

Melt 1 tablespoon of the ghee or butter in a small skillet. Add the hing if desired and the dried herbs if using and sauté over low heat for 1 minute, stirring constantly. Blend the mixture into the remaining butter in a food processor or by hand. If using fresh herbs, process or mix them in as well. Add salt to taste.

VARIATION

Add 2 tablespoons lemon or lime juice—delicious with cilantro. If you add it using fresh parsley as your herb, you have made a French classic, ghee or butter *Maître d' Hôtel.*

FRESH STRAWBERRY GHEE OR BUTTER

1⅔ cups (370 g)

Perfect for spreading on pancakes, muffins, croissants, and other breakfast rolls. Substitute 1 cup (215 g) chopped fresh mangoes or apricots for a golden version, or use cherries, blueberries, peaches, or other soft, juicy fruits.

STEP ONE

1 cup (155 g) *thinly sliced*	2 tablespoons water
strawberries	½ teaspoon orange zest
2 tablespoons sugar	½ teaspoon ground cardamom

STEP TWO

1 cup (230 g) *ghee or unsalted*
   butter, softened

1. Place the strawberries, sugar, water, orange zest, and cardamom in a small saucepan. Simmer, uncovered, over low heat, stirring occasionally, for about 10 minutes, until the berries are tender and the mixture is jamlike.
2. Blend the berry mixture into the ghee or butter in a food processor or blender. At room temperature, it has the consistency of whipped cream; chilled, it hardens.

VARIATION
   Substitute ½ cup (230 g) cream cheese for the butter.

CREAM

The word *cream* comes from the Greek *chriein* or *chrisma*, meaning "unguent." Christ, "the anointed," comes from the same root. In Ayurvedic cooking, cream is regarded as a wonderful, life-supporting substance. It is balancing for Vata and in lesser amounts for Pitta. It must be treated in the same manner as milk, served separately from all other tastes except sweet. In savory dishes it is better to substitute crème fraîche, sour cream, or thick coconut milk.

❖ Avoid *sterilized* or *ultra-pasteurized cream* if possible. They are heated with 280°F (138°C) steam, and the water created by the steam is then vacuumed away—along with the exquisite flavor. This allows them to last for a long time, and therefore they may be quite old by the time they reach you. At any age their flavor is inferior to that of fresh, untreated cream.

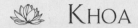 # KHOA

About ¾ cup (180 ml)

A thick, condensed milk paste used for preparing Indian desserts. It takes a long time to make but is unlike anything else. Khoa will last for a few days in a covered container in the refrigerator.

½ gallon (2 l) whole milk

1. Bring the milk to a boil in a heavy pot with high sides. Be careful not to scorch.
2. Cook the milk at as vigorous a boil as is possible without boiling over for 1 to 1½ hours, stirring frequently.
3. When the milk begins to thicken, stir constantly until it forms a thick paste that pulls slightly away from the sides of the pot. This can take up to 30 minutes. Be very careful that the milk doesn't burn. Let cool to thicken completely. If the khoa is yellowish, it was not boiled at a high enough heat, but the flavor will be fine.

CULTURED MILK PRODUCTS

Specific bacterial cultures are added to milk at optimum temperatures to transform the milk into a variety of products: yogurt, buttermilk, and certain cheeses. The bacteria in these foods aid digestion, making them a valuable addition to one's diet. Many people drink yogurt Lassi (pp. 489–91) with every meal. Those who have trouble digesting milk can often eat cultured milk products without difficulty. The sour flavor of cultured milk products is balancing to Vata but not to Pitta and Kapha. Ayurveda recommends eating all cultured milk products, with the exception of lassi, in the morning and afternoon only. They can block the shrotas and create toxins, ama, when eaten in the evening. Ayurvedic texts particularly identify imperfectly formed curds ("curds" refers to any food made by culturing or curdling milk, including yogurt and cheese) as the most ama-producing food, so when in doubt about the age or goodness of a particular batch of a cultured milk product, you know what to do with it.

Yogurt

Yogurt is an important Ayurvedic food. Ayurveda favors eating freshly made yogurt because it is easier to digest. Fresh homemade yogurt has a sweet, mild flavor and custardlike texture completely unlike most commercial yogurts. It is easy to make, economical, and its wonderful qualities leave even the best commercial products miles behind. So why not? If you drink lassi or otherwise eat yogurt on a daily basis, you can set up your equipment and adopt a yogurt-making routine that takes a few enjoyable minutes each evening and in the morning yields the most wholesome and delicious yogurt you've ever tasted. If you still want to pluck yours off a supermarket shelf after reading the above, look for "organic" yogurt prepared with active cultures and without gelatin or stabilizers. *Kosher* or *pareve* yogurt usually contains no additives and definitely doesn't contain gelatin.

❖ Yogurt can be prepared with anything from nonfat milk to cream, depending on the richness you desire. For creamy yogurt, boil milk for 10 minutes or more to evaporate some of its water content, or use half-and-half or a mixture of milk and heavy (whipping) cream for your base.

❖ Raw milk must first be boiled because it contains an enzyme that inhibits the bacterial culture; boiling neutralizes this enzyme.

 # Yogurt

1 quart (1 l)

Don't get put off by the following lengthy commentary—making yogurt is a lot easier than describing how to make it! There are several methods of incubation described here for you to choose from. If you have an electric yogurt maker with individual 1-cup (240 ml) containers, use the recipe for "The Vaidya's Yogurt" (opposite).

STEP ONE

1 quart (1 l) milk
One or two ¼-inch (6 mm) slices fresh ginger (optional)

STEP THREE

1 cup (240 ml) unflavored yogurt
   (*make sure it has active cultures*)

1. Place the milk in a saucepan with the ginger and bring to a boil. If you are short on time, stop here. Ideally, reduce the heat and simmer for 10 minutes.

2. Allow the milk to cool to 110° to 115°F (43° to 46°C). If testing without a thermometer, remember that this is just a little above body temperature.

3. Mix the yogurt thoroughly into the milk with a whisk. Incubate by any of the following methods:

   ❖ Pour the yogurt mixture into a 1-quart (1 l) thermos. Replace the cover and wrap a towel around the thermos for added insulation. This is an excellent method, though it's more difficult to clean a thermos than other containers.

   ❖ Use a heating pad on the medium setting, covered with a towel. Place the yogurt mixture in a 1-quart (1 l) glass container, cover, and set on the heating pad. Cover the entire setup with another towel for insulation.

   ❖ Turn the oven on for a minute or two until it is just warm. Place the yogurt in a 1-quart (1 l) ceramic or Pyrex container, cover, place in the oven, and turn it off. Do not open the oven door for at least 4 hours. This method is the least accurate, but it will work.

❖ Finally, if you live in a hot climate, place the yogurt mixture in a 1-quart (1 l) glass container, cover, and set in a warm place where it won't be disturbed.

4. You can incubate yogurt anywhere from 4 to 12 hours. The less time it sits, the sweeter and runnier it will be. Under average conditions, 6 hours is usually just about the right amount of time. However, all the variables of temperature, strength of the yogurt culture, etc., can alter the time it takes for an individual batch to set.

5. Store the finished yogurt in the refrigerator to stop incubation. Save 1 cup (240 ml) of yogurt to start the next batch. However, yogurt is often more successful if you use a fresh commercial yogurt as a starter once a week.

May this Earth, replete with seas, rivers and water sources, excellent foodgrain from agriculture, prolific vegetation and abundant living creatures, bestow upon us munificent nutrition. —ATHARVA VEDA, PRITHIVI SUKTA

 # THE VAIDYA'S YOGURT

1 quart (1 l)

Here's a way to make mild-flavored, easily digested yogurt on a daily basis. It requires an electric yogurt maker with four individual cups. Boiling milk for 10 minutes with a slice of fresh ginger renders it most digestible for use in yogurt. You can also add a pinch of black pepper and/or turmeric to the milk to increase its digestibility.

STEP ONE

1 quart plus ½ cup (1.1 l) whole milk

One ¼-inch (6 mm) slice fresh ginger

STEP THREE

4 teaspoons unflavored yogurt

1. At about 9:00 P.M. the evening before you wish to use the yogurt, boil the milk with the slice of ginger for 10 minutes.
2. Allow the milk to cool to 110° to 115°F (43° to 46°C).
3. Pour the milk into the 4 individual cups of an electric yogurt maker. Add about 1 teaspoon of the yogurt to each cup. Do not stir.
4. Incubate the yogurt overnight. Check on it first thing in the morning.

HUNG YOGURT, YOGURT CHEESE, OR LABAN

About 1½ cups (360 ml)

Hung yogurt is thick and creamy, with a consistency somewhere between sour cream and cream cheese. It can be used as a spread, as a substitute for sour cream, or sweetened to make frosting and desserts.

1 quart (1 l) thick yogurt

1. Place the yogurt in a muslin cloth or a clean pillowcase. Tie shut and hang it over the sink or a receptacle to catch the whey as it drains off.
2. Allow to hang overnight. In the morning, squeeze out the last drops of whey, untie the bag, and remove the thick hung yogurt with a rubber spatula. For best flavor and effects, use the same day. However, you can store it in the refrigerator in an airtight container.

OTHER CULTURED MILK PRODUCTS

 ## SOUR CREAM

1 pint (480 ml)

Homemade sour cream is easy and delicious and doesn't contain the stabilizers and gelatin that are found in many commercial brands.

STEP ONE

1 pint (480 ml) heavy (whipping) cream

STEP TWO

¼ cup (60 ml) cultured buttermilk

1. Bring the cream to a boil over low heat, stirring occasionally to avoid burning. Let cool to room temperature.
2. Stir the buttermilk thoroughly into the cream. Cover and allow to stand in a dark, draft-free place at room temperature for about 36 hours, until thick. Store in the refrigerator in an airtight container, where it can last up to a week.

 ## CRÈME FRAÎCHE

1¼ cups (300 ml)

A lightly cultured, slightly soured cream found throughout France. Unlike other cultured milk products, crème fraîche does not separate when heated. You can use it in place of cream in dishes containing salt and/or mixed tastes, such as cream soups and creamy sauces for vegetables. It is marvelous spooned over fruit salads and desserts.

STEP ONE

1 cup (240 ml) heavy (whipping) cream

STEP TWO

¼ cup (60 ml) cultured buttermilk

1. Bring the cream to a boil over low heat, stirring occasionally to avoid burning. Let cool until lukewarm (90° to 100°F/32° to 38°C). If too hot, it will curdle when the buttermilk is added.
2. Mix thoroughly with the buttermilk and pour into a nonreactive container, such as a glass jar. Cover and allow to stand in a dark, draft-free place at room temperature for 24 to 36 hours, until slightly thickened and soured. Store in the refrigerator in an airtight container, where it can last up to a week.

BUTTERMILK

A little over 1 quart (1 l)

True and original buttermilk is the whey left over from making butter. The cultured milk product we all know today as buttermilk is made by an entirely different process. Buttermilk can be made from either whole or nonfat milk. Buttermilk is balancing for Vata. If you prepare buttermilk from unhomogenized milk, a wonderful golden-tinged sour cream forms on the top.

STEP ONE

1 quart (1 l) milk

STEP TWO

¼ cup (60 ml) cultured buttermilk

1. Bring the milk to a boil. Allow to cool to room temperature.
2. Mix the milk and buttermilk together thoroughly in a nonreactive container, such as a glass jar. Cover and place in a dark, draft-free place at room temperature for 24 to 36 hours. Taste-test for doneness.
3. Store in the refrigerator. Reserve ¼ cup (60 ml) of each batch to start the next batch. If the buttermilk gets too strong after making a number of batches, use commercial buttermilk as a starter.

 ## KEFIR

1 quart (1 l)

Kefir has been enjoyed in the Middle East and the Caucasus Mountains for centuries. Nomadic tribes incubated it in their saddlebags, where it could be transported without refrigeration. Kefir can be served plain or used as a substitute for yogurt or buttermilk. Kefir grains can be obtained from natural foods stores. This recipe for kefir is fairly flexible; use a larger amount of grains and a longer incubation period for a stronger flavor.

If you are not going to use your kefir grains again immediately, you can store them in the refrigerator immersed in milk or water for up to 10 days. The kefir culture will double about every 2 months, so you'll have a nice gift for friends, or else you can proceed gradually into mass production.

STEP ONE

1 quart (1 l) milk

STEP TWO

3 tablespoons kefir grains

1. Bring the milk to a boil. Let cool to room temperature.
2. Mix the kefir grains into the milk. Cover and allow to stand at room temperature for 24 hours, until the milk seems to gel. There may be some slight separation.
3. Strain, pressing with the back of a spoon to separate the milk curds from the kefir grains. Store the kefir in the refrigerator in an airtight container for up to a week. Rinse the kefir grains and start the next batch of kefir.

Cheese

Cheese—milk's leap toward immortality.   —Clifton Fadiman

The word *cheese* encompasses an enormous range of products, with varying effects on the mind-body system. Ayurveda exercises a good deal of caution when it comes to cheeses. In general, cheeses, particularly when aged, have great potential for blocking the microcirculatory channels, or shrotas. Fresh cheeses eaten the day they are made, such as homemade panir and ricotta, are fine for Ayurvedic cooking. Fresh, soft cheeses such as cottage cheese, cream cheese, soft chèvre, and quark are the next best. Semisoft cheeses that under the best of circumstances are only "aged" for a few days at most, such as feta, fresh mozzarella, and teleme, are borderline. Aged, hard cheeses such as cheddar and Parmesan are the most problematical, and many adherents to Ayurvedic principles refrain from eating them at all. (One Ayurvedic expert refers to aged cheese as "rotten milk.") I have included a handful of recipes that include hard cheeses because they are familiar and well-loved foods to many and would be sorely missed if eliminated immediately and totally. See how you feel about eating hard cheese less frequently, and be alert to the following points, which help lessen the undesirable effects of all cheeses:

❖ As with all curds, it is advisable to eat cheeses at lunchtime rather than with the evening meal.
❖ Serve cheese dishes with digestive spices, particularly black pepper.
❖ Cheese has a predominantly sour taste, making it most balancing for Vata and aggravating to Pitta and Kapha.
❖ Cow's milk cheeses are generally the most nourishing. Goat's milk cheese is all right, but sheep's milk has less favorable effects, and buffalo milk is identified as inducing sleep. (Avoid *mozzarella di bufala* before taking the bar exam!)
❖ Purchased cheeses may contain *rennet*, a nonvegetarian coagulant. The good news is that a vegetable enzyme that does the same job has been widely adopted by cheese makers. Cheeses labeled "made with vegetable enzymes," "enzymes," "kosher," "pareve," or "made with kosher enzymes," are free from rennet.

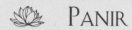 PANIR

INDIA/MIDDLE EAST   *About 1¾ cups (350 g)*

Panir can be made using either yogurt or lemon juice. One vaidya recommends yogurt as being more "natural" for the process. In my experience it makes a better textured and flavored product as well. Panir is somewhat unpredictable; how it turns out depends on the fat content of the milk, the sourness of the yogurt, the timing and temperatures of just about everything involved in the process, the sun, moon, and stars. . . . Very occasionally I've prepared panir under what appeared to be ideal conditions, only to watch in mute horror as the milk separated into tiny granules and disappeared through the sieve and down the drain! The best policy is to accept that there will be variations among the final results—and a once-in-a-blue-moon washout. That's the story of, that's the glory of . . .

½ gallon (1.9 l) whole milk
1 cup (240 ml) yogurt or
lemon juice

1. Bring the milk to a full boil. Gently stir in the yogurt or lemon juice. Do not stir for more than a few seconds. After a few more seconds, the curds and whey will separate. Separation is complete when white curds are floating in yellowish whey. If the liquid remains milky, stir in more yogurt or lemon juice and wait another few seconds.
2. *For soft or medium panir:* Pour the entire contents of the pot through a sieve or a colander. Scrape off any remaining panir in the bottom of the pot. Allow to drain just until the whey is gone, but for no more than 1 hour.
   For hard panir: Continue to simmer the coagulated panir for 10 minutes. Remove the pot from the heat, cover, and allow to stand for no less than 10 minutes. Line a sieve or colander with cheesecloth or unbleached muslin, allowing the edges to drape over the sides. Very gently ladle the curds into it without breaking them up and scrape off the panir at the bottom of the pot. Bring up the edges of the cloth over the cheese. Cover with something flat, like a pie pan. Place a weight on it, such as a brick or a jar of beans. Allow to drain for several hours or overnight.
3. Ideally, serve panir the day you prepare it or at lunch following an overnight draining. It will, however, last 2 to 3 days in the refrigerator if well wrapped.

Their tables were stor'd full, to glad the sight
And not so much to feed on as delight.   —WILLIAM SHAKESPEARE

RICOTTA

ITALY   *About 2 cups (410 g)*

Ricotta was originally made from the whey of sheep's milk. Homemade ricotta from whole cow's milk is wonderfully fresh and sweet. It is also quite simple to prepare—most of the time you just leave it alone.

½ gallon (1.9 l) milk
2 cups (480 ml) cultured buttermilk

1. Mix the milk and buttermilk together in a large pot. Heat the mixture over low heat until it is just barely simmering. The top of the milk should hardly be moving. This will take 25 to 30 minutes. Do not stir the mixture at any time.
2. Turn the heat to the very lowest setting and allow the mixture to continue just barely simmering for 25 to 45 minutes. The lesser time is for a soft cheese. The longer time yields firmer ricotta. The curds will separate from the whey at some point, but *do not stir*.
3. Line a sieve or colander with a piece of cheesecloth or muslin. Set it in the sink and very gently ladle the mixture into it so that the curds don't break up.
4. Allow the cheese to drain for 30 minutes. Gently remove it from the cloth with a rubber scraper and store in an airtight container in the refrigerator for no more than a few days. The flavor and effects are optimum if the cheese is eaten the day it is made.

TVOROG (FARMER'S CHEESE)

UKRAINE/RUSSIA   *About 2 cups (400 g)*

A buttermilk-based cheese found in farmers' markets throughout Ukraine and western Russia, *tvorog* resembles the dry cottage cheese called *farmer's cheese* or *baker's cheese* in the United States. It can replace ricotta in recipes and is ideal for making blintzes.

½ gallon (1.9 l) buttermilk

1. Pour the buttermilk into two 1-quart (1 l) wide-mouthed jars with tight-fitting lids. Place in a large soup pot and fill with water until the jars are immersed. If you don't have a tall stockpot, use 2 separate pots and lay the jars on their sides.
2. Bring the water to a full boil. Turn off the heat and allow the water to cool to room temperature with the jars undisturbed. The whey should have separated and the curds formed into a mass.

3. Line a colander with a clean piece of unbleached muslin or cheesecloth. Carefully strain the contents of the jars through the cloth, trying to leave the curds as whole as possible.
4. Tie up the corners of the cloth to form a sack enclosing the curds. Hang the bag over the sink or a bowl for 5 hours or overnight.
5. Place the sack in a cheese drainer or colander. Place a heavy, even weight over it, such as a flat-bottomed pot filled with water, for about 8 hours.
6. The cheese should be very crumbly. Ukrainians rub it through a sieve for a finely grained, crumbly cheese resembling dry ricotta. You can grind it in a food processor for the same effect. Store in the refrigerator for not more than a few days.

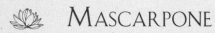

MASCARPONE

ITALY   *1¼ cups (290 g)*

A rich, luxurious cheese with the flavor of sour cream and the texture of cream cheese.

2 cups (480 ml) heavy (whipping)   ¼ cup (60 ml) buttermilk
  cream

1. Mix the buttermilk and cream in a saucepan and heat until just barely lukewarm (90°F/32°C). Do not overheat, or the cream will curdle.
2. Pour the cream into a glass or ceramic container. Place in a warm spot in the kitchen. Cover with a towel and allow to stand for 24 to 36 hours, until thickened.
3. Place a piece of wet cheesecloth or muslin in a sieve and set over a bowl. Gently spoon the cheese into it, cover, and allow to drain overnight in the refrigerator.
4. Remove the cheese from the cloth. You may have to scrape it off with a knife. Store in an airtight container in the refrigerator for no more than a few days. The flavor and effects are optimum if you eat mascarpone the day it is made.

> *Heaven is to be at peace with all things.*
>
> —GEORGE SANTAYANA, *Sonnets*

Basic Ingredients for a Heavenly Banquet

God has distributed His benefits in such a manner that there is no area on the earth so rich that it does not lack all sorts of goods. It appears that God did this in order to induce all the subjects of His Republic to entertain friendly relations with one another.   —JEAN BODIN, 1568

Knowledge is power—in the pantry as much as anywhere else. Finding the finest ingredients is a major consideration in Ayurvedic cooking and one that requires a modicum of information and, in this day and age, a bit of Sherlock Holmes's detective abilities as well. Unfortunately, a good ingredient can be hard to find without knowing exactly what to look for. Priorities in today's wide world of food engineering such as "shelf life," "eye candy," and "marketing" can work against the desires of an Ayurvedic cook in search of fresh, nourishing, tasty food that does no harm to anyone or anything. Food today is not always the plain and simple fare of yore, when Ayurvedic texts were first expounded. This chapter contains information to help you navigate the market aisles for real food, good food, the ideal raw materials for creating heavenly Ayurvedic banquets.

Food is an important part of a balanced diet.   —FRAN LEBOWITZ

FLOURS

❖ The more freshly ground, the better. The whole grains themselves can be older; in fact, Ayurveda recommends eating rice that has been stored for one year. European master bakers prefer older grains, recognizing subtle differences in flours milled from fresh wheat berries and those that have been stored for several months. However, once grains are ground into flour, they become susceptible to

541

rancidity. Flours milled from whole grains contain the germ of the grain and are therefore particularly perishable. Store in airtight containers in the refrigerator or freezer. Try not to store flours for more than two months.

❖ The freshest flour is obtained by grinding whole grains at home with a flour mill just before using. If you do a lot of leisurely baking and want to reap the ideal nutritional and culinary rewards, a flour mill would be a practical investment.

❖ The next best thing, which is the more likely option for most of us is to purchase high-quality flours milled from organically grown grains. These are available in natural foods stores. Check the pull date ("Purchase by . . .") on the package. Two months is about as old as flour should get—and remember, it may have sat in a warehouse before arriving at the store. *Stone-ground flour* is superior to that ground by metal mills. Metal heats up from the high-speed friction of volume grinding done by commercial mills, and the heat alters the texture and nutritional value of the flour. Stones, on the other hand, stay cool.

Unbleached white flour is refined but not bleached or otherwise chemically treated. Look for organic unbleached white flour in natural foods stores.

Whole wheat flour contains the whole wheat kernel. It is not necessary to sift whole wheat flour. *Graham flour,* named for Dr. Sylvester Graham, an American health food crusader and innovator, is a coarse version of whole wheat flour and is usually used in bread baking. *Kamut* and *Spelt flours* are ground from ancient varieties of durum (hard) wheat, both with high nutritional profiles.

Nonwheat Flours

Nonwheat flours have a wide range of applications, flavors, and physiological effects. However, for use in baking, there is one universal consideration: they have little or no gluten and therefore little or no ability to rise and make baked goods light. Nonwheat flours are perishable; unless otherwise noted, store in airtight containers in the refrigerator or freezer for no more than two months.

Amaranth flour has a sweet, nutty taste and a moist quality. It is high in fat and therefore quite perishable. Always store in the refrigerator or freezer.

Barley flour makes baked goods moist and tender. It has outstanding flavor when lightly toasted.

Bean flours: *Chickpea flour,* or *besan,* is used frequently in Middle Eastern and Indian cooking. Besan can be found in Indian markets, and a close relative, *garbanzo flour,* is available in natural foods stores. *Soy flour* can be used interchangeably with chickpea flour in Western baking.

Buckwheat flour comes in light and dark varieties; the dark contains more hull material and nutrients. Anything you cook with buckwheat will come out tasting essentially like buckwheat. Buckwheat flour stores quite well. Keep in a cool, dark place for 2 to 3 months.

Chestnut flour is heavy, dense, and tasty. It is used in European bread baking and is delicious in small amounts in cakes and pastries. It is available in gourmet foods stores.

Millet flour is quite bland but adds a pleasant crunchy texture when added in small amounts to breads and crackers. Its close relation, purple-gray *teff flour*, is the basis of *injera*, the staple flatbread of Ethiopia. Add in small amounts to Western baked goods, but be aware of the color you are adding.

Oat flour is a thickening and binding agent. It also makes baked goods moist. Although it produces soft, crumbly results when used by itself in baking, it is probably one of the best wheat flour replacers for those with allergies.

Quinoa flour makes baked goods moist and tender. It has a high fat content and is therefore quite perishable. Store in the refrigerator or freezer.

Rice flour is a standard ingredient in south India and in parts of Africa where wheat is not indigenous. It is also gourmet fare in Europe for the special delicate texture it imparts when used as a thickener for sauces and puddings. Both brown and white rice flours are available, the former in natural foods stores and the latter in Asian and Hispanic markets. Store on a cool, dark shelf.

Rye Flour, once the only flour available in eastern Europe, has a distinctive flavor that lends itself best to breads and crackers. Rye flour comes in light, medium, and dark varieties. Both light and medium are refined, while dark contains the germ and bran.

LEAVENINGS

> *The kingdom of heaven is like unto leaven, which a woman took, and hid in three measures of meal, till the whole was leavened.* —MATTHEW 13.33

Leavenings produce gases, chiefly carbon dioxide, in moist batters or doughs that cause them to rise and lighten during baking or cooking. Leavenings can be affected by hard water and high altitudes.

Baking powder, known as *chemical leavening* by professionals, is a quick-acting leaven that generally contains baking soda plus some type of acid in salt crystal form, along with a starch to absorb any atmospheric moisture that might set off its reaction. Chemical leavenings are not discussed in the Ayurvedic texts and cannot really be called an Ayurvedic ingredient. However, the small amount of chemical leavening used in baked goods is considered negligible by many vaidyas.

❖ Use a baking powder that does not contain aluminum, such as *tartrate* baking powders and baking powders made with *calcium acid phosphate*. A characteristic of some nonaluminum baking powders is that they are *single acting*: they start their leavening action as soon as they come into contact with moisture. (Double acting baking powders contain a second chemical that is heat activated, coming to life only when placed in the oven.) For this reason they should be stored away from moisture, and a batter should be baked as soon as the baking powder has been stirred in to make full use of its leavening action. The longer the batter stands, the weaker the leavening.

❖ *To make single-acting baking powder at home*: For each teaspoon of baking powder required, mix together ¼ teaspoon baking soda, ¼ teaspoon arrowroot or cornstarch, and ½ teaspoon cream of tartar. Be advised that cream of tartar is a by-product of wine making, so it has been subjected to fermentation.

Baking soda is highly alkaline, and its meeting with an acid liquid causes a strong acid-alkaline reaction that leavens a batter or dough. Ingredients such as buttermilk, yogurt, lemon juice, and molasses must be used to trigger the leavening action of baking soda. Baking soda can be used alone, but for best taste use a small amount as an adjunct to baking powder.

Baker's yeast is made of living microorganisms. They feed on sugars in the flour and added sweeteners in the dough, producing bubbles of carbon dioxide in the process, which are trapped between the gluten strands in the dough to leaven it. Yeast is alive, and you are essentially feeding and nurturing it, then kissing it good-bye. Under such circumstances, understandably, it can be a bit touchy. Yeast begins to activate at about 60°F (16°C), thrives between 70° and 80°F (21° and 27°C), and dies between 138° and 143°F (59° and 62°C). The amount of time that yeast is allowed to feed on dough also affects it: too little and it is underfed and fails to produce carbon dioxide. Left to work overtime, it experiences something akin to executive burnout and ceases to function effectively on the job.

> *Yeast performs wonders and the levitating powers of yeast can make magicians of us all.*   —BETTY FUSSELL, *In Good Season*

Dry yeast comes in two forms: *conventional,* or *traditional*, and *quick rising*. They are two separate strains of yeast and cannot be used interchangeably in baking. The recipes in *Heaven's Banquet* use conventional yeast. Quick-rising yeast is more unstable; it leavens with only one rising and then rapidly burns out. *Yeast in jars or large packages*, which are repeatedly opened and shut, should be stored tightly closed in the refrigerator. *Packaged yeast* is vacuum sealed and thus well protected. Conventional yeast can be stored for about six months without refrigeration, and packaged quick-rising yeast will last for one year.

Compressed yeast, moist yeast sold in cakes, is slightly less processed than dry yeast. It requires refrigeration at all times—even before it reaches you. Depending on how it was treated before you met it will last for 3 to 8 weeks in the refrigerator. It is very sensitive to moisture, highly perishable, and best used only if you bake bread and purchase fresh yeast on a regular basis. If you store yeast for occasional use, it's better to go with dry yeast. One-third of a 2-ounce cake equals one package dry yeast.

Nuts and Seeds

The word *nut* comes from the Latin *nutriens,* "to nourish." Many nuts are native to two or three different continents—and are some of the most ancient flora that grace the earth today. All nuts are essentially fruits—of a different stripe than the soft, luscious orbs we think of as fruits, but nevertheless the crest jewel of a tree's growth that it graciously offers to us.

❖ Like all other fruits, nuts are harvested seasonally. They are freshest in autumn and winter. They have built-in ideal storage containers—their shells. However, if cracking and shelling them is too arduous and time-consuming, the best shelled nuts are the raw, unsalted types found in natural foods stores and ethnic markets. Packaged roasted nuts often contain added oil, preservatives, and too much salt to make them practical for general cooking.

❖ Nuts contain large amounts of oil, making them subject to rancidity. They stay fresh for varying amounts of time, depending on how much oil they contain. For safety, purchase small amounts and keep them in the freezer. Follow this general rule of thumb for storage:

> Up to 2 months in a dark, cool, dry place
> Up to 3 months in the refrigerator
> Up to 1 year in the freezer

Blanched nuts: Nuts are blanched in order to remove their skins.

1. Drop nuts into boiling water. Remove from the heat and allow to stand for 1 minute. Drain.
2. Let the nuts cool just until you can handle them. Slip the skins off by rubbing them briskly between your fingers or squeezing at one end. Careful—they're slippery little critters.

Toasted/roasted nuts: Toasting nuts brings out their full flavor potential, and the fragrance of nuts as they toast is a particular delight. Blanch and remove the skins before toasting for the most sumptuous result. Different nuts take different amounts of time to cook, so don't attempt to toast a mixed batch—you'll end up with some still raw while others are burning. Pecans, pine nuts, and cashews cook much more quickly than walnuts and almonds.

- ❖ *Oven method:* Nuts can be dry roasted, or you can lightly coat them with melted ghee or oil before roasting. Scatter raw or blanched nuts on a baking sheet. Sprinkle lightly with salt if desired. Roast in a 350°F (180°C) oven for 15 to 20 minutes. Stir every 5 minutes, being careful to chase them out of the corners of the pan, where they brown most quickly. Remove immediately when the nuts are browned; they proceed from perfectly done to burned at a rapid pace.
- ❖ *Skillet method:* Whole nuts do not brown evenly by this method as their uneven surfaces only partially touch the pan. Slivered and chopped nuts and sunflower seeds, which have flat surfaces, fare better. Melt 1 tablespoon of ghee or oil for every 2 cups of nuts in a heavy skillet on a low heat. Add only enough nuts to cover the bottom of the skillet, and stir often until they are browned.

 ## NUT BUTTER

Homemade nut butters are absolutely divine. They can be made from raw, blanched, or toasted nuts, depending on the flavor you desire. Toasted almonds, cashews, walnuts, and hazelnuts make delicious nut butters. For unabashed luxury, try macadamia and pistachio butters. Store homemade nut butters in airtight containers in the refrigerator.

Grinder method: A grinder crushes nuts to a paste, producing a pure nut product. The texture can be smooth or chunky, depending on how finely you grind the nuts. Grind raw, blanched, or toasted nuts in a nut grinder or a meat grinder. You may have to put them through the grinder more than once to achieve a smooth texture. Add salt if desired.

Food processor method: The result will have a chunky texture; it is not possible to make it completely smooth. Using the metal blade, process raw, blanched, or toasted nuts as finely as possible. Add melted ghee or oil a little at a time until the desired consistency is achieved. Add salt to taste if desired.

Blender method (2½ cups/600 ml): Ghee makes the tastiest nut butter; combine it with blanched, toasted almonds for a taste of heaven. You can toast the nuts in the minimum amount of ghee or oil listed below.

2½ cups nuts (275 g) (raw, blanched, or toasted)
½ to ¾ cup (120 to 180 ml) melted ghee or butter or mild-flavored oil
Salt (optional)

Combine the nuts and oil in a blender on low speed to form a smooth paste, adding only as much oil as necessary. It will take about 3 minutes of blending to achieve a smooth texture. Add salt to taste if desired.

A Glossary of Nuts and Seeds

Almonds were known throughout ancient India and the Middle East. Some vaidyas recommend eating several blanched, peeled almonds daily. Ayurveda recommends blanching and peeling almonds because the skins are slightly toxic.

❖ *Golden almonds:* Light-colored nuts such as cashews and pine nuts can also be dyed this way. Soak a pinch of saffron in hot water until the water is bright yellow. Immerse blanched almonds in the water and soak for several hours or overnight. Drain and allow the nuts to dry.

Brazil nuts: Enormous Brazil nut trees flourish in the steamiest climes of South America and wither away even in subtropical Florida. About two dozen Brazil nuts grow inside an enormous fruit, and pickers must wear protective headgear, lest one fall on them. Brazil nuts are one of the oiliest of all nuts and therefore quite perishable. For best results, buy in season (autumn and winter) in small amounts and store in their shells or in the freezer. Brazil nuts are generally used raw but can also be blanched and toasted. Because of their size, sliver them before adding to dishes.

❖ *Brazil nut curls:* For decorating desserts and garnishing soups, pasta, and vegetable dishes. Blanch and peel Brazil nuts. When dry, shave off thin curls along the wide edge of the nut with a sharp paring knife. Gently spread the curls on a baking sheet and roast in a 350°F (180°C) oven, stirring every few minutes, until golden brown. Be very careful not to burn.

Cashew trees grow in tropical countries; presently India provides 90 percent of the world's harvest. The nut grows in an unusual position, dangling at the bottom of the cashew fruit. Fresh cashews contain *cardol*, a chemical that can cause burns on the skin. All cashews that come to market have been toasted, shelled, then heat-treated again to remove the cardol. In other words, "raw" cashews are in reality thoroughly cooked.

❖ Ground cashews have an almost creamy consistency, making them ideal for Nut Milk and for sauces such as Cashew Mayonnaise.
❖ Cashews contain less fat than other nuts and are therefore less perishable.

Chestnuts are available fresh in the autumn. They are perishable and should be stored in the refrigerator for no more than a month or two. Chestnuts must always be cooked and shelled before they are added to other foods. Whole chestnuts, chestnut purée, and chestnut flour are used in European and Japanese sweets. Sweetened chestnut purée is used in cake and pastry fillings, often lightened by folding into whipped cream.

❖ You can occasionally find dried, shelled chestnuts in Japanese markets and gourmet foods stores. To reconstitute, soak overnight in water and then simmer in water to cover until tender.

Boiled chestnuts
1. With a sharp knife, make deep crosscuts on the flat side of the shell.
2. Place in a pot and fill with water to cover. Bring the water to a boil, reduce the heat, and simmer for 15 to 25 minutes.
3. Drain, and as soon as the chestnuts are cool enough to handle, remove the shells and the brown inner skin. This skin is difficult to remove once the chestnuts have cooled.

Oven-roasted chestnuts
1. With a sharp knife, make deep crosscuts on the flat side of the shell.
2. Coat the chestnuts with oil and spread out in a single layer on a baking sheet.
3. Roast in a 375°F (190°C) oven for 30 to 40 minutes, until the shells can be removed easily.
4. As soon as the chestnuts are cool enough to handle, peel off the shells and brown inner skins.

Pan-toasted chestnuts: True to nostalgic form, chestnuts can be toasted in a pan over an open fire.

1. With a sharp knife, make deep crosscuts on the flat side of the shell.
2. Coat the chestnuts with oil. Place them in a heavy skillet, preferably with a long handle.
3. Toast them over a fire, shaking the pan frequently, until the shells can be removed easily.
4. As soon as the chestnuts are cool enough to handle, peel off the shells and the brown inner skins.

You can also do this procedure on a stove, but if you have already abandoned the thought of using your fireplace, you might want to throw romantic notions completely to the wind and opt for the more thorough oven-roasting method.

Chia seeds, cousins of the sage plant, are native to the Americas. When boiled in water or fruit juice chia seeds produce a type of gelatin that can be sweetened, mixed with fruits, and served as a dessert. You can find them in natural foods stores.

Coconuts are essential food for much of the world family. Cooling to Pitta, they are a naturally balancing food for eating in the tropical climates in which they grow.
Coconuts take a full year to mature. After six months the flesh is jellylike and can be eaten with a spoon. Mature coconuts, the only type available in the West, yield a hard, white flesh used in cooking and for its rich oil.

❖ Dried grated coconut (sometimes called *desiccated coconut*) and coconut chips can be found in natural foods stores. Use the unsweetened type; the moist, sweetened variety is chemically treated to stay soft. Store in an airtight container in the refrigerator for up to one month or in the freezer for up to one year.

Toasted coconut: Scatter grated fresh or dried coconut on a baking sheet or in a skillet.

❖ **Oven method:** Place in a 350°F (180°C) oven for 5 to 10 minutes, stirring frequently. When it is light brown, remove immediately to a bowl, or it will burn.
❖ **Skillet method:** Place on a medium flame for a minute or two, stirring constantly until light brown. Remove immediately to a bowl, or it will burn.

To open a fresh coconut:

1. Pierce with a screwdriver or drill holes in the "eyes," the dark round indented marks on one end. Drain out the liquid. You can drink this liquid, but it is not used in cooking. It is quite perishable and must be stored in the refrigerator. (Miriam's impatient alternative to Step 1: Forget the juice—don't drill any holes and proceed to Step 2 immediately.)
2. To remove the meat most easily from the shell, place the coconut in a 400°F (200°C) oven for 15 minutes. Break the coconut open with a hammer or smash against a hard surface. (I take it outside and smash it on the sidewalk.) Pry out the meat with a knife and carefully pare off the brown inner skin.

Coconut chips

1. Shave off wafer-thin chips from the meat of a fresh coconut with a sharp paring knife.
2. Scatter on a baking sheet. Place in a 350°F (180°C) oven and stir frequently until the chips are golden brown. Remove immediately to a bowl, or they will burn.

Hazelnuts or filberts: To the Celts, hazelnut trees were symbolic of justice and also love and reconciliation. Today hazelnuts are used frequently in European cooking. Their exquisite, assertive flavor tends to dominate the foods to which they are added and intensifies further with toasting.

Macadamia nuts, though most often exported from Hawaii, are actually native to Australia. They are sold shelled, as they tend to mold inside their rock-hard shells. Macadamia nuts are very perishable. Purchase in small amounts and store in the refrigerator or freezer. A luxury food, macadamias are best employed where you can show them off. They are particularly delicious in desserts.

Pecans: The name *pecan* is a Native American word. They are grown almost solely in the United States, and those exported are almost solely sent to Canada. Pecans have a high fat content, making them very rich and also quite perishable. Pecans can be used interchangeably with walnuts, although they toast more quickly and their flavor is different.

Pine nuts, pignolias, or piñons: Pine nuts grow in the cones of the piñon tree of the Americas and of the *Pinus pineas* tree of the Mediterranean region. Besides their native habitats, they are prized in the cuisines of the Middle East, India, China, and Korea. Pine nuts are highly perishable. Buy in small quantities and store in the refrigerator or freezer. Pine nuts are eaten raw, but light toasting enhances their delicate flavor. Be careful—they burn easily.

Pistachios belong to the cashew and mango family and are used in the cuisines of the Middle East, India, and in European desserts. They are usually found raw and shelled or roasted in their shells. Choose pistachios with undyed (beige, not red) shells. Pistachios may be blanched to remove their skins. Split in half, they make colorful decorations, and a garnish of chopped pistachios can offer a striking color contrast.

Poppy seeds: It was not until medieval times in Europe that poppy seeds gained popularity for use in baking, which is mostly how they are used in the West today. Poppy seeds can be sprinkled into bread doughs and cake batters and sprinkled on rolls for accent. Buy in bulk in natural foods stores rather than in the little jars sold with the spices in supermarkets.

❖ *Khus,* white poppy seeds, are particularly nourishing and can be found in Indian markets. They are toasted, ground, and used to thicken and flavor dishes.

Pumpkin seeds or pepitas, have a beautiful green color that can be employed to contrast with other foods. Since Aztec times, ground pumpkin seeds have been used to thicken Mexican sauces.

Sesame seeds are a particularly prized food in Ayurveda for their life-supporting qualities. They are one of the oldest cultivated foods in history. Buy sesame seeds in bulk in natural foods stores—the tiny jars sold in supermarkets are expensive and the amounts far too small for most of the recipes in this book. Sesame seeds store quite well and can be kept for several months in a cool, dry place. *Brown, unhulled sesame seeds* are excellent for general use. You may wish to keep some *white, hulled seeds* on hand for garnishes; when toasted, they take on a warm, red-brown hue. *Black sesame seeds* are available in Indian and Chinese markets and add a lively color accent.

Sunflower seeds were first brought to Europe from Central America by Spanish explorers. They are quite perishable and should be stored in the refrigerator or freezer. Besides using whole, they can be ground into meal to enrich baked goods and thicken sauces.

Walnuts were called *karuon basilikon*, "kingly nut," by the ancient Greeks. Walnuts are native to the Himalayas, where they still grow wild. The most common variety is the *English walnut*, sometimes called the *Persian walnut. Black walnuts*, native to America, have a stronger flavor that is preferred by many. However, they are more difficult to shell and hull. Rare and highly prized by aficionados are *butternuts*.

OILS

In remote villages of the world, people bring their own seeds, nuts, and olives to a person operating an oil press and walk away with their own produce transformed into bottles of freshly pressed, completely natural oil. Woe to the rest of us who can only walk away with bottles of oil from the market, blissfully ignorant of how they got there and what happened to them between the field and the check-out counter. When they are good for you, they are very very good, and when they are bad, they are horrid: harbingers of free radicals, chemical residues, and other travesties that wreak havoc on health. Most of us are accustomed to bland, characterless, refined oils—and what refinement! Many oil-giving plants have been genetically engineered, particularly canola, soy, and corn. Oils are either extracted with hexane solvent or heated and expeller pressed. From there they are bleached, degummed, and deodorized to remove any last vestiges of flavor and color. Sometimes preservatives are added on top of all that. If the oils are then partially or fully hydrogenated, not only are health-giving properties effectively eliminated, but health-destroying substances are abundantly created. A strong statement, but this is serious stuff. A good oil is hard to find.

❖ The most nourishing and best-tasting oils used in Ayurvedic cooking are *organic* and *unrefined*. They have darker colors and occasionally a small amount of sediment at the bottom of the bottle. Their aromas and flavors are pronounced and individual, reflecting the foods from which they have been pressed. However, such oils usually have very low "smoking points," the temperatures at which their molecular structures break down, eliminating all healthy properties. This means that they are best used in lower-temperature cooking and in uncooked foods. Unrefined oils can be found in natural foods stores and sometimes in gourmet foods stores.

❖ Some oils are *partially refined* or *conditioned*. This is not necessarily the most terrible thing if they have been refined by natural processes that don't involve solvent extraction. They can be used for high-heat cooking, such as stir-frying. Not all oil-producing foods are organically grown, and the refining process helps remove pesticides. Other oils have an unpleasant taste when completely unrefined. There also are *refined oils made by natural means*: expeller pressed rather than solvent extracted, and bleached and deodorized with nontoxic materials.

❖ Be wary of the terms "cold pressed," "cold processed," and "expeller pressed." They have no legal significance. Any oil that has a light color and indistinct flavor has probably received its unfair share of processing. Train your taste buds to enjoy the wonderful and varied flavors of unrefined oils. Flavor, after all, is a desirable quality in food!

❖ Rancid oils are harbingers of free radicals and are highly compromising to health. You will taste something "off" in any rancid oil. Purchase oils in small amounts that you can use up within a month or two. Store in the freezer, the refrigerator, or in a cool, dark area. As a general rule, store opened bottles of unrefined oils in the refrigerator for no more than six months. Refined oils last for up to a year. Olive oil, palm oil, and coconut oil are best stored in a cool, dark place because they become semisolid when chilled.

❖ Do not reuse cooking oil. Repeated heating up and cooling down can break down the structure of the oil, making it very hard to digest.

❖ Heating oil until it smokes also breaks down its structure. If oil starts smoking, throw it out and start again. Your tummy will thank you.

Oils Frequently Used in Ayurvedic Cooking

Sesame oil, when unrefined, is a light, excellent, all-purpose oil, especially balancing for Vata and Kapha. *Charaka Samhita* calls it the best among oils. It is used frequently in Ayurveda as a massage oil as well as for cooking. Sesame oil stores particularly well because it contains natural antioxidants.

❖ *Toasted sesame oil* is pressed from toasted sesame seeds. It has a stronger flavor and is used as a garnish in Chinese cooking. Organic, unrefined, toasted sesame oil is available in natural foods stores.

Olive oil: Throughout history olives have represented all that is beautiful, peaceful, and holy. Olive oil has a low smoking point of 280°F (138°C); however, its moisture content makes it suitable for most cooking, including low-temperature deep-frying. Olive oil comes in three grades. *Extra virgin,* recommended for Ayurvedic cooking, comes from the first pressing and is one of the handful of truly cold-pressed oils in the world. However, know ye this: Some companies are playing fast and loose with the grading system. Buy from a source you trust. *Virgin* oil is extracted from second and third pressings. *Pure* olive oil is extracted next with chemical solvents; at best, some higher-quality oil has been mixed in to give it more flavor. Some variations in color and flavor among olive oils are caused by the different geographical conditions where the olives were grown. They are more or less the same quality; they're just different.

Sunflower oil and high-oleic sunflower oil are tri-doshic all-purpose oils for dishes requiring a mild-flavored medium. High-oleic sunflower oil has a higher smoking point than conventional sunflower oil and also a longer shelf life. When refined, its smoking point is 450°F (232°C). Unrefined, both should be used for lower-temperature cooking.

Pumpkin seed oil is tri-doshic and can be found unrefined in natural foods stores. It is delightful for low-heat cooking and in uncooked foods.

Almond oil, when unrefined, has a delicate but pronounced flavor that has been prized in fine French cooking for centuries. It is excellent for balancing Vata and Kapha. It is sensitive to heat and best used in uncooked foods. It is also highly perishable, so make sure it is fresh.

Corn oil is balancing for Kapha and suitable for most lower-temperature cooking and uncooked foods. Look for organic, unrefined corn oil.

HERBS AND SPICES

I can think of no dish, offhand, whose message cannot be heightened and refined by the magic of some spice or herb. —CROSBY GAIGE

The art of seasoning foods is one of the most essential and subtle aspects of Ayurvedic cooking. The Ayurvedic cook who seasons dishes that make your whole body sing a blissful song is a highly skilled cook indeed. You can utilize herbs and spices not only for adding exquisite flavors but for promoting health-enhancing effects such as balancing the doshas, kindling the digestive fire, Agni, eliminating impurities, ama, and adding the six tastes. Because you need to use only a small amount, you can add one, several, or even all six tastes to a dish with a few well-chosen seasonings.

What is paradise? but a garden, an orchard of trees and herbs full of pleasure and nothing there but delights. —WILLIAM LAWSON, 1687

❖ To awaken the flavor of *dried herbs,* sauté them in a little oil or lightly toast them in a dry pan to release their oils before adding to a dish.
❖ A general rule is that ½ teaspoon of crumbled dried herbs equals 1 tablespoon of minced fresh herbs.
❖ Purchase nonirradiated and, if possible, organically grown herbs and spices. Irradiation is a highly questionable practice involving the use of nuclear waste products to lengthen the shelf life of foods. Unfortunately, some spice-exporting countries are embracing it wholeheartedly as a means to increase their volume of exportable goods. Natural foods stores generally carry nonirradiated spices, and organically grown herbs and spices are becoming increasingly available.
❖ Spices retain the greatest amount of their flavorful oils when purchased whole and ground in a mortar and pestle or a small electric grinder just before using. Electric coffee grinders work well for grinding spices.
❖ Purchase spices in small quantities and store in airtight containers on a cool, dark shelf.

FRESH HERBS

Nothing compares with the flavor of fresh herbs. Lightly bruise fresh herbs to release their flavor by rubbing between your fingers. From there you can chop them if necessary. Add most fresh herbs to cooked dishes just before serving. Only a few fresh herbs, such as rosemary and parsley, can hold up during long cooking. Herb flowers add an intense flavor of their herb and look lovely strewn on top of soups, pasta, and salads. However, they usually disappear if you mix them into a dish.

[Medicinal plants and herbs], Mothers [of humankind], a hundred are your applications, a thousand-fold is your growth; do you who fulfill a hundred functions make my people free from disease.   —RIK VEDA X.8.7

Warming Herbs and Spices

Most herbs and spices have a warming quality that stimulates digestion. Warming spices in general are balancing for Kapha and, if not too pungent and taken in smaller amounts, for Vata. They can aggravate Pitta when used frequently and in large amounts. There is a handful of warming spices that are identified as being particularly effective digestive aids and are employed in Ayurvedic cooking to assist in the assimilation of a dish. These spices kindle the digestive fire, Agni, and also help remove toxins, ama. Fortunately, they also add wonderful flavors.

Ajwain or ajowan (*Carum ajowan*) are tiny seeds used in Indian and Middle Eastern cooking that could easily find themselves at home in Western dishes. Ajwain has the flavor of thyme but is actually related to cumin. It is available in Indian and Middle Eastern markets.

Cardamom (*Elettaria cardamomum*) is lauded in Ayurvedic texts. It can be enjoyed by all three doshas, with Pitta types using a bit less of it. Cardamom is commonly used in Indian sweets and curries, Middle Eastern desserts and coffee, and German and Scandinavian baked goods. It also enhances fruits and fruit salads, and the seeds can be chewed as a breath freshener. In India cardamom pods (which are naturally green, but are often bleached with sulphur dioxide until straw colored) are cracked open and cooked whole in rice dishes. For most other dishes the seeds are removed from the pods and ground to a coarse powder. The powder loses flavor quickly; it is better to buy *whole decorticated seeds* (whole seeds removed from the pod) in small amounts and grind them just before cooking. If you don't have a mortar and pestle, a simple method is to spread the seeds on a cutting board and run a rolling pin over them a few times while bearing down on it. If you are an unhurried purist, purchase whole green pods and remove and grind the seeds as needed.

❖ *Brown cardamom,* which has a large, brown pod, is not actually true cardamom. Its flavor is quite different from the genuine article.

Ginger (*Zingiber officinale*) is called "the best among tubers" by the *Charaka Samhita* and often referred to as "the universal medicine" in Ayurveda. Ginger was considered beneficial—and available—enough during the Revolutionary War to be a standard ration for George Washington's troops.

❖ *Fresh ginger* is used for both its flavor and its pungent qualities in all the cuisines of Asia. Raw ginger adds sharpness and heat to a dish in the manner of chilies. However, it is less aggravating to the digestive tract. When sautéed, it mellows and adds wonderful flavor to dishes of all ethnic persuasions—even those not normally flavored with ginger. To use fresh ginger, slice off the necessary amount, peel, and mince fine. A garlic press is great for mincing ginger. *Young ginger*, sometimes available in Asian markets, is less flavorful than the mature root and has no advantage over conventional ginger other than its novelty. Store fresh ginger root in the refrigerator away from moisture.

❖ *Dried ground ginger* is more concentrated in its flavor and its effects and is used in baked goods and desserts. *Crystallized ginger* is found in Chinese dishes, chutneys, jams, and desserts. It is also a candy in itself.

❖ The three types do not give an equal effect—fresh ginger can never really replace ground ginger, and vice versa. Nevertheless, in a pinch, 1 teaspoon minced fresh ginger equals ¼ teaspoon ground ginger *or* 2 teaspoons crystallized ginger with the sugar rinsed off.

Ginger pickle: Sprinkle a thin, peeled slice of ginger with lemon juice and salt (black salt is best). Eat about 30 minutes before a meal to help kindle the digestive fire, Agni.

Hing or asafoetida (*Ferula asafoetida*), the dried resin obtained from several related plants native to India, has a unique flavor that substitutes well for onions and garlic. *Charaka Samhita* states, "Hing is the best among appetizers." Hing's fetid odor when sniffed straight from the jar does not do justice to the magic it works when added in tiny amounts to savory dishes. You can find hing in Indian markets, and some herb and spice companies market it as "asafoetida." The purest hing comes in a hard lump from which you break off the amount needed with a knife. It is sold more commonly in powdered form, usually cut with rice flour or cornstarch.

❖ Hing must be sautéed in oil before it is added to a dish—it is bitter when uncooked. It is difficult to specify exact amounts of hing for each recipe, as it comes in a wide range of strengths and qualities. I specify "a pinch of hing" in the recipes. If you have a highly diluted batch, you may need to add considerably more. However, don't overdo—it won't help you win points for flavor or for health.

Pepper (*Piper nigrum*) was the king of spices of the ancient world. Pepper can be enjoyed by people of all doshas, while Pitta types might want to eat a bit less. For best flavor, effects, and shelf life, purchase whole peppercorns and grind them as needed. Stored in an airtight container in a dry place, whole peppercorns last a long time. However, it does not take long for stored ground pepper to end up tasting like dust.

> *Pepper is small in quantity and great in virtue.*   —PLATO

❖ *Black pepper* is the unripe, cured berry of the pepper tree.
❖ *White pepper* is the ripe berry with its husk removed. It adds a pleasant flavor along with a milder pungency.
❖ *Long pepper or pippali* (*Piper longum*), is a mildly pungent black pepper mentioned frequently in Ayurvedic texts. Long pepper was the prevalent black pepper of the ancient world and was considered superior to the more common type used today. It can sometimes be found in Indian markets.
❖ *Cubebs* (*Piper cubeba*), like black pepper, are the unripe, dried fruits of a type of pepper that is used in Ayurvedic medecine. They have a subtle, complex flavor, and can be obtained from medicinal herbs sources.

Cooling Herbs and Spices

Although most digestion-aiding spices have a warming effect, there are some notable exceptions that are cooling for Pitta and balancing for all three doshas.

Cilantro or fresh coriander leaf (*Coriandrum sativum*), also enjoys wide popularity throughout Asia (with the exception of Japan), in Mexico, and among the Zuni tribe of the southwestern United States. Cilantro leaves are usually served uncooked or are chopped and stirred into cooked dishes just before serving. Any amount of cooking changes their characteristic flavor. However, they are often cooked into Mexican soups and sauces to achieve a different flavor from that offered by the raw leaves. Cilantro root is ground with other spices for Thai curries.

Coriander seeds (*Coriandrum sativum*) boast a Latin name that comes from *koris*, Greek for—bedbug! Never fear: this appellation refers to the odor of the foliage. The praises of coriander seeds have been sung since ancient times in Ayurvedic texts, Egyptian manuscripts, the Bible, and by Hippocrates. Coriander seeds can be used whole but are usually used in ground form. They are most often found in the foods of India and Mexico. Ground coriander can be added to vegetable and bean dishes and chutneys. Indians mix ground coriander with sugar and serve the powder as a cooling sweet.

*And in the house of Israel called the name thereof Manna: and it was like
coriander seed, white; and the taste of it was like wafers made with honey.*

—EXODUS 16.31

Cumin seed (*Cuminum cyminum*) is most frequently found today in the cuisines of
Mexico, India, and the Middle East. It is an excellent tri-doshic digestive aid that helps
remove toxins, or ama, without aggravating the digestive fire, Agni. A pinch of ground
cumin and ginger mixed with warm water and taken first thing in the morning helps
remove ama. Cumin seeds can be used whole or ground. They need toasting for their flavor
to awaken. Either sautée in ghee or oil as the first step in cooking a dish or, when sprinkling
onto foods like raitas and uncooked vegetables, toast in a dry skillet until fragrant.

Fennel (*Foeniculum vulgare*) was a significant spice in ancient Asia and Europe. The
herb was sacred to the Saxons. Like its cousin, dill, fennel possesses both seeds and a
feathery top, which are both used to impart dishes with a slightly licorice taste.

❖ Fennel is an excellent digestive aid that kindles Agni, the digestive fire, without
   aggravating Pitta. In India toasted fennel seeds are mixed with a little rock sugar
   and chewed following a meal.

*Down by a little path I fond
Of mintes full and fennell greene.*   —CHAUCER

Mint (*Mentha*) is named for the nymph Minthes, who was turned into a mint plant
by Pluto's jealous wife, Proserpina. There are many varieties of mint, *spearmint* and *pep-
permint* being the most common today. Mint was introduced to America by the Puritans
and now grows wild throughout most of the United States. It is used extensively in the
cooking of India and the Middle East and is used throughout Southeast Asia in chutneys
and sauces. In Morocco sweet mint tea is the beverage of hospitality, and business trans-
actions are sweetened and tempered by cups of Pitta-pacifying mint tea.

❖ By all means, cook with fresh mint whenever possible. Unlike many other green
   herbs, mint holds up well in cooking. It is one of the easiest herbs to grow at
   home; it thrives and spreads lavishly without much encouragement. However, if
   only dried mint is available, purchase it as a loose-leaf tea at a natural foods store
   rather than in the little spice jars sold in supermarkets. I have been known to rip
   open mint tea bags and empty out their contents when nothing else was available.

The Ayurvedic Herbs and Spice Box

Almost all culinary herbs and spices can be utilized in an Ayurvedic kitchen. Some are
particularly lauded in Ayurvedic texts for their health-giving effects, which are noted in
their descriptions. Unless otherwise described, the following herbs and spices are
heating and increase Pitta while balancing Vata and Kapha.

Happiness is a row of fragrant herbs on a sunny windowsill and a rack of pungent, aromatic dried herbs and spices. For here we have the elements of good cooking, the elements which transform the primitive gratification of hunger into a pleasurable aesthetic experience.   —NIKA HAZELTON

Allspice (*Pimenta officinalis*), a native of the Americas, is prized for its complex flavor resembling a combination of cinnamon, juniper, nutmeg, and cloves. Ground allspice is used most successfully in desserts and baked goods. It can also be added, whole or ground, to chutneys and grain dishes.

Anise (*Pimpinella anisum*) is a member of the parsley family. It was a popular digestive aid in ancient Rome. The licorice-flavored seeds can be added to baked goods and Indian-style spiced vegetables.

Annatto (*Bixa orellana*) is used to add a golden color to foods in the Caribbean, Mexico, and Central and South America. It is added to cooking oils, which are used to mimic the way *dendê*, or palm oil, colors dishes.

Basil (*Ocymum basilicum*), a member of the mint family, is indigenous to both Asia and Africa. Fresh basil is balancing to all three doshas, albeit in smaller amounts for Pitta. Basil is commonly associated with Italian cooking, but Thais exceed Italians in their use of it. There is no comparison between the flavors of the fresh and dried leaves. Do not cut them far in advance or cover then in advance with salad dressing: they turn black.

❖ *Thai basil*, sometimes known as *licorice basil*, has a somewhat different flavor from the *sweet basil* most commonly found in the West. It is used throughout Southeast Asia and can be purchased in Asian markets. Varieties of basil used in European cooking include *sweet, cinnamon, lemon, camphor,* and *purple basil*, each having a subtly different flavor. Ethiopian cuisine features *tulsi*, or *holy basil*.

If I had to choose just one plant for the whole herb garden, I should be content with basil.   —ELIZABETH DAVID

Bay leaves (*Laurus nobilis*) from the evergreen bay laurel tree were used in early Greek ceremonies dedicated to Apollo. Bay leaf garlands crowned both champion athletes and revered scholars. Such noble leaves are added whole to soups, sauces, curries, and stews and are removed before serving. Only the leaves of *Laurus nobilis* have culinary value; other types of bay leaves can be toxic.

Caraway seeds (*Carum carvi*) were known in Asia as "Roman cumin" or "foreign cumin," suggesting that, for once, a spice was imported from west to east! Today the seeds are commonly found in German and European cooking. They are good in cabbage and potato dishes and can be sprinkled in or on top of breads, crackers, and rolls.

Caraway seeds are responsible for the definitive flavor of rye bread—almost more than the rye flour itself. Caraway seeds can become bitter if cooked more than half an hour, so add them to dishes toward the end of cooking.

Celery seeds (*Apium graveolens*) is indigenous to southern Europe and was utilized by the ancient Greeks and Romans for its medicinal properties. Celery seeds are usually ground before using and impart a strong celery flavor to soups, stews, and vegetable dishes. Add sparingly.

Chervil (*Anthriscus cerefolium*) is another relative of parsley. Its Greek name, *chairéphyllon*, translates as "herb of joy." Today it is mostly cultivated and used in France, where it is one of the classic *fines herbes*. Chervil can be added to green salads and combines well with spinach. However, its flavor diminishes when cooked.

Cinnamon (*Cinnamomum zeylanicum*), a tree bark, is almost always replaced by its near relative, *Cinnamomum cassia* and should technically be referred to as cassia. Both cinnamon and cassia are referred to in Ayurvedic texts, and with Pitta eating a little less, can be enjoyed by all three doshas. Cinnamon is used in Ayurvedic herbal formulas to aid in the absorption of the other herbs. Cinnamon is one of the most widely used and versatile dessert spices. It is also used in the savory dishes of India and the Middle East.

❖ Cinnamon can be purchased ground or in tight curls of bark known as *cinnamon sticks*. The sticks are an aesthetic addition to beverages and grain dishes, but attempts to grind them can produce as many wood splinters as powder—don't try this at home!

Cloves (*Eugenia aromatica*) are the unopened buds of a tree that now grows mostly in Zanzibar. Cloves have long been chewed to freshen the breath. *Ground cloves* can be added in small amounts to most sweet baked goods and desserts, and *whole cloves* can be added where they can later be removed, to puddings, beverages, and so forth.

Curry leaves (*Murraya koenigii*) are used in Indian cooking and are available, usually in dried form, in Indian markets. Use fresh leaves, if you can find them. Add whole to savory dishes in the manner of bay leaves. They are usually left in the dish for serving but are not eaten.

Dill (*Anethum graveolens*) grows wild throughout western Europe and the United States and is balancing for all three doshas.

❖ *Dill seeds* are used to flavor burgers, casseroles, and grain dishes.
❖ Feathery dill tops are used in Middle Eastern, Scandinavian, and Russian cuisines. Add dill to salads, soups, stews, and vegetable dishes, and sprinkle over dishes for a decorative effect.

The pot finds its own herbs.   —CATULLUS, 57 B.C.

Epazote (*Chenopodium ambrosioides*) is a spicy green herb used in Mexican and Central American cooking. You can purchase it from Hispanic markets and add it to savory dishes.

Fenugreek (*Trigonella foenum-graecum*) seeds can be boiled into a Kapha-reducing tea. They are a major ingredient in curry powder. Sauté either whole or ground seeds in oil before adding to dishes. Ethiopians eat fenugreek leaves as a vegetable. Sometimes the flavorful leaves are available from farmers' markets; add them to savory dishes.

Filé or sassafras leaves (*Sassafras albidium*) are an important seasoning in gumbos, properly used by crumbling and sprinkling on at the table to add seasoning and thickening.

Galangal or thai ginger (*Alipine officinarum*) was imported to Europe from Asia in the Middle Ages and used in a powdered dried form. In this century it is virtually unknown outside South Asia, though it is more popular than ginger in Thailand. Galangal has a pungent, powerful flavor that is not suitable for eating straight up. Slice it into soups and stews, then remove before serving, or grind it and sauté a small amount in oil to add to vegetable dishes and stews.

Horseradish (*Amoracia rusticana*) is a potent member of the mustard family, used as a condiment and flavoring in eastern Europe and Russia. It is quite aggravating to Pitta and is best used in tiny amounts. Mix into sour cream, mayonnaise, and other sauces. Approach horseradish carefully: do not touch your eyes or other mucous membranes after handling until you have thoroughly washed your hands. *Wasabi* is a radish similar to horseradish in flavor that is dried and powdered in Japan for a pungent seasoning. You can purchase it in Japanese markets. Soak in hot water for ten minutes to bring out its flavor and add very sparingly to soups, savory dishes, and sauces. It's not for nothing that *wasabi* means "tears."

Juniper berries (*Juniperus communis*) are common in European cooking. Add whole to soup stocks and strain out, or add to vegetable and bean stews.

Kaffir lime leaves look like two Siamese twin leaves attached end-to-end. They are, in fact, found in Siam. You can occasionally find them fresh in Thai markets, but more often they are found in their dried form, which has much less flavor. Add kaffir lime leaves whole to Thai vegetable and rice dishes and remove before serving.

Kalonji or nigella (*Nigella sativa*), are the tiny, aromatic black seeds of the love-in-a-mist plant. They were used in Europe prior to the seventeenth century and today are used in Indian and Middle Eastern dishes, particularly in pickles and in breads. They are available in Indian markets, often incorrectly called *onion seeds*. Middle Eastern markets sell them as *black seeds* or *siya daneh*. Toast for best flavor.

Lemon grass (*Cymbopogon citratus*) is used in the cooking of Southeast Asia. Fresh lemon grass is used in cooking; when dried, it is suitable only for tea. Fresh lemon grass adds a subtle, lemony flavor particularly characteristic of Thai and Indonesian cooking. Trim off the upper two-thirds of the stalks, then pound the white ends and lower part of the green stalk in a mortar and pestle. Add to soups, rice dishes, and vegetable dishes and remove before serving. If it is very fresh and tender, you can mince it and leave in the dish.

Mustard seeds (*Brassica juncea*, brown; *Brassica nigra*, black; *Brassica hirta* or *alba*, yellow) have been found in the ancient ruins at Narrappá and Mohenjo Daro.

❖ *Black mustard seeds* are found in Indian cooking. However, today we mostly get *brown mustard seeds* in their place. Sauté the seeds in oil until they "dance," or begin to pop, before adding to foods.

❖ *Yellow mustard seeds* are found in Western cooking, most commonly used as a pickling spice, or ground for mustard à la ballpark. The whole seeds give a lively color accent and a burst of pungency when added in *small* amounts to sauces and salad dressings. *Mustard powder* or *mustard flour*, made from hulled, sifted, and ground yellow mustard seeds, adds pungent flavor to savory dishes and salad dressings. It is more nose-tingling than the whole seeds, as the seeds must be broken and exposed to moisture to form their volatile oils.

The kingdom of heaven is like to a grain of mustard seed, which a man took, and sowed in his field: which indeed is the least of all seeds: but when it is grown, it is the greatest among herbs, and becometh a tree, so that the birds of the air come and lodge in the branches thereof.   —MATTHEW 13.31–32

Nutmeg and mace (*Myristica fragrans*) come from the same fruit: nutmeg is the inner core and is covered by mace, the dried membrane that separates the seed from the fruit, known as a "blade." Vaidyas recommend drinking warm milk with nutmeg before bed as a sleep aid. Ground nutmeg and mace can be added to desserts and sweet baked goods. Nutmeg marries particularly well with spinach and is a classic flavoring for Béchamel Sauce.

❖ The flavor of *freshly grated nutmeg* is infinitely superior to purchased *ground nutmeg*. Grate whole nutmeg on a fine grater just before using. There are very fine graters made specifically for nutmeg sold in specialty kitchen stores, but for very occasional use, an ordinary grater does just fine.

Oregano (*Origanum vulgare*) *and marjoram* (*Marjorana*): The name *marjoram* covers a number of herbs. Some botanists consider oregano to be a type of marjoram. In any case, the herb was symbolic of bliss to the ancient Greeks, who wove bridal wreaths of the herb to symbolize wedded bliss. Marjoram and oregano are used largely in the cuisines of Italy and Greece, and both can be added to vegetables, soups, stews, salad dressings, and sauces.

> *Indeed, sir, she was the sweet marjoram of the sallet, or, rather, the herb of grace.*   —WILLIAM SHAKESPEARE, *All's Well That Ends Well*

Paprika (*Capsicum annuum*) is made from dried ground capsicums, which were developed in Hungary from the more fiery chilies brought from the New World. Hot paprika contains the stalks and seeds. Small amounts of sweet paprika are more appropriate for Ayurvedic cooking. Paprika is used as much for its fiery orange color as for its flavor. Sprinkle it over savory dishes as a decorative garnish after cooking—it scorches and turns brown when exposed to high temperatures.

Parsley (*Petroselinum crispum*) is utilized in Ayurvedic cooking for all three doshas, with Pitta eating a little less. Fresh parsley is so widely available that there is no earthly reason to use tasteless dried parsley flakes. Parsley has an excellent flavor that comes into its own when the herb is added to sauces, soups, stews, and vegetable dishes or added raw to salads. *Italian flat-leaf parsley* has a more tender texture than curly parsley and is preferred by many cooks.

Rose petals (*Rosa*) are very helpful for balancing Pitta. Look for organically grown, unsprayed, undyed petals. Bright red petals have the most flavor. Cut off the white base of each petal, which can be bitter. Distilled rose essence can be found in natural foods stores and Indian and Middle Eastern markets. Highly concentrated, a few drops add the flavor and perfume of the flower. Less concentrated is rose water, which can be sprinkled on more lavishly. Add at the end of cooking to delicately flavored puddings, halvas, ice cream, and sweet sauces, as well as to Sweet Lassi and milk beverages.

> *Nature laughs in flowers.*   —RALPH WALDO EMERSON

Rosemary (*Rosmarinus officinalis*) became known as "the troubadour's herb" in the Middle Ages, after the custom of the traveling bards to present rosemary sprigs to the ladies whose charms they extolled in song. Rosemary's own charms were perhaps best extolled by Madame de Sevigne, who rhapsodized, "I use it every day, I always have some in my pocket, I find it excellent against sadness." Rosemary leaves can be used whole or ground. They are very potent, and small amounts enhance soups, stews, and vegetable dishes. It is best to sauté them in oil before adding to dishes.

Saffron (*Crocus sativus*) can be enjoyed by all three doshas and is used extensively in Ayurvedic cooking for delicately flavoring and coloring desserts, grains, soups, sauces, and vegetable dishes. Saffron-colored robes have been worn since antiquity by the swamis of India to symbolize the fire of knowledge that destroys ignorance. Soak saffron threads in hot water for 5 to 10 minutes to bring out their delicate flavor and golden color. Powdered saffron does not need to be soaked. However, it is better to purchase the whole stigmas, known as *saffron threads*, as they retain their flavor longer and also are less easy to adulterate.

❖ There is an inexpensive product called "saffron tea" that in actuality is safflower. Accept no such substitutes! Unfortunately, if it isn't expensive, it isn't saffron.

Sage (*Salvia officinalis*) was known as a healing herb throughout the ancient world. Its Latin name, *Salvia,* comes from *salvere,* "to heal." Add small amounts of crushed sage to soups, stews, and casseroles. A very little goes a very long way—too much imparts a soapy flavor. Sautéing sage in oil enhances its flavor.

❖ If you are ever in the high desert country of the American Southwest, gather ye sage leaves while ye may! If you are not, purchase fresh sage. If you can't find it, whole dried sage leaves will have to do; rubbed (ground) sage is vastly inferior to all the above.

> *Why should a man die who grows sage in his garden?*
> —SALERNO, ITALY, MEDICAL SCHOOL, 12TH CENTURY

Summer savory (*Satureia montana*) **and winter savory** (*Satureia hortensis*): In Europe the peppery flavor of savory is primarily used to flavor bean dishes. Summer savory is the most common type and can be added to potatoes, salad dressings, and beans. Winter savory has a more assertive flavor that works well in combination with other green herbs in bean and vegetable dishes.

Tarragon (*Artemisia dracunculus*) gets its name from *Tarkhun,* "dragon" in Arabic. What is available to us commercially is *Russian,* or *false, tarragon,* which is virtually tasteless compared to the genuine article, which can sometimes be purchased fresh in farmers' markets. Tarragon adds a unique flavor to salads, savory dishes, and sauces. The flavor of tarragon, in my opinion, works best as a solo act. The only other herb I mix it with is fresh parsley.

Thyme (*Thymus vulgaris*) comes in more than one hundred varieties. Thyme is associated with bravery: in ancient Greece, to tell a man that he "smelled of thyme" was to offer high praise. Thyme is a popular herb in the cooking of Italy, where it is often teamed up with basil and rosemary. In Sweden it is a classic in yellow split pea soup. Thyme is also featured in Creole cooking.

Turmeric (*Curcuma longa*) is a major Ayurvedic spice. It can be enjoyed by all three doshas. Applied externally, turmeric is good for the skin and is used in Ayurvedic topical creams and ointments. Although heat brings out the flavor of turmeric, the spice is also sensitive to long cooking. Do not sauté turmeric in oil; sprinkle it directly into vegetable dishes as they cook and add it to long-simmering dishes such as dal soup at the end of cooking. A pinch of turmeric adds golden color to cracker and bread doughs. A pinch or two added to the cooking water for rice or other light-colored grains gives them a yellow hue. Be careful: it's easy to overdo it and produce a stoplight yellow.

> *Rare spices, esoteric blends, dried herbs in leaf, stalk and powder, private mixtures and essences as precious as phrases from Keats or poems from the Chinese.*
> —CROSBY GAIGE

Herb and Spice Blends

In my opinion, blending individual herbs and spices for each dish you cook at the time you are cooking it is a more sensitive way to season foods than relying on generic seasoning blends. However, there are some classic combinations, usually with specific ethnic associations and often with a large number of ingredients, that you may wish to keep ready-mixed for some of your creations. Commercial spice blends are convenient, but they may be old and therefore less potent. You may prefer different proportions of the ingredients, or you may not want *all* the ingredients, such as chilies, onions, and garlic.

 ## FIVE-SPICE POWDER (WU XIANG)

CHINA   *About 7½ tablespoons*

Besides ginger and cilantro, these are just about the only spices found in Chinese cooking—and they are usually used only in this mixture. Star anise and Sichuan pepper can be found in Asian markets. You can replace the Sichuan pepper with black pepper.

2 tablespoons ground star anise
1 tablespoon ground cloves
1 teaspoon ground cinnamon

2 tablespoons ground fennel seeds
2 tablespoons ground Sichuan
 pepper

Mix the ingredients together.

 ## ZAARTAR

LEBANON   *6 tablespoons*

A blend to add to savory dishes or to mix with ghee or olive oil and spread on bread before toasting. Bright red sumac berries (*Rhus coriaria*) are used in Middle Eastern,

Georgian, and Moroccan cooking to add a sour flavor. You can find ground sumac in Middle Eastern markets.

STEP ONE

2 tablespoons besan (chickpea flour)

STEP TWO

1½ teaspoons dried oregano   *1½ teaspoons dried thyme*
2 tablespoons ground sumac   *1 tablespoon sesame seeds, toasted*

Place the besan in a dry skillet and toast over low heat, stirring constantly, until it darkens slightly. After it cools, grind the spices with the flour.

 # Curry Powder

About 7 tablespoons

Curry powder is not used frequently in India, where traditionally a *masala*, or spice mixture, is prepared individually to suit each particular dish. That having been said, a good curry powder can certainly be added to all types of sauces, vegetable dishes, and salad dressings for a specific "curry" flavor that many people enjoy. If you add a very small amount to a dish, it provides an indefinable, interesting undertone. Use whole spices as much as possible and grind them to a powder.

2 tablespoons ground cumin   *1 teaspoon ground fenugreek*
Pinch of hing   *1 teaspoon ground black pepper*
3 tablespoons ground coriander   *1 tablespoon turmeric*

Toast all the spices except the turmeric in a dry pan over low heat, stirring constantly, until fragrant and smoking slightly. Stir in the turmeric and remove from the heat.

VARIATIONS

 Add ¼ teaspoon ground ginger and ⅛ teaspoon ground cloves.
 Add ground dried curry leaves.

❧ Garam Masala

INDIA   *About ¼ cup (60 ml)*

Garam masala, "hot spice mixture," is designed to be added to Indian-style vegetable dishes and soups in the last few minutes of cooking. There are many versions of garam masala—many Indian cooks have their own family recipe.

2 teaspoons each: ground coriander, cinnamon, cardamom	*1 teaspoon ground mace*
	1 teaspoon black pepper
	1 tablespoon ground, toasted cumin
1½ teaspoons ground cloves	

Mix all the ingredients together.

Churnas: Maharishi Ayur-Veda dosha-specific Vata churna, Pitta churna, and Kapha churna are high-quality spice mixtures specifically designed to provide all six tastes while at the same time emphasizing those that balance one particular dosha. They are designed to be sprinkled on food just before serving to provide flavor and help keep the doshas in balance. They are available from the sources listed in Appendix B.

Herb teas: Herb teas add fine flavor when used as the liquid in Sweet-and-Sour Sauce, chutneys, fruit desserts, and creamy desserts. Mint, rose hip, lemon balm, and hibiscus teas are especially successful flavor additions.

Herb- and Spice-Infused Oils, Ghee, and Butter

An excellent method of adding subtle flavors to dishes is to use cooking oils infused with herbs and spices. The techniques are simple and the amounts of flavorings very flexible.

1. Place oil, ghee, or butter and the desired herbs or spices in a pot on the stove and gently bring to a simmer. Simmer for about 1 minute. Remove from the heat and let cool to room temperature.
2. For maximum flavor, allow the herbs or spices to stand in the oil for at least one day in an airtight glass container, preferably in a sunny window so they continue to stay warm. Strain if desired, and store in airtight glass containers.

Note: You can add herbs and spices to ghee while it is being prepared, and strain them out with the milk solids.

Herbs for infused oils (use dried leaves unless indicated otherwise)

Rosemary	Marjoram
Basil	Oregano
Thyme	Tarragon
Bay	Sage

Spices for infused oils

Whole cumin seeds	Peppercorns
Cloves	Fennel seeds
Coriander	Caraway seeds
Cinnamon sticks	Fresh ginger, peeled and sliced

 # SESAME-FLAVORED OIL (ZHIMA YOU)

CHINA   *1 cup (240 ml)*

This has a mild taste suitable for general cooking.

1 cup (240 ml) mild-flavored oil   *½ cup (70 g) sesame seeds*

1. Place the oil and sesame seeds in a skillet and cook over medium heat until the seeds are lightly toasted. Remove from the heat and allow to cool.
2. Place in a blender and blend until smooth. Strain the oil through a fine sieve, pressing it out of the remaining sesame paste. Store in the refrigerator. The sesame paste can be served as tahini.

 # GINGER-FLAVORED OIL (JIANG YOU)

CHINA

Peel and mince a piece of fresh ginger (the amount is to your taste). Place in a heavy pot with a mild-flavored oil and cook over medium heat until the ginger turns brown. Let the oil cool to room temperature, then strain out the ginger bits and discard them. Store in the refrigerator.

ROSEMARY OIL

ITALY

As for rosemary, I let it run all over my garden walls, not only because my bees love it, but because it is the herb sacred to remembrance and to friendship, whence a sprig hath a dumb language.   —SIR THOMAS MORE

Olive oil is the best medium for this treatment. Rosemary oil is delicious in salad dressings, vegetable dishes, pasta, and for sopping up with crusty pieces of Italian bread.

1. Pick a sprig of fresh rosemary. Place on a cutting board and bruise the leaves slightly with a pestle or clean hammer.
2. Place the leaves in a skillet and cover with oil. Heat just until the oil becomes hot.
3. Remove from the heat and let cool to room temperature. Store the oil, rosemary and all, in a jar or bottle.

 # LEMON-PEPPER OIL

ITALY   *2 cups (480 ml)*

This treatment is exceptionally good with olive oil. You can use it as a salad dressing, adding only a sprinkling of salt. When peeling the lemons, it is important to obtain only the yellow zest—none of the white. Use a sharp paring knife or a sharp vegetable peeler.

⅔ cup (75 g) lemon zest cut into strips   *2 cups (480 ml) oil*
  (about 3 large lemons)
1 teaspoon cracked black
  peppercorns

Place all the ingredients in a saucepan. Heat just until the oil is very warm to the touch. Transfer the mixture to a glass jar. Place in a sunny window for 3 days. You can either strain the oil or leave in the peel and pepper to intensify the flavors over time.

FLAVORINGS AND SEASONINGS

HERB SALTS AND SEASONED SALTS

For extra flavor, salt can be mixed with powdered herbs and dried vegetables. Read the labels on commercial seasoned salts to make sure that they do not contain monosodium glutamate or other unwanted additives. You can easily make your own seasoned salt by grinding herbs, spices, and salt together in a blender or spice grinder. Use approximately 1 part salt for 7 to 10 parts flavorings. Try different combinations of the following:

Allspice	Dried parsley
Basil	Pepper
Mace	Rosemary
Oregano	Thyme
Coriander	Toasted sunflower, sesame, or pumpkin seeds
Marjoram	Curry powder
Mustard seeds	Celery, caraway, and dill seeds
Nutmeg	Toasted cumin
Paprika	Black salt

 ## SEASONED SALT

About ⅓ cup (90 g)

¼ cup (75 g) salt
½ teaspoon each: dried rosemary, basil, sage
1 teaspoon each: paprika, ground coriander, celery seeds

4 teaspoons sesame seeds, toasted
½ teaspoon curry powder

Grind all the ingredients together in a blender or spice grinder.

 ## GOMASIO (SESAME-FLAVORED SALT)

JAPAN   *About ¾ cup (180 ml)*

A delicious, low-sodium seasoning.

⅔ cup (90 g) sesame seeds

1 tablespoon salt

Toast the sesame seeds and salt together in a skillet over medium heat, stirring frequently, until the seeds are golden and begin to pop. Grind the mixture, a little at a time, in a blender or spice grinder. Store in an airtight container in a cool place.

Fruit and Vegetable Seasonings

Amchur powder, made from dried green mangoes, is used in Indian cooking to add a sweet-and-sour flavor to dal, chutneys, and savory dishes. Sprinkle amchur powder into dishes as they cook. It is available in Indian markets.

Broth powders are commercially prepared mixtures of dried vegetables and herbs blended to a powder and mixed with salt. They are good for seasoning savory dishes, soups, salad dressings, and sauces.

Grated lemon and orange zests can be added to both savory dishes and sweet puddings, sauces, and baked goods to add a fresh, tart flavor. Use only fresh rinds from undyed, unsprayed fruits, and scrub them under running lukewarm water to help remove any bitterness. Grate the colored part on a fine grater, or use a *zester* to cut very thin strips, which serve as decorative garnishes as well as flavorings.

Liquid seasonings: The only commercially prepared sauces I use consistently are either Dr. Bronner's Balanced Mineral Bouillon or Dr. Bragg's Liquid Aminos. Both are concentrated dark brown liquids resembling soy sauce, made from fruits and natural flavorings. Unlike soy sauce, they are not fermented. Though these types of seasonings are not mentioned in the Ayurvedic texts and are therefore not technically "Ayurvedic," for the many people who wish to add more flavor, they are a better option than fermented soy sauce, and their salt content is already partially absorbed. You can find liquid seasonings in natural foods stores.

Tamarind is a pod of an enormous tree that grows in India, the Middle East, Africa, Latin America, and Southeast Asia. It is used in traditional Ayurvedic cooking for balancing Vata with its sweet-and-sour flavor. It is used to season soups, dal, and chutneys. Although the fruit is eaten fresh and you can purchase whole pods in Hispanic markets, tamarind is more commonly found dried or in a paste form in Indian markets.

❖ *Tamarind paste* is ready to use. It is highly concentrated; a little goes a long way.
❖ *Dried tamarind* comes pressed into 1-pound rectangular blocks. It must be prepared for cooking in the following manner.

TAMARIND WATER

For flavoring dishes to serve 4 to 6 people

2 ounces (30 g) dried tamarind ½ *cup (120 ml) very hot water*
 (⅛ of a 1-pound/500 g block)

1. Soak the tamarind in the water for about 15 minutes.
2. Break up the tamarind and squish with your fingers in the water to release its flavor.
3. Strain the mixture into a bowl, pressing as much of the liquid and softened fruit through the strainer as possible. There will be very little fruit; you will have mostly hard fibers to be discarded. Scrape the puréed fruit off the underside of the strainer and mix into the water. Use for cooking.

SWEETENERS

Sugar

Sugar originated in India, where the juice of sugar cane was first extracted and processed. *Raw sugar* is generally the most highly recommended by Ayurvedic doctors. It is balancing for Vata and Pitta, and gives energy, particularly in very hot weather. Sugar in general is less balancing to Kapha.

Substituting sugar for honey and molasses: Increase the amount by one-third and add 3 to 4 tablespoons of liquid per cup.

Granulated white sugar adds sweetness but not flavor to foods. In general, Ayurveda recommends raw sugar over white sugar, but white sugar can be used occasionally in Ayurvedic cooking. Ayurveda recommends cane sugar over beet sugar. *Rock sugar candy*, clear, crystallized sugar made by a process of distillation, is used in Ayurvedic medicinal preparations, and is considered a better option than granulated white sugar.

Jaggery or gur, the most ancient type of raw sugar, has a similar flavor and texture to dark brown sugar, making it both delicious and easy to incorporate into existing recipes. Jaggery can be found in Indian markets and comes either in sticky lumps that can be broken up in a food processor or in dried solid pieces that must be either grated or pulverized with a hammer. *Piloncillo*, raw sugar from Mexico that is dried into cone shapes, is identical to dry jaggery and can be found in Hispanic markets. (The names *jaggery* and *gur* are also occasionally applied to palm sugar, so check with the grocer to determine which is which. Palm sugar, which is also wonderful for Ayurvedic cooking, has a lighter, blond color.)

The least refined form of raw sugar is *dried sugar cane juice*, marketed in the United States under the brand name *Sucanat*. It is available in natural foods stores. It is less sweet than refined white sugar. Those who find Sucanat's flavor too strong for baking, as I do, can mix it with a gentler raw sugar such as turbinado. Sucanat weighs 25 percent less than other sugars: 1 cup Sucanat equals 150 grams.

Turbinado, sometimes called *demarara sugar*, is the most widely marketed form of raw sugar. It is the unrefined crystals remaining after the molasses has been extracted. It is useful in dishes calling for white sugar.

Honey

> *What is sweeter than honey?*   —JUDGES 14.18

Ayurveda considers honey to be one of the most beneficial foods when in its natural, unheated, uncooked state. Honey is the only sweetener that is balancing for Kapha, and it is an excellent Kapha reducer. It is less balancing for Vata and Pitta.

❖ The importance of eating only unheated, uncooked honey cannot be overemphasized. While uncooked honey is considered a *rasayana*, a rejuvenator, cooked honey is considered to act as a very undesirable toxin. Don't even stir it into hot tea, only warm liquids. It is entirely worth it to check labels and reject anything that has been cooked with honey, such as breads and cakes. Also, look for the word "unheated" on the labels on jars of honey.

❖ The variation in color and flavor among different honeys is largely the result of the type of flowers from which they were made. Dark honeys, such as buckwheat honey, contain more acid and generally have a more intense flavor than light ones like clover honey.

❖ While it is fine to mix honey and ghee together, Ayurvedic texts state that it is best not to mix them in equal amounts.

Substituting honey for other sweeteners: Substitute ¾ cup (180 ml) honey for 1 cup (210 g) of sugar and reduce the liquid in the recipe by 3 to 4 tablespoons per cup. Substitute honey cup for cup for molasses.

Molasses

Molasses is balancing for Vata and less balancing for Pitta and Kapha. It is best to use unsulphured molasses both for taste and for health. The label will tell you if the product contains sulfur. *Dark molasses* is slightly less refined than light and is recommended for the recipes in this book.

❖ *Blackstrap molasses*, a by-product of sugar making, has a very strong flavor which is not particularly sweet and is actually slightly bitter. Use in very small amounts in bread, or tone it down by combining it with sugar. It does not substitute for conventional molasses in recipes.

Substituting molasses for other sweeteners: Substitute ¾ cup (180 ml) molasses for 1 cup (210 g) of sugar and reduce the liquid in the recipe by 3 to 4 tablespoons per cup. Substitute molasses cup for cup for honey.

CORN SWEETENERS

Corn syrup is an extremely sweet, horrifically refined product that is used in candy making for its thickening properties. *Fructose* has been marketed as the Great White Hope of all sugar substitutes; be aware that it is basically powdered corn syrup! Fructose can be found, ironically, in natural foods stores. I don't recommend it for Ayurvedic cooking.

Malted Sweeteners: Rice Malt and Barley Malt Syrups

Maltose is the type of sugar found in sprouted grains. Grain is first moistened and sprouted, then dried to produce malted sweeteners. They are balancing for Vata and Pitta, and though sugar and honey are more usual in Ayurvedic cooking, they are fine to use. Barley malt syrup and rice malt syrup have a rich flavor resembling molasses. Rice malt syrup is slightly sweeter and milder than barley malt syrup, and substitutions can basically be made with the proportions for molasses, with adjustments to be judged by taste. Refrigerate malt syrups during warm weather to prevent fermentation. Malted syrups can be found in natural foods stores.

Fruit Sweeteners

Fresh fruit adds a sweetness milder than that of concentrated sweeteners. Mashed bananas, grated or sliced apples, crushed ripe juicy fruits, fruit juices, and even some vegetables such as grated beets and carrots add some degree of sweetness to dishes.

Sweet fruit juices, particularly apple and grape, are good for stewing fruits and making fruit sauces. Different juices have different amounts of sweetness. *Concentrated fruit juice sweeteners* can be found in natural foods stores.

Dried fruit can be effective for adding concentrated sweetness to foods. One method is to simmer dried fruit in water or fruit juice until it is soft and then purée it. Puréed raisins and dates are particularly sweet. You can also purchase syrups made this way from natural foods stores: fig syrup, date syrup, and raisin syrup.

❖ *Date sugar* is dried, pulverized dates and looks something like brown sugar. It can be used to replace cane sugar except in dishes in which the sugar must caramelize or dissolve. Date sugar gives roughly half the sweetness of sugar to dishes. However, it is better to go by taste than by a set proportion.

THICKENERS

Thickeners add body to liquids. Most thickeners contain starches that absorb the liquid and expand their own volume.

Agar agar or kanten is extracted from a sea vegetable and produces an effect similar to that of gelatin. Agar agar comes in bundles, bars, and flakes; the flakes are easy to use and can be found in most natural foods stores. Read package directions: different amounts of agar agar are recommended for different brands.

❖ One standard agar agar bar thickens 3 cups (720 ml) liquid. Break up the bar and simmer in the liquid for 15 minutes, stirring occasionally.

ARROWROOT VS. CORNSTARCH

Arrowroot, grown on St. Vincent in the West Indies, is processed in a natural way. Cornstarch is a relatively new substance, as corn must be subjected to a stupefying amount of processing to extract it. In the end, cornstarch has very little to do with corn. Arrowroot has more nutritive value than cornstarch and also less flavor. Arrowroot and cornstarch can be used interchangeably to thicken sauces, puddings, and pie fillings. They can also be employed as emulsifiers for frozen desserts and ice cream and as substitutes for the binding properties of eggs. One tablespoon of arrowroot or cornstarch thickens 1 cup (240 ml) of liquid.

Before cornstarch's test tube birth in the nineteenth century, East Asians used *water chestnut flour*, made of sun-dried, ground water chestnuts. You can sometimes find it in Asian markets.

Ground nuts: Nuts ground to a powder can be used to thicken puddings, sauces, and vegetable dishes. Unlike other thickeners, they do not absorb liquids and expand in size; rather, they "fill in" thin liquids.

Kudzu or kuzu powder comes from a starchy vine plant native to East Asia, where it enjoys both medicinal and culinary uses. Kuzu is processed in a natural way and thickens foods in the manner of arrowroot and cornstarch. When simmered for a few minutes, it becomes transparent, like an agar agar gel. It comes in nuggets that must be crushed in a spice grinder or mortar and pestle. One to two teaspoons kuzu thickens 1 cup (240 ml) liquid.

A man can receive nothing, except it be given him from heaven.   —JOHN III.27

BAKING WITHOUT EGGS

The properties of eggs in Western cuisine are not entirely replaceable. However, they are also not absolutely necessary. It is not a matter of trying to *replace* eggs but rather of finding other ingredients and cooking techniques to use *instead of* them. Eggs provide four things in baked goods: *liquid, leavening, binding,* and *lightness.* When eggs are omitted from a recipe, all four qualities must be replaced.

COMMERCIAL EGG REPLACERS

The liquid types found in supermarkets contain additives and often egg whites, as they are designed for people trying to avoid the cholesterol found in the yolks. There is no mystery about powdered egg replacers found in natural foods stores; they are mixtures of starches designed to replace eggs' binding properties and can be easily replicated at home.

Liquid: One "large" egg contains approximately ¼ cup (60 ml) liquid. However, eggless cake batters must be thicker than egg batters to rise evenly, so add extra liquid cautiously.

Leavening: Eggs leaven batters by introducing air into them. There is no substance I have found to date that easily mimics this property. Therefore, to produce the extra leavening that is necessary in the absence of eggs, the effectiveness of the chemical leavening must be increased.

❖ It is not desirable, in the interests of both health and flavor, to greatly increase the amounts of baking powder and soda. Instead, the combination of an acid liquid with baking powder and soda together is very effective. Baking powder's acid-alkaline ratio is designed to work with sweet milk. When combined with an acid liquid, its alkaline level must be increased by the addition of baking soda. You can use yogurt or buttermilk for the liquid. Sour cream is also effective.

❖ Unbleached white flour, or a mixture of white flour and whole wheat flour, should be used for smooth and even rising. Adding a little whole wheat flour to a bleached white flour batter ensures that you won't have to face the topographical map of a mountain range within a cake pan.

Binding: Binders keep baked goods from crumbling. They are not absolutely necessary in all baked goods, but the reasons some need one and others don't are often complex. For simplicity's sake, I advise using binders in all recipes from which you are omitting eggs.

❖ *Homemade binder:* Use 2 tablespoons binder per omitted egg, mixed in with the dry ingredients. *Arrowroot* and *cornstarch* are the best general binders. You can also mix any of the following starches into a base of arrowroot or cornstarch and store the mixture in an airtight container to use as necessary:

Kuzu   Barley flour
Tapioca flour   Oat flour

Lightness

❖ Mix your batter only enough to blend all the ingredients. Overbeating develops the gluten in the flour and toughens the final product.
❖ Creaming the butter and sugar together as the first step in making cakes, cookies, and pastries helps give a lighter effect. Creaming incorporates air into the butter, and the sugar crystals make tiny cuts in the butter, which form minuscule air pockets. For the same reason, the use of a liquid fat, such as ghee or oil, makes a cake heavier and denser, as no air can be incorporated into it.
❖ Milk and other dairy products, rather than water alone, make the final result more tender. Cultured milk products produce the tenderest baked goods. Buttermilk is ideal.
❖ Unbleached white flour gives a lighter result than whole wheat and other whole grain flours.
❖ Excessive sugar makes a cake more dense and heavy.

Food is the form of the soul, the Atman, for life consists of food.
—MAITRI UPANISHAD

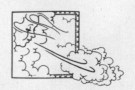

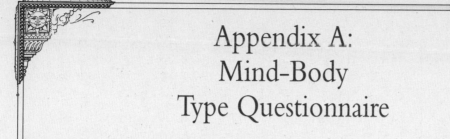

Appendix A:
Mind-Body
Type Questionnaire

Filling out the Mind-Body Type Questionnaire will help you learn some of the basic characteristics of your mind-body type.

After you answer all the questions, add the total number of answers under Vata, Pitta, and Kapha, respectively. The column(s) with the highest total(s) indicate which of these fundamental principles of nature (Vata, Pitta, and Kapha) are dominant in your psychophysiology. This is a preliminary indication; for a comprehensive evaluation, please consult a health care practitioner trained in Maharishi Ayur-Veda.

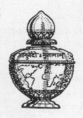

Discover Your Dosha: A Mind-Body Questionnaire

Instructions: For each trait, mark an "X" by the description that applies to you. If more than one description applies, then place your "X" by the one that describes you best.

	VATA	PITTA	KAPHA
TEXTURE OF HAIR	__ Coarse	__ Thin	__ Thick
AMOUNT OF HAIR	__ Average	__ Thinning	__ Thick
TYPE OF HAIR	__ Dry	__ Medium	__ Oily
COLOR OF HAIR	__ Light brown	__ Red/Auburn	__ Dark brown
APPEARANCE OF HAIR	__ Kinky, curly	__ Fine with curls	__ Straight or wavy
EYES	__ Small	__ Medium	__ Large
WHITES OF THE EYES	__ Ash-colored	__ Yellow or red	__ White or glossy
SKIN	__ Dry, rough	__ Soft, medium oily	__ Oily, moist
COMPLEXION	__ Darker	__ Pink to red	__ Pale, white
TEETH	__ Crooked	__ Yellowish	__ White, strong
SIZE OF TEETH	__ Small or very large	__ Small to medium	__ Medium to large
VOICE	__ High pitch, fast	__ Medium pitch, clear	__ Low pitch, deep, resonating
BODY SIZE	__ Small frame	__ Medium frame	__ Large frame
WEIGHT	__ Thin, hard to gain	__ Medium	__ Heavy, easy to gain
HUNGER	__ Irregular	__ Sharp, needs food	__ Can easily miss meals
FOOD & DRINK	__ Prefers warm	__ Prefers cold	__ Prefers dry and warm
EAT	__ Quickly	__ Medium speed	__ Slowly

	VATA	PITTA	KAPHA
MENTAL ACTIVITY	— Quick mind, restless	— Sharp intellect, aggressive	— Calm, steady, stable
MEMORY	— Short term is best	— Good general memory	— Long term is best
SLEEP	— Light, interrupted	— Sound, medium length	— Sound, heavy, long
DREAMS	— Fearful, flying, running	— Anger, fiery, violent	— Water, clouds, romance
MOODS	— Changes quickly	— Changes slowly	— Steady, unchanging
RESTING PULSE RATE *(BEATS/MIN.)*			
WOMEN	— 80–100	— 70–80	— 60–70
MEN	— 70–90	— 60–70	— 50–60
PERFORMANCE	— Performs quickly	— Tends to be precise	— Slow and relaxed
REACTION TO STRESS	— Worries, excites quickly	— Angers easily, quick temper	— Slow to get irritated
EXERCISE TOLERANCE	— Low	— Medium	— High
WALK	— Fast	— Average	— Slow and steady
ENDURANCE	— Poor	— Good	— Excellent
STRENGTH	— Poor	— Good	— Excellent
FINANCIAL	— Doesn't save, spends quickly	— Saves but big spender	— Saves regularly
WEATHER	— Aversion to cold	— Aversion to hot	— Aversion to damp, cool
SEX DRIVE	— Variable, irregular	— Moderate	— Strong
ELIMINATION	— Dry, hard, constipation	— Many, soft to normal	— Heavy, slow, thick, regular

Totals: VATA _____ PITTA _____ KAPHA _____

DIETING, WEIGHT LOSS, AND MAHARISHI AYUR-VEDA

A waist is a terrible thing to mind.   —ZIGGY BY TOM WILSON

Ayurvedic texts states that suppression of natural physiological urges like sneezing, yawning, and sleeping is dangerous for health and can actually shorten one's life. Among those natural urges are hunger and thirst. Nothing—repeat, nothing—we would want in our lives can come out of starvation dieting or suppression of appetite by use of diet pills. Furthermore, Ayurveda has the eminently sensible view that different mind-body types have different physical characteristics. The tall, slim contemporary ideal of beauty is a classic Vata physique. A predominantly Pitta type has a medium height, weight, and structure, and a classic Kapha type has a larger frame enrobed with more padding. People with a large proportion of Kapha in their constitutions will never be able to achieve the lithe look of the Vata—not, at least, without efforts that can cause misery and health problems somewhere down the line. It's ridiculous to uphold an ideal that only certain members of one mind-body type can ever come by honestly. So why not expand our perception of beauty to include all mind-body types rather than only one particular physiological configuration? If society won't do it for us, at least we can do it for ourselves and refuse to try to be something we are not.

That being said, true obesity—not borderline *zaftig* tendencies but the real thing—does represent a health hazard, and it is right and good to want to do something about it. It is often an imbalance of Kapha causing the problem, but there are also Vata disorders, Pitta-based digestive problems, and imbalances among the dhatus that can cause weight to climb. Ama is often involved as well. What to do? Follow the guidelines for balanced eating given in this book—in some cases that's enough. However, I strongly recommend a consultation with a health care practitioner trained in Maharishi Ayur-Veda to determine the underlying causes of your overweight body. Such a person can design a health program that addresses your personal needs, including a sane plan of eating choices among a variety of recommendations for restoring balance.

Appendix B:
Sources of Information on
Maharishi Ayur-Veda

M aharishi Ayur-Veda universities, colleges, and schools and Maharishi Ayur-Veda health centers, which are being established in all major cities, offer treatment programs for most common diseases, as well as programs for prevention of disease and promotion of ideal health. In addition, many physicians have been trained to integrate Maharishi Ayur-Veda into their daily medical practice. For information on Maharishi Ayur-Veda programs or products or the name of a physician practicing Maharishi Ayur-Veda in your area, please write or call the following, or visit the website: mapi.com.

United States

Maharishi Ayur-Veda Information Service
P. O. Box 49667
Colorado Springs, CO 80949-9667
(800) ALL-VEDA [255-8332]

Maharishi Ayur-Veda Medical Center
679 George Hill Rd.
Lancaster, Massachusetts 01523
(800) 290-6702

Maharishi Ayur-Veda Health Center
The Raj
1734 Jasmine Ave.
Fairfield, Iowa 52556
(800) 248-9050

Canada

Maharishi Ayur-Veda Products Canada
4965 Stanley Ave.
Niagara Falls
Ontario, Canada L2E 5A1
(800) 461-9685

Europe

MTC
Maharishi Ayur-Veda Products
Postbus 8811
6063 ZG Vlodrop
The Netherlands
    31-475-404060; fax 404055
E-mail: mtc@ayurveda.nl

South Africa

Ambrosia Import and Export (PTY) Ltd.
P.O. Box 29564
0132 Sunnyside, Republic of South Africa
27-12-321-5443 or 328-4211;
   fax 326-8840
E-mail: ambrosia@mweb.co.za

Australia

Maharishi Ayur-Ved Products
P.O. Box 81, Bundoora
Victoria 3083, Australia
61-03-9467-4633

United Kingdom

Maharishi Ayur-Ved Products
Beacon House, Willow Walk
Skelmersdale, Lancashire WN8 6UR
England
44-1695-51015

Holland

Maharishi Technology Corporation B.V.
Tussen De Bruggen 10
NL-6063 NA Vlodrop
The Netherlands
31-475-404060

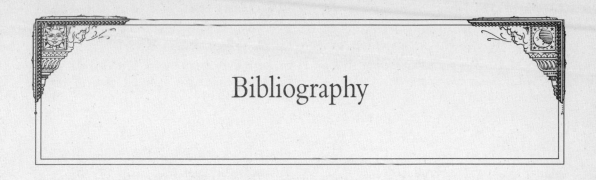

Bibliography

The American Heritage Cookbook and Illustrated History of American Eating and Drinking. American Heritage, 1974.

Anderson, Jean. *The New Doubleday Cookbook.* Doubleday, 1985.

Atlas, Nava. *The Wholefood Catalog.* Ballantine, 1988.

Batmangli, Namieh. *Food of Life.* Mage, 1986.

Behr, Edward. *The Artful Eater: A Gourmet Investigates the Ingredients of Great Food.* Atlantic Monthly Press, 1992.

Bothwell, Don and Patricia. *Food in Antiquity: A Survey of the Diet of Early Peoples.* Frederick A. Praeger, 1969.

Charaka. *Charaka Samhita.* 4 vols. Ed. and trans. by Prof. Priyabrat Sharma. Chaukhamba Orientalia, 1983.

Chirinian, Linda. *Secrets of Cooking, Armenian, Lebanese, Persian.* Lionhart, 1987.

Coe, Sophie D., and Michael D. *America's First Cuisines.* Thames & Hudson, 1994.

Crosby, Alfred W., Jr. *The Columbian Exchange: Biological and Cultural Consequences of 1492.* Greenwood, 1972.

Devi, Yamuna. *Lord Krishna's Cuisine: The Art of Indian Vegetarian Cooking.* Bala Books, Dutton, 1987.

———. *Yamuna's Table.* Dutton, 1992.

Elkort, Martin. *The Secret Life of Food.* Jeremy P. Tarcher, Putnam, 1991.

Ferrary, Jeanette, and Louise Fiszer. *The California-American Cookbook.* Simon and Schuster, 1989.

Fisher, M. F. K., and the editors of Time-Life. *Foods of the World: The Cooking of Provincial France.* Time-Life Books, 1968.

Franklin, Benjamin. *Benjamin Franklin on the Art of Eating together with the Rules of Health and Long Life and the Rules to find out a fit Measure of Meat and Drink.* American Philosophical Society, Princeton University Press, 1958.

Friedlander, Barbara. *The Secrets of the Seed, Vegetables, Fruits and Nuts.* Grosset and Dunlap, 1974.

Fussell, Betty. *Food in Good Season.* Alfred A. Knopf, 1988.

———. *I Hear America Cooking: A Journey of Discovery from Alaska to Florida—The Cooks, the Recipes, and the Unique Flavors of Our National Cuisine.* Elizabeth Sifton Books, Viking, 1986.

———. *The Story of Corn.* Alfred A. Knopf, 1992.

Greene, Burt. *The Grains Cookbook.* Workman, 1988.

———. *Greene on Greens.* Workman, 1984.

Harris, Jessica B. *Iron Pots and Wooden Spoons, Africa's Gifts to New World Cooking.* Macmillan, Atheneum, 1989.

Hazan, Marcella. *Essentials of Classic Italian Cooking.* Alfred A. Knopf, 1992.

Hazelton, Nika. *The Regional Italian Kitchen.* M. Evans and Co., 1978.

———. and the Editors of Time-Life. *Foods of the World: The Cooking of Germany.* Time-Life Books, 1969.

Jones, Evan, ed. *A Food Lover's Companion.* Harper and Row, 1979.

Kasin, Miriam (Miriam Kasin Hospodar). *The Age of Enlightenment Cookbook.* Arco, 1980.

Lewis, Edna. *In Pursuit of Flavor.* Alfred A. Knopf, 1988.

Lonsdorf, Nancy, M.D., Valerie Butler, M.D., and Melanie Brown, Ph.D. *A Woman's Best Medicine: Health, Happiness, and Long Life Through Maharishi Ayur-Veda.* Jeremy P. Tarcher, Putnam, 1993.

Lovelock, Yann. *The Vegetable Book: An Unnatural History.* George Allen and Unwin, 1972.

McGee, Harold. *On Food and Cooking: The Science and Lore of the Kitchen.* Charles Scribner's Sons, 1984.

Nader, Tony, M.D., Ph.D. *Human Physiology: Expression of Veda and the Vedic Literature.* 2nd ed. Maharishi Vedic University, 1995.

Norman, Jill. *The Complete Book of Spices.* Viking Penguin, 1991.

The Picayune Creole Cookbook (1901). Dover, 1971.

Robertson, Laurel, Carol Flinders, and Bronwen Godfrey. *Laurel's Kitchen Bread Book: A Guide to Whole-Grain Breadmaking.* Random House, 1984.

Roden, Claudia. *The Book of Jewish Food: An Odyssey from Samarkand to New York.* Alfred A. Knopf, 1997.

Rombauer, Irma S., and Marion Rombauer Becker. *The Joy of Cooking.* Bobbs-Merrill, 1975.

Root, Waverly. *Food.* Simon and Schuster, 1980.

———. *Herbs and Spices: The Pursuit of Flavor.* McGraw-Hill, 1980.

———. and Richard de Rochemont. *Eating in America: A History.* William Morrow, 1976.

Rosengarten Jr., Frederic. *The Book of Spices*. Livingston, 1969.

Shosteck, Patti. *A Lexicon of Jewish Cooking*. Contemporary Books, 1979.

Shurtleff, William, and Akiko Aoyagi. *The Book of Kudzu: A Culinary and Healing Guide*. Avery, 1985.

———. *The Book of Tofu*. Autumn, 1983.

Schutz, Philip Stephen. *As American as Apple Pie*. Simon and Schuster, 1990.

Sohoni, Shrinivas, trans. *Hymn to the Earth: The Prithvi Sukta*. Sterling, 1991.

Sokolov, Raymond. *Why We Eat What We Eat: How the Encounter Between the New World and the Old Changed the Way Everyone on the Planet Eats*. Summit Books, Simon and Schuster, 1991.

Stone, Sally and Martin. *The Brilliant Bean*. Bantam, 1988.

Sunset Magazine, Editors of. *Fresh Produce from A to Z*. Lane, 1987.

Sushruta. *Sushruta Samhita*. 3 vols. Ed. and trans. by Kaviraj Kunjalal Bhishagratna. Chowkhamba, 1991.

Tannahill, Reay. *Food in History*. Crown, 1988.

Theoharous, Anne. *Cooking and Baking the Greek Way*. Holt, Reinhart and Winston, 1977.

Tropp, Barbara, *The Modern Art of Chinese Cooking*. William Morrow, 1982.

Tsuji, Shizuo. *Japanese Cooking: A Simple Art*. Kodansha, 1980.

The Upanishads. 2 vols. Trans. by F. Max Müller. Dover, 1962.

Vagbhata. *Astanga Hrdayam*. 2 vols. Trans. by Prof. K. R. Srikanthu Murthy. Krishnadas Academy, 1991.

Van der Post, Laurens, and the Editors of Time-Life. *Foods of the World: African Cooking*. Time-Life Books, 1970.

Visser, Mary. *Much Depends on Dinner*. Grove, 1986.

Volokh, Anne. *The Art of Russian Cuisine*. Macmillan, 1983.

Wallace, Robert Keith, Ph.D., *The Physiology of Consciousness*. M.I.U. Press, 1993.

Wason, Betty. *Cooks, Gluttons and Gourmets: A History of Cookery*. Doubleday, 1962.

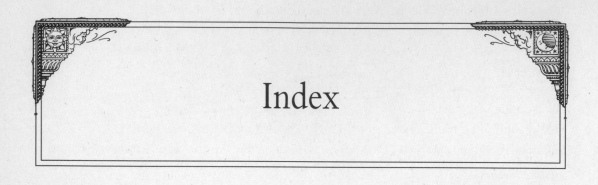

Index